PHARMACOLOGY FOR HEALTH PROFESSIONALS

Second Edition

W. RENÉE ACOSTA, RPH, MS

College of Pharmacy
University of Texas at Austin

Wolters Kluwer | Lippincott Williams & Wilkins
Health
Philadelphia • Baltimore • New York • London
Buenos Aires • Hong Kong • Sydney • Tokyo

Executive Editor: David B. Troy
Product Manager: Matt Hauber
Art Director: Jennifer Clements
Vendor Manager: Cynthia Rudy
Design Coordinator: Stephen Druding
Manufacturing Coordinator: Margie Orzech
Developmental Editor: Rose Foltz
Production Services/Compositor: SPi Global

Library of Congress Cataloging-in-Publication Data
Acosta, W. Renée.
  Pharmacology for health professionals. — 2nd ed. / W. Renée Acosta.
     p. ; cm.
  Rev. ed. of: Pharmacology for health professionals / Sally Roach. 1st ed. c2005.
  Includes bibliographical references and index.
  ISBN 978-1-60831-575-8
 I. Roach, Sally S. Pharmacology for health professionals. II. Title.
  [DNLM: 1. Pharmaceutical Preparations. 2. Pharmacology. QV 55]
  615′.1—dc23
                                                                          2011048150

Care has been taken to confirm the accuracy of the information presented and to describe generally accepted practices. However, the authors, editors, and publisher are not responsible for errors or omissions or for any consequences from application of the information in this book and make no warranty, expressed or implied, with respect to the currency, completeness, or accuracy of the contents of the publication. Application of the information in a particular situation remains the professional responsibility of the practitioner.

 The authors, editors, and publisher have exerted every effort to ensure that drug selection and dosage set forth in this text are in accordance with current recommendations and practice at the time of publication. However, in view of ongoing research, changes in government regulations, and the constant flow of information relating to drug therapy and drug reactions, the reader is urged to check the package insert for each drug for any change in indications and dosage and for added warnings and precautions. This is particularly important when the recommended agent is a new or infrequently employed drug.

 Some drugs and medical devices presented in the publication have Food and Drug Administration (FDA) clearance for limited use in restricted research settings. It is the responsibility of the health care provider to ascertain the FDA status of each drug or device planned for use in their clinical practice.

To purchase additional copies of this book, call our customer service department at (800) 638-3030 or fax orders to (301) 223-2320. International customers should call (301) 223-2300.

Visit Lippincott Williams & Wilkins on the Internet: at LWW.com. Lippincott Williams & Wilkins customer service representatives are available from 8:30 am to 6 pm, EST.

Preface

The second edition of *Pharmacology for Health Professionals* reflects the ever-changing science of pharmacology and the roles of health professionals related to pharmacologic agents. All information has been revised and updated according to the latest available information. The text prepares health care workers directly or indirectly involved in patient care to understand the uses of and issues related to most medications.

Purpose

This text is designed to provide a clear, concise introduction to pharmacology for students entering health professions programs. The basic explanations presented in this text are not intended to suggest that pharmacology is an easy subject. Drug therapy is one of the most important and complicated treatment modalities in modern health care. Because of its importance and complexity, and the frequent additions and changes in the field of pharmacology, it is imperative that health care professionals constantly review and update their knowledge.

Current Drug Information

The drug information in this text has been updated to include new drugs, uses, adverse reactions, and other information. The fully updated Summary Drug Tables throughout the text list current drugs by generic and trade name for each drug class.

Students and practitioners should remember that information about drugs, such as dosages and new forms, is constantly changing. Likewise, there may be new drugs on the market that were not approved by the Food and Drug Administration (FDA) at the time of publication of this text. The reader may find that certain drugs or drug dosages available when this textbook was published may no longer be available. For the most current drug information and dosages, references should be consulted, such as the most current *Physician's Desk Reference* or *Facts and Comparison* and the package inserts that accompany most drugs. Pharmacists or physicians can also be contacted for information concerning a specific drug, including dosage, adverse reactions, contraindications, precautions, interactions, or administration.

Special Features

A number of features have proven useful for students in health professions programs in their study of basic pharmacology. The features listed below appear in this text. Please see the User's Guide for more detailed information.

- Chapter Overview
- Chapter Objectives
- Key Terms
- Fact Check Questions
- Key Concepts Boxes
- Alerts
- Lifespan Considerations Boxes
- Signs and Symptoms Boxes
- Facts About Boxes
- Complementary and Alternative Medicine Boxes
- Key Points
- Critical Thinking Case Study Exercises
- Review Questions
- thePoint Resources
- Web Activities
- Summary Drug Tables

New to This Edition

Numerous new chapters and features have been added to this edition:

- **Chapter 2, The Administration of Drugs,** enhances student understanding of drug administration, including new tables on commonly used medication abbreviations and abbreviations that should be avoided, new Alert boxes, and new photographs.
- **Chapter 3, Math Review,** focuses on a review of basic math, including fractions, decimals percents, ratios and proportions, systems of measurement, conversions, and dosage calculations for adults and children. In-text examples are provided, and over 50 exercises are included in the Practice Problems section at the end of the chapter.
- **Chapter 46, Complementary and Alternative Medicine,** covers the use complementary and alternative medicine and discusses the uses, adverse reactions, and special considerations regarding herbal substances, vitamins, minerals and other natural remedies.
- **Chapter Overview** lists drug classes covered in each chapter and provides page numbers for the Summary Drug Tables for quick and easy reference.
- **Key Drug Concepts Boxes** emphasize important content or provide concise explanations of essential concepts that are critical for student understanding.
- **Lifespan Considerations Boxes** describe specific problems for which older adults and infants/children are at increased risk.
- **Signs and Symptoms Boxes** provide information on the signs and symptoms of various disorders or adverse reactions related to drugs covered in the chapter.
- **Complementary and Alternative Medicine Boxes** highlight key information about natural and alternative remedies that are proven effective for disorders treated by specific drugs or drug classes covered in the chapter.

- **Fact Check Questions** offer brief questions to quiz students on key points covered in the chapter. They reinforce learning and help students review as they read.
- **Chapter Review Elements** have been updated to include Critical Thinking Case Studies with open-ended questions, Review Questions that include a mix of multiple choice, true or false, fill in the blanks, and short answer exercises, and new and revised Web Activities.
- **Pregnancy Category** is included for drugs, where relevant.

The enhanced art program includes new figures to provide a refresher on anatomy and physiology and promote understanding of pharmacological concepts.

For easier instruction and better student understanding, several multi-topic chapters have been broken out into single-topic chapters. Adrenergic and Cholinergic Drugs is now covered in four chapters – Chapter 11: Adrenergic Drugs; Chapter 12: Adrenergic Blocking Drugs; Chapter 13: Cholinergic Drugs; and Chapter 14: Cholinergic Blocking Drugs. CNS and PNS drugs are now covered in two units (Unit II and Unit III), Urinary and GI drugs are also covered in two units (Unit VI and Unit VII), and Anti-Infective drugs, which were previously grouped with Immune drugs, are covered separately (Unit IX).

Organization

The text contains 46 chapters organized in 12 units. The organization is based on the teaching method most commonly used for pharmacology: drugs affecting the different body systems. Although pharmacological agents are presented in specific units, a disease may be treated with more than one type of drug, which may require consulting one or more units.

- **Unit I** presents a foundation for the study of pharmacology. These chapters cover the general principles of pharmacology, drug forms and methods of administration, and a review of basic math concepts, including concrete examples and student practice problems.
- **Unit II** contains seven chapters that present drugs that affect the central nervous system, grouped according to common classifications. Included are the various types of drugs used to manage pain.
- **Unit III** contains four chapters on drugs that affect the peripheral nervous system.
- **Unit IV** contains three chapters on drugs that affect the respiratory system.
- **Unit V** contains seven chapters on drugs that affect the cardiovascular system, including drugs for heart conditions and those related to the blood.
- **Unit VI** has three chapters covering drugs that affect the urinary system. Diuretic drugs are included here because of their primary effects on the urinary system.
- **Unit VII** covers drugs that affect the gastrointestinal system.
- **Unit VIII** contains five chapters that cover drugs that affect the endocrine and reproductive systems.
- **Unit IX** contains five chapters on anti-infective drugs.
- **Unit X** deals with drugs that affect the immune system, including antineoplastic agents.

- **Unit XI** has four chapters addressing drugs that affect other body systems, including the musculoskeletal system, skin, ears, and eyes, as well as fluids and electrolytes.
- **Unit XII** includes a new chapter on complementary and alternative medicine.

Appendices at the end of the book include the following:

- *Glossary*—key terms and other drug-related terms are listed and defined in Appendix A.
- *Answers to Fact Check Questions*—appear in Appendix B to help students assess their responses to these exercises.
- *Drugs and Health Care Information Sources on the World Wide Web*—are provided in Appendix E as a resource listing for more information about pharmacological issues.
- *Vaccine Adverse Event Reporting System (VAERS)* and *Med-Watch Forms* are included in Appendix C and Appendix D.
- *Abbreviations*—important pharmacological and general medical abbreviations that health care professionals need to know, related to drug therapy, are spelled out in Appendix F.

Chapter Content

The body of each chapter focuses on the actions, uses, adverse reactions, contraindications, precautions, and interactions of drug classes or types along with patient management issues and patient and family education. The information is intended to be introductory and at a level appropriate for students in health professions who may not administer drugs directly to patients but who may be directly or indirectly involved in patient care or otherwise need to understand basic pharmacological principles and information about drug classes.

- *Actions*—a basic explanation of how the drug accomplishes its intended activity.
- *Uses*—the more common uses of the drug class or type are provided. No unlabeled or experimental uses of drugs are given in the text (unless specifically identified as an unlabeled use) because the FDA does not approve these uses. Students should be reminded that under certain circumstances, some physicians may prescribe drugs for a condition not approved by the FDA or may prescribe an experimental drug.
- *Adverse Reactions*—the most common adverse drug reactions are listed under this heading.
- *Contraindications/Precautions/Interactions*—contraindications for use of the drug or drugs discussed in the chapter; precautions that should be taken before, during, or after drug administration; and the most common interactions between the drug(s) discussed in the chapter and other drugs or substances.
- *Patient Management Issues*—includes assessments that need to be made of the patient related to the administration of the drugs discussed in the chapter. In addition, information is provided related to promoting an optimal response to therapy, and monitoring and managing adverse reactions are included.
- *Educating the Patient and Family*—includes information that the patient and family members should know regarding the expected effects and adverse reactions associated with drug therapy. In addition, precautions or special instructions that the patient or family should know related to drug administration and the course of therapy are noted.

Summary Drug Tables appear at the end of each drug chapter. They list commonly used drugs representative of the class of drugs discussed in the chapter. In these tables, generic names are followed by trade names; when a drug is available under several trade names, several of the available trade names are given. To avoid interrupting the flow of the text, the exhaustive and complete Summary Drug Table for each of the drug category chapters is provided to students and faculty on the companion website, http://thepoint.lww.com/pharmacologyHP2e. In these tables, the more common or serious adverse reactions associated with the drug are listed in the adverse reaction section. It should be noted that any patient might exhibit adverse reactions not listed. Because of this possibility, any sign or symptom should be considered a possible adverse reaction until the primary health care provider determines the cause of the problem. The dose ranges for the drug follow the adverse reactions. In most cases, the adult dose ranges are given in these tables because space does not permit the inclusion of all possible dosages for various types of disorders. Pediatric dose ranges are not included because of the complexity of determining the pediatric dose. Many drugs given to children are determined on the basis of body weight or body surface area and have a variety of dosage schedules.

Teaching/Learning Package

Ancillary resources for students and faculty are available on the text's companion website on thePoint, http://thePoint.lww.com/AcostaPharmHP2e. They include the following:

Resources for Students:

- Free Access to online E-Book version of the complete text
- Comprehensive Summary Drug Tables, by chapter
- Pharmacology Animations
- Lippincott's Interactive Tutorials and Case Studies
- Dosage Calculation Quizzes
- Interactive Exercises for Study and Review
- Monographs of Most Commonly Prescribed Drugs

Additional Resources for Instructors:

- Answers to Case Study and Review Questions
- PowerPoint Slides
- Test Generator
- Image Bank

In addition, a companion print *Study Guide for Pharmacology for Health Professionals*, Second Edition, is also available.

User's Guide

About the Author

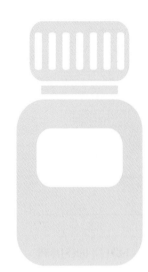

A pharmacist for more than 20 years, W. Renée Acosta, RPh, MS, currently teaches in the College of Pharmacy at the University of Texas at Austin. She was formerly the Department Chair for the Pharmacy Technician Training Program at Austin Community College. She has taught medication aides and has conducted a continuing education program on new drugs for nurses, EMTs, massage therapists, and other healthcare professionals for 10 years. She is the author of two textbooks in LWW's Foundations Series: *LWW's Foundations in Pharmacology for Pharmacy Technicians* and *LWW's Foundations in Sterile Products for Pharmacy Technicians*.

P harmacology for Health Professionals, second edition, addresses pharmacology topics that are essential for students entering health professions programs. This User's Guide introduces you to the special features of this text, which are designed to fully engage you in the learning process and enhance your understanding of the material.

Chapter Opening Elements

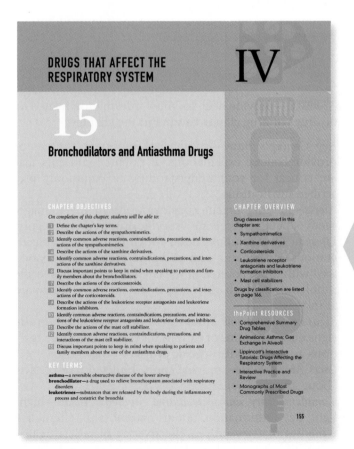

CHAPTER OVERVIEW —lists drug classes covered in each chapter. For quick and easy reference, page numbers for the Drug Summary Tables are also included.

CHAPTER OBJECTIVES —clarify what information you are expected to learn while reading and studying each chapter. Read these before beginning the chapter, then review them after completing the chapter to assess your comprehension.

KEY TERMS —provide a list of important new words used in the chapter and their definitions. These terms are boldfaced at their first use in the chapter to remind you of the earlier definitions. Study these terms to help build your vocabulary, so you can communicate more effectively with other health care professionals or patients.

THEPOINT RESOURCES —lists resources on the companion website on thePoint.

Chapter Features

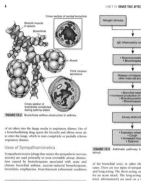

FULL-COLOR ILLUSTRATIONS —highlight and explain important pharmacologic concepts. In addition, detailed images of relevant anatomy and physiology provide a quick refresher before you learn about drug actions and uses for particular body systems.

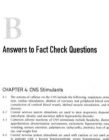

FACT CHECK QUESTIONS —test and reinforce your understanding of key facts to ensure learning objectives are met. Assess your understanding by checking the answers in Appendix B.

FEATURE BOXES —provide need-to-know information related to specific drugs or drug classes covered in the chapters.

- *Key Concepts Boxes*—emphasize important content or provide concise explanations of essential concepts that are critical for your understanding of commonly prescribed medications.
- *Alerts*—identify urgent considerations in the management of patients receiving a specific drug or drug category.
- *Lifespan Considerations Boxes*—highlight special considerations for geriatric and pediatric populations associated with drugs covered in the chapter, including specific problems for which older adults and infants/children are at increased risk.
- *Signs and Symptoms Boxes*—provide information on the signs and symptoms of various disorders or adverse reactions associated with specific drugs or drug classes
- *Facts About Boxes*—provide short, bulleted lists of facts about specific disorders.
- *Complementary and Alternative Medicine Boxes*—highlight key information about natural and alternative remedies that are proven effective for disorders treated by specific drugs or drug classes covered in the chapter.

Chapter Closing Features

KEY POINTS —provide a bulleted summary of critical information covered in the chapter.

CRITICAL THINKING CASE STUDY EXERCISE —presents a realistic patient situation followed by multiple-choice and open-ended questions to help you recall and apply information learned in the chapter.

REVIEW QUESTIONS —include a mix of multiple-choice, true or false, fill in the blanks, and short answer questions to help you review key chapter content and assess your learning.

WEB ACTIVITIES —encourage you to use the Internet as a resource to obtain additional information about drugs and patient care related to pharmacology therapy.

SUMMARY DRUG TABLES —contain generic and brand names of commonly used drugs representative of the class of drugs discussed in the chapter. Comprehensive Summary Drug Tables, including the generic name, pronunciation guide for generic names, trade names, uses, adverse reactions, dosage ranges, and pregnancy categories, are provided on the companion website, http://thepoint.lww.com/pharmacologyHP2e.

---

166   UNIT IV Drugs That Affect the Respiratory System

SUMMARY DRUG TABLE Bronchodilators
(left, generic; right, trade)
Comprehensive Summary Drug Tables, including uses, adverse effects, dosages, and pregnancy classifications, are provided on the companion website, http://thePoint.lww.com/PharmacologyHP2e

Sympathomimetics	
albuterol sulfate *al-byoo'-ter-ole*	Proventil HFA, Ventolin HFA, ProAir HFA, VoSpire ER, AccuNeb, *generic*
arformoterol *ar-for-moe'-ter-ol*	Brovana
ephedrine sulfate *e-fed'-rin*	*generic*
epinephrine *ep-i-nef'-rin*	Adrenalin (Rx), *generic* (Rx)
formoterol fumarate *for-moh'-te-rol*	Foradil Aerolizer
isoproterenol HCl *eye-soe-proe-ter'-a-nole*	Isuprel
levalbuterol HCl *lev-al-byoo'-ter-ole*	Xopenex
metaproterenol sulfate *met-a-proe-ter'-e-nole*	*generic*
pirbuterol acetate *peer-byoo'-ter-ole*	Maxair Autohaler
salmeterol *sal-mee'-ter-ol*	Serevent
terbutaline sulfate *ter-byoo'-ta-leen*	Brethine, *generic*
Xanthine Derivatives	
aminophylline *am-in-off'-i-lin*	*generic*
dyphylline *dye'-fi-lin*	Lufyllin
theophylline *thee-off-i-lin*	Theo-24, Theochron, Uniphyl, *generic*
Anticholinergic	
ipratropium bromide *ih-prah-trow'-pea- um*	Atrovent, Atrovent HFA, *generic*

SUMMARY DRUG TABLE Antiasthma Drugs
(left, generic; right, trade)
Comprehensive Summary Drug Tables, including uses, adverse effects, dosages, and pregnancy classifications, are provided on the companion website, http://thePoint.lww.com/PharmacologyHP2e

Corticosteroids	
beclomethasone dipropionate *be-kloe-meth'-a-sone*	Beconase AQ, QVAR
budesonide *bue-des'-oh-nide*	Pulmicort Flexhaler, Rhinicort Aqua, *generic*
ciclesonide *sye-kles'-oh-nide*	Alvesco
flunisolide *floo-niss'-oh-lide*	AeroBid, AeroBid-M, Nasarel, *generic*
fluticasone propionate *flew-tick'-ah-sone pro'-pee-oh-nate*	FloVent Diskus, FloVent HFA, Flonase, Veramyst
mometasone *moe-met'-a-sone*	Asmanex
Leukotriene Receptor Antagonists	
montelukast sodium *mon-tell-oo'-kast*	Singulair
zafirlukast *zah-fir'-luh-kast*	Accolate
Leukotriene Formation Inhibitors	
zileuton *zye-loot'-on*	Zyflo, Zyflo CR
Mast Cell Stabilizers	
cromolyn *kroe'-moe-lin*	Nasalcrom (OTC), *generic*

Teaching/Learning Package

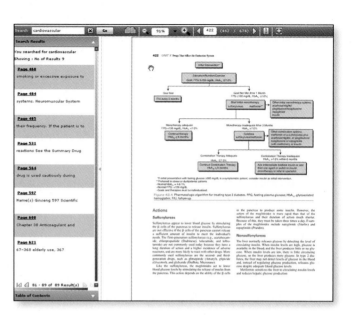

Ancillary resources for students and faculty are available on the text's companion website on thePoint, **http://thePoint.lww.com/PharmacologyHP2e.**

RESOURCES FOR STUDENTS

- Free E-Book Version of the Complete Text
- Comprehensive Summary Drug Tables, by chapter
- Pharmacology Animations
- Lippincott's Interactive Tutorials and Case Studies
- Dosage Calculation Quizzes
- Interactive Exercises for Study and Review
- Monographs of Most Commonly Prescribed Drugs

ADDITIONAL RESOURCES FOR INSTRUCTORS

- Answers to Case Study and Review Questions
- PowerPoint Slides
- Test Generator
- Image Bank

In addition, a companion print *Study Guide for Pharmacology for Health Professionals*, Second Edition, is also available.

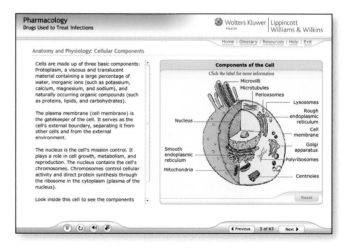

Reviewers

Esther Brown
Brown Mackie College

P. David Falkenstein, MS, PA-C
Northern Virginia Community College

Terry Forrest, MBA
Gwinnett Technical College

Kay Frieze
College of the Mainland

Ellen Wruble Hakim, DScPT, PT, MS, CWS, FAACWS
University of Maryland School of Medicine

Betty Klein, MS, RN
Ivy Tech Community College of Indiana

Randy De Kler, MS
Miami Dade College

Richelle Laipply, PhD
University of Akron

Stephanie LaPuma, MAM, MBA, CRTT
Hamilton College

Mary Larsen
Academy of Professional Careers

Marisa Maron, CPhT
Institute of Technology, Inc.

Patricia A. Moody, RN
Athens Technical College

Melyssa Munch
Star Technical Institute

Georgette Rosenfeld, PhD
Indian River State College

Stephen Scott, RN, PhD
University of Kansas School of Nursing

Janet Stringer, MD, PhD
Baylor College of Medicine

Tonia Watson
Lincoln Technical Institute

Figure Credits

8-1, 12-1, 20-2, 20-3, 30-1	Acosta WR. LWW's Foundations in Pharmacology for Pharmacy Technicians. Baltimore: Lippincott Williams & Wilkins, 2010.
p. 276	With permission from American Association of Poison Control Centers.
16-2, 20-1, 22-1, 29-2	Anatomical Chart Company.
p. 41	Ansel HC. Pharmaceutical Calculations. 13th Edition. Baltimore: Lippincott Williams & Wilkins, 2010.
43-1	Bickley LS. Bates' Guide to Physical Examination and History Taking. 10th Ed. Philadelphia: Lippincott Williams & Wilkins, 2009.
38-1	DPDx - CDC Parasitology Diagnostic Web Site, Centers for Disease Control.
40-2, 42-1	Cohen BJ. Medical Terminology: An Illustrated Guide. 6th ed. Baltimore: Lippincott Williams & Wilkins, 2011.
15-1, 33-1, 33-3	Cohen BJ. Memmler's The Human Body in Health and Disease. 11th Edition. Baltimore: Lippincott Williams & Wilkins, 2009.
37-2	Engleberg NC, Dermody T, DiRita V. Schaecter's Mechanisms of Microbial Disease, 4th Edition. Baltimore: Lippincott Williams & Wilkins, 2007.
1-1	FDA/Center for Drug Evaluation and Research
1-2, 2-3, 5-1, 7-1, 8-2, 9-1, 11-3, 11-5, 14-1, 15-2, 19-1, 19-2, 21-1, 23-1, 25-1, 31-1, 31-2, 35-1, 37-1, 38-2, 40-3, 41-2, 44-1, 44-3	Ford SM, Roach SS. Roach's Introductory Clinical Pharmacology. Philadelphia: Lippincott Williams & Wilkins, 2010.
43-5	Goodheart HP. Goodheart's Photoguide to Common Skin Disorders: Diagnosis and Management. 3rd Ed. Philadelphia: Lippincott Williams & Wilkins, 2009.
p. 40	Buchholz S. Henke's Med-Math Dosage Calculation, Preparation & Administration. 7th Ed. Philadelphia: Lippincott Williams & Wilkins, 2012.
1-3, 1-5	Karch AM. Focus on Nursing Pharmacology. 5th Ed. Philadelphia: Lippincott Williams & Wilkins, 2005.
2-1, 2-2, 2-5, 30-2	Lynn P. Lippincott's Photo Atlas of Medication Administration. 4th Ed. Philadelphia: Lippincott Williams & Wilkins, 2011.
4-1	McConnell TH, Hull KL. Human Form, Human Function: Essentials of Anatomy & Physiology. Baltimore: Lippincott Williams & Wilkins, 2011.
2-6	Photo by Rick Brady.
40-1, 44-2	Pillitteri A. Maternal and Child Nursing. 6th Ed., Philadelphia: Lippincott Williams & Wilkins, 2010.
34-1	Premkumar K. Anatomy & Physiology: The Massage Connection. 3rd Ed. Baltimore: Lippincott Williams & Wilkins, 2012.
42-2, 42-3, 28-1	Rubin R, Strayer DS, Rubin E. Rubin's Pathology: Clinicopathologic Foundations of Medicine. 6th Ed. Philadelphia: Lippincott Williams & Wilkins, 2012.
43-4	National Pressure Ulcer Advisory Panel, Reston, VA.
38-3	McConnell TM. The Nature of Disease: Pathology for the Health Professions. Baltimore: Lippincott Williams & Wilkins, 2008.
18-2	Willis MC. Medical Terminology: The Language of Health Care. 2nd Ed. Baltimore: Lippincott Williams & Wilkins, 2006.
4-2, 29-1, 33-2	Willis MC. A Programmed Learning Approach to the Language of Health Care. 2nd Ed. Baltimore: Lippincott Williams & Wilkins, 2008.

Other figures drawn by Kim Battista.

Table of Contents

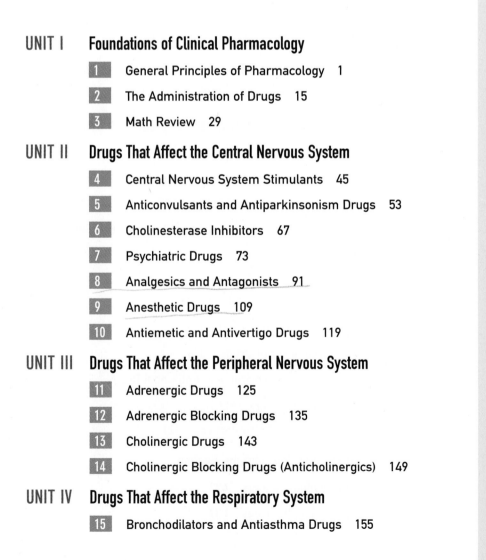

1

General Principles of Pharmacology

CHAPTER OBJECTIVES

On completion of this chapter, students will be able to:

1. Define the chapter's key terms.
2. Describe the drug development process.
3. Identify the different names assigned to drugs.
4. Distinguish between prescription drugs, nonprescription drugs, and controlled substances.
5. Discuss federal laws regarding drug distribution and administration.
6. Discuss the pharmacokinetic phase.
7. Discuss the concepts of biotransformation, first-pass effect, and clearance.
8. Discuss the difference between an agonist and an antagonist.
9. Discuss the types of drug reactions and interactions that may occur.
10. Identify the different factors that affect the way a patient responds or reacts to a drug.
11. Identify different types of allergic drug reactions.

KEY TERMS

additive drug reaction—a reaction that occurs when the combined effect of two drugs is equal to the sum of each drug given alone
adverse reaction—undesirable drug effect; also called adverse effect
agonist—a drug that binds with a receptor to produce a therapeutic response
allergic reaction—a drug reaction that occurs because the individual's immune system views the drug as a foreign substance; also called adverse effect or reaction
anaphylactic shock—an extremely serious allergic drug reaction
antagonist—a drug that joins with a receptor to prevent the action of an agonist at that receptor
antibodies—immune system molecules produced in reaction to an antigen
antigen—a substance that the immune system perceives as foreign and that causes production of antibodies

thePOINT RESOURCES

- Animations: Drug Absorption; Drug Binding; Drug Distribution; Drug Excretion
- Lippincott's Interactive Tutorials: Pharmacology Basics
- Interactive Practice and Review
- Monographs of Most Commonly Prescribed Drugs

biotransformation—chemical alteration of a substance in the body occurring at some point between absorption into the general circulation and renal elimination

clearance—a measure of the body's ability to eliminate a substance or drug

controlled substances—drugs with a high potential for abuse and dependence that are regulated by the Drug Enforcement Agency (DEA)

cumulative drug effect—a drug effect that occurs when the body has not fully metabolized a dose of a drug before the next dose is given

drug idiosyncrasy—any unusual or abnormal reaction to a drug

drug tolerance—a decreased response to a drug, requiring an increase in dosage to achieve the desired effect

first-pass effect—a process that may limit a drug's bio-availability whereby the drug is absorbed intact and transported to the liver via the portal circulation where it undergoes extensive metabolism

half-life—time required for the body to eliminate 50% of the drug

hypersensitivity—being allergic to a drug

nonprescription drugs—drugs designated by the Food and Drug Administration (FDA) to be obtained without a prescription

pharmaceutic phase—the dissolution of the drug

pharmacodynamics—a drug's actions and effects within the body

pharmacogenetic disorder—a genetically determined abnormal response to normal doses of a drug

pharmacokinetics—activities occurring within the body after a drug is administered, including absorption, distribution, metabolism, and excretion; the body's effect on the drug

pharmacology—the study of drugs and their action on living organisms

physical dependence—a compulsive need to use a substance repeatedly to avoid mild to severe withdrawal symptoms

polypharmacy—the taking of numerous drugs that can potentially react with one another

prescription drugs—drugs the FDA has designated as potentially harmful unless supervised by a licensed health care provider

psychological dependence—a compulsion to use a substance to obtain a pleasurable experience

receptor—a specialized macromolecule that binds to the drug molecule, altering the function of the cell and producing the therapeutic response

synergism—a drug interaction that occurs when drugs produce an effect that is greater than the sum of their separate actions

teratogen—any substance that causes abnormal development of the fetus

therapeutic response—the intended (beneficial) effect of a drug

toxic reaction—harmful drug effect

Pharmacology is the study of drugs and their actions on living organisms. A sound knowledge of basic pharmacologic principles is essential for most health care professionals, especially those who interact with patients who receive medications. This chapter gives a basic overview of pharmacologic principles, drug development, and federal legislation affecting the dispensing and use of drugs.

Drug Development

Drug development is a long and arduous process, which takes anywhere from 7 to 12 years, and sometimes even longer. The United States Food and Drug Administration (FDA) has the responsibility of approving new drugs and monitoring drugs for adverse or toxic reactions. The development of a new drug is divided into the pre-FDA phase and the FDA phase (Fig. 1-1). During the pre-FDA phase, a manufacturer develops a drug that looks promising. *In vitro* testing (testing in an environment outside the body, such as in a test tube) is performed using animal and human cells. This testing is followed by studies in live animals. The manufacturer then applies to the FDA for investigational new drug (IND) status.

With IND status, clinical testing of the new drug begins. Clinical testing involves three phases, each involving a larger number of people. All pharmacologic and biologic effects are noted. Phase I lasts 4 to 6 weeks and involves 20 to 100 individuals who are either "normal" volunteers or individuals in the intended treatment population. If phase I studies are successful, the testing moves to phase II and, if those results are positive, to phase III. Each successive phase has a larger subject

population. Phase III studies generate more information on dosing and safety. The three phases last anywhere from 2 to 10 years, with an average of 5 years.

A new drug application (NDA) is submitted after the investigation of the drug in phases I, II, and III is complete and the drug is found to be safe and effective. With the NDA, the manufacturer submits all data collected during the clinical trials. A panel of experts, including pharmacologists, chemists, physicians, and other professionals, reviews the application and makes a recommendation to the FDA. The FDA then either approves or disapproves the drug for use. This process of review takes approximately 2 years, although some drugs are reviewed and approved more quickly while others take longer.

After FDA approval, continued surveillance is performed to ensure safety after the manufacturer places the drug on the market. During this surveillance, which is also referred to as phase IV, an ongoing review of the drug occurs with particular attention given to adverse reactions. Health care professionals are encouraged to help with this surveillance by reporting adverse effects of both prescription and nonprescription drugs to the FDA by using the MedWatch system.

A drug must be used and studied for many years before all of its adverse reactions are identified. The FDA established a reporting program called MedWatch, by which health care professionals can report observations of serious adverse drug effects using a standard form (see Appendix D for a sample form). The FDA protects the identity of those who voluntarily report adverse reactions. This form is also used to report an undesirable experience associated with the use of medical products (e.g., latex gloves, pacemakers, infusion pumps, anaphylaxis, blood, blood

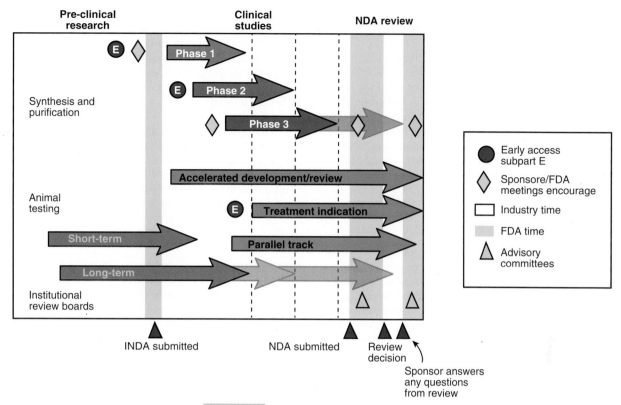

FIGURE 1-1 Phases of drug development.

components, etc).The FDA considers serious adverse reactions as those that may result in death, life-threatening illness, hospitalization, disability, or those that may require medical or surgical intervention. Adverse drug reactions may be reported to the FDA by mail, fax, or e-mail. For more information, go to this Web site: www.fda.gov/medwatch/index.html

Special FDA Programs

Although it takes considerable time for most drugs to get FDA approval, the FDA has special programs to meet certain needs, such as the orphan drug program, accelerated programs for urgent needs, and compassionate use programs.

Orphan Drug Program

The Orphan Drug Act of 1983 was passed to encourage the development and marketing of products used to treat rare diseases. The act defines a "rare disease" as a condition affecting fewer than 200,000 individuals in the United States. The National Organization of Rare Disorders reports that there are nearly 7000 rare disorders that affect a total of approximately 25 million individuals. Examples of rare disorders include Tourette syndrome, acquired immunodeficiency syndrome (AIDS), Huntington disease, and certain forms of leukemia.

The Orphan Drug Act provides for incentives, such as research grants, protocol assistance by the FDA, and special tax credits, to encourage manufacturers to develop orphan drugs. If the drug is approved, then the manufacturer has 7 years of exclusive marketing rights. More than 300 new drugs and products have received FDA approval since the law was passed. Examples of orphan drugs include thalidomide for leprosy,

triptorelin pamoate for ovarian cancer, tetrabenazine for Huntington disease, and zidovudine for AIDS.

Accelerated Programs

Accelerated approval of drugs is offered by the FDA as a means to make promising products for life-threatening diseases available on the market, based on preliminary evidence, before complete testing has demonstrated benefits for patients. A "provisional approval" may be granted, with a written commitment from the pharmaceutical company to complete clinical studies that formally demonstrate patient benefit. This program seeks to make life-saving investigational drugs available to treat diseases that pose a significant health threat to the public. One example of a disease that qualifies as posing a significant health threat is AIDS. Because AIDS is so devastating to the individuals affected, and because of the danger the disease poses to public health, the FDA and pharmaceutical companies are working together to shorten the IND approval process for some drugs that show promise in treating AIDS. This accelerated process allows health care providers to administer a drug with positive results in early phase I and II clinical trials, rather than wait until final approval is granted. If the drug continues to prove beneficial, then the process of approval is accelerated.

Compassionate Access to Unapproved Drugs

The compassionate access program allows patients to receive drugs that have not yet been approved by the FDA. This program provides experimental drugs for patients who could benefit from new treatments but who probably would die before the drug is approved for use. These patients are often too sick to participate in controlled studies. Drug manufacturers make a proposal to the FDA to target patients with the disease. The company then provides the drug free to these patients. The pharmaceutical company analyzes and presents to the FDA data about this treatment. This program can be beneficial but is not without problems. Because the drug is not in full production, quantities may be limited; the number of patients may be limited, and patients may be selected at random. Because patients receiving compassionate access often are sicker, they have an increased risk for toxic reactions. Thus, a newly developed drug may gain a bad reputation even before marketing begins.

Drug Names

Throughout the process of development, drugs may have several names: a chemical name, a generic (nonproprietary) name, an official name, and a trade or brand name. These names can be confusing without a clear understanding of the different names used. Table 1-1 identifies the different names and explains each.

A need still exists to standardize the naming of drugs. The RxNorm system was developed by the National Library of Medicine to coordinate information among the various forms of drug nomenclatures through the use of the Unified Medical Language System, a computerized metathesaurus. Even if only one name of a drug is known, any information about the drug can be located using this system.

Drug Categories

After approving a drug, the FDA assigns it to one of the following categories: prescription, nonprescription, or controlled substance.

Prescription Drugs

Prescription drugs are drugs that the federal government has designated to be potentially harmful unless their use is supervised by a licensed health care provider, such as a nurse practitioner, physician, or dentist. Although these drugs have

been tested for safety and therapeutic effect, prescription drugs may cause different reactions in some individuals.

In hospitals and other institutional settings, patients are monitored for the therapeutic effect and adverse reactions of the drugs they are given. Some drugs have the potential to be toxic (harmful). When these drugs are prescribed to be taken at home, the patient and/or family members are educated about the drug.

Prescription drugs, also called legend drugs, are the largest category of drugs. Prescription drugs must be prescribed by a licensed health care provider. The prescription (Fig. 1-2) contains the name of the drug, the dosage, the method and times of administration, and the signature of the licensed health care provider prescribing the drug, along with other information.

Nonprescription Drugs

Nonprescription drugs are drugs that are designated by the FDA to be safe without supervision by a health care provider if taken as directed. They can be obtained without a prescription. These drugs are also referred to as over-the-counter (OTC) drugs and are available in many different settings, such as a pharmacy, drugstore, or supermarket. OTC drugs include those taken for symptoms of the common cold, headaches, constipation, diarrhea, and upset stomach.

Even nonprescription drugs, however, carry some risk and may produce adverse reactions. For example, acetylsalicylic acid, commonly known as aspirin, is potentially harmful and can cause gastrointestinal bleeding and salicylism (see Chapter 8). Product labels must give consumers important information regarding the drug, dosage, contraindications, precautions, and adverse reactions. Consumers are urged to read the directions carefully before taking OTC drugs.

Controlled Substances

Controlled substances are the most carefully monitored of all drugs. These drugs have a high potential for abuse and may cause physical or psychological dependence. **Physical dependence** is a compulsive need to use a substance repeatedly to avoid mild to severe withdrawal symptoms; it is the body's dependence on repeated administration of a drug.

TABLE 1-1 **Drug Names**

Drug Name and Example	Explanation
Chemical name Example: ethyl 4-(8-chloro-5,6-dihydro-11*H*-benzo[5,6] cyclohepta[1,2-*b*]-pyridin-11-ylidene)-1-piperidinecarboxylate	Gives the exact chemical makeup of the drug and placing of the atoms or molecular structure; it is not capitalized
Generic name (nonproprietary) Example: loratadine	Name given to a drug before it becomes official; may be used in all countries, by all manufacturers; it is not capitalized
Official name Example: loratadine	Name listed in *The United States Pharmacopeia-National Formulary*; may be the same as the generic name
Trade name (brand name) Example: Claritin	Name that is registered by the manufacturer and is followed by the trademark symbol; the name can be used only by the manufacturer; a drug may have several trade names, depending on the number of manufacturers; the first letter of the name is capitalized

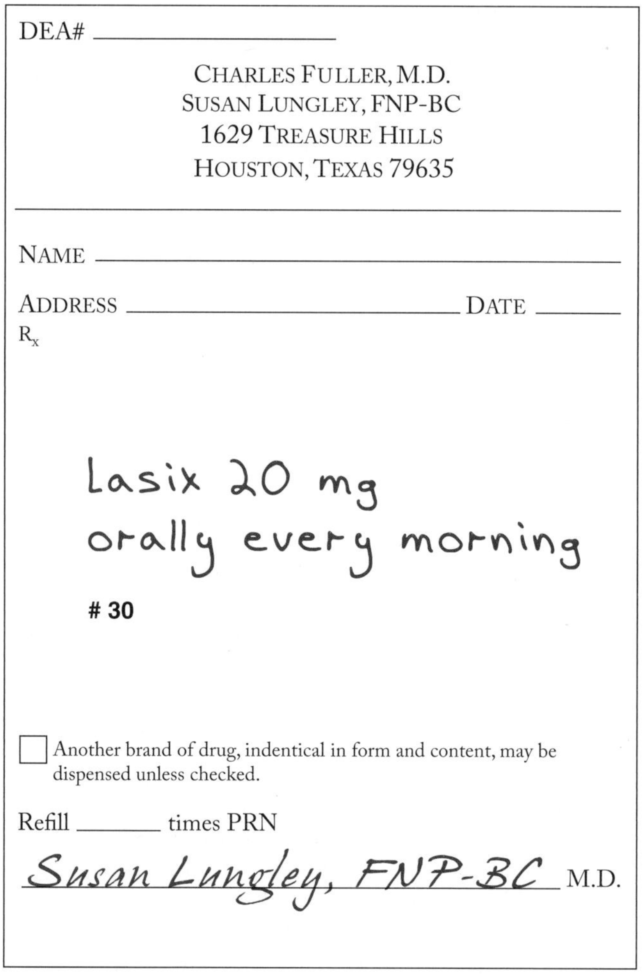

DEA# _____

CHARLES FULLER, M.D.
SUSAN LUNGLEY, FNP-BC
1629 TREASURE HILLS
HOUSTON, TEXAS 79635

_____

NAME _____

ADDRESS _____ DATE _____

R_x

Lasix 20 mg
orally every morning

30

☐ Another brand of drug, indentical in form and content, may be
dispensed unless checked.

Refill _____ times PRN

Susan Lungley, FNP-BC M.D.

FIGURE 1-2 Example of a prescription form.

KEY CONCEPTS

1-1 Schedules of Controlled Substances

Schedule I (C–I)
- High abuse potential
- No accepted medical use in the United States
- Examples: heroin, marijuana, lysergic acid diethylamide, peyote

Schedule II (C–II)
- Potential for high abuse with severe physical or psychological dependence
- Examples: narcotics such as meperidine, methadone, morphine, oxycodone; amphetamines; and barbiturates

Schedule III (C–III)
- Less abuse potential than schedule II drugs
- Potential for moderate physical or psychological dependence
- Examples: nonbarbiturate sedatives, nonamphetamine stimulants, limited amounts of certain narcotics

Schedule IV (C–IV)
- Less abuse potential than schedule III drugs
- Limited dependence potential
- Examples: some sedatives and anxiety agents, nonnarcotic analgesics

Schedule V (C–V)*
- Limited abuse potential
- Examples: small amounts of narcotics (codeine) used as antitussives or antidiarrheals

*Under federal law, limited quantities of certain schedule V drugs may be purchased without a prescription directly from a pharmacist if allowed under state law. The purchaser must be at least 18 years of age and must furnish identification. All such transactions must be recorded by the dispensing pharmacist.

Psychological dependence is a compulsion to use a substance to obtain a pleasurable experience; it is the mind's dependence on the repeated administration of a drug. One type of dependence may lead to the other.

The Controlled Substances Act of 1970 regulates the manufacture, distribution, and dispensing of drugs that have abuse potential. Drugs under the Controlled Substances Act are categorized in five schedules, based on their potential for abuse and physical and psychological dependence. Key Concepts 1-1 describes the five schedules.

Prescriptions for controlled substances must be written in ink and include the name and address of the patient and the Drug Enforcement Agency (DEA) number of the health care provider. Prescriptions for these drugs cannot be filled more than 6 months after the prescription was written and cannot be refilled more than five times. Under federal law, limited quantities of certain schedule C-V drugs may be purchased without a prescription, with the purchase recorded by the dispensing pharmacist. In some cases, state laws are more restrictive than federal laws and impose additional requirements for the sale and distribution of controlled substances. In hospitals or other agencies that dispense controlled substances, scheduled drugs are counted every 8 to 12 hours to account for each ampule, tablet, or other form of the drug. Any discrepancy in the number of drugs must be investigated and explained immediately.

The Drug Enforcement Administration within the U.S. Department of Justice is the chief federal agency responsible for enforcing the Controlled Substances Act. Failure to comply with the Controlled Substances Act is punishable by fine and/or imprisonment. With drug abuse so prevalent, all health care workers must diligently adhere to DEA, FDA, and state regulations.

Federal Drug Legislation and Enforcement

Many laws regarding drug distribution and administration have been enacted during the past century, including the Pure Food and Drug Act; Harrison Narcotic Act; Pure Food, Drug, and Cosmetic Act; the Comprehensive Drug Abuse Prevention and Control Act; the Dietary Supplement Health Education Act; and the Health Insurance Portability and Accountability Act (HIPAA).

These laws control the use of prescription and nonprescription drugs, supplements, and controlled substances.

Pure Food and Drug Act

The Pure Food and Drug Act, passed in 1906, was the first attempt by the government to regulate and control the manufacture, distribution, and sale of drugs. Before 1906, any substance could be called a drug, and no testing or research was required before placing a drug on the market. Before this time, the potency and purity of many drugs were questionable, and some were even dangerous for human use.

Harrison Narcotic Act

The Harrison Narcotic Act, passed in 1914, regulated the sale of narcotic drugs. Before the passage of this act, any narcotic could be purchased without a prescription. This law was amended many times. In 1970, the Harrison Narcotic Act was replaced by the Comprehensive Drug Abuse Prevention and Control Act.

Food, Drug, and Cosmetic Act

In 1938, Congress passed the Food, Drug, and Cosmetic Act, which gave the FDA control over the manufacture and sale of drugs, food, and cosmetics. Previously, some drugs, as well as foods and cosmetics, contained chemicals that were often harmful to humans. This law requires that these substances are safe for human use. It also requires pharmaceutical companies to perform toxicology tests before submitting a new drug to the FDA for approval. After FDA review of the tests performed on animals and other research data, approval may be given to market the drug, as described earlier.

Comprehensive Drug Abuse Prevention and Control Act

Congress passed the Comprehensive Drug Abuse Prevention and Control Act in 1970 because of the growing problem of drug abuse. It regulates the manufacture, distribution, and dispensation of drugs with a potential for abuse. Title II of this law, the Controlled Substances Act, deals with control and enforcement. The DEA within the U.S. Department of Justice is the leading federal agency responsible for the enforcement of this act.

Dietary Supplement Health and Education Act of 1994

This law allows the DEA limited oversight of vitamins, minerals, herbs, and nutritional supplements. The DEA may investigate "false claims" advertising and may require manufacturers to provide research and proof to back up their claims of product efficacy.

Health Insurance Portability and Accountability Act of 1996

HIPAA has many provisions that have directly impacted all health care facilities and primarily affects the confidentiality of patient medical records. All health care facilities must provide information to the patient and document how they protect the patient's health information.

KEY CONCEPTS

1-2   Pregnancy Categories

Category	Risk Level
A	No risk
B	Risk can't be ruled out
C	Caution is advised
D	Definite risk
X	Do not use

Drug Use and Pregnancy

The use of any prescription or nonprescription medication carries a risk of causing birth defects in a developing fetus. Drugs administered to pregnant women, particularly during the first trimester (3 months), may cause teratogenic effects. A **teratogen** is any substance that causes abnormal development of the fetus, which may lead to a severely deformed fetus.

In an effort to prevent teratogenic effects, the FDA has established five drug categories based on the potential of a drug for causing birth defects. Key Concepts 1-2 outlines these categories. Information regarding the pregnancy category of a specific drug is found in reliable drug literature, such as the inserts accompanying drugs and drug reference books. In general, most drugs are contraindicated during pregnancy or lactation unless the potential benefits of taking the drug outweigh the risks to the fetus or infant.

During pregnancy, no woman should consider taking any drug, legal or illegal, prescription or nonprescription, unless the drug is prescribed or recommended by her health care provider. Smoking and drinking alcoholic beverages also carry risks, such as low birth weight, premature birth, and fetal alcohol syndrome. Children born to mothers using addictive drugs, such as cocaine or heroin, often are born with an addiction to the drug, along with other health problems.

Drug Actions within the Body

Drugs act in various ways in the body. Drugs taken by mouth (except liquids) go through three phases: the pharmaceutic phase, pharmacokinetic phase, and pharmacodynamic phase. Liquid and parenteral drugs (drugs given by injection) go through the latter two phases only.

Pharmaceutic Phase

The **pharmaceutic phase** of drug action is the dissolution of the drug. Drugs must be in solution to be absorbed. Drugs that are liquid or drugs given by injection (parenteral drugs) do not go through the pharmaceutic phase because they are already in solution. A tablet or capsule (solid forms of a drug) goes through this phase as it disintegrates into small particles and dissolves into body fluids within the gastrointestinal tract. Enteric-coated tablets do not disintegrate until reaching the alkaline environment of the small intestine.

Pharmacokinetic Phase

Pharmacokinetics refers to metabolic activities involving the drug within the body after it is administered. These activities include absorption, bioavailability and distribution, metabolism, and excretion. Another pharmacokinetic component, the drug's half-life, is a measure of the rate at which it is removed from the body.

Absorption

Absorption follows administration and is the process by which a drug becomes available for use in the body. It occurs after dissolution of a solid form of the drug or after the administration of a liquid or parenteral drug. In this process of absorption, drug particles are moved into body fluids. This movement can be accomplished in several ways: active absorption, passive absorption, and pinocytosis. In active absorption, a carrier molecule such as a protein or enzyme actively moves the drug across a membrane. Passive absorption occurs by diffusion (movement from a higher concentration to a lower concentration). In pinocytosis, cells engulf the drug particle causing movement across the cell.

As the body transfers the drug from body fluids to tissue sites, absorption into body tissues occurs. Several factors influence the rate of absorption, including the route of administration, the solubility of the drug, and certain body conditions. Drugs are most rapidly absorbed when given by the intravenous route directly into the bloodstream, followed by the intramuscular route (injection into muscle tissue), the subcutaneous (injection under the skin), and, lastly, the oral route. Some drugs are more soluble and thus are absorbed more rapidly than others. For example, water-soluble drugs are readily absorbed into the systemic circulation. Some body conditions, such as developing lipodystrophy (atrophy of the subcutaneous tissue) caused by repeated subcutaneous injections, inhibit absorption of a drug given in the site of lipodystrophy. Also, the presence of food in the stomach can affect the absorption of orally administered medications.

Bioavailability and Drug Distribution

Bioavailability is the term used to describe the fraction of the drug that reaches systemic circulation (blood flow throughout the body) chemically unchanged. The systemic circulation distributes drugs to various body tissues or target sites. There, drugs interact with specific receptors. Some drugs travel through the bloodstream by binding to protein (albumin) in the blood. Drugs bound to protein are pharmacologically inactive. Only when the protein molecules release the drug can it diffuse into the tissues, interact with receptors, and produce a therapeutic effect.

As the drug circulates in the blood, a certain blood level must be maintained for it to be effective. When the blood level decreases to below the therapeutic level, the drug will not produce the desired effect. Should the blood level increase significantly above the therapeutic level, toxic symptoms may develop.

Metabolism

Metabolism, sometimes called **biotransformation**, is the process of chemical reactions by which the liver converts a drug to inactive compounds. The process called **first-pass effect** applies to drugs absorbed across the cell membranes of the small intestines that are first transported to the liver via portal circulation where they undergo liver metabolism before release into the systemic circulation. The first-pass effect can decrease bioavailability of the drug. Only drugs administered orally undergo the first-pass effect. Frequent liver function tests are necessary when a patient has liver disease. The kidneys, lungs, plasma, and intestinal mucosa also aid in the metabolism of drugs.

Excretion

The elimination of drugs from the body is called **clearance**. It occurs primarily through renal excretion. After the liver renders a drug inactive, the kidneys excrete the inactive compounds from the body in the urine. Some drugs are excreted unchanged by the kidney without liver involvement. Patients with kidney disease may require a lower dosage and careful monitoring of their kidney function. The concept of renal clearance is a way to measure the rate of drug elimination by the kidneys in relation to the drug concentration in the blood. Other drugs are eliminated from the body through sweat, breast milk, breathing, feces, or bile (Fig. 1-3).

Half-Life

Half-life is the time required for the body to eliminate 50% of the drug. Drugs with a short half-life (2–4 hours) need to be administered frequently, whereas a drug with a long half-life (21–24 hours) requires less frequent dosing. For example, digoxin (Lanoxin) has a long half-life (36 hours) and requires once-daily dosing. However, aspirin has a short half-life and requires frequent dosing. It takes five to six half-lives to eliminate approximately 98% of a drug from the body. Although a drug's half-life is the same in most people, patients with liver or kidney disease may have problems excreting a drug; this increases its half-life and increases the risk of toxicity. Older patients or patients with impaired

---

ALERT Rx

Liver Disease

Because drugs are primarily metabolized by the liver, patients with liver disease may require lower dosages of a drug, or the health care provider may select a drug that does not undergo biotransformation in the liver.

CONSIDERATIONS

LIFESPAN

Kidney Function

Because children have immature kidney function, they may require dosage reduction and kidney function tests. Similarly, older adults have diminished kidney function and require careful monitoring and lower dosages.

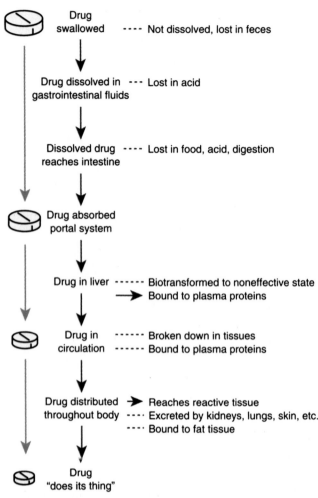

FIGURE 1-3   Pharmacokinetics affect the amount of a drug reaching reactive tissues. Very little of an oral dose of a drug actually reaches reactive sites.

kidney or liver function require frequent diagnostic tests of their renal or hepatic function.

Pharmacodynamic Phase

Pharmacodynamics are the drug's actions and effects within the body. Key Concepts 1-3 summarizes the difference between pharmacokinetics and pharmacodynamics. After administration, most drugs enter the systemic circulation and expose almost all body tissues to their possible effects. All drugs produce more than one effect in the body. The primary effect of a

drug is the desired or therapeutic effect. Secondary effects are all other effects, whether desirable or undesirable, produced by the drug.

Most drugs have an affinity for certain organs or tissues and exert their greatest action at the cellular level in those specific areas, which are called target sites. The two main mechanisms of action are an alteration in cellular environment or cellular function.

Alteration in Cellular Environment

Some drugs act on the body by changing the cellular environment physically or chemically. Physical changes in the cellular environment include changes in osmotic pressures, lubrication, absorption, or conditions on the surface of the cell membrane. An example of a drug that changes osmotic pressure is mannitol, which produces a change in the osmotic pressure in brain cells, reducing cerebral edema. A drug that acts by altering the cellular environment by lubrication is sunscreen. An example of a drug that acts by altering absorption is activated charcoal, which is administered orally to absorb a toxic chemical ingested into the gastrointestinal tract. The stool softener docusate is an example of a drug that acts by altering the surface of the cellular membrane. Docusate has emulsifying and lubricating activity that causes a lowering of the surface tension in the cells of the bowel, permitting water and fats to enter the stool. This softens the fecal mass, allowing easier passage of the stool.

Chemical changes in the cellular environment include inactivation of cellular functions or an alteration of the chemical components of body fluid, such as a change in the pH. For example, antacids neutralize gastric acidity in patients with peptic ulcers.

Alteration in Cellular Function

Most drugs act on the body by altering cellular function. A drug cannot completely change the function of a cell, but it can alter its function. A drug that alters cellular function can increase or decrease certain physiologic functions, for example, increase heart rate, decrease blood pressure, or increase urine output.

Receptor-Mediated Drug Action

The function of a cell alters when a drug interacts with a receptor. A **receptor** is a specialized macromolecule (a large group of molecules linked together) that attaches or binds to the drug molecule. This alters the function of the cell and produces the drug's **therapeutic response**. For a drug–receptor reaction to occur, a drug must be attracted to a particular receptor. Drugs bind to a receptor much like a piece of a puzzle. The closer the shape, the better the fit, and the better the therapeutic response. The intensity of a drug response is related to how good the "fit" of the drug molecule is and the number of receptor sites occupied.

Agonists are drugs that bind with a receptor to produce a therapeutic response. Drugs that bind only partially to the receptor generally have only a slight therapeutic response. Figure 1-4 identifies the different drug–receptor interactions. Partial agonists are drugs that have some drug receptor fit and produce a response but inhibit other responses.

Antagonists join with a receptor and thereby prevent the action of an agonist. When the antagonist binds more tightly

KEY CONCEPTS

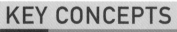

| 1-3 | **Understanding Pharmacokinetics and Pharmacodynamics** |

Pharmacokinetics are the body's effects on the drug. Pharmacodynamics are the drug's effects on the body.

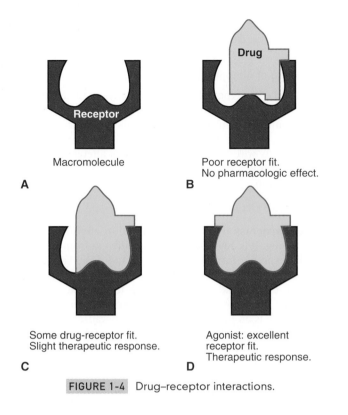

FIGURE 1-4 Drug–receptor interactions.

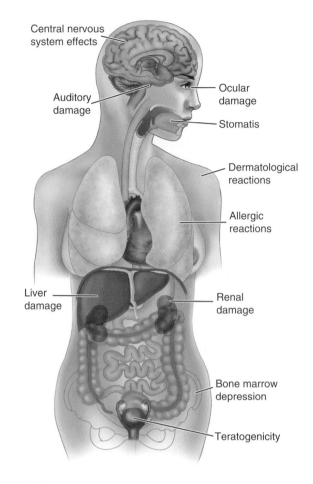

FIGURE 1-5 Various adverse effects may occur with drug use.

than the agonist to the receptor, the action of the antagonist is strong. Drugs that act as antagonists produce no pharmacologic effect. An example of an antagonist is Narcan (naloxone), a narcotic antagonist that completely blocks the effects of morphine. This drug is useful in reversing the effects of an overdose of narcotics (see Chapter 8).

Receptor-Mediated Drug Effects

The number of available receptor sites influences the effects of a drug. If a drug occupies only a few receptor sites when many sites are available, then the response will be small. If the drug dose is increased, then more receptor sites are involved and the response increases. If only a few receptor sites are available, then the response does not increase if more of the drug is administered. However, not all receptors on a cell need to be occupied for a drug to be effective. Some extremely potent drugs are effective even when the drug occupies few receptor sites.

Drug Reactions

Drugs produce many reactions in the body. The following sections discuss adverse drug reactions, allergic drug reactions, drug idiosyncrasy, drug tolerance, cumulative drug effect, toxic reactions, and pharmacogenetic reactions.

Adverse Drug Reactions

Patients may experience one or more adverse reactions when they are given a drug (Fig. 1-5). **Adverse reactions** are undesirable drug effects. Adverse reactions may be common or rare. They may be mild, severe, or life threatening. They may occur after the first dose, after several doses, or after many doses. An adverse reaction often is unpredictable, although

some drugs are known to cause certain adverse reactions in many patients. For example, drugs used in the treatment of cancer are very toxic and are known to produce adverse reactions in many patients receiving them. Other drugs produce adverse reactions in fewer patients. Some adverse reactions are predictable, but many adverse drug reactions occur without warning.

Some texts use both the terms "side effect" and "adverse reaction." Often "side effects" refers to mild, common, and nontoxic reactions; "adverse reactions" refers to more severe or life-threatening reactions. In this text, only the term "adverse reaction" is used, referring to reactions that may be mild, severe, or life threatening.

Allergic Drug Reactions

An **allergic reaction** also is called a **hypersensitivity** reaction. Allergy to a drug usually begins to occur after more than one dose of the drug has been given. Sometimes an allergic reaction may occur the first time a drug is given.

A drug allergy occurs because the individual's immune system views the drug as a foreign substance, or **antigen**. The recognition of an antigen stimulates the antigen–antibody response that prompts the body to produce **antibodies**, which are immune system molecules that react with the antigen. If the patient takes the drug after the antigen–antibody response has occurred, then an allergic reaction results.

Even a mild allergic reaction can produce serious effects if it goes unnoticed and the drug is given again. Any indication of an allergic reaction must be reported to the health care provider before the next dose of the drug is given. Serious allergic reactions must be reported immediately because emergency treatment may be necessary.

Some allergic reactions occur within minutes (even seconds) after the drug is given; others may be delayed for hours or days. Allergic reactions that occur immediately are often the most serious.

Allergic reactions cause a variety of signs and symptoms that may be observed by health care workers or reported by the patient. Examples of some allergic signs and symptoms include itching, skin rashes, and hives (urticaria). Other signs and symptoms include difficulty breathing, wheezing, cyanosis, a sudden loss of consciousness, and swelling of the eyes, lips, or tongue.

Anaphylactic shock is an extremely serious allergic drug reaction that usually occurs soon after the administration of a drug to which the individual is sensitive. This type of allergic reaction requires immediate medical attention. The signs and symptoms of anaphylactic shock are listed in Table 1-2. All or only some of these signs and symptoms may be present. Anaphylactic shock can be fatal if it is not recognized and treated immediately. Key Concepts 1-4 explains how patients can ensure drug allergies are recognized during an emergency situation.

Angioedema (angioneurotic edema) is another type of allergic drug reaction. It is manifested by the collection of fluid in subcutaneous tissues. The most commonly affected areas are the eyelids, lips, mouth, and throat, although other areas also may be affected. Angioedema can be dangerous when the mouth is affected because the swelling may block the airway causing asphyxia. Difficulty breathing or swelling in any area of the body should be reported immediately to the health care provider.

Misreporting of Allergies by Patients

Patients will often report that they are allergic to medications. It is the responsibility of the health care provider to interpret if the reaction the patient had was a true allergy. Erythromycin, for example, will upset the stomach when taken orally. As a result, patients will often state that they are allergic to erythromycin. An upset stomach, while uncomfortable, is not an allergic reaction.

Drug Idiosyncrasy

Drug idiosyncrasy refers to any unusual or abnormal reaction to a drug. It is any reaction that is different from the one normally expected from a specific drug and dose. For example, a patient may be given a drug to promote sleep (e.g., a hypnotic), but instead of falling asleep the patient remains wide awake and shows signs of nervousness or excitement. This response is an idiosyncratic response because it is different from what normally occurs with this type of drug. Another patient may receive the same drug and dose, fall asleep, and after 10 hours be difficult to awaken. This, too, is an abnormal overresponse to the drug.

The cause of drug idiosyncrasies is not clear. They are believed to occur because of a genetic deficiency that makes a patient unable to tolerate certain chemicals, including drugs.

Drug Tolerance

Drug tolerance is a decreased response to a drug, requiring an increase in dosage to achieve the desired effect. Drug tolerance may develop when a patient takes a certain drug, such as a narcotic or tranquilizer, for a long time. Someone who takes the drug at home may increase the dose when the expected effect does not occur. Drug tolerance is a sign of drug dependence. Drug tolerance may also occur in hospitalized patients. When a patient receives a narcotic for more than 10 to 14 days, drug tolerance (and possibly drug dependence) may be occurring. The patient may also begin to ask for the drug more frequently.

Cumulative Drug Effect

A **cumulative drug effect** may occur in patients with liver or kidney disease because these organs are the major sites for the breakdown and excretion of most drugs. This drug effect occurs when the body does not metabolize and excrete one

TABLE 1-2   Signs and Symptoms of Anaphylactic Shock

Respiratory	Bronchospasm
	Dyspnea (difficult breathing)
	Feeling of fullness in the throat
	Cough
	Wheezing
Cardiovascular	Extremely low blood pressure
	Tachycardia (heart rate >100 bpm)
	Palpations
	Syncope (fainting)
	Cardiac arrest
Integumentary	Urticaria (rash)
	Angioedema
	Pruritus (itching)
	Sweating
Gastrointestinal	Nausea
	Vomiting
	Abdominal pain

KEY CONCEPTS

1-4   Drug Allergy ID

Patients who have had an anaphylactic reaction to a medication should be instructed to wear some sort of identification, either a necklace or a bracelet, that indicates their allergy. In an emergency situation, health care providers will look for Medical ID Alert jewelry.

(normal) dose of a drug before the next dose is given. Thus, if a second dose of this drug is given, some drug from the first dose remains active in the body. A cumulative drug effect can be serious because too much of the drug can accumulate in the body and lead to toxicity.

Toxic Reactions

Most drugs can produce **toxic reactions,** or harmful reactions, if administered in large dosages or when blood concentration levels exceed the therapeutic level. Toxic levels may also build if the patient's kidneys are not functioning properly and cannot excrete the drug. Some toxic effects are immediately visible; others may not be seen for weeks or months. Some drugs, such as lithium or digoxin, have a narrow margin of safety, even when given in recommended dosages. It is important to monitor these drugs closely to avoid toxicity.

Drug toxicity can be reversible or irreversible, depending on the organs involved. Damage to the liver may be reversible because liver cells can regenerate. An example of irreversible damage is hearing loss caused by damage to the eighth cranial nerve caused by toxic reaction to the anti-infective drug streptomycin. Sometimes drug toxicity can be reversed by the administration of another drug that acts as an antidote. For example, in serious instances of digitalis toxicity, the drug Digibind (digoxin immune fab) may be given to counteract the effect of digoxin toxicity.

Because some drugs can cause toxic reactions even in recommended doses, health care workers involved in direct patient care should be aware of the signs and symptoms of toxicity of commonly prescribed drugs.

Pharmacogenetic Reactions

A **pharmacogenetic disorder** is a genetically caused abnormal response to normal doses of a drug. This abnormal response occurs because of inherited traits that cause abnormal metabolism of a drug. For example, individuals with glucose-6-phosphate dehydrogenase (G6PD) deficiency have abnormal reactions to a number of drugs.

These patients experience varying degrees of hemolysis (destruction of red blood cells) if they take these drugs. More than 100 million people are affected by this disorder. Examples of drugs that cause hemolysis in patients with a G6PD deficiency include aspirin, chloramphenicol, and the sulfonamides.

Drug Interactions

Health care workers involved in patient care should be aware of the various drug interactions that can occur, most importantly drug–drug interactions and drug–food interactions. The following sections give a brief overview of drug interactions. Specific drug–drug and drug–food interactions are discussed in later chapters.

Drug–Drug Interactions

A drug–drug interaction occurs when one drug interacts with or interferes with the action of another drug. For example, taking an antacid with oral tetracycline causes a decrease in the effectiveness of the tetracycline. The antacid chemically interacts with the tetracycline and impairs its absorption into the bloodstream, thus reducing the effectiveness of the tetracycline. Drugs known to cause interactions include oral anticoagulants, oral hypoglycemics, anti-infectives, antiarrhythmics, cardiac glycosides, and alcohol. Drug–drug interactions can produce effects that are additive, synergistic, or antagonistic.

Additive Drug Reaction

An **additive drug reaction** occurs when the combined effect of two drugs is equal to the sum of each drug given alone. For example, taking the drug heparin with alcohol will increase bleeding. The equation "one + one = two" is sometimes used to illustrate the additive effect of drugs.

Synergistic Drug Reaction

Drug **synergism** occurs when drugs interact with each other and produce an effect that is greater than the sum of their separate actions. The equation "one + one = four" illustrates synergism. An example of drug synergism occurs when a person takes both a hypnotic and alcohol. When alcohol is taken simultaneously or soon before or after the hypnotic is taken, the action of the hypnotic increases. The individual experiences a drug effect that is much greater than that of either drug taken alone.

ALERT ℞

Treatment of Anaphylactic Shock

Anaphylactic shock is a life-threatening situation that requires immediate action. Treatment involves raising the patient's blood pressure, improving breathing, restoring cardiac function, and treating other problems as they occur. Epinephrine (adrenalin) may be given by subcutaneous or intramuscular injection. Hypotension and shock may be treated with fluids and vasopressors. Bronchodilators are given to relax the smooth muscles of the bronchial tubes to improve breathing. Antihistamines may also be given to block the effects of histamine. Patients who are allergic to things in the environment, such as bee stings or peanuts, will often carry an emergency form of epinephrine with them at all times.

ALERT ℞

Cumulative Drug Effect with Liver or Kidney Disease

Patients with liver or kidney disease are usually given drugs with caution because a cumulative drug effect may occur. When the patient is unable to excrete the drug at a normal rate, the drug accumulates in the body, causing a toxic reaction. Sometimes the health care provider lowers the dose of the drug to prevent a toxic drug reaction.

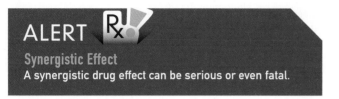

ALERT ℞

Synergistic Effect

A synergistic drug effect can be serious or even fatal.

Antagonistic Drug Reaction

An antagonistic drug reaction occurs when one drug interferes with the action of another, causing neutralization or a decrease in the effect of one drug. For example, protamine sulfate is a heparin antagonist. This means that the administration of protamine sulfate completely neutralizes the effects of heparin in the body.

Drug–Food Interactions

When a drug is given orally, food may impair or enhance its absorption. A drug taken on an empty stomach is absorbed into the bloodstream at a faster rate than when taken with food in the stomach. Some drugs must be taken on an empty stomach to achieve an optimal effect. Drugs that should be taken on an empty stomach are taken 1 hour before or 2 hours after meals. Other drugs, especially drugs that irritate the stomach, result in nausea or vomiting, or cause epigastric distress, are best given with food or meals to minimize gastric irritation. The nonsteroidal anti-inflammatory drugs and salicylates are examples of drugs given with food to decrease epigastric distress. Still other drugs combine with a food, forming an insoluble food–drug mixture. For example, when tetracycline is administered with dairy products, a drug–food mixture is formed that is unabsorbable by the body. When a drug cannot be absorbed by the body, no pharmacologic effect occurs.

Factors Influencing Drug Response

Various factors may influence a patient's drug response, including age, weight, gender, disease, and the route of administration.

Age

The age of the patient may influence the effects of a drug. Infants and children usually require smaller doses of a drug than adults do. Immature organ function, particularly the liver and kidneys, can affect the ability of infants and young children to metabolize drugs. An infant's immature kidneys are less able to eliminate drugs in the urine. Liver function is poorly developed in infants and young children. Drugs metabolized by the liver may produce more intense effects for longer periods. Parents must be taught the potential problems associated with administering drugs to their children. For example, a safe dose of a nonprescription drug for a 4-year-old child may be dangerous for a 6-month-old infant.

Elderly patients may also require smaller doses, although this depends also on the type of drug administered. For example, an elderly patient may take the same dose of an antibiotic as a younger adult. However, the same older adult may require a smaller dose of a drug that depresses the central nervous system, such as a narcotic. Changes that occur with aging affect the pharmacokinetics (absorption, distribution, metabolism, and excretion) of a drug. Any of these processes may be altered because of the physiologic changes of aging.

Table 1-3 summarizes body system changes that occur in children and in the elderly and possible pharmacokinetic effects.

Weight

In general, dosages are based on an average weight of approximately 150 lb for both men and women. A drug dose may sometimes be increased or decreased because the patient's weight is significantly higher or lower than this average. With narcotics, for example, higher or lower dosages may be necessary to produce relief of pain, depending on the patient's weight.

Gender

The person's gender may influence the action of some drugs. Women may require a smaller dose of some drugs than men

TABLE 1-3   Factors Altering Drug Response in Children and Elders

Body System Changes	Children/Infants	Elderly
Gastric acidity	Higher pH—slower gastric emptying resulting in delayed absorption	Higher pH—slower gastric emptying resulting in delayed absorption
Skin changes	Less cutaneous fat and greater surface area—faster absorption of topical drugs	Decreased fat content—decreased absorption of transdermal drugs
Body water content	Increased body water content—greater dilution of drug in tissues	Decreased body water content—greater concentration of drug in tissues
Serum protein	Less protein—less protein binding creating more circulating drug	Less protein—less protein binding creating more circulating drug
Liver function	Immature function—increased half-life of drugs and less first-pass effect	Decreased blood flow to liver—delayed and decreased metabolism of drug
Kidney function	Immature kidney function—decreased elimination, potential for toxicity at lower drug levels	Decreased renal mass and glomerular filtration rate—increased serum levels of drugs

From Ford SM, Roach SS. *Introductory Clinical Pharmacology*, 9th ed. Baltimore, MD: Lippincott Williams & Wilkins; 2010.

CONSIDERATIONS Older adults

LIFESPAN

Polypharmacy

Polypharmacy is the taking of multiple drugs, which can potentially react with one another. When practiced by the elderly, polypharmacy leads to an increased potential for adverse reactions. Although multiple drug therapy is necessary to treat certain disease states, it always increases the possibility of adverse reactions.

because women have a body fat and water ratio different from that of men.

Disease

The presence of disease may influence the action of some drugs. Sometimes disease is a reason for not prescribing a drug or for reducing the dose of a certain drug. Both hepatic (liver) and renal (kidney) disease can greatly affect drug response.

In liver disease, for example, the ability to metabolize or detoxify a drug may be impaired. If the normal dose of the drug is given, then the liver may be unable to metabolize it at a normal rate. Consequently, the drug may be excreted from the body at a much slower rate than normal. The health care provider may then prescribe a lower dose and lengthen the time between doses.

Patients with kidney disease may experience drug toxicity and a longer duration of drug action. The dosage of drugs may be reduced to prevent the accumulation of toxic levels in the blood or further injury to the kidney.

Route of Administration

Intravenous administration of a drug produces the most rapid drug action. Next in order of time of action is the intramuscular route, followed by the subcutaneous route. Giving a drug orally usually produces the slowest drug action.

Some drugs can be given only by one route; for example, antacids are given only orally. Other drugs are available in oral and parenteral forms. The health care provider selects the route of administration based on many factors, including the desired rate of action. For example, a patient with a severe cardiac problem may require intravenous administration of a drug that affects the heart. Another patient with a mild cardiac problem may have a good response to oral administration of the same drug.

Chapter Review

KEY POINTS

- Federal and sometimes state laws govern the development and sale of drugs to ensure public safety and to control prescription drugs and controlled substances whose effects could be harmful. Health care professionals are an important part of this process by monitoring patients' responses to drugs and reporting adverse reactions.
- Drugs may have several names: a chemical name, a generic (nonproprietary) name, an official name, and a trade or brand name.
- Drugs are categorized in a number of ways: (1) as prescription or nonprescription drugs; (2) in different classes of controlled substances; and (3) by pregnancy categories.
- After absorption and distribution in the body, drugs have therapeutic effects by binding to specific receptors on cells and altering cellular environment or function. Then the drug is metabolized and excreted.
- Possible drug reactions include adverse reactions, allergic reactions, idiosyncratic reactions, tolerance, cumulative drug effect, toxic reactions, and pharmacogenetic reactions. All such observed patient responses should be reported to the health care provider.
- Drug interactions include additive reactions, synergistic reactions, antagonist reactions, and interactions with food.

- How an individual patient responds to a drug depends on factors such as age, weight, gender, disease conditions present, and the route of administration. Dose size and frequency may have to be adjusted for the individual.

CRITICAL THINKING CASE STUDY

Antibiotic Reaction

Cassidy Daniels, age 43, started taking a prescription of amoxicillin 7 days ago. She has 3 days of therapy left. When she woke up this morning, she noticed a red rash on her body and is wondering what is going on.

1. What is Ms. Daniels experiencing?
   a. Allergic reaction
   b. Anaphylactic shock
   c. Drug idiosyncrasy
   d. Drug tolerance
2. What should Ms. Daniels do?
3. The pharmacist recommended that Ms. Daniels start taking diphenhydramine to help with the allergic reaction but also warned her that the medication may make her drowsy. However, since starting the diphenhydramine, she is having trouble sleeping. What type of reaction is she experiencing?
   a. Drug idiosyncrasy
   b. Drug tolerance
   c. Drug dependence
   d. Allergic reaction

Review Questions

MULTIPLE CHOICE

1. Mr. Carter has a rash and pruritus. You suspect an allergic drug reaction. Which of the following questions would be most important to ask Mr. Carter?
   a. Are you having any difficulty breathing?
   b. Have you noticed any blood in your stool?
   c. Do you have a headache?
   d. Are you having difficulty with your vision?
2. Mr. Jones, a newly admitted patient, has a history of liver disease. Drug dosages must be based on the consideration that liver disease may result in a(n)
   a. increase in the excretion rate of a drug
   b. impaired ability to metabolize or detoxify a drug
   c. necessity to increase the dosage of a drug
   d. decrease in the rate of drug absorption
3. A drug that blocks the effect of another drug by binding to its receptors is called a(n)
   a. mediator
   b. receiver
   c. antagonist
   d. agonist
4. If you think a patient is experiencing anaphylactic shock, you should
   a. write this in the patient's chart at the end of your shift
   b. ask the patient to call you in an hour if he/she feels the same
   c. report this to the health care provider as soon as you have a free moment
   d. call for help immediately

MATCHING

_____ 5. schedule I
_____ 6. schedule II
_____ 7. prescription drug
_____ 8. nonprescription drug

a. available without a prescription
b. high abuse potential; no accepted medical use in the United States
c. potentially harmful unless supervised by a licensed health care provider
d. Potential for high abuse with severe physical or psychological dependence

TRUE OR FALSE

_____ 9. If a patient takes a drug on an empty stomach, the drug will be absorbed more slowly than if taken with food.

_____ 10. Drug tolerance is a compulsive need to use a substance repeatedly to avoid mild to severe withdrawal symptoms.
_____ 11. A teratogen is a drug that causes an abnormal development of a fetus.
_____ 12. A drug's effect will occur most quickly if it is administered intravenously.

FILL IN THE BLANKS

13. A patient asks you what a hypersensitivity reaction is. You begin your response by explaining that a hypersensitivity reaction is also called a(n) _____.
14. A synergistic drug effect may be defined as _____ _____.
15. _____ is the measure of the body's ability to eliminate a substance or drug from the body.
16. The _____ is the chief federal agency responsible for enforcing the Controlled Substances Act.

SHORT ANSWERS

17. What are the four phases of activities of pharmacokinetics?
18. What two organs if impaired will often require a dosage adjustment?
19. What is the first-pass effect? Which routes avoid it?
20. What is the difference between an additive drug reaction and a synergistic drug reaction?

Web Activities

1. Go to the MedWatch Web site http://www.fda.gov/Safety/MedWatch/default.htm Navigate to the section on "Safety Information" and look for "Drug Safety Labeling Changes." This information is organized by year; find the list of drugs for which safety alerts have been issued in the current year. Read the alerts for several different drugs and consider the following questions:
   a. Find a drug safety alert for which new adverse reactions are being reported. Look up that drug in this text or a drug reference such as the PDR. Does the alert add significant new information to what you would have known about the drug from only looking at this text or the reference?
   b. Explain the value of the alert for a health care provider who is prescribing this drug for a new patient.
2. Go to the U.S. Department of Health and Human Services Web site (www.hhs.gov/ocr/privacy/) and navigate to "Understanding HIPAA Privacy." Read the section labeled "For Consumers" and respond to the following questions:
   a. What information is protected?
   b. How is that information to be protected?

2

The Administration of Drugs

CHAPTER OBJECTIVES

On completion of this chapter, students will be able to:

1. Define the chapter's key terms.
2. Name the six rights of drug administration.
3. Identify the different types of medication orders.
4. Describe the various types of medication dispensing systems.
5. List the various routes by which a drug may be given.
6. Describe the administration of oral and parenteral drugs.
7. Describe the administration of drugs through the skin and mucous membranes.

KEY TERMS

buccal—between the cheek and gum

drug error—any incident in which a patient receives the wrong dose, the wrong drug, a drug by the wrong route, or a drug given at the incorrect time

extravasation—the escape of fluid from a blood vessel into surrounding tissues

infiltration—the collection of fluid in a tissue

inhalation—route of administration in which drug droplets, vapor, or gas is inhaled and absorbed through the mucous membranes of the respiratory tract

intradermal—route of administration in which the drug is injected into skin tissue

intramuscular—route of administration in which the drug is injected into muscle tissue

intravenous—route of administration in which the drug is injected into a vein

parenteral—a general term for drug administration in which the drug is injected inside the body

Standard (Universal) Precautions—a set of actions, such as wearing gloves or using other protective gear, recommended by CDC for preventing contact with potentially infectious blood or body fluids

subcutaneous—route of administration in which the drug is injected just below the layer of skin

sublingual—route of administration in which the drug is placed under the tongue for absorption

thePOINT RESOURCES

- Animations: Administering Oral Medications; Administering a Subcutaneous Injection; Administering an Intramuscular Injection; Administering IV Medications by Piggyback Infusion; Intramuscular Injection; Intravenous Injection; Medications: The Three Checks and Five Rights of Medication Administration; The Rights of Medication Administration; Preventing Medication Errors

- Lippincott's Interactive Tutorials: Pharmacology Basics

- Interactive Practice and Review

- Monographs of Most Commonly Prescribed Drugs

topical—route of administration in which the drug affects only the area of skin or mucous membranes on which it is applied

transdermal—route of administration in which the drug is absorbed through the skin from a patch

unit dose—a single dose of a drug packaged ready for patient use

Z-track—a technique of intramuscular injection used with drugs that are irritating to subcutaneous tissues

All health professionals who work with patients should understand the basics of drug administration to help ensure patient safety. The patient, and often family members as well, need to understand how drugs are administered safely.

The Medication Order

Preparation for administering medication to a patient begins with the medication order, usually written by a physician. Dentists, nurse practitioners, and physician assistants are also authorized to write specified drug orders although the laws vary from state to state. The medication order is kept with the patient's medical records. Common orders include the standing order, the single order, the PRN order, and the STAT order. Key Concepts 2-1 explains these types of orders.

A medication order is used in an inpatient setting. A prescription, as discussed in Chapter 1, is used in an outpatient setting. A medication order is for a drug to be administered, while a prescription is for a drug to be dispensed.

The Six Rights of Drug Administration

Six "rights" in the administration of drugs ensure that patients receive ordered medications correctly and safely:

- Right patient
- Right drug
- Right dose
- Right route
- Right time
- Right documentation

Right Patient

The health care professional administering a drug must be certain that the patient receiving the drug is the patient for whom the drug has been ordered. With a hospitalized patient, this is accomplished by checking the patient's wristband containing the patient's name and birth date. In pharmacies, the patient name, date of birth, address, and phone number may all be used to verify the prescription is going to the right patient.

Right Drug

Drug names can be confused, especially when the names sound similar or the spellings are similar. Someone who hurriedly prepares a drug for administration or who fails to look up a questionable drug is more likely to administer the wrong drug. Table 2-1 gives examples of drugs that can easily be confused. The person administering the drug should compare the medication, container label, and medication record (Fig. 2-1).

Right Dose, Route, and Time

As noted above, the health care professional prescribing drugs for patients should write an order for the administration of all drugs. This written order must include the patient's name, the drug name, the dosage form and route, the dosage to be administered, and the frequency of administration. The health care provider must sign the drug order. In an emergency, a nurse or other qualified health care professional may administer a drug with a verbal order from the health care provider, who must then write and sign the order as soon as the emergency is over.

The caregiver administering the medication must ensure that the patient is receiving the right dose. Many medications are available in more than one strength. Other times, the patient may be taking more than one tablet at a time to get the correct dose. Liquids and injectables should be double-checked to ensure that the correct volume is being administered.

The caregiver administering the medication must ensure that the patient is receiving the medication by the right route. Some medications can be given by a variety of different routes. Sometimes, a medication is being given by a different route than normal. For example, an eye drop can be administered otically (in the ear). However, an ear drop should never be administered ophthalmically (in the eye).

Finally, the caregiver administering the medication must ensure that the patient is receiving the medication at the right time. Medications should not be given too soon, but they also should not be given too far apart. It is important to ensure that the dosage intervals are consistent.

KEY CONCEPTS

2-1   Types of Medication Orders

Standing order: This type of order is written when the patient is to receive the prescribed drug on a regular basis. The drug is administered until the physician discontinues it. Occasionally a drug may be ordered for a specified number of days, or in some cases, a drug can only be given for a specified number of days before the order needs to be renewed.
Example: Lanoxin 0.25 mg PO once per day
Single order: An order to administer the drug one time only.
Example: Valium 10 mg IV Push at 10.00 AM.
PRN order: An order to administer the drug as needed.
Example: Demerol 100 mg IM q4h PRN for pain.
STAT order: A one-time order given as soon as possible.
Example: Morphine 10 mg IV STAT.

TABLE 2-1   Examples of Easily Confused Drugs

Accupril	Accutane
Albuterol	atenolol
Alupent	Atrovent
Amikin	Amicar
Bentyl	Aventyl
Capitrol	captopril
Cefzil	Ceftin
Celebrex	Celexa
DiaBeta	Zebeta
dobutamine	dopamine
Elavil	Mellaril
Eurax	Serax
Flomax	Fosamax
Inderal	Isordil
K-Dur	Imdur
Klonopin	clonidine
Lodine	codeine
Nicobid	Nitro-Bid
nifedipine	nicardipine
prednisolone	prednisone
Prilosec	Prozac
Retrovir	ritonavir
Taxol	Paxil
TobraDex	Tobrex
Versed	VePesid
Zocor	Zoloft

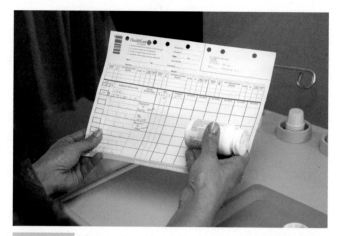

FIGURE 2-1   Comparing the medication label with the medication record.

Considerations in Drug Administration

Health professionals who are responsible for administering medications play an important role in ensuring the safety and quality of patient care. For example, they must possess knowledge about the drugs to be given, understand why the drugs are being given and their usual mechanisms of action, and recognize the most common adverse reactions that might be expected. They also need to know about any special precautions associated with administering the drugs and the typical doses. By reading approved references for current drug information, health professionals administering drugs can gain this understanding.

Drug Errors

Drug errors are any occurrence that can cause a patient to receive the wrong dose, the wrong drug, a drug by the wrong route, or a drug given at the incorrect time. Errors may occur in transcribing drug orders, dispensing the drug, or administering the drug. Mix-ups between frequently used abbreviations can also lead to errors. In fact, certain abbreviations that are

Right Documentation

After any drug is administered, the health care professional who administered it must record the process immediately (Fig. 2-2). Immediate documentation is particularly important when drugs are given on an as-needed basis (PRN drugs). For example, most analgesics require 20 to 30 minutes before the drug begins to relieve pain. Patients may forget that they received a drug for pain, may not have been told that the administered drug was for pain, or may not know that pain relief is not immediate—and may then ask another health care worker for the drug. If the first administration of the analgesic had not been recorded, then the patient might receive a second dose soon after the first dose. This kind of situation can be extremely serious, especially with narcotics or other central nervous system depressants. Immediate documentation prevents accidental administration of a drug by another individual. Proper documentation is essential to the process of administering drugs correctly.

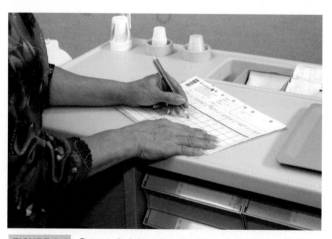

FIGURE 2-2   Drug administration must be documented immediately on the patient's medical record.

TABLE 2-2   Official "Do Not Use" List.

Do Not Use	Potential Problem	Use Instead
U (unit)	Mistaken for "0" (zero), the number "4" (four) or "cc"	Write "unit"
IU (International Unit)	Mistaken for IV (intravenous) or the number 10 (ten)	Write "International Unit"
Q.D., QD, q.d., qd (daily)	Mistaken for each other	Write "daily"
Q.O.D., QOD, q.o.d, qod (every other day)	Period after the Q mistaken for "I" and the "O" mistaken for "I"	Write "every other day"
Trailing zero (X.0 mg)*	Decimal point is missed	Write X mg
Lack of leading zero (.X mg)		Write 0.X mg
MS	Can mean morphine sulfate or magnesium sulfate	Write "morphine sulfate"
MSO$_4$ and MgSO$_4$	Confused for one another	Write "magnesium sulfate"

¹Applies to all orders and all medication-related documentation that is handwritten (including free-text computer entry) or on pre-printed forms.
*Exception: A "trailing zero" may be used only where required to demonstrate the level of precision of the value being reported, such as for laboratory results, imaging studies that report size of lesions, or catheter/tube sizes It may not be used in medication orders or other medication-related documentation.

Additional Abbreviations, Acronyms and Symbols (For *possible* future inclusion in the Official "Do Not Use" List)		
Do Not Use	**Potential Problem**	**Use Instead**
> (greater than)	Misinterpreted as the number "7" (seven) or the letter "L"	Write "greater than"
< (less than)	Confused for one another	Write "less than"
Abbreviations for drug names	Misinterpreted due to similar abbreviations for multiple drugs	Write drug names in full
Apothecary units	Unfamiliar to many practitioners Confused with metric units	Use metric units
@	Mistaken for the number "2" (two)	Write "at"
cc	Mistaken for U (units) when poorly written	Write "ml" or "milliliters"
μg	Mistaken for mg (milligrams) resulting in one thousand-fold overdose	Write "mcg" or "micrograms"

© 2007, The Joint Commission. Reprinted with permission.

easily confused or misunderstood are considered dangerous by the Joint Commission and should be avoided; these are listed in Table 2-2. Table 2-3 lists abbreviations that are commonly used in medication orders and their meanings. Health professionals who administer drugs will need to carefully learn these to avoid errors.

Drug errors occur when one or more of the six "rights" has not been followed. Each time a drug is prepared and administered, the six rights must be a part of the procedure. In addition to consistently practicing the six rights, the person administering the drug should follow these precautions to help prevent drug errors:

- Confirm any questionable orders.
- When a dosage calculation is necessary, verify it with another person.
- Listen to the patient when he or she questions a drug, the dosage, or the drug regimen. Never administer the drug until the patient's questions have been adequately researched.
- Concentrate on only one task at a time.

Many drug errors are made during administration. The most common errors are a failure to administer a drug that has been ordered, administration of the wrong dose or strength of the drug, or administration of the wrong drug. Errors commonly occur, for example, with insulin and heparin.

ALERT Rx

Reporting Drug Errors
When a drug error occurs, it must be reported immediately so that any necessary steps can be taken to counteract the action of the drug or observe the patient for adverse effects. The caregiver who made the drug error can be held legally liable if the patient is harmed. However, even if the patient suffers no harm, it is important that errors are reported.

TABLE 2-3 Commonly Used Medication Abbreviations

Abbreviation	Meaning	Abbreviation	Meaning
ac	Before meals	NKA	No known allergies
ad lib	As desired	Noc	Night
ADL	Activities of daily living	NPO	Nothing by mouth
AM, a.m., A.M.	Morning	NS	Normal saline
amp	Ampule	OD	Right eye
amt	Amount	OS	Left eye
aq	Aqueous	OU	Both eyes
bid	Twice a day	Os	Mouth
BM	Bowel movement	Oz	Ounce
BRP	Bathroom privileges	P	After
c̄	With	Pc	After meals
cap	Capsule	PM, p.m., P.M.	Afternoon or evening
DC,disc,d/c	Discontinue	po, PO	By mouth
disp	Dispense	prn, PRN	Whenever necessary
DW	Distilled water	Pt	Print or patient
EDC	Estimated date of confinement (date baby is due)	Q Qh q2h	Every Every hour Every 2 hours
et	And	q3h	Every 3 hours
ext	Extract	qid	Four times a day
FGW	Full glass of water	Qt	Quart
FU	Follow up	R	Right, rectal
g, gm	Gram	RTW	Return to work
gr	Grain	Rx	Take, prescribe
gt(t)	Drop(s)	s̄	Without
h, hr	Hour	SC, subcu, subq, S/Q, SQ	Subcutaneously
hs, HS	Hour of sleep	Sig	Label
Id, ID	Intradermal	SL	Sublingual
IM	Intramuscular	sol	Solution
IV	Intravenous	SOS	Once if necessary
Kg	Kilogram	ss	One-half
L, l	Liter	stat, STAT	Immediately
lb	Pound	supp	Suppository
LMP	Last menstrual period	syr	Syrup
mcg, μg	Microgram	tab	Tablet
mEq	Milliequivalent	T, tb, tbs, tbsp	Tablespoon
ml, mL	Milliliter	t, tsp	Teaspoon
N	Normal	tid	Three times a day
NaCl	Sodium chloride	WNL	Within normal limits
NH	Nursing home		

From Holly J. *LWW's Medical Assisting Made Incredibly Easy: Pharmacology.* Baltimore, MD: Lippincott Williams & Wilkins, 2009.

Periodic Drug Dosing

Some drugs are available in once-per-week, once-per-month, or once-per-year forms. These are designed to replace daily doses of drugs. For example, two strengths for alendronate (Fosamax), a drug used to treat osteoporosis (see Chapter 42), may be given once per week. The 70-mg tablet is used to treat postmenopausal osteoporosis, and the 35-mg tablet is used for prevention of postmenopausal osteoporosis. Clinical trials showed that the once-per-week dosing caused no greater adverse reactions than the once-daily regimen. Once-per-week dosing may prove beneficial for those experiencing mild adverse reactions because they would experience the reactions only once per week rather than every day. In addition, ibandronate (Boniva) is a once-per-month drug used to treat or prevent postmenopausal osteoporosis and zoledronic acid (Reclast) is a once-per-year intravenous (IV) infusion of the drug used to treat postmenopausal osteoporosis.

Drug Dispensing Systems

A number of drug dispensing systems are used to dispense medications after they have been ordered for patients. A brief description of three methods follows.

Computerized Dispensing System

Automated or computerized dispensing systems are used in many hospitals and other agencies dispensing drugs. Drugs are dispensed in the pharmacy for drug orders sent from the individual floors or units. Each floor or unit has a medication cart in which medications are placed for individual patients. Medication orders are filled in the hospital pharmacy and are placed in the drug dispensing cart. When orders are filled, the cart is delivered to the unit. The dispensing of the drugs is automatically recorded in the computerized system. After drugs are dispensed, the cart goes back to the pharmacy to be refilled and for new drug orders to be placed.

Unit Dose System

In the **unit dose** system, drug orders are filled and medications dispensed to fill each patient's medication order(s) for a 24-hour period. The pharmacist dispenses each dose (unit) in a package that is labeled with the drug name and dosage. The drug(s) are placed in drawers in a portable medication cart with a drawer for each patient. Many drugs are packaged by their manufacturers in unit doses; each package is labeled by the manufacturer and contains one tablet or capsule, a premeasured amount of a liquid drug, a prefilled syringe, or one suppository. Hospital pharmacists also may prepare unit doses. The pharmacist restocks the cart each day with the drugs patients need for the next 24-hour period (Fig. 2-3). Each unit dose package contains a bar code that uniquely identifies that medication.

Some hospitals use a bar code scanner in the administration of unit dose drugs. A bar code is placed on the patient's hospital identification band when the patient is admitted to the hospital. This bar code, along with bar codes on the drug unit dose packages, is used to identify the patient and to record and charge routine and PRN drugs. The scanner also keeps an ongoing inventory of controlled substances, which eliminates the need for narcotic counts at the end of each shift.

If a bar code is not used, then the caregiver administering the medication must record each dose administered

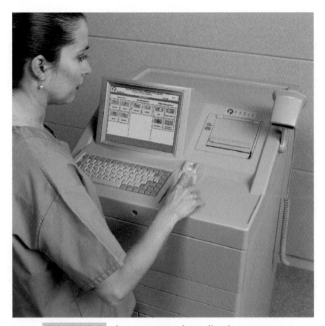

FIGURE 2-3　An automated medication system.

in the medication administration record (MAR). The MAR documents each dose administration and helps prevent errors.

Floor Stock

Some agencies, such as nursing homes or small hospitals, use a floor stock method to dispense drugs. Some special units in hospitals, such as the emergency department, may use this method. In this system, the drugs most frequently prescribed are kept on the unit in containers in a designated medication room or at the nurses' station. Medications are taken from the appropriate containers and administered to patients and recorded in each patient's medication administration record.

General Principles of Drug Administration

Health care professionals involved in drug administration and patient care should know about each drug given, the reasons the drug is used, the drug's general action, its more common adverse reactions, special precautions in administration (if any), and the normal dose ranges.

With commonly used drugs, health care workers often become familiar with their pharmacologic properties. With less commonly used or new drugs, information can be obtained from reliable sources, such as the drug package insert or the hospital pharmacy.

Patient considerations are also important, such as allergy history, previous adverse reactions, the patient's comments, and any change in the patient's condition. Before a patient is given any drug for the first time, he or she should be asked about any known allergies and any family history of allergies. This includes allergies not only to drugs but also to food, pollen, animals, and so on. Patients with a personal or family history of allergies are more likely to experience additional allergies and must be monitored closely.

If the patient makes any statement about the drug or if the patient's condition changes, then the situation is carefully considered before the drug is given. Examples of such situations include

- Problems that may be associated with the drug, such as nausea, dizziness, ringing in the ears, and difficulty walking. Any comments made by the patient may indicate the occurrence of an adverse reaction.
- A patient's comment that the drug looks different from the one previously received, that the drug was just given by someone else, or that the health care provider had discontinued the drug therapy.
- A change in the patient's condition, a change in one or more vital signs (pulse, respiration, blood pressure, or temperature), or the appearance of new symptoms. Depending on the drug being given and the patient's diagnosis, such a change may indicate that the drug should be withheld and the health care provider contacted.

Preparing a Drug for Administration

Health care professionals involved in preparing a drug for administration should follow these guidelines:

- The health care provider's written orders should be checked and any questions answered.
- Drugs should be prepared in a quiet, well-lit area.
- The label of the drug should be checked three times: (1) when the drug is taken from its storage area; (2) immediately before removing the drug from the container; and (3) before returning the drug to its storage area.
- A drug should never be removed from an unlabeled container or from a container whose label is illegible.
- The person preparing a drug for administration should wash hands immediately before the procedure.
- Capsules and tablets should not be touched with one's hands. The correct number of tablets or capsules is shaken into the cap of the container and from there into the medicine cup.
- Aseptic technique must be followed when handling syringes and needles.
- Drug names must be checked carefully. Some drugs have names that sound alike but are very different. Giving one drug when another is ordered could cause serious consequences. For example, digoxin and digitoxin sound alike but are different drugs.
- The caps of drug containers should be replaced immediately after the drug is removed.
- Drugs requiring special storage must be returned to the storage area immediately after being prepared for administration. This rule applies mainly to the refrigeration of drugs but may also apply to drugs that must be protected from exposure to light or heat.
- Tablets must never be crushed or capsules opened without first checking with the pharmacist. Some tablets can be crushed or capsules opened and the contents added to water or a tube feeding when the patient cannot swallow a whole tablet or capsule. Some tablets have a special coating that delays the absorption of the drug. Crushing the tablet may destroy this drug property and result in problems such as improper absorption of the drug or gastric irritation. Capsules are made of gelatin and dissolve on contact with a liquid. The contents of some capsules do not mix well with water and therefore are best left in the capsule. If the patient cannot take an oral tablet or capsule, then the health care provider should be consulted because the drug may be available in liquid form.
- With a unit dose system, the wrappings of the unit dose should not be removed until the drug reaches the bedside of the patient who is to receive it. After the drug is administered, it is charted immediately on the unit dose drug form.

Administration of Drugs by the Oral Route

The oral route is the most frequent route of drug administration and rarely causes physical discomfort in patients. Oral drug forms include tablets, capsules, and liquids. Some capsules and tablets contain sustained-release drugs, which dissolve over an extended period of time. Administration of oral drugs is relatively easy for patients who are alert and can swallow.

Patient Care Considerations for Oral Drug Administration

- The patient should be in an upright position. It is difficult, as well as dangerous, to swallow a solid or liquid when lying down.
- A full glass of water should be available to the patient.
- The patient may need help removing the tablet or capsule from the container, holding the container, holding a medicine cup, or holding a glass of water. Some patients with physical disabilities cannot handle or hold these objects and may require assistance.
- The patient should be advised to take a few sips of water before placing a tablet or capsule in the mouth.
- The patient is instructed to place the pill or capsule on the back of the tongue and tilt the head back to swallow a tablet or slightly forward to swallow a capsule. The patient is encouraged to take a few sips of water to move the drug down the esophagus and into the stomach, and then to finish the whole glass.
- The patient is given any special instructions, such as drinking extra fluids or remaining in bed, that are pertinent to the drug being administered.
- A drug is never left at the patient's bedside to be taken later unless the health care provider has ordered this. A few drugs (e.g., antacids and nitroglycerin tablets) may be ordered to be left at the bedside.
- Patients with a nasogastric feeding tube may be given their oral drugs through the tube. Liquid drugs are diluted and then flushed through the tube. Tablets are crushed and dissolved in water before administering them through the tube. The tube should be checked first for correct placement. Afterwards, the tube is flushed with water to completely clear the tubing.
- The patient is instructed to place a **buccal** drug against the mucous membranes of the cheek in either the upper or lower jaw. These drugs are given for a systemic effect. They are absorbed slowly from the mucous membranes of the mouth. An example of a drug given bucally is nicotine gum which is chewed and then parked bucally for absorption.

- Certain drugs are given by the **sublingual** route (placed under the tongue). These drugs must not be swallowed or chewed and must be dissolved completely before the patient eats or drinks. Nitroglycerin is commonly given sublingually.

Administration of Drugs by the Parenteral Route

Parenteral drug administration means the giving of a drug by the **subcutaneous, intramuscular** (IM), **intravenous** (IV), or **intradermal** route. Other routes of parenteral administration include intra-arterial (into an artery), intracardiac (into the heart), and intra-articular (into a joint).

Patient Care Considerations for Parenteral Drug Administration

- Gloves must be worn for protection from a potential blood spill when giving parenteral drugs. The risk of exposure to infected blood is increasing for all health care workers. The Centers for Disease Control and Prevention (CDC) recommends that gloves be worn when touching blood or body fluids, mucous membranes, or any broken skin area. This recommendation is one of the **Standard Precautions**, which combine the Universal Precautions for Blood and Body Fluids with Body Substance Isolation guidelines.
- At the site for injection, the skin is cleansed. Most hospitals and medical offices have a policy regarding the type of skin antiseptic used for cleansing the skin before parenteral drug administration. The skin is cleansed with a circular motion, starting at an inner point and moving outward.
- After the needle is inserted for IM administration, the syringe barrel is pulled back to aspirate the drug. If blood appears in the syringe, the needle is removed so that the drug is not injected. The drug, needle, and syringe are discarded, and another injection prepared. If no blood appears in the syringe, the drug is injected. Aspiration is not necessary when giving an intradermal or subcutaneous injection.
- Syringes are not recapped but are disposed of according to agency policy. Needles and syringes are discarded into clearly marked, appropriate containers. Most agencies have a "sharps" container located in each room for immediate disposal of needles and syringes after use (Fig. 2-4).
- Most hospitals and medical offices use needles designed to prevent accidental needle sticks. This needle has a plastic guard that slips over the needle as it is withdrawn from the injection site. The guard locks in place and eliminates the need to recap the syringe. Other models are available as well. These newer types of methods for administering parenteral fluids provide a greater margin of safety (see Occupational Safety and Health Administration [OSHA] Guidelines).

Occupational Safety and Health Administration Guidelines

Occupational Safety and Health Administration estimates that 5.6 million workers in the health care industry are at risk of occupational exposure to blood-borne pathogens. The CDC

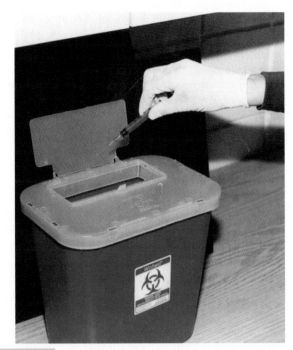

FIGURE 2-4   A sharps container for disposal of used hypodermic needles.

estimates about 400,000 health care workers experience a needlestick or sharps injury each year, which may expose them to the hepatitis B, hepatitis C, or the HIV viruses.

Other infections, such as tuberculosis, syphilis, and malaria, also can be transmitted through needlesticks. Most needlestick or sharps injuries can be prevented with the use of safe medical devices.

In 2001, the OSHA announced new guidelines for needlestick prevention. The revisions clarify the need for employers to select safer needle devices as they become available and to involve employees in identifying and choosing the devices. Employers with 11 or more employees must also maintain a Sharps Injury Log to help employees and employers track all needlestick incidents to help identify problem areas. In addition, employers must have a written Exposure Control Plan that is updated annually. As new safer devices become available, they should be adopted for use in the agency. The new OSHA guidelines help reduce needlestick injuries among health care workers and others who handle medical sharps. Safety-engineered devices such as self-sheathing needles and needleless systems are now commonly used.

Administration of Drugs by the Subcutaneous Route

A subcutaneous injection places the drug into the tissues between the skin and the muscle. Drugs administered in this manner are absorbed more slowly than are IM injections. Heparin and insulin are two drugs most commonly given by the subcutaneous route.

Patient Care Considerations for Subcutaneous Drug Administration

- A small volume of 0.5 to 1 mL is used for subcutaneous injection. Larger volumes are best given as IM injections.

- The sites for subcutaneous injection are the upper arms, the upper abdomen, and the upper back. Injection sites are rotated to ensure proper absorption and to minimize tissue damage.

Administration of Drugs by the Intramuscular Route

An intramuscular (IM) injection is the administration of a drug into a muscle. Drugs that are irritating to subcutaneous tissue can be given via IM injection. Drugs given by this route are absorbed more rapidly than drugs given by the subcutaneous route because of the rich blood supply in the muscle. In addition, a larger volume (1–3 mL) of drug can be given at one site.

Patient Care Considerations for Intramuscular Drug Administration

- With a large drug volume, the drug is divided and given as two separate injections. Volumes larger than 3 mL will not be absorbed properly at one site.
- The sites for IM administration are the deltoid muscle (upper arm), the ventrogluteal or dorsogluteal sites (hip), and the vastus lateralis (thigh). The vastus lateralis site is frequently used for infants and small children because it is more developed than the gluteal or deltoid sites. In children who have been walking for more than 2 years, the ventrogluteal site may be used.
- The **Z-track** method of IM injection is used when a drug is highly irritating to subcutaneous tissues or may permanently stain the skin. In this technique, the skin and subcutaneous tissues are pulled to one side before the injection, and an air bubble is injected from the syringe after the drug. This technique prevents the drug from oozing up through the small pathway created by the needle into the subcutaneous tissue.

Administration of Drugs by the Intravenous Route

A drug administered by the IV route is given directly into the blood by a needle inserted into a vein. Drug action occurs almost immediately. Drugs administered via the IV route may be given in a number of ways:

- Slowly, over 1 or more minutes
- Rapidly (IV push, or IVP)
- By piggyback infusions (IVPB, drugs are mixed with a compatible IV fluid and administered over 20 to 60 minutes piggybacked onto the primary IV line)
- Into an existing IV line (the IV port)
- Into an intermittent venous access device called a heparin lock (a small IV catheter in the patient's vein connected to a small fluid reservoir with a rubber cap through which the needle is inserted to administer the drug)
- By being added to an IV solution and allowed to infuse into the vein over a longer period

Some drugs are added to an IV solution, such as 1000 mL of dextrose 5% and water (D5W) or 0.9% sodium chloride (normal saline). Whenever a drug is added to an IV fluid, the bottle or bag must have an attached label indicating the drug and drug dose added to the IV fluid.

Intravenous Infusion Controllers and Pumps

Electronic infusion devices include infusion controllers and infusion pumps. The primary difference between the two is that an infusion pump administers the infused drug under pressure, whereas an infusion controller does not add pressure. An infusion pump can be set to deliver the desired number of drops of medication per minute. An alarm sounds if the IV rate is more than or less than the preset rate. Controllers and pumps have detectors and alarms that alert health care workers to problems such as air in the line, an occlusion, a low battery, the completion of an infusion, or an inability to deliver the drug at the preset rate. Whenever an alarm is activated, the device must be checked.

Patient Care Considerations for Intravenous Drug Administration

- After an IV infusion is started, the type of IV fluid and the drug added to the IV solution are documented in the patient's chart.
- The infusion rate must be checked regularly.
- The needle site is inspected for signs of redness, swelling, or other problems. Swelling around the needle may indicate extravasation or infiltration. **Extravasation** is the escape of fluid from a blood vessel into surrounding tissues while the needle or catheter is in the vein. **Infiltration** is the collection of fluid in tissues (usually subcutaneous tissue) when the needle or catheter is out of the vein. Either problem necessitates stopping the infusion and inserting an IV line in another vein.

Administration of Drugs by the Intradermal Route

The intradermal route is usually used for sensitivity tests (e.g., the tuberculin test or allergy skin testing). Absorption is slow from this route, providing good results when testing for allergies or administering local anesthetics. The needle is inserted between the upper layers of the skin. Injection produces a small wheal (raised area) on the outer surface of the skin (Fig. 2-5). If a wheal does not appear, then the drug may have entered the subcutaneous tissue, making test results inaccurate.

Patient Care Considerations for Intradermal Drug Administration

- The inner part of the forearm and the upper back are used for intradermal injections. A hairless area should be chosen; areas near moles, scars, or pigmented skin

ALERT Rx

Avoiding Tissue Damage
Some IV drugs can cause severe tissue damage if extravasation or infiltration occurs. All health professionals, including those who do not administer medications, should be alert for this critical situation. The health care provider should be contacted if such a drug escapes into the tissues surrounding the needle insertion site.

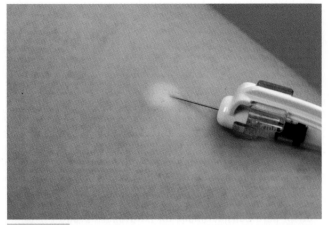

FIGURE 2-5 Observing for wheal while injecting medication by the intradermal route.

areas should be avoided. The area is cleansed in the same manner as for subcutaneous and IM injections.

- Small volumes (usually <0.1 mL) are used for intradermal injections.

Other Parenteral Routes of Drug Administration

The health care provider may administer a drug by the intracardiac, intra-arterial, or intra-articular routes. Special devices and materials are required for these routes of administration.

Venous access ports are implanted self-sealing ports attached to a catheter leading to a large vessel, usually the vena cava. These devices are most commonly used for chemotherapy or other long-term therapy. They require surgical insertion and removal. Drugs are administered through injections made into the portal through the skin.

Administration of Drugs through the Skin and Mucous Membranes

Drugs may be applied to the skin and mucous membranes using several routes: **topically** (affecting only the area of the skin or mucous membranes on which it is applied), **transdermally** through a patch in which the drug has been implanted, or inhaled through the membranes of the upper respiratory tract.

Administration of Drugs by the Topical Route

Most topical drugs act on the skin but are not absorbed through the skin. These drugs are used to soften, disinfect, or lubricate the skin. A few topical drugs are enzymes that remove superficial debris, such as the dead skin and purulent matter present in skin ulcerations. Other topical drugs are used to treat minor superficial skin infections. The various forms of topical applications are described in Key Concepts 2-2.

Patient Care Considerations for Topical Drug Administration

- The health care provider may write special instructions for the application of a topical drug, such as to apply the drug in a thin even layer or to cover the area after the drug is applied to the skin.

KEY CONCEPTS

2-2 Topical and Mucous Membrane Applications

Topical
- Creams, lotions, or ointments

Sprays
- Continuous or intermittent wet dressings applied to skin surfaces
- Liquids, creams, or ointments applied to the scalp

Eye
- Ophthalmic ointments applied to the eyelids or dropped into the lower conjunctival sac
- Liquid drops

Ear
- Liquid drops

Mouth
- Solids (e.g., tablets, lozenges, troches) dissolved in the mouth
- Spray
- Liquid

Nose
- Spray

Lungs
- Sprays or mists inhaled into the lungs

Vagina
- Cream
- Solids (e.g., suppositories, tablets), foams, liquids, and creams inserted into the vagina
- Suppository or tablet

Rectal
- Solids (e.g., suppositories), liquids, or foams inserted into the rectum

Other
- Liquids inserted into the bladder or urethra
- Solids (e.g., suppositories) or jellies inserted into the urethra
- Liquids inserted into body cavities, such as fistulas

- The manufacturer sometimes provides special instructions for drug administration. All such instructions are important because drug action may depend on correct administration of the drug.

Administration of Drugs by the Transdermal Route

Drugs administered by the transdermal route are readily absorbed from the skin and have systemic effects. The drug dose is implanted in a small patch-type bandage. The backing is removed, and the patch is applied to the skin, where the drug is gradually absorbed into the systemic circulation. This drug administration system maintains a relatively constant commonly used sites. The area of application should not be shaved because this may cause skin irritation.

- Ointments are sometimes used. They come with a special paper marked in inches. The correct length of ointment is measured onto the paper, and the paper is placed with the drug ointment side down on the skin and secured with tape. Before the next dose, the paper and tape are removed and the skin cleansed. Nitroglycerin is administered this way.

Administration of Drugs through Inhalation

Drug droplets, vapor, and gas are administered through the mucous membranes of the respiratory tract. The patient breathes the drug in through a face mask, a nebulizer, or a positive-pressure breathing machine. Examples of drugs administered through **inhalation** include bronchodilators, mucolytics, and some anti-inflammatory drugs. These drugs primarily have a local effect in the lungs.

Patient Care Considerations for Drug Administration by Inhalation

The patient must be provided with proper instructions for taking the drug. For example, many patients with asthma use a metered-dose inhaler to dilate the bronchi and make breathing easier. Without proper instruction on how to use the inhaler, much of the drug may be deposited on the tongue rather than in the respiratory tract; this would decrease the therapeutic effect of the drug. The specific instructions are provided with the inhaler. Figure 2-6 illustrates the proper use of one type of inhaler.

Patient Care Considerations after Drug Administration

- The administration of a drug to a patient is always documented. This should be performed as soon as possible.
- Other information concerning the administration of the drug is also often recorded, including information such as the IV flow rate, the site used for parenteral administra-

tion, any problems with administration, and the patient's vital signs taken immediately before administration.

- The patient's response to the drug is monitored and, when applicable, recorded. This evaluation may include such facts as relief of pain, decrease in body temperature, relief of itching, and decrease in the number of stools passed.
- The patient is observed for adverse reactions. The frequency of observation depends on the drug administered. All suspected adverse reactions are documented and reported to the health care provider. Serious adverse reactions must be reported immediately.

Administration of Drugs in the Home

Often drugs are taken by patients in their homes or are administered by family members acting as caregivers. The patient or caregivers need to understand the treatment regimen and to be able to ask questions about their drug therapy, such as why the drug was prescribed, how to give or take it, and possible adverse reactions that may occur. Key Concepts 2-3 gives guidelines for drug use in the home by the patient or caregiver rather than by health care providers.

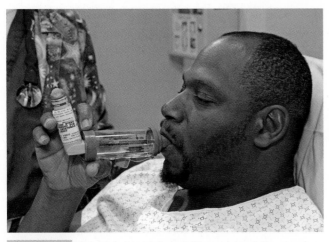

FIGURE 2-6 A respiratory inhalant is used to deliver a drug directly into the lungs. To deliver a dose of the drug, the patient takes a slow, deep breath while depressing the top of the canister. (See Chapter 15 for more information on drugs given by inhalation.) (Photo by Rick Brady.)

KEY CONCEPTS

2-3 Administering Drugs Safely in the Home

Patients are often prescribed drugs to be taken at home. Because the home environment is not as controlled as a health care facility, the following aspects of the patient's home environment should be considered:

- Does the home have a space that is relatively free of clutter and easily accessible to the patient or a caregiver?
- Do any small children live in or visit the home? If so, is there a place where drugs can be stored safely out of their reach?
- Does the drug require refrigeration? If so, does the refrigerator work?
- Does the patient need special equipment, such as needles and syringes? If so, where and how can the equipment be stored for safety and convenience? Does the patient have an appropriate disposal container? Will disposed items be safe from children and pets? Plastic storage containers with snap-on lids or clean, dry glass jars with screw tops can be used for needle disposal. A plastic milk jug with a lid or a heavy-duty, clean, cardboard milk or juice carton may be used if necessary. Patients should understand the importance of precautions to make sure discarded needles do not puncture the container.
- If the patient needs several drugs, can the patient or caregiver identify which drugs are used and when? Do they know how to use them and why?

Chapter Review

KEY POINTS

- Six "rights" in the administration of drugs ensure that patients receive medications correctly and safely: right patient, right drug, right dose, right route, right time, and right documentation.
- Drug errors are any occurrence that can cause a patient to receive the wrong dose, the wrong drug, a drug by the wrong route, or a drug given at the incorrect time. Errors may occur in transcribing drug orders, dispensing the drug, or administering the drug. When a drug error occurs, it must be reported immediately.
- Common medication orders include the standing order, the single order, the PRN order, and the STAT order.
- Drug dispensing systems include computerized dispensing systems, unit dose systems, and floor stock systems.
- Health care professionals involved in drug administration and patient care should know about each drug given, the reasons the drug is used, the drug's general action, its more common adverse reactions, special precautions in administration, and the normal dose ranges.
- In drug administration, patient considerations are important, such as allergy history, previous adverse reactions, the patient's comments, and any change in the patient's condition.
- Drugs may be administered by any of the following routes, each with its own patient care considerations: the oral, parenteral (subcutaneous, IM, IV, or intradermal), topical, transdermal, and inhalation routes.
- When drugs are taken by patients in their homes, the patients or caregivers need to understand the treatment regimen, such as why the drug was prescribed, how to give or take it, and possible adverse reactions that may occur.

CRITICAL THINKING CASE STUDY

Needlestick Injuries

The clinic where you work has a sharps-resistant container for disposing of used needles and syringes located in a room where immunizations are usually administered. Occasionally, however, patients in other examining rooms need injections. After caregivers administer the injections, they recap the needles and carry the used syringes to the other room to dispose of them in the sharps container.

1. What agency has established guidelines for needlestick prevention?
    a. Centers for Disease Control and Prevention (CDC)
    b. The Joint Commission
    c. Occupational Safety and Health Administration (OSHA)
    d. Food and Drug Administration (FDA)

2. Is this practice acceptable?
    a. Yes, as long as they are disposed of correctly.
    b. No, they should recap the needle, but the sharps container should be in the same room in which they are administering immunizations.
    c. No, they should not recap prior to carrying the used syringes to the other room.
    d. No, they should not recap or carry the used syringes to the other room.

3. What should be done differently in your clinic to minimize the risk of exposure to blood-borne infections via a needlestick injury?

Review Questions

MULTIPLE CHOICE

1. To ensure a drug is given correctly, it should be administered
    a. to the right patient
    b. at the right time
    c. by the right route
    d. all of the above

2. If a patient reports that the pill just given to him/her is a different color from the last one he/she received, you should
    a. explain they should not worry because many pills come in different colors
    b. pretend you will check on it so he/she stops worrying
    c. report this to the health care provider
    d. try to get the patient to vomit up the pill as quickly as possible

3. A STAT medication order means the drug should be given
    a. as soon as possible
    b. whenever the patient is having symptoms and requests it
    c. first thing in the morning
    d. following the daily staff meeting

4. Why do health care workers watch patients for potential allergic reactions?
    a. Allergic reactions can be uncomfortable for patients.
    b. A different drug may need to be prescribed.
    c. Allergic reactions can be life threatening.
    d. All of the above.

MATCHING

_____ 5. buccal
_____ 6. sublingual
_____ 7. transdermal
_____ 8. parenteral

a. under the tongue
b. absorbed through the skin
c. injected inside body
d. between the cheek and gum

TRUE OR FALSE

_____ 9. Reviewing medications with the patient may help reduce medication errors.

_____ 10. The administration of topical medications need not follow the "six rights" of medication administration because the medication can be wiped off the skin if given incorrectly.

_____ 11. The floor stock system involves medications that are packaged in individual unit of use packaging for one patient.

_____ 12. Medications that are available in tablet form may be crushed or chewed for patients who cannot swallow the tablet whole.

FILL IN THE BLANKS

13. Needles are dropped into a _____ container without touching the inside of the container. Needles should never be pushed or forced into the container, as damage to the container and/or needlestick injuries may result.

14. In the _____ _____ system, drug orders are filled and medications dispensed to fill each patient's medication order(s) for a 24-hour period.

15. Drugs administered through _____, such as bronchodilators, have a local effect in the lungs.

16. The administration of a drug must always be _____ as soon as possible to prevent medication errors.

SHORT ANSWERS

17. Six rights of drug administration have been discussed in this chapter. Can you list them?

18. If a patient is scheduled to be given a medication at 7.00 am and 7.00 pm, but the 7.00 am dose is not given until 10.00 am, is this considered a medication error? Explain your answer.

19. Name and briefly describe the four types of parenteral drug administration discussed in this chapter.

20. What are the components of a drug order?

Web Activities

1. Go to the Web site of the U.S. Department of Labor Occupational Safety & Health Administration (OSHA) (http://www.osha.gov/) and the section on Bloodborne Pathogens. Explore this page and find the OSHA material addressing the question: "What are some examples of possible solutions for workplace hazards?" Write up the key points that would need to be discussed during an in-service for health care professionals regarding OSHA's Bloodborne Pathogens Standard.

2. Go to the website of the institute for safe medication practices (http://www.ismp.org).
   a. Find their list of Confused Drug Names.
   b. Find their Error-Prone abbreviation list.

3

Math Review

CHAPTER OBJECTIVES

On completion of this chapter, students will be able to:

1 Define the chapter's key terms.
2 Factor a number.
3 Add and subtract fractions.
4 Multiply and divide fractions.
5 Convert fractions to decimals and percentages.
6 Convert decimals to fractions and percentages.
7 Convert Arabic numbers to Roman numerals.
8 Convert Roman numerals to Arabic numbers.
9 Convert percentages to decimals and fractions.
10 Convert within and between different systems of measurements.
11 Convert times between a 12-hour clock and a 24-hour clock.
12 Convert temperatures from Fahrenheit to Celsius.
13 Convert temperatures from Celsius to Fahrenheit.
14 Understand and apply the techniques of ratio and proportion and dimensional analysis.
15 Calculate correct dosages for adults and children.

KEY TERMS

biological standard unit—a specific amount of biologically active substance that is used pharmacologically or therapeutically
common (proper) fraction—a fraction with the numerator smaller than the denominator
denominator—the divisor of a fraction written in the bottom half of a common fraction
factors—any numbers multiplied together to form a product

thePOINT RESOURCES

- Drug Calculations Review
- Interactive Practice and Review

fraction—a part of a whole containing a numerator and denominator

improper fraction—fractions with the numerator larger than the denominator

mixed number—fractions preceded by a whole number

nomogram—a chart that is made up of several lines marked off to scale and arranged so that by using a straightedge to connect known values on two lines, an unknown value can be read at the point of intersection with another line; used to calculate body surface area using a patient's height and weight

numerator—the top portion of a fraction

percent—a portion of a whole divided into 100 parts, means "per 100"

proportion—two ratios that are equal to each other

ratio—a comparison of two amounts that represents a constant relationship between two values; may be written with a color or as a fraction

reciprocal—the inverse of a fraction

word factors—the units used in a mathematical term

This chapter reviews basic mathematical skills needed for calculating medication dosages. Calculating the right dosage of medication administered to a patient is a patient right and is a first step in preventing medication errors. Regardless of your area of practice within health care, it is very important that you are able to apply basic math skills.

Fractions

A **fraction** is a part of a whole. Every fraction is written with three parts: a numerator, a denominator, and a division line. The **numerator** is the top number and indicates how many parts of the whole used. The **denominator** is the bottom number and indicates how many total parts make up the whole. The division line separates the numerator from the denominator. Example: What fraction indicates the number of shaded portions in the square?

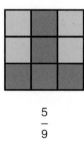

$$\frac{5}{9}$$

There are 9 total boxes, and 5 boxes are shaded. The fraction indicating the number of shaded portions would be

$$5 \leftarrow \text{Numerator}$$
$$- \leftarrow \text{Division Line}$$
$$9 \leftarrow \text{Denominator}$$

A **common fraction,** also called a proper fraction, is written when the numerator is smaller than the denominator.

Example: $\frac{1}{2}, \frac{2}{3}$, and $\frac{4}{5}$ are all common fractions.

Fractions preceded by a whole number are called **mixed numbers**.

Example: $4\frac{2}{3}, 7\frac{7}{8}$, and $10\frac{3}{5}$ are mixed numbers.

Improper fractions are written with the numerator larger than the denominator.

Example: $\frac{8}{5}, \frac{11}{7}$, and $\frac{21}{13}$ are all improper fractions.

Principles of Fractions

Several standard principles of fractions must be understood in order to accurately calculate fractions in a problem. The list below represents the eight most common principles of fractions:

1. The denominator of any fraction is never zero.

$$\frac{5}{0} = \text{undefined}$$

2. A fraction with a zero in the numerator is always equal to zero.

$$\frac{0}{23} = 0$$

3. The division line separates the numerator from the denominator, indicating that the entire expression above the division line is the numerator, and the entire expression below is the denominator.

$$\text{Correct}: \frac{(1+2)}{(2+5)} = \frac{3}{7} \quad \text{Incorrect}: \frac{(1+2)}{(2+5)} \neq \frac{1}{2} + \frac{2}{5}$$

4. A minus sign placed in front of either the numerator, the denominator, or the entire fraction indicates that the fraction is negative.

$$\text{Negative Fraction}: \frac{-2}{3} = \frac{2}{-3} = -\frac{2}{3}$$

5. A minus sign placed in front of both the numerator and the denominator indicates that the fraction is positive.

$$\text{Positive Fraction}: \frac{-2}{-3} = \frac{2}{3}$$

6. Multiplying *or* dividing a number by 1 does not change the value of the number.

$$6 \times 1 = 6 \qquad \frac{6}{1} = 6$$

7. The number 1 can have different forms as a fraction. When the numerator of a fraction is the same or equivalent to the denominator, the fraction is equal to 1, and the equivalent fraction can be substituted for the number 1.

$$\frac{6}{6} = 1 \quad \text{and} \quad \frac{3+3}{6} = 1$$

8. A number (integer) can be expressed as a fraction by simply dividing by 1. An integer can also be expressed as a fraction by selecting a numerator and denominator so the overall value of the fraction is equal to the integer.

$$12 = \frac{12}{1} \qquad 12 = \frac{24}{2} = \frac{36}{3}$$

Factoring Numbers

A **factor** is a portion or a piece of a number. When two numbers are multiplied together, each number is a factor of the product. A factor can divide evenly into a whole number with no remainder. To factor an integer, break it down into the groups of numbers whose product equals the original number. The number 1 and the number itself will be a factor for every number.
Example: Find the factors of 12.
Start with the lowest whole number and determine if it can be multiplied to form a product.

F_{12}
$1 \times 12 = 12$
$2 \times 6 = 12$ The factors of 12 are 1, 2, 3, 4, 6, and 12.
$3 \times 4 = 12$
$4 \times 3 = 12$
$5 \times$ No Factors

Order of Operations

Specific mathematical operations must be done first in order to eliminate errors in calculation. Following an order of operations will allow for correct calculations. The standard steps of mathematical calculations follow the rules below:

1. Solve within parentheses and brackets.
2. Solve exponents, powers, and roots.
3. Multiply and divide from left to right.
4. Add and subtract in order from left to right.

Example: Simplify the expression following the correct order of operations.

$$(6 + 8 \div 2) - 8 + 4(3)^2 + (5 \times 4 + 8)$$

Follow the correct order of operations and simplify each portion of the expression one step at a time to simplify.

$$(6 + 8 \div 2) - 8 + 4(3)^2 + (5 \times 4 + 8)$$
$$= (6 + 4) - 8 + 4(9) + (20 + 8)$$
$$= (10) - 8 + 36 + (28)$$
$$= 2 + 36 + (28)$$
$$= 38 + (28)$$
$$= 66$$

Reciprocal Numbers

Every mathematical expression other than zero has an inverse expression that can be multiplied to give a product of 1. This matching expression is called its **reciprocal**. To determine the reciprocal of a number, first create a fraction; then, invert the fraction.

Example: Find the reciprocal of $\frac{3}{4}$.

Invert $\frac{3}{4}$ to create its reciprocal $\frac{4}{3}$. We can check that $\frac{4}{3}$ is the Correct reciprocal by multiplying the two factors together. The product should be equal to 1.

$$\frac{3}{4} \times \frac{4}{3} = \frac{12}{12} = 1$$

Reducing Fractions

Fractions in different forms can be equal each other. These types of fractions are called equivalent fractions.
Example: Write the fraction for the shaded portion in each shape.

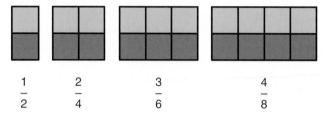

$$\frac{1}{2} \qquad \frac{2}{4} \qquad \frac{3}{6} \qquad \frac{4}{8}$$

Each fraction indicates that exactly half of the boxes in each shape are shaded. These fractions are all equivalent and have the same value. To reduce a fraction, divide both terms of the fraction by a common factor. Common factors in the numerator and the denominator can be canceled out.

Example: Reduce $\frac{4}{6}$ to lowest terms.

$$\frac{4}{6} = \frac{2 \times 2}{3 \times 2} = \frac{2}{3} \times 1 = \frac{2}{3}$$

Converting Mixed Numbers to Improper Fractions

To convert a mixed number to an improper fraction, multiply the denominator by the whole number, and add the product to the numerator. This value becomes the numerator, and the denominator remains the same.

Example: Convert $5\frac{3}{4}$ to an improper fraction.

$$5\frac{3}{4} = \frac{[(5 \times 4) + 3]}{4} = \frac{(20 + 3)}{4} = \frac{23}{4}$$

Converting Improper Fractions to Mixed Numbers

An improper fraction can be converted into a mixed fraction by dividing the numerator by the denominator. The quotient becomes the whole number, while the remainder becomes the numerator for the mixed fraction, and the denominator remains the same.

$$\frac{31}{8} = \frac{\begin{array}{r} 3 \\ 8\overline{)31} \\ -24 \\ \hline 7 \end{array}}{} = 3\frac{7}{8}$$

Constructing Fractions

Constructing a fraction is the opposite of reducing the fraction. Equivalent fractions can be constructed by multiplying a fraction by another fraction that is equal to 1.

Example: Create equivalent fractions of $\frac{1}{3}$ by multiplying by $\frac{2}{2}, \frac{3}{3}$, and $\frac{4}{4}$.

Since $\frac{2}{2}, \frac{3}{3}$, and $\frac{4}{4}$ are equal to 1, multiplying them by $\frac{1}{3}$ does not change the value of the fraction we are constructing. An equivalent form of the fraction is created.

$$\frac{1}{3} \times \frac{2}{2} = \frac{2}{6} \qquad \frac{1}{3} \times \frac{3}{3} = \frac{3}{9} \qquad \frac{1}{3} \times \frac{4}{4} = \frac{4}{12}$$

Example: Create a fraction with 12 in the denominator that is equivalent to $\frac{2}{3}$.

First, determine the factors of 12 to determine what number multiplied by 3 will equal 12. Since the denominator is equal to 3, and 3 times 4 is equal to 12, we can use the fraction $\frac{4}{4}$. Since $\frac{4}{4} = 1$, the value is not changing, but we are creating an equivalent form of the fraction.

$$\frac{2}{3} \times 1 = \frac{2}{3} \times \frac{4}{4} = \frac{8}{12}.$$

We have now created a fraction with a denominator equal to 12 that is an equivalent to $\frac{2}{3}$.

Finding a Common Denominator

Constructing fractions allows us to find common denominators between fractions. To find a common denominator between fractions, you must determine the least common multiple of the denominators. The least common multiple is the smallest number in which both numbers share a common factor.
Example: Find the least common multiple of 5 and 6.

Begin by listing multiples of each number. Begin by multiplying by 1, then by 2, and continue until you have found the common multiple.

Multiples of 5 = [5, 10, 15, 20, 25, 30, 35, 40]

Multiples of 6 = [6, 12, 18, 24, 30, 36, 42]

Both numbers have 30 as a common multiple. After finding the least common multiple to be used as the denominator, convert each fraction into an equivalent form with a denominator of 30.

Example: Convert $\frac{2}{5}$ and $\frac{1}{6}$ to equivalent fractions with a common denominator.

$$\frac{2}{5} \times 1 = \frac{2}{5} \times \frac{6}{6} = \frac{12}{30} \qquad \frac{1}{6} \times 1 = \frac{1}{6} \times \frac{5}{5} = \frac{5}{30}$$

Adding Fractions

Fractions can only be added together when their denominators are the same. A common denominator must be found first before adding fractions. When adding fractions, the numerators are added together, and the common denominator stays the same.

$$\text{Example : Add } \frac{3}{4} \text{ and } \frac{6}{7}.$$

First, find a common denominator between the two fractions.

Multiples of 4 = [4, 8, 12, 16, 20, 24, 28, 32]

Multiples of 7 = [7, 14, 21, 28, 35]

After determining that the least common multiple is 28, convert both fractions into equivalent forms with 28 as the denominator.

$$\frac{3}{4} \times 1 = \frac{3}{4} \times \frac{7}{7} = \frac{21}{28} \qquad \frac{6}{7} \times 1 = \frac{6}{7} \times \frac{4}{4} = \frac{24}{28}$$

Next, add the fractions by adding the numerators while keeping the denominators the same.

$$\frac{21}{28} + \frac{24}{28} = \frac{(21+24)}{28} = \frac{45}{28}$$

In your answers, it is common to convert improper fractions to mixed numbers and reduce fractions to lowest terms when possible.

$$\frac{45}{28} = \begin{array}{r} 1 \\ 28\overline{)45} \\ -28 \\ \hline 17 \end{array} = 1\frac{17}{28}$$

Subtracting Fractions

To subtract fractions, the same principles apply as in addition. A common denominator must be found, then the numerators are subtracted, and the denominators remain the same.

$$\text{Example: Subtract } \frac{10}{11} \text{ and } \frac{3}{5}.$$

$$\frac{10}{11} \times 1 = \frac{10}{11} \times \frac{5}{5} = \frac{50}{55}$$

$$\frac{3}{5} \times 1 = \frac{3}{5} \times \frac{11}{11} = \frac{33}{55}$$

$$\frac{10}{11} - \frac{3}{5} = \frac{50}{55} - \frac{33}{55} = \frac{(50-33)}{55} = \frac{17}{55}$$

Multiplying Fractions

Multiplication and division of fractions are performed differently than addition and subtraction. To multiply fractions, the numerators are multiplied together, and the denominators are multiplied together. Then, the product is reduced to lowest terms.

Example: Multiply and write the product in lowest terms. $\frac{5}{8} \times \frac{2}{5}$

$$\frac{5}{8} \times \frac{2}{5} = \frac{(5 \times 2)}{(8 \times 5)} = \frac{10}{40}$$

Reduce to lowest terms by finding the common factors in the numerator and the denominator.

$$\frac{10}{40} = \frac{(5 \times 2)}{(8 \times 5)} = \frac{(2 \times 5)}{(8 \times 5)} = \frac{(1 \times 2 \times 5)}{(4 \times 2 \times 5)} = \frac{1}{4} \times \frac{2}{2} \times \frac{5}{5} = \frac{1}{4} \times 1 \times 1 = \frac{1}{4}$$

Canceling in Multiplication

In order to avoid reducing to lowest terms of large multiplication, canceling can be done before multiplying. In order to cancel, common factors in the numerator and the denominator can be found in either fraction and eliminated before multiplication.

Example : Multiply $-\frac{5}{8} \times \frac{2}{5}$.

To multiply, cancel common factors in each term first.

$$\frac{5}{8} \times \frac{2}{5} = \frac{\cancel{5}^1}{8} \times \frac{2}{\cancel{5}^1} = \frac{1}{8} \times \frac{2}{1} = \frac{1}{\cancel{8}^4} \times \frac{\cancel{2}^1}{1} = \frac{1}{4} \times \frac{1}{1} = \frac{1}{4}$$

After canceling and multiplying, our product is in lowest terms and does not have to be reduced.

Multiplying Mixed Numbers

Before multiplying mixed numbers, each must be changed to an improper fraction before multiplying.

Example: Multiply $4\frac{2}{5}$ and $6\frac{7}{8}$.

First, change both numbers to improper fractions.

$$4\frac{2}{5} = \frac{(4 \times 5) + 2}{5} = \frac{22}{5} \qquad 6\frac{7}{8} = \frac{(6 \times 8) + 7}{8} = \frac{55}{8}$$

Next, multiply the numerators and the denominators, canceling first when possible.

$$\frac{22}{5} \times \frac{55}{8} = \frac{\cancel{22}^{11}}{\cancel{5}^1} \times \frac{\cancel{55}^{11}}{\cancel{8}^4} = \frac{121}{4} = 30\frac{1}{4}$$

Multiplying Fractions by Whole Numbers

Before multiplying a whole number and a fraction, change the whole number to an equivalent fraction to multiply.

Example: Multiply $\frac{2}{7} \times 9$.

A whole number can be converted to a fraction by placing the whole number in the numerator and setting the denominator to 1.

$$9 = \frac{9}{1}$$

Now multiply the fractions as normal.

$$\frac{2}{7} \times \frac{9}{1} = \frac{18}{7} = 2\frac{4}{7}$$

Dividing Fractions

Division is the inverse of multiplication. To divide by a fraction, *multiply* by the inverse of the second fraction (reciprocal).

Example: Divide $\frac{4}{7} \div \frac{5}{6}$.

The reciprocal of $\frac{5}{6}$ is $\frac{6}{5}$. Now, multiply $\frac{4}{7}$ by $\frac{6}{5}$.

$$\frac{4}{7} \div \frac{5}{6} = \frac{4}{7} \times \frac{6}{5} = \frac{24}{35}$$

Just as in multiplication, cancel common factors out before multiplying to avoid reducing at the end.

Example: Divide $\frac{8}{15} \div \frac{2}{5}$. Reduce to lowest terms.

$$\frac{8}{15} \div \frac{2}{5} = \frac{8}{15} \times \frac{5}{2} = \frac{\cancel{8}^4}{\cancel{15}^3} \times \frac{\cancel{5}^1}{\cancel{2}^1} = \frac{4}{3} \times \frac{1}{1} = \frac{4}{3} = 1\frac{1}{3}$$

Dividing Mixed Numbers

To divide mixed numbers, first convert the mixed number to an improper fraction. Be sure to remember to multiply by the reciprocal of the second term.

Example: Divide $5\frac{1}{3}$ by $2\frac{1}{4}$.

$$5\frac{1}{3} \div 2\frac{1}{4} = \frac{16}{3} \div \frac{9}{4} = \frac{16}{3} \times \frac{4}{9} = \frac{64}{27} = 2\frac{10}{27}$$

Dividing Whole Numbers

To divide a fraction and a whole number, convert the whole number to its equivalent fraction before dividing.
Example:

Divide 5 by $\frac{2}{3}$.

$$5 \div \frac{2}{3} = \frac{5}{1} \div \frac{2}{3} = \frac{5}{1} \times \frac{3}{2} = \frac{15}{2} = 7\frac{1}{2}$$

Decimals

Decimals are numbers that represent parts of a whole. A decimal has decimal point with digits to the right. Numbers to the left of the decimal point represent the tens, hundreds, and thousands places, while numbers to the right of the decimal point represent fractions of numbers such as tenths, hundredths, and thousandths. Fractions and decimals are related because both can be used to represent values that are smaller than one.

Reading Decimals

The place or position of a digit in a number written in standard form determines the value that is given to the digit. Table 3-1 shows place values for various positions.

Writing Decimals

Decimals represent fractions. The fraction $\frac{2}{5}$ can be written as 0.4. If a decimal is less than 1, a zero is normally placed in front of the decimal.

Example: Convert $\frac{1}{4}$ to a decimal.

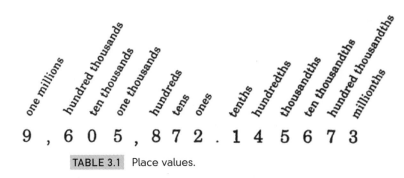

TABLE 3.1 Place values.

To convert to a decimal, divide the numerator by the denominator.

$$\frac{1}{4} = 4\overline{)1} = 4\overline{)1.00}^{\,0.25}$$

If a decimal is less than 1, a zero is placed to the left of the decimal point.

Adding Decimals

To add decimals, be sure to line up the decimal points. The decimal point in the sum should also be placed so that it lines up with the others. Adding zeros after the decimal point may be necessary to correctly line up the decimal points. Adding zeros to the right of the decimal point does not change the value. Example: Add 3.61 + 4.59.

$$\begin{array}{r} 3.61 \\ +4.59 \\ \hline 8.20 \end{array}$$ Line up the decimal points and add as normal.

Subtracting Decimals

Subtracting decimals is the opposite of addition. In order to correctly subtract decimals, line up the decimal points just as in addition and subtraction. Example: Subtract 64.52 – 45.23

$$\begin{array}{r} 64.52 \\ -45.23 \\ \hline 19.29 \end{array}$$ Remember to line up the decimal points.

Multiplying Decimals

Multiply decimals the same way you multiply whole numbers. You do not have to line up the decimal points. The number of decimal places in the product is equal to the sum of the decimal places in the factors. Remember, if one of the factors is negative, the product will be negative, and if both factors are negative, the product will be positive. Example: Multiply 8.98 × 4.5.

$$\begin{array}{r} 8.98 \\ \times\ 4.5 \\ \hline 40.410 \end{array}$$

Dividing Decimals

To divide decimals using long division, follow the same method as dividing whole numbers. Place the decimal point in the quotient above the decimal point in the dividend. If the divisor also has a decimal point, shift the decimal point of the divisor to make a whole number. Shift the decimal the same number of places in the dividend and divide as normal. If the quotient is a repeating decimal, draw a bar over the repeating decimal pattern. Dividing with negative numbers follows the same principle as multiplication. If one of the values is negative, the quotient will be negative, and if both dividend and divisor are negative, the quotient will be positive. Example: Divide 5.98 by 4.

$$\begin{array}{r} 1.495 \\ 4\overline{)5.980} \\ -4 \\ \hline 19 \\ -16 \\ \hline 38 \\ -36 \\ \hline 20 \\ -20 \\ \hline 0 \end{array}$$

Converting Decimals to Fractions

To convert a decimal to a fraction, first create a fraction by putting a 1 in the denominator. Multiply the numerator and denominator by a multiple of 10 (100, 1000, 10,000, etc.) to remove the decimal point. Then reduce the fraction to its lowest terms. Hint: The number of zeros in the denominator will be equal to the number of decimal places. Example: Convert 0.25 to a fraction.

$$0.25 = \frac{0.25}{1} = \frac{0.25}{1} \times 1 = \frac{0.25}{1} \times \frac{100}{100} = \frac{25}{100} = \frac{1}{4}$$

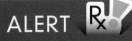

ALERT

Leading and Trailing Zero

To prevent errors with medication doses, a leading zero is placed before the decimal point if the decimal is less than 1. Correct example: 0.2 mg. If the decimal is a whole number, avoid placing a trailing zero after the decimal point. Correct example: 2 mg. Incorrect use of a leading or trailing zero may cause the decimal point to be missed, leading to a dosage error.

Converting Fractions to Decimals

To convert a fraction to a decimal, the numerator is the dividend, and the denominator is the divisor. Divide the numerator by the denominator.

Example: Convert $\frac{5}{8}$ to a decimal.

$$
\begin{array}{r}
0.625 \\
8\overline{)5.000} \\
-0 \\
\hline
50 \\
-48 \\
\hline
20 \\
-16 \\
\hline
40 \\
-40 \\
\hline
0
\end{array}
$$

Rounding of Decimals

Decimals may be rounded. The accuracy that you are seeking will determine at what point you should round. For example, if you complete a dosage calculation that results in the number 374.89 mg, you are not going to be able to give the patient exactly that amount. You will need to round in this case to the nearest whole number. If the number to the right of the decimal is greater than or equal to 0.5, then round up to the next number. If the number to the right of the decimal is less than 5, then delete the remaining numbers and leave the number as is. In the example above, 374.89 will round to 375 because 8 is larger than 5.

Arabic Number and Roman Numerals

Most medication dosages are ordered and administered using Arabic numbers called digits (i.e., 1, 2, 3). However, on occasion, you may see an order or a prescription drug bottle that uses Roman numerals, which are symbols that represent numbers. It is important that you are able to convert between Arabic numbers and Roman numerals with ease.
Roman numerals use seven basic symbols.

Roman Numerals	Arabic Numbers
I	1
V	5
X	10
L	50
C	100
D	500
M	1000

The combination of Roman numeral symbols are based on a few principles:

1. Symbols are used to construct a number, but a symbol may not be used more than three times in a row. The exception is 5 (V) since VV is the same as X (10).

Example : III $=$ $(1+1+1)$ $=$ 3

XXX $=$ $(10\ +\ 10\ +\ 10)$ $=$ 30

2. When a symbol of lesser value follows a symbol of greater value, they are added together to determine the number.

Example : XIII $=$ $(10+1+1+1)$ $=$ 13

XXVII $=$ $(10\ +\ 10\ +\ 5\ +\ 1\ +\ 1)$ $=$ 27

3. When a symbol of lesser value precedes a symbol of greater values, the symbol of lesser value is subtracted from the symbol of greater value to determine the number.

Example : IV $=$ $(1\ \text{and}\ 5)$ $=$ $(5-1)$ $=$ 4

IX $=$ $(1\ \text{and}\ 10)$ $=$ $(10-1)$ $=$ 9

To convert an Arabic number to a Roman numeral, the number must be separated into numbers that can be represented using the symbols. For example, 24 would be separated into 20 and 4, each of which can then be written using the Roman numeral symbols. 20 is XX and 4 is IV, so 24 can be written XXIV.

Percentages

A **percent** describes a whole per 100 parts. A percentage should be thought of as a whole number divided by 100. 50% represents 50 parts out of 100 total parts. Medications are expressed as weight/volume, weight/weight, or volume/volume. The weight is expressed in grams. The volume is expressed in milliliters. Weight/volume as a percentage is the number of grams per 100 milliliters of solution. For example, normal saline is 0.9% sodium chloride, which means there are 0.9 g of sodium chloride in every 100 mL of solution.

Converting a Ratio to a Percent

To find a percentage, divide the part of the whole by the total number of parts and multiply by 100.

Example: Convert $\frac{3}{4}$ to a percentage value.

$$\frac{3}{4} = 0.75 \times 100 = 75\%$$

Converting Percents to Decimals

To calculate a decimal from a percentage, simply divide the percentage by 100.
Example: Convert 65% to a decimal.

$$65\% = \frac{65}{100} = 0.65$$

Systems of Measurement

Three systems of measurement are commonly used for medication dosage administration: the metric system, the apothecary system, and the household system.

Metric System

The metric system is a decimal system for both weights and measures based on units of ten. The basic units of measure are as follows:

Gram $=$ weight

Meter $=$ length

Liter $=$ volume

Weight

The most frequently used metric units of weight are kilogram (kg), gram (g), milligram (mg), and microgram (mcg).

It is important that you are able to convert between the different units of weight. The relationship between the units of weight is a multiple of 1000 as you move from one unit to the next.

0.001	1	1,000	1,000,000
kg	g	mg	mcg

To convert 1 g to a kilogram, you would move the decimal three places to the left. This means that there is 0.001 kg in each gram because the kilogram is a larger unit of weight than the gram.

To convert 1 g to milligrams, you would move the decimal three places to the right. This means that there are 1,000 mg in each gram because the milligram is a smaller unit of weight than the gram.

Volume

The most frequently used metric units of volume are liter (L) and milliliter (mL).

It is important that you are able to convert between liters and milliliters.

1	1,000
L	mL

Like the units of weight, the relationship between the units of volume is also a multiple of 1000. 1 L is equal to 1000 mL, which means that there are 1000 mL in each liter.

To convert a liter to a milliliter, multiply by 1000 or move the decimal 3 places to the right. For example, a 3-L TPN (total parenteral nutrition) bag contains 3000 mL of fluid.

To convert a milliliter to a liter, divide by 1000 or move the decimal 3 places to the left. For example, a 250-mL IV bag contains 0.25 L of fluid.

Make note that a milliliter and a cubic centimeter (cc) are the same and are often used interchangeably, especially when referring to syringes and injections.

Apothecary System

The Apothecary system is the system that was used to weigh and measure medications prior to being replaced by the metric system. Although it has largely been replaced, it is important to understand because some physicians continue to order medications using the apothecary system, often combined with Roman numerals.

Weight

The units of weight in the apothecary system are the pound (lb), ounce (oz), dram (dr), and grain (gr).

1 lb	16 oz
1 oz	8 dr
1 dr	60 gr

Volume

The units of volume in the apothecary system include gallon (gal), quart (qt), pint (pt), fluid ounce (fl oz), fluid dram (fl dr), and minim (M).

1 gal	4 qt
1 qt	2 pt
1 pt	16 fl oz
1 fl oz	8 fl dr
1 fl dr	60 M

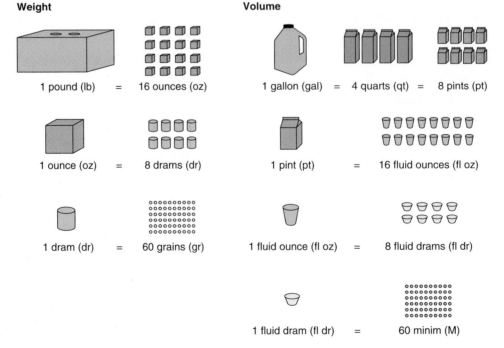

Apothecary system conversions.

Household Measurement System

The household measurement system is considered inaccurate for medication dosages because of the varying sizes of cups, glasses, and measuring spoons. However, as a patient moves from the hospital to the home setting, it is important to understand the household measurement system and be able to use and educate patients and their families on the system.

The common units of measure in the household system are cup, tablespoon (Tbsp), teaspoon (tsp), and drop (gtt).

1 cup	8 oz
2 Tbsp	1 oz
3 tsp	1 Tbsp
1 tsp	60 gtts

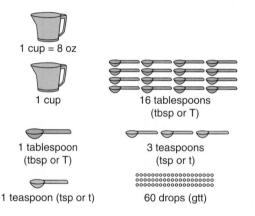

1 cup = 8 oz

1 cup

16 tablespoons (tbsp or T)

1 tablespoon (tbsp or T)

3 teaspoons (tsp or t)

1 teaspoon (tsp or t)

60 drops (gtt)

For most situations where the household measurement system is used, a conversion to the metric system is the easiest way to ensure that the patient receives the correct amount of medication.

1 oz	30 mL
1 Tbsp	15 mL
1 tsp	5 mL
15 gtts	1 mL

To demonstrate how these would be used in medication administration, a few examples are provided.

If a patient is to take 1 tsp of a medication, the medication label may read "take 5 mL" or "take 1 teaspoonful." In either case, the most accurate form of measurement is 5 mL using a dosing cup or syringe that is marked in milliliters.

There are times when a household spoon might be used, such as a powder laxative that must be mixed in a glass of water. Then, a household tablespoon or teaspoon might be used to measure the powder and mix in a full glass of water, which is considered to be 8 oz of water.

Drops may be used to measure some liquid medications. But the most common situation in which drops are used involves otic and ophthalmic preparations. The pharmacy will use the conversion of 1 mL = 15 gtts to determine how long an ophthalmic or otic bottle will last. For example, if a patient is using 2 gtts in each eye twice daily, then the patient uses 8 gtts a day. If the patient's ophthalmic bottle contains 15 mL, the pharmacy would convert that to drops and determine that the bottle contains approximately 225 gtts in it. If the patient is using 8 gtts per day, then the bottle will last approximately 28 days.

The table below lists some common conversions between the different systems of measure that are useful when dealing with medications:

Volumes		
1 gal	128 fl oz	3840 mL
1 qt	32 fl oz	960 mL
1 pt	16 fl oz	480 mL
1 cup	8 fl oz	240 mL
1 Tbsp	½ fl oz	15 mL
1 tsp	1/6 fl oz	5 mL
Weights		
1 lb	16 oz	480 g
	1 oz	30 g

Temperature Coversions

Fahrenheit formula: $F = \frac{9}{5}C + 32$ or F = (C × 1.8) divided by 32

Celsius formula: $C = \frac{5}{9}(F - 32)$ or C = F − 32 + 1.8

Example: Convert 98.6°F (normal body temperature) to °C.
Example: Convert 85°C to °F.

$$C = \frac{5}{9}(F - 32) \qquad F = \frac{9}{5}C + 32$$

$$C = \frac{5}{9}(140 - 32) \qquad F = \frac{9}{5}(85) + 32$$

$$C = \frac{5}{9}(108) \qquad F = \frac{765}{5} + 32$$

$$C = \frac{540}{9} \qquad F = 153 + 32$$

$$C = 60 \qquad F = 185$$

or   or

C = (98.6 − 32) divided by 1.8   F = 85 × 1.8 + 32

C = 108 divided by 1.8   F = 185

C = 37

Ratios and Proportions

Ratios and proportions are used to compare numbers and to describe the relationship between the numbers. Ratios and proportions can be used to compare equivalencies between numbers with different units. Ratios and proportions are very

KEY CONCEPTS

| 3-1 | **24-Hour Time** |

Another conversion that you must be able to make is the conversion from standard time to military time, which runs on a 24-hour clock. The 24-hour clock is a time keeping method in which the day runs from midnight to midnight and is divided into 24 hours, numbered from 0 to 23. This system is the most commonly used time notation in the world today. The 24-hour clock avoids confusion between AM and PM administration of meds.

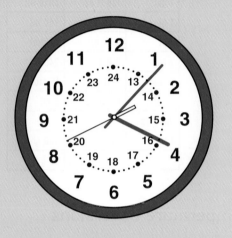

12-Hour	24-Hour	12-Hour	24-Hour
12 Midnight	0	12 Noon	1200
1:00 AM	100	1:00 PM	1300
2:00 AM	200	2:00 PM	1400
3:00 AM	300	3:00 PM	1500
4:00 AM	400	4:00 PM	1600
5:00 AM	500	5:00 PM	1700
6:00 AM	600	6:00 PM	1800
7:00 AM	700	7:00 PM	1900
8:00 AM	800	8:00 PM	2000
9:00 AM	900	9:00 PM	2100
10:00 AM	1000	10:00 PM	2200
11:00 AM	1100	11:00 PM	2300

useful in real-life scenarios and in the medical field to calculate dosages based on factors such as age or weight.

Ratios

A **ratio** represents a constant relationship between two values and may be written with a colon between the two values or as a fraction. A constant ratio indicates that the relationship does not change. Ratios are used to calculate related values with different units.

KEY CONCEPTS

| 3-2 | **Temperature Conversions** |

There are two common temperature systems used in the United States, the Fahrenheit scale and the Celcius scale. The Fahrenheit scale places 180 degrees between the freezing point at 32°F and the boiling point at 212°F. The Celsius scale, which is used around the world and in SI and metric measurements, places 100 degrees between the freezing 0°C and the boiling point at 100°C. Equations are listed below that can be used to convert between the two temperature scales:

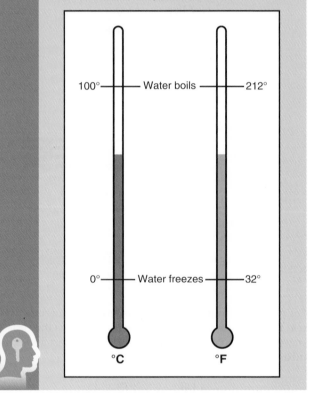

Example: Write a ratio comparing the units of hours and minutes.

$$60 \text{ minutes} : 1 \text{ hour} \quad \text{or} \quad \frac{60 \text{ minutes}}{1 \text{ hour}}$$

Example: In a hospital, there are 500 male patients and 300 female. What is the ratio of male to female patients?

$$500 : 300 \quad \text{OR} \quad \frac{500 \text{ male}}{300 \text{ female}}$$

The ratio can also indicate the total. To find the total number, add each portion of the ratio together. The total may also be used to determine the ratio.

Example: There are 50 vials of red and blue solutions. What is the ratio of red to blue solutions if there are 30 red vials of solution?

50 Total Vials = 30 Red Vials + x Blue Vials
x Blue Vials = 50 Total Vials − 30 Red Vials
Blue Vials = 20
Red to Blue Ratio = 30 : 20

Proportions

Proportions are used to show that two ratios are equal to each other. Proportions can be written either with colon (Box 3-1) or as a fraction, which is discussed below.

$$\text{Fraction Form}: \frac{a}{b} = \frac{c}{d}$$

Proportions can be used to compare two ratios or to make equivalent fractions. By cross-multiplying the proportion, we can see that both sides of the equation are equal to each other. To find the cross product, multiply the numerator of the left side by the denominator on the right side; then multiply the numerator of the right side by the denominator on the left side. The two products will be equal.

Example: Cross-multiply and show that the proportion

$\frac{5}{8} = \frac{40}{64}$ is equal.

$$5 \times 64 = 40 \times 8$$
$$320 = 320$$

We can use the cross products to find an unknown in a proportion.

Example: Solve the proportion for x.

$$\frac{10}{11} = \frac{x}{88}$$
$$88 \times 10 = 11x$$
$$x = \frac{88 \times 10}{11}$$
$$x = 80$$

BOX 3.1

Proportions may also be written in colon form, as shown below:

$$a : b = c : d$$

Solving Problems Using Dimensional Analysis

Dimensional analysis is a problem-solving method that allows for any number of mathematical expressions to be multiplied together. Dimensional analysis is also called the factor–label method or the unit–factor method. The word "dimensional" means that there is a *unit of measure* attached to the number. Units can be anything. The method progresses from what you *already* know about a problem to what is unknown about the problem. Factors can also be words. Units in mathematical terms are called **word factors**. In the expression 24 hours, the word *hours* is a factor. If there is no number in front of a word factor, it always has an implied value of 1.

For example: $x = 1x$; mL = 1 mL; $oz = 1\ oz$

To multiply with a word factor, place the unit in the numerator; and to divide by a word factor, place the unit in the denominator. Addition and subtraction can only be done with expressions that have the same word factors. Word factors are normally referred to as units in mathematical problems. It is important to recognize whether or not word factors are in the numerator or

denominator. For example, in the expression 10 mL per minute, mL is in the numerator and minute is in the denominator.

There are five steps involved in the basic dimensional analysis problem:

Step 1: Write down the *given quantity* and knowns from the problem.
Step 2: Write down the *wanted quantity* and unknowns from the problem.
Step 3: Establish a *unit path* to take you from the given quantity to the wanted quantity.
Step 4: Set up *conversion factors* to allow for cancellation of units that are not needed.
Step 5: Multiply numerators and denominators; divide the product of the numerators by the product of the denominators to give the numerical value of the wanted quantity.

Example: How many milliliters are equal to 3 qt?

Step 1: The known quantity is 3 qt.
Step 2: The unknown quantity is x mL.
Step 3: The unit path from the given quantity to the unknown quantity is to convert quarts to liters and liters to milliliters.
Step 4: Set up conversion factors 1 qt = 1 L and 1 L = 1,000 mL.
Step 5: Set up dimensional analysis.

$$3\ \text{qt} \times \frac{1\ \text{L}}{1\ \text{qt}} \times \frac{1,000\ \text{mL}}{1\ \text{L}} = x\ \text{mL}$$

$$3\ \cancel{\text{qt}} \times \frac{1\ \cancel{\text{L}}}{1\ \cancel{\text{qt}}} \times \frac{1,000\ \text{mL}}{1\ \cancel{\text{L}}} = x\ \text{mL}$$

$$\frac{3 \times 1 \times 1,000}{1 \times 1} = 3,000\ \text{mL}$$

Example: The dosage prescribed for a painkiller is 0.4 mg/kg. How many milligrams should be given for a patient weighing 225 lb?

Step 1: The known quantities are dosage $= 0.4\ \dfrac{\text{mg}}{\text{kg}}$ and patient = 225 lb.
Step 2: The unknown quantity is dosage = x mg.
Step 3: The unit path taken will be to convert kilograms to pounds.
Step 4: The conversion factor from kilograms to pounds is 1 kg = 2.2 lb.
Step 5: Set up dimensional analysis, so numerators and denominators cancel and result in milligrams for units.

BOX 3.2

Note: This problem could also be solved using ratio and proportion.

$$\frac{0.4\ \text{mg}}{1\ \text{kg}} = \frac{X\ \text{mg}}{225\ \text{lb}}$$

Restate, changing either the kilograms to pounds or the pounds to kilograms.

$$\frac{0.4\ \text{mg}}{2.2\ \text{lb}} = \frac{X\ \text{mg}}{225\ \text{lb}}$$

$$X = 40.9\ \text{mg}$$

Example: The recommended dosage for acetaminophen for pain relief is 7 mg/lb every 4 hours. How many milligrams can a child weighing 76 lb take in regular doses in 1 day?

Step 1: The known quantities are $dosage = 7\frac{mg}{kg}$ per 4 hours and child = 76 lb.

Step 2: The unknown quantity is dosage = x mg in 24 hours.

Step 3: The unit path taken will be to convert kilograms to pounds and every 4 hours to 24 hours.

Step 4: The conversion factors from kilograms to pound is 1 kg = 2.2 lb and 24 hours in 1 day.

Step 5: Set up dimensional analysis, so numerators and denominators cancel and we are left with milligrams for units.

$$dosage = 7\frac{mg}{kg \cdot 4\,hours} \times \frac{1\,kg}{2.2\,lbs} \times 76\,lbs \times \frac{24\,hours}{1\,day} = x\frac{mg}{day}$$

$$dosage = 7\frac{mg}{kg \cdot 4\,hours} \times \frac{1\,kg}{2.2\,lbs} \times 76\,lbs \times \frac{24\,hours}{1\,day} = x\frac{mg}{day}$$

$$dosage = \frac{7 \times 1 \times 76 \times 24}{4 \times 2.2 \times 1} = x\frac{mg}{day}$$

$$dosage = 1,450\,\frac{mg}{day}$$

Drug Dosages in Standardized Units

A **biological standard unit** is a specific amount of a biologically active substance that is used pharmacologically or therapeutically, such as some antibiotics, heparin, and insulin.

Antibiotics Dosages

A few antibiotics are administered using standard units. Examples include nystatin, polymyxin B sulfate, and penicillin G potassium. These may be prepared for injection as a specified number of units per milliliter. Antibiotics are also available as lyophilized powder that must first be reconstituted with water or another diluent.

To find the desired concentration of an antibiotic, find the volume of diluent needed:

Step 1: Write a proportion using the fraction or colon method; state the *wanted concentration* as the first two terms of the proportion.

Step 2: Write the total number of units in the vial as the third term of the proportion, and write the unknown volume of diluent as the fourth term of the proportion.

Step 3: Solve for the unknown volume.

Example: A vial of penicillin G contains 1,000,000 units of lyophilized powder. How much diluent should be added to obtain a solution that contains 100,000 units/mL?

$$\frac{100,000\,units}{1\,mL} = \frac{1,000,000\,units}{x\,mL}$$
$$x\,mL = \frac{1,000,000\,units\,(1\,mL)}{100,000\,units}$$

Therefore, 10 mL of diluent must be added to the vial of lyophilized penicillin G.

Example: If a 1,000,000 unit vial of penicillin powder is reconstituted with 10 mL of diluent, how many units will it contain per milliliter?

$$x{:}1\,mL = 1,000,000\,units : 10\,mL$$
$$10\,mL \cdot x = 1,000,000\,units \cdot 1\,mL$$
$$x = \frac{1,000,000\,units \cdot 1\,mL}{10\,mL}$$
$$x = 100,000\,units$$

Heparin Dosages

Heparin anticoagulant helps to prevent the formation of blood clots. It is sometimes called a blood thinner even though heparin does not really thin the blood. It also does not dissolve a blood clot once it has been formed.

Example: A vial of heparin sodium contains 5000 units/mL in a 10-mL vial. How many mL are needed to give a 7,500 unit dose?

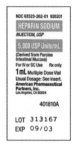

$$\frac{5000\,units}{1\,mL} = \frac{7,500\,units}{x\,mL}$$
$$x\,mL = \frac{7,500\,units(1\,mL)}{10,000\,units}$$
$$x = 1.5\,mL$$

Insulin Dosages

Insulin helps control how much glucose is in the bloodstream. Millions of patients with diabetes need to take insulin. Insulin from cows (bovine insulin) and pigs (porcine insulin) has been used since the early 1900s to treat diabetes. Now, human insulin can be mass-produced through genetic engineering processes that use special non–disease-producing strains of *Escherichia coli* bacteria. The resulting insulin is called human insulin. Insulin is given with insulin syringes. These syringes are already calibrated in units and the desired dose can be read directly on the syringe. If a tuberculin syringe must be used, the unit dosage for insulin can be converted to the equivalent number of milliliters by calculating proportions.

Example: Give 70 units of insulin using 100-U insulin and a tuberculin syringe. Convert to the equivalent number of milliliters.

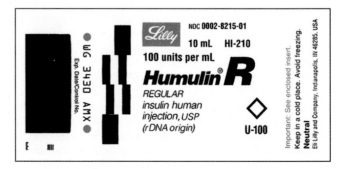

$$\frac{100\,\text{units}}{1\,\text{mL}} = \frac{70\,\text{units}}{x\,\text{mL}}$$

$$x\,\text{mL} = \frac{70\,\text{units}(1\,\text{mL})}{100\,\text{units}}$$

$$x\,\text{mL} = 0.7\,\text{mL}$$

Drug Dosages for Children

Children cannot tolerate adult doses of drugs. Different formulas are used to calculate dosages for infants and children, based variously on the child's height, weight, or age. Some physicians prefer to use the "body surface area" method that takes into account both the child's height and weight.

The Body Surface Area Nomogram

Another formula for calculating drug dosage is by using a body surface area (BSA) nomogram. A **nomogram** chart is used to compare the height and weight of a patient and deliver the BSA of the patient. The specific BSA is then used to determine the dosage. A figure used to display a normal BSA nomogram is shown below:

Nomogram for Determination of Body Surface Area From Height and Weight

Example:

BSA for a
15-kg. child,
100 cm. tall =
0.64 M²

From the formula of Du Bots and Du Bots, *Arch Intern Med* 17, 863 (1916): $S = W^{0.425} \times H^{0.725} \times 71.84$, or
$\log S = \log W \times 0.425 + \log H \times 0.725 + 1.8564$ (S = body surface in cm², W = weight in kg, H = height in cm).

To manually calculate a patient's BSA, use the following formula:

$$BSA(m^2) = \sqrt{\frac{Weight(kg) \times Height(cm)}{3,600}}$$

Example: Calculate a child's BSA who weighs 10 kg and whose height is 70 cm. Verify your answer by drawing a line connecting known values on the nomogram. The unknown value will be intersected by the straight line on the nomogram.

$$BSA(m^2) = \sqrt{\frac{Weight(kg) \times Height(cm)}{3,600}}$$
$$Weight(kg) = 10 \text{ kg}$$
$$Height(cm) = 70 \text{ cm}$$
$$BSA(m^2) = \sqrt{\frac{10(kg) \times 70(cm)}{3,600}}$$
$$BSA(m^2) = \sqrt{\frac{700}{3,600}}$$
$$BSA(m^2) = \sqrt{0.194}$$
$$BSA(m^2) = 0.44 m^2$$

The formula for calculating a patient's dosage is given based on their BSA. The formula for calculating the proper dosage is shown below:

$$Dosage(mg) = \frac{BSA(m^2)}{1.73 m^2} \times Dose\ Level(mg)$$

Example: Calculate the correct dosage for a 250 mg dose level with a BSA of 2.10 m².

$$Dosage(mg) = \frac{BSA(m^2)}{1.73 m^2} \times Dose\ Level(mg)$$
$$Dose\ Level(mg) = 250 \text{ mg}$$
$$BSA(m^2) = 2.10 \text{ m}^2$$
$$Dosage(mg) = \frac{2.10\ m^2}{1.73\ m^2} \times 250 \text{ mg}$$
$$Dosage(mg) = \frac{2.10\ m^2}{1.73\ m^2} \times 250 \text{ mg}$$
$$Dosage(mg) = 303.5 \text{ mg}$$

Dosage Calculations Based on Weight

Many medications for children and adults alike are based on the patient's weight. This dosage is often written as milligrams/kilogram.

Calculate the dosage for a patient who weighs 10 kg if the dose is 50 mg/kg.

$$\frac{50\,mg}{1\,kg} = \frac{X\,mg}{10\,kg}$$
$$X = 500 \text{ mg}$$

Using the same problem from above, calculate the dosage for a patient who weighs 22 lb if the dose is 50 mg/kg. Note: This problem may be solved using either ratio and proportion or dimensional analysis. Since the above example used ratio and proportion, this example will use dimensional analysis.

$$X\,mg = \frac{50\ mg}{1\,\cancel{kg}} \times \frac{1\,\cancel{kg}}{2.2\,\cancel{lbs}} \times 22\,\cancel{lbs}$$
$$= \frac{50 \times 1 \times 22}{2.2}$$
$$= 500 \text{ mg}$$

As previously stated, the dosage may be written as a daily dose that should then be divided into one or more daily doses. Or, the dosage may be written as a dose that should then be given one or more times a day. Using the same example as above, calculate the daily dosage for a patient who weighs 10 kg if the dose is 50 mg/kg/day in two divided doses.
The daily dosage would be

$$X\,mg = \frac{50\ mg}{1\,kg} \times 10\,kg$$
$$= 500 \text{ mg}$$

The amount given per dose would be

$$500 \text{ mg divided by } 2 = 250 \text{ mg}$$

It is very important to carefully read the prescription or medication order to ensure that the dosage is calculated correctly or it may be prepared, dispensed, and/or administered incorrectly.

Chapter Review

KEY POINTS

This chapter focused on reviewing mathematical examples for pharmacology. Upon completion of this chapter, the student should have a working knowledge of the major units of measure, conversions between systems, and an understanding of dimensional analysis in solving medication dosage problems. The key points to this chapter are summarized in the following list:

- Fraction mathematics
- Factoring
- Conversions between fractions, decimals, and percentages

- Systems of measurement
- Dimensional analysis
- Conversions of temperature scales
- Ratios and proportions
- Using the 24-hour clock
- Determining dosages for adults and children based on height, weight, and body surface area

CRITICAL THINKING CASE STUDY
Calculating Dosages

Two patients are sharing a hospital room; patient A has a height of 5½ ft and a weight of 145 lbs and has been prescribed tetracycline. A normal dose is 500 mg twice daily. Patient B with a height of 6 ft 2 in and a weight of 215 lb has been prescribed 1000 mg of ceftriaxone four times per day. Based on their surface area, how many milligrams of each prescribed drug should they take daily?

Practice Problems

FACTORING

Write the factors for each number.

1. 98
2. 125
3. 44

Reduce the fractions to lowest terms.

4. $\dfrac{9}{45}$

5. $\dfrac{85}{100}$

6. $\dfrac{79}{196}$

Equivalent fractions

7. Write a fraction with 18 in the denominator that is equivalent to the fraction $\dfrac{2}{9}$.
8. Write a fraction with 210 in the denominator that is equivalent to the fraction $\dfrac{3}{5}$.
9. Write a fraction with 48 in the denominator that is equivalent to the fraction $\dfrac{5}{12}$.

Convert the following mixed numbers to improper fractions:

10. $8\dfrac{8}{9}$

11. $10\dfrac{1}{2}$

12. $47\dfrac{2}{9}$

Convert the following improper fractions to mixed numbers:

13. $\dfrac{91}{5}$

14. $\dfrac{149}{33}$

15. $\dfrac{69}{10}$

Add the following fractions, reduce if necessary.

16. $\dfrac{2}{3}+\dfrac{2}{3}=$

17. $\dfrac{6}{11}+\dfrac{2}{11}=$

18. $\dfrac{12}{15}+\dfrac{4}{30}=$

Subtracting fractions

19. $\dfrac{4}{5}-\dfrac{2}{5}=$

20. $\dfrac{24}{32}-\dfrac{3}{8}=$

21. $\dfrac{13}{15}-\dfrac{9}{15}=$

Multiplying fractions

22. $\dfrac{1}{2}\times\dfrac{2}{5}=$

23. $\dfrac{6}{16}\times\dfrac{2}{3}=$

24. $1\dfrac{3}{8}\times\dfrac{1}{2}=$

Dividing fractions

25. $\dfrac{1}{2}\div\dfrac{2}{5}=$

26. $\dfrac{4}{7}\div\dfrac{1}{3}=$

27. $\dfrac{7}{8}\div\dfrac{3}{5}=$

Adding decimals

28. 12.59 + 4.5 =
29. 65.002 + 25.26 =
30. 0.5897 + 0.4897 =

Subtracting decimals

31. 42.348 − 24.978 =
32. 36 − 0.857
33. 125.78 − 450.254

Multiplying decimals

34. 65.25 × 0.158 =
35. 45.67 × 12.25 =
36. −85.759 × 0.578 =

Dividing decimals (round to 3 decimal places)

37. 5.2 ÷ 2.4 =
38. 12.6 ÷ 1.2 =
39. 1.2 ÷ 12.6 =

Converting fractions to decimals

40. $\dfrac{3}{8}=$

41. $\dfrac{9}{10}=$

42. $\dfrac{4}{7} =$

Converting decimals to fractions

43. 1.8 =
44. 0.75 =
45. 0.96 =

Calculating ratios and proportions

46. There are 12 hospital beds and 50 waiting room chairs. What is the ratio of beds to chairs?
47. Of 45 patients, 16 are on dialysis, and the rest have heart monitors. What is the ratio of heart monitors to patients on dialysis?
48. The ratio of X-ray machines to MRI machines 6:5. If there are 18 X-ray machines, how many MRI machines are there?

Calculate the percentages from the following numbers:

49. 0.78
50. 1.85
51. $\dfrac{7}{8}$

Systems of measurements

52. Convert 750 mL to liters.
53. Convert 250 mL to grams.
54. If the hospital clock reads 1400 hours, and you are about to start an 18-hour shift, what time will it be when you get off work?
55. Convert 39°C to °F.
56. Convert 150°F to °C.

Dosage calculation

57. If a patient is to take 250 mg of amoxicillin liquid every 8 hours for 10 days, how may milliliters would the patient take per dose if the concentration is 125 mg/5 mL? How many milliliters would the patient need for the entire 10 days?
58. If the recommended dosage for rosuvastatin is 4 mg/kg/day in 3 divided doses per day. How many milligrams should be given per dose for a patient weighing 121 kg?
59. A vial of penicillin G contains 500,000 units of lyophilized powder. How many milliliters of diluent should be added to obtain a solution that contains 100,000 units/mL?
60. Calculate a patient's correct dosage level for a 300-mg prescription if the patient's height is 110 cm and weights 65 kg.
61. A patient is to take 10 units of insulin with breakfast, 30 units with lunch, and 20 units with dinner. How many units will the patient take per day? How long will one 10-mL vial of U-100 insulin last? How many 10-mL vials of U-100 insulin will the patient need for a month?

Web Activities

1. Go to http://www.mathplayground.com/matching_fraction_percent.html and try the matching game for selecting fractions and their equivalent percentages. Record your best time.
2. Go to http://www.quia.com/jg/67993.html and play the Dosage Calculation Conversion Matching Game. Attempt the game at least three times and record the best time of your attempts.
3. Go to http://www.cut-the-knot.org/arithmetic/rapid/index.shtml. Read the section on "Fast Arithmetic Tips." How can these tips be applied to multiplying decimals?
4. Take the Tablet Dosage Quiz at http://www.testandcalc.com/quiz/testtab.htm. Try the quiz first using a calculator; then try the quiz a second time without a calculator.

4

Central Nervous System Stimulants

CHAPTER OBJECTIVES

On completion of this chapter, students will be able to:

1. Define the chapter's key terms.
2. Identify the uses and actions of central nervous system stimulants.
3. Describe the common adverse reactions to expect when taking a central nervous system stimulant.
4. Describe the common contraindications, precautions, and interactions of central nervous system stimulants.
5. Discuss important points to keep in mind when educating the patient and family members about central nervous system stimulants for narcolepsy, attention deficit hyperactivity disorder, and obesity.

KEY TERMS

analeptics—drugs that stimulate the respiratory center

anorexiants—drugs used to suppress the appetite

attention deficit hyperactivity disorder—a disorder manifested by a short attention span, hyperactivity, impulsiveness, and emotional lability

narcolepsy—disorder causing an uncontrollable desire to sleep during normal waking hours

CHAPTER OVERVIEW

Drug classes covered in this chapter are:

- Analeptics
- Amphetamines
- Anorexiants

Drugs by classification are listed on page 52.

thePOINT RESOURCES

- Comprehensive Summary Drug Tables
- Animations: Nerve Synapse
- Lippincott's Interactive Tutorials: Drugs Affecting the Central Nervous System
- Interactive Practice and Review
- Monographs of Most Commonly Prescribed Drugs

The central nervous system (CNS) is composed of the brain and the spinal cord (Fig. 4-1). The CNS processes information to and from the peripheral nervous system and is the center of coordination and control for the entire body.

The functional cells of the nervous system are called neurons. Each neuron is made up of a soma (the body of the neuron), dendrites, and an axon (Fig. 4-2) Terminals called synapses link neurons and allow information to be passed from one cell to another. Neurons carry out one of three functions:

- Conduct electrical impulses to the spinal cord and brain
- Carry impulses from the CNS to the body's muscles and glands
- Relay information within the CNS

The nervous system works by means of electrical impulses sent along neuron fibers and transmitted from cell to cell at the synapse, across a tiny gap between the cells. Information usually crosses the gap in the form of a chemical known as a neurotransmitter.

Neurotransmitters are chemical substances called neurohormones. They are released at the nerve endings to help transmit nerve impulses. Electron microscopes show a minuscule space between nerve endings and the effector organ (e.g., the muscle, cell, or gland) that the nerve innervates (controls).

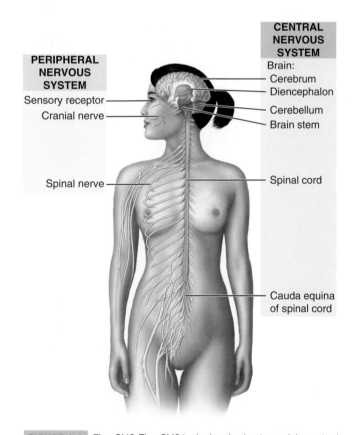

FIGURE 4-1 The CNS. The CNS includes the brain and the spinal cord. The PNS includes the sensory receptors as well as the cranial and spinal nerves. In order to affect the CNS, drugs must be able to enter the brain or the spinal cord.

For a nerve impulse to be transmitted from the nerve ending across the space to the effector organ, a neurohormone is needed. The neurohormones (neurotransmitters) of the CNS are acetylcholine, norepinephrine, serotonin, and dopamine.

Many drugs stimulate the CNS, but only a few are used therapeutically. This chapter discusses drugs that stimulate the CNS

Central Nervous System Stimulants

Central nervous system stimulants include **analeptics**, drugs that stimulate the respiratory center; amphetamines, drugs with a high abuse potential because of their ability to produce euphoria and wakefulness; and **anorexiants**, drugs used to suppress the appetite.

Actions of Central Nervous System Stimulants

Actions of Analeptics

Doxapram (Dopram) and caffeine (a combination of caffeine and sodium benzoate) are two analeptics used in medicine. Doxapram increases the depth of respirations by stimulating receptors located in the carotid arteries and upper aorta. These special receptors, called chemoreceptors, are sensitive to the amount of oxygen in arterial blood. Stimulation of these receptors results in an increase in the depth of the respirations. In larger doses, doxapram increases the respiratory rate by stimulating the medulla.

Caffeine is a mild to potent CNS stimulant. The extent of its stimulating effect depends on the dose. Caffeine stimulates the CNS at all levels, including the cerebral cortex, the medulla, and the spinal cord. Caffeine also has mild analeptic (respiratory stimulating) activity. Other actions include cardiac stimulation (which may lead to tachycardia), dilation of coronary and peripheral blood vessels, constriction of cerebral blood vessels, and skeletal muscle stimulation. Caffeine also has mild diuretic (promoting urination) activity. Figure 4-3 shows caffeine's effects on various body systems.

Modafinil's exact mechanism of action is not known, but the drug is thought to bind to dopamine reuptake carrier sites, increasing alpha activity in the brain and decreasing delta, theta, and beta activity, thereby reducing the number of sleepiness episodes. Modafinil does not cause the same cardiac and other systemic stimulatory effects as other CNS stimulants.

Actions of Amphetamines

Amphetamine, dextroamphetamine (Dexedrine), and methamphetamine (Desoxyn) are sympathomimetic (adrenergic) drugs that stimulate the CNS (see Chapter 11). Their action raises blood pressure, causes wakefulness, and may increase or decrease the pulse rate. Their anorexiant effect of suppressing the appetite is thought to be caused by their action on the appetite center in the hypothalamus.

Actions of Anorexiants

Anorexiants, such as phentermine and phendimetrazine, are nonamphetamine drugs that are pharmacologically similar to the amphetamines. Like the amphetamines, they are thought

NEURON

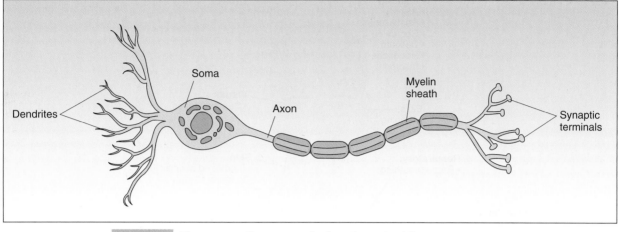

FIGURE 4-2 Neurons are the communication channels of the nervous system.

to suppress the appetite because of their action on the appetite center in the hypothalamus.

FACT CHECK

4-1   Caffeine is a common CNS stimulant that many patients consume on a daily basis. What are the actions of caffeine on the CNS?

Uses of Central Nervous System Stimulants

CNS stimulants have limited medical use. Primary uses are described in the following sections.

Uses of Analeptics

Doxapram is used to treat drug-induced CNS depression and to temporarily treat respiratory depression in patients with chronic pulmonary disease. This drug also may be used during the postanesthesia period when respiratory depression results from the anesthesia. It also is used to stimulate deep breathing in patients after anesthesia.

Caffeine and sodium benzoate are administered intramuscularly or intravenously as part of the treatment of respiratory depression caused by CNS depressants, such as narcotic analgesics and alcohol. Because caffeine also has other effects, such as constriction of cerebral arteries and stimulation of skeletal muscles, it is seldom used now for this purpose. Instead, narcotic antagonists are used for respiratory depression caused by narcotic overdose, and other drugs with greater analeptic activity (e.g., doxapram) are used more commonly. Orally, caffeine ingested as a beverage (coffee, tea) or taken in nonprescription tablet form is used by some individuals to relieve fatigue. Caffeine is also an ingredient in some nonprescription and prescription analgesics.

Modafinil is used to treat **narcolepsy** and decreases the number of sleepiness episodes during the day. It is also used to treat obstructive sleep apnea (OSA)/hypopnea syndrome, which is a disorder that involves a breathing blockage during sleep. In addition, modafinil is useful for patients who suffer from shift work sleep disorders.

Uses of Amphetamines

Amphetamines may be used in the short-term treatment of exogenous obesity (obesity caused by eating more than needed by the body). This use of amphetamines has declined, however, because long-term use carries the potential for addiction and abuse.

These drugs are also sometimes used for narcolepsy. An individual with narcolepsy may fall asleep for a few minutes to a few hours many times in one day. This disorder begins in adolescence or young adulthood and persists throughout life.

Amphetamines are also used to manage **attention deficit hyperactivity disorder** (ADHD) in children and adults. Children with this disorder have a short attention span, hyperactivity, impulsiveness, and emotional lability. The condition is more common in boys than in girls and causes problems with school and learning, although these children usually have normal or above average intelligence. How amphetamines, which are CNS stimulants, calm a hyperactive child is unknown. These drugs reduce motor restlessness, increase mental alertness, elevate mood and produce mild euphoria, and reduce feelings of fatigue. In addition, children with ADHD also commonly receive psychotherapeutic counseling.

Uses of Anorexiants

Phendimetrazine and phentermine are chemically related to amphetamines and are also used for short-term treatment of exogenous obesity. These prescription drugs have addiction and abuse potential.

FACT CHECK

4-2   CNS stimulants are used to treat what disorders?

Adverse Reactions of Central Nervous System Stimulants

While the adverse reactions of the CNS stimulants will vary in degree and intensity depending on the specific drug and dosage and the patient, many of the adverse reactions are

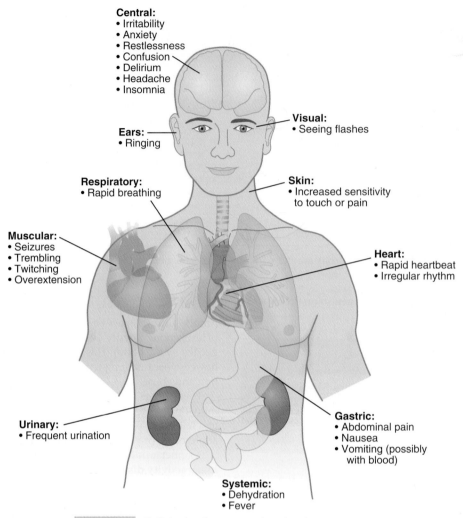

Central:
• Irritability
• Anxiety
• Restlessness
• Confusion
• Delirium
• Headache
• Insomnia

Visual:
• Seeing flashes

Ears:
• Ringing

Respiratory:
• Rapid breathing

Skin:
• Increased sensitivity
  to touch or pain

Muscular:
• Seizures
• Trembling
• Twitching
• Overextension

Heart
• Rapid heartbeat
• Irregular rhythm

Urinary:
• Frequent urination

Gastric:
• Abdominal pain
• Nausea
• Vomiting (possibly
  with blood)

Systemic:
• Dehydration
• Fever

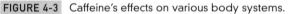

FIGURE 4-3   Caffeine's effects on various body systems.

common for all drugs in the category. It is common for a patient to experience excessive CNS stimulation, causing headache, dizziness, apprehension, disorientation, nervousness, excitement, and hyperactivity. Other adverse reactions include nausea, vomiting, urinary retention, and variations in heart rate (palpitations and tachycardia). Since many of the agents are used to treat exogenous obesity, it is not a surprise that anorexia, loss of appetite, and weight loss are also common.

Contraindications, Precautions, and Interactions of Central Nervous System Stimulants

- Central nervous system stimulants are contraindicated in patients with a known hypersensitivity or severe hypertension, in newborns, and in patients with epilepsy or convulsive states, pneumothorax, acute bronchial asthma, head injury, or stroke.
- Amphetamines are contraindicated in patients with hyperthyroidism or glaucoma.
- These drugs are given with caution in all patients because of the risk of physical dependence. Some individuals are especially sensitive to the effects of CNS stimulants.

- Analeptics and amphetamines are used only with extreme caution in patients with cardiovascular disease and in women during the early stages of pregnancy.
- Amphetamines and anorexiants should not be given during or within 14 days after giving a monoamine oxidase inhibitor (see Chapter 7) because the patient may experience a hypertensive crisis and intracranial hemorrhage.
- When guanethidine is administered with an amphetamine or anorexiant, the antihypertensive effect of guanethidine may be diminished.
- Administration of an amphetamine or anorexiant with a tricyclic antidepressant may decrease the effects of the amphetamine or anorexiant.

FACT CHECK

4-3   Central nervous system stimulants have a number of adverse reactions that are common to the class of drugs. What are these adverse reactions?

4-4   In which patients would you expect CNS stimulants to be used with caution or not used at all?

FACTS ABOUT . . .

Attention Deficit Hyperactivity Disorder

- ADHD, one of the most common mental disorders in children and adolescents, also affects an estimated 4.1% of adults, ages 18 to 44, in a given year.
- ADHD usually becomes evident in preschool or early elementary years. The median age of onset of ADHD is seven years, although the disorder can persist into adolescence and occasionally into adulthood.

Source: The National Institute of Mental Health.

Patient Management Issues with Central Nervous System Stimulants

When a CNS stimulant is prescribed for respiratory depression, the patient's blood pressure, pulse, and respiratory rate are first measured. Oxygen is usually given before, during, and after the drug administration. The patient's respiratory rate and pattern are then carefully monitored until they return to normal. The patient is observed for any adverse drug reactions, which are reported immediately to the health care provider.

When an amphetamine is prescribed for any reason, the patient is weighed and the blood pressure, pulse, and respiratory rate are measured before starting drug therapy. A child with ADHD is observed for abnormal behavior, which is recorded in the patient's chart for comparison with changes that later occur during therapy. The drug regimen is periodically interrupted to determine if the child still has the symptoms of ADHD.

When an anorexiant or amphetamine is used to treat obesity, the drug is usually prescribed for outpatient use. Before

ALERT ℞

Addiction with Central Nervous System Stimulants

Amphetamines and anorexiants may be abused and can result in addiction. Long-term use of amphetamines may result in tolerance to the drug and a tendency to increase the dose. Extreme psychological dependence may also occur.

Amphetamines and anorexiants are recommended only for short-term use in selected patients for the treatment of exogenous obesity. When used in children to treat ADHD, long-term use must be followed by gradual withdrawal of the drug.

When a CNS stimulant causes insomnia, the drug should be taken early in the day (when possible) to diminish sleep disturbances. The patient is encouraged not to nap during the day. The patient should avoid other stimulants, such as coffee, tea, or cola drinks. Some patients may experience nervousness, restlessness, and palpitations. Often these adverse reactions diminish with continued use as tolerance develops. If tolerance develops, then the dosage is not increased.

CONSIDERATIONS Infants & Children

LIFESPAN

Drugs for ADHD

Children with ADHD may respond differently to the same medication. For example, a drug that works well for one child may be ineffective or produce adverse effects in another. Consequently, prescribers may need to try different drugs and dosages before determining what works. It is important to closely monitor any child taking these kinds of medications.

therapy is started, the patient's blood pressure, pulse, respiratory rate, and weight are measured and recorded. Thereafter, the patient's weight and vital signs are measured at each outpatient visit.

Educating the Patient and Family about Central Nervous System Stimulants

The information given to the patient and family depends on the specific drug and the reason for its use. It is important to emphasize the need to follow the recommended dosage schedule. Following are key points about CNS stimulants the patient or family members should know.

Attention Deficit Hyperactivity Disorder

- Take the drug in the morning 30 to 45 minutes before breakfast and before lunch. Do not take the drug in the afternoon.
- Insomnia and anorexia usually disappear during continued therapy.
- Write a daily summary of the child's behavior, including periods of hyperactivity, general pattern of behavior, socialization with others, and attention span. Bring this record to each health care provider visit because the drug dosage may need to be adjusted or additional treatments given.
- The health care provider may prescribe the drug to be given only on school days when high levels of attention and performance are necessary.

Narcolepsy

- Keep a record of the number of times per day that periods of sleepiness occur, and bring this record to each visit to the health care provider.

CONSIDERATIONS Older adults

LIFESPAN

Central Nervous System Stimulants

Older adults are especially sensitive to the effects of CNS stimulants and may experience excessive anxiety, nervousness, insomnia, and mental confusion. Cardiovascular disorders, which are more common in older adults, may be worsened by these drugs. Careful monitoring is important because such reactions may require discontinuing the drug.

Amphetamines and Anorexiants

- Take the drug early in the day to avoid insomnia.
- Do not increase the dose or take the drug more frequently, except on the advice of your health care provider.
- These drugs may impair your ability to drive or perform hazardous tasks and may mask extreme fatigue.
- Avoid or decrease your use of coffee, tea, and carbonated beverages containing caffeine (see Key Concepts 4-1).

Caffeine (Oral, Nonprescription)

- Do not use products with caffeine to stay awake if you have a history of heart disease, high blood pressure, or stomach ulcers.
- These products are intended for occasional use and should not be used if you experience heart palpitations, dizziness, or light-headedness.

FACT CHECK

4-5   CN stimulants cause insomnia. How does this affect the patient's timing of when to take the medication?

KEY CONCEPTS

4-1   Using Anorexiants for Weight Loss

It is important to take the drug exactly as prescribed. Do not increase the dose or take it more frequently unless your health care provider so instructs.

This drug is for short-term therapy only. It can lead to possible addiction, drug tolerance, or psychological dependency.

Notify your health care provider immediately should any adverse reaction occur.

Take the drug early in the day to prevent insomnia.

Do not drive or perform hazardous tasks if you feel dizzy or disoriented.

Avoid other stimulants, including those containing caffeine such as coffee, tea, and cola drinks.

Read the labels of foods and nonprescription drugs you are taking to avoid other possible stimulants.

Follow your prescribed dietary and exercise program for weight reduction.

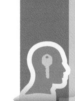

Chapter Review

KEY POINTS

- Central nervous system stimulants act in various ways to stimulate different parts of the CNS, including actions involving respiration, cardiac and cardiovascular effects, skeletal muscle stimulation, and appetite suppression.
- Many of these drugs have a potential for dependence.
- CNS stimulants are used to treat CNS depression, narcolepsy, ADHD, and obesity.
- CNS stimulants will increase the depth of respirations and respiratory rate, wakefulness, cardiac stimulation (which may lead to tachycardia), dilation of coronary and peripheral blood vessels, constriction of cerebral blood vessels, and skeletal muscle stimulation.
- Patient management and teaching for all of these drugs focus on the need for strict dosage control and the management of adverse reactions, many of which are severe.

CRITICAL THINKING CASE STUDY
ADHD Drug Therapy

Ms. Basinger's son has been diagnosed with ADHD and has been prescribed methylphenidate HCL (Concerta). Ms. Basinger is anxious about how the medication will work and what adverse effects her son may experience.

1. When should her son be taking his Concerta?
    a. In the morning
    b. At lunch
    c. After shool
    d. At night

2. The next time you see Ms. Basinger, she tells you that her son is doing well on the Concerta, but she is concerned that her son does not seem to be eating well. What should you tell her?
    a. This is a normal adverse effect and she should not be concerned.
    b. This is a normal adverse effect but she might want to talk with the prescriber if her son is not eating well and is losing weight.
    c. This is not a normal adverse effect and she should contact the prescriber immediately.
    d. This is not a normal adverse effect and she should stop the medication immediately.

3. During your conversation, Ms. Basinger expresses concern that her son may not remember to take his medication everyday. What could you tell her?

Review Questions

MULTIPLE CHOICE

1. The adverse drug reactions of doxapram given for chronic pulmonary disease may include
    a. headache, dizziness, nausea
    b. diarrhea, drowsiness, hypotension
    c. decreased respiratory rate, weight gain, bradycardia
    d. fever, dysuria, constipation

2. A patient with narcolepsy who is receiving an amphetamine should be instructed to
   a. record the times of the day the medication is taken
   b. take the medication at bedtime as well as in the morning
   c. take the drug with meals
   d. keep a record of how often periods of sleepiness occur
3. Which of the following is used to treat both ADHD and narcolepsy?
   a. Dexmethylphenidate
   b. Doxapram
   c. Dextroamphetamine
   d. Diethylpropion

MATCHING

_____ 4.   adderall
_____ 5.   dexedrine
_____ 6.   adipex-P
_____ 7.   desoxyn
_____ 8.   dopram
_____ 9.   focalin

a. phentermine
b. dexmethylphenidate
c. amphetamine mixtures
d. dextroamphetamine
e. doxapram
f. methamphetamine

TRUE OR FALSE

_____ 10. Amphetamines have the potential for abuse and addiction.
_____ 11. Taking a CNS stimulant early in the day will help reduce the adverse effect of insomnia.
_____ 12. The amphetamines and anorexiants are all schedule II controlled substances.

FILL IN THE BLANKS

13. The central nervous system is composed of the _____ and the _____ _____.
14. An anorexiant suppresses the _____ center of the hypothalamus.
15. ADHD stands for _____ _____ _____ disorder.

SHORT ANSWERS

16. What should a patient taking a CNS stimulant do if the drug is causing insomnia?
17. Why must older adults who take CNS stimulants be carefully monitored?
18. What information should be documented in the patient's chart before anorexiant therapy is initiated and at each outpatient visit?

Web Activities

1. Go to the Mayo Clinic's public health website (http://www.mayoclinic.com) and navigate to "Caffeine" section. Which coffee, tea, and soft drinks have the most caffeine? How much caffeine do they each have?
2. Go to the National Institute of Mental Health website (http://www.nimh.nih.gov) and conduct a search for "Attention Deficit Hyperactivity Disorder." What are the symptoms of ADHD in children?

SUMMARY DRUG TABLE: Central Nervous System Stimulants (left, generic; right, trade)

Comprehensive Summary Drug Tables, including uses, adverses effects, dosages, and pregnancy classifications, are provided on the companion website, http://thePoint.lww.com/PharmacologyHP2e

Analeptics		methylphenidate HCL	Concerta (CII), Metadate ER/
caffeine	Cafcit, No-Doz Maximum	*meh-thyl-fen'-ih-date*	Metadate CD (CII), Ritalin/ Ritalin
kaf-een'	Strength (OTC), Vivarin (OTC), *generic*		LA//Ritalin SR (CII); Methylin/ Methylin ER (CII), Daytrana (CII), *generic*
doxapram HCL	Dopram	**MISC ADHD Treatment**	
docks'-a-pram		atomoxetine	Strattera
modafinil	Provigil (CIV)	*at'-oh-mox-e-teen*	
moe-daf'-in-ill			
Amphetamines		**Anorexiants**	
amphetamine mixtures	Adderall/ Adderall XR (CII),	benzphetamine HCL	Didrex (CIII)
am-fet'-a-meen	*generic*	*benz-fe-ta-meen*	
dexmethylphenidate	Focalin/ Focalin XR (CII)	diethylpropion HCl	*generic* (CIV)
dex-meth-thyl-fen-i-date		*die-eth'-uhl-pro'-pee-ahn*	
dextroamphetamine sulfate	Dexedrine (CII), ProCentra (CII),	phendimetrazine	Bontril/Bontril PDM (CIII),
dex-troe-am-fet'-a-meen	*generic*	*fen-dye-me'-tra-zeen*	*generic*
lisdexamfetamine dimesylate	Vyvanse (CII)	phentermine HCl	Adipex-P (CIV), *generic*
lis-dex-am-fet'-a-meen		*fen-ter'-meen*	
methamphetamine	Desoxyn (CII), *generic*		
meth-am-fet'-a-meen			

*The term generic indicates the drug is available in generic form.

5

Anticonvulsants and Antiparkinsonism Drugs

CHAPTER OBJECTIVES

On completion of this chapter, students will be able to:

1. Define the chapter's key terms.
2. Identify the actions and uses of anticonvulsants.
3. Describe common adverse reactions, contraindications, precautions, and interactions of anticonvulsants.
4. Discuss important points to keep in mind when educating the patient and family members about the use of anticonvulsants.
5. Identify the signs and symptoms of Parkinson disease.
6. Identify medications commonly used to treat Parkinson disease and how they work.
7. Describe common adverse reactions, contraindications, precautions, and interactions of drugs used to treat Parkinson disease.
8. Discuss important points to keep in mind when educating the patient and family members about the use of drugs for Parkinson disease.

KEY TERMS

absence seizures—previously referred to as petit mal seizures; are characterized by a brief loss of consciousness, during which physical activity ceases, and may last a few seconds and happen multiple times a day

anticonvulsants—drugs used for the management of convulsive disorders

ataxia—a loss of control of voluntary movements, especially producing an unsteady gait

blood–brain barrier—a meshwork of tightly packed cells in the walls of the brain's capillaries that screen out certain substances

choreiform movements—the involuntary twitching of the limbs or facial muscles

convulsion—another term for seizure

CHAPTER OVERVIEW

Drug classes covered in this chapter are:

- Anticonvulsants
- Antiparkinsonism drugs

Drugs by classification are listed on page 66.

thePOINT RESOURCES

- Comprehensive Summary Drug Tables
- Lippincott's Interactive Tutorials: Drugs Affecting the Central Nervous System
- Interactive Practice and Review
- Monographs of Most Commonly Prescribed Drugs

dyscrasia—a morbid general state resulting from the presence of abnormal material in the blood

dystonic movements—muscular spasms most often affecting the tongue, jaw, eyes, and neck

epilepsy—a permanent, recurrent seizure disorder

gingival hyperplasia—overgrowth of gum tissue

jacksonian seizure—a focal seizure that begins with an uncontrolled stiffening or jerking of the body such as the finger, mouth, hand, or foot that may progress to a generalized seizure

myoclonic seizures—sudden, forceful contractions involving the musculature of the trunk, neck, and extremities

nystagmus—constant, involuntary movement of the eyeball

on–off phenomenon—associated with long-term levodopa treatment, a patient may alternate suddenly between improved clinical status and loss of therapeutic effect

parkinsonism— refers to the symptoms of Parkinson disease, as well as Parkinson-like symptoms that may be seen with the use of certain drugs, head injuries, and encephalitis

Parkinson disease—a degenerative disorder of the central nervous system; also known as paralysis agitans

psychomotor seizures—most often occur in children younger than 3 years of age through adolescence; may involve an aura with perceptual alterations, such as hallucinations or a strong sense of fear

seizure—a periodic attack of disturbed cerebral function

status epilepticus—an emergency situation characterized by continual seizure activity with no interruptions

tonic–clonic seizure—an alternate contraction (tonic phase) and relaxation (clonic phase) of muscles, a loss of consciousness, and abnormal behavior

---

The terms **convulsion** and seizure are often used interchangeably and basically have the same meaning. A **seizure** is a periodic attack of disturbed cerebral function. A seizure may also be described as an abnormal disturbance in the electrical activity in one or more areas of the brain. Seizures may be classified as partial (focal) or generalized. Each different type of seizure disorder is characterized by a specific pattern of events as well as a different pattern of motor or sensory manifestation (Key Concepts 5-1).

Partial or focal seizures arise from a localized area in the brain and cause specific symptoms. A partial seizure can spread to the entire brain and cause a generalized seizure. Partial seizures include simple seizures in which consciousness is not impaired, **jacksonian seizures** (a focal seizure that begins with an uncontrolled stiffening or jerking in one part of the body such as finger, mouth, hand, or foot that may progress to a generalized seizure) and psychomotor seizures.

Psychomotor seizures occur most often in children 3 years of age through adolescence. The individual may experience an aura with perceptual alterations, such as hallucinations or a strong sense of fear. Repeated coordinated but inappropriate movements, such as clutching, kicking, picking at clothes, walking in circles, and licking are characteristic. The most common motor symptom is drawing or jerking of the mouth and face.

Generalized seizures include absence, myoclonic, and tonic–clonics. Manifestations of a generalized **tonic–clonic** seizure include alternate contraction (tonic phase) and relaxation (clonic phase) of muscles, a loss of consciousness, and abnormal behavior. **Myoclonic seizures** involve sudden, forceful contractions involving the musculature of the trunk, neck, and extremities. **Absence seizures**, previously referred to as petit mal seizures, are seizures characterized by a brief loss of consciousness during which physical activity ceases. The seizures typically last a few seconds, occur many times per day, and may go unnoticed by others.

Epilepsy is a permanent, recurrent seizure disorder. Examples of the known causes of epilepsy include brain injury at birth, head injuries, and inborn errors of metabolism. In some patients, the cause of epilepsy is never determined.

Anticonvulsants

Drugs used for the management of convulsive disorders are called **anticonvulsants**. Most anticonvulsants have specific uses; that is, they are of value only in the treatment of certain types of seizure disorders. There are four categories of drugs used as anticonvulsants: barbiturates, benzodiazepines, hydantoins, and the succinimides. In addition, many miscellaneous drugs are used as anticonvulsants. All can depress abnormal neural discharges in the central nervous system (CNS), resulting in an inhibition of seizure activity. Drugs that control generalized tonic–clonic seizures are not effective for absence (petit mal) seizures. If both conditions are present, then combined drug therapy is required.

Actions of Anticonvulsants

Generally, anticonvulsants reduce the excitability of the neurons (nerve cells) of the brain. When neuron excitability is decreased, seizures are theoretically reduced in intensity and frequency of occurrence or, in some instances, are virtually eliminated. For some patients, only partial control of the seizure disorder may be obtained with anticonvulsant drug therapy.

KEY CONCEPTS

5-1　Categorizing Seizure Disorders

Seizure disorders are generally categorized as idiopathic or acquired. Idiopathic seizures have no known cause; acquired seizure disorders have a known cause, including high fever, electrolyte imbalances, uremia, hypoglycemia, hypoxia, brain tumors, and some drug withdrawal reactions. Once the cause is removed (if it can be removed), the seizures theoretically cease.

Uses of Anticonvulsants

Drugs for the more common types of seizures, which respond to a specific anticonvulsant, are listed in the Summary Drug Table: Anticonvulsants. In some cases, the patient does not respond well to one drug, and another drug or a combination of anticonvulsants must be tried. Dosage increases and decreases are often necessary during the initial period of treatment. Dosage adjustment also may be necessary during times of stress, severe illness, or when other drugs are being taken for treatment of conditions other than a seizure disorder. The miscellaneous anticonvulsants are adjuncts to the more widely used anticonvulsants. They are used in patients who have an inadequate response to other anticonvulsants.

Occasionally, **status epilepticus** (an emergency situation characterized by continual seizure activity with no interruptions) can occur. Diazepam (Valium) is most often the initial drug prescribed for this condition. However, because the effects of diazepam last less than 1 hour, a longer-lasting anticonvulsant, such as phenytoin or phenobarbital, also must be given to control the seizure activity.

FACT CHECK

5-1 How do anticonvulsants work?

5-2 When anticonvulsant therapy is initiated, will the starting drug and dosage be the same for all patients with a particular type of seizure?

Adverse Reactions of Anticonvulsants

Adverse Reactions of Barbiturates

The most common adverse reaction associated with phenobarbital is sedation, which can range from mild sleepiness or drowsiness to somnolence. Agitation, rather than sedation, may occur in some patients. Some of the adverse effects may be reduced or eliminated as therapy continues. Occasionally, a slight dosage reduction, without reducing the ability of the drug to control the seizures, will reduce or eliminate some of the adverse reactions. The barbiturates can produce a hypersensitivity rash. Should a skin rash occur, the health care provider must be notified immediately because he or she may choose to discontinue the drug.

Adverse Reactions of Benzodiazepines

As with the barbiturates, the most common adverse reaction seen with the use of clonazepam (Klonopin), clorazepate (Tranxene), and diazepam (Valium) is sedation in varying degrees. Additional adverse effects may include anorexia, constipation, or diarrhea. Some adverse reactions are dose dependent, whereas others may diminish in intensity or cause few problems after several weeks of therapy. Unusual bruising or unusual bleeding, fever, sore throat, rash, or mouth ulcers sometimes occur with the use of benzodiazepines and should be reported to the health care provider.

Adverse Reactions of Hydantoins

Phenytoin is the most commonly prescribed anticonvulsant. Many adverse reactions are associated with the use of phenytoin (Dilantin). The most common adverse reactions associated with the hydantoins are related to the CNS and include **nystagmus** (constant, involuntary movement of the eyeball), **ataxia** (loss of control of voluntary movements, especially gait), slurred speech, and mental changes. Other adverse reactions include various types of skin rashes, nausea, vomiting, **gingival hyperplasia** (overgrowth of gum tissue), hematologic changes (changes relating to the blood or blood-forming tissue), and hepatotoxicity. Some of these adverse reactions diminish with continuous use of the hydantoins.

Signs of blood **dyscrasias**, such as sore throat, fever, general malaise, bleeding of the mucous membranes, epistaxis (bleeding from the nose), and easy bruising are serious reactions that must be reported to the health care provider immediately. When a blood dyscrasia is present, the skin and mucous membranes are protected from bleeding and easy bruising by using a soft-bristled toothbrush, and the extremities are protected from trauma or injury.

Hypersensitivity reactions and Stevens–Johnson syndrome (a serious, sometimes fatal inflammatory disease) have been reported with the use of phenytoin.

The health care provider should be notified immediately if a skin rash occurs. The use of phenytoin is usually discontinued if a skin rash occurs. If the rash is exfoliative (red rash with scaling of the skin), purpuric (small hemorrhages or bruising on the skin), or bullous (skin vesicle filled with fluid, i.e., a blister), then use of the drug is not resumed. If the rash is milder (e.g., measles-like), then therapy may be resumed after the rash has completely disappeared.

Signs of phenytoin drug toxicity include slurred speech, ataxia, lethargy, dizziness, nausea, and vomiting, and at concentrations greater than 30 mcg/mL, ataxia and mental changes are usually seen. These symptoms must be reported to the health care provider as well.

The hydantoins may affect the blood glucose levels. In some patients, these drugs have an inhibitory effect on the release of insulin in the body, causing hyperglycemia. Blood glucose

---

ALERT ℞

Anticonvulsants in Pregnancy

Research suggests an association between the use of anticonvulsants by pregnant women with epilepsy and an increased incidence of birth defects in children born to these women. The use of anticonvulsants generally is not discontinued in pregnant women with a history of major seizures because of the danger of precipitating status epilepticus. However, when seizure activity poses no serious threat to the pregnant woman, the health care provider will consider discontinuing use of the drug during pregnancy.

levels must be closely monitored, particularly in patients with diabetes. Any abnormalities are reported to the health care provider.

Long-term administration of the hydantoins can cause gingivitis and gingival hyperplasia (overgrowth of gum tissue). It is important that the teeth and gums of patients in a hospital or long-term clinical setting who are receiving one of these drugs have an oral examination periodically. Any changes in the gums or teeth are reported to the health care provider. In outpatient settings, it is important that oral care be given after each meal and that the mouth and gums be inspected routinely.

Adverse Reactions of Succinimides

Gastrointestinal symptoms occur frequently with the administration of ethosuximide (Zarontin) and methsuximide (Celontin). Mental confusion and other personality changes, pruritus, urticaria, urinary frequency, weight loss, and hematologic changes may also be seen.

The succinimides are particularly toxic. Signs of blood dyscrasias, such as the presence of fever, sore throat, and general malaise should be reported immediately because fatal blood dyscrasias have occurred. Routine blood tests may be performed, such as complete blood counts and differential counts.

Adverse Reactions of Miscellaneous Anticonvulsants

A severe and potentially fatal rash can occur in patients taking lamotrigine. Before the next dose is due, any rash must be reported to the health care provider. Discontinuation of the drug may be required.

Contraindications, Precautions, and Interactions of Anticonvulsants

Contraindications, Precautions, and Interactions of Barbiturates

- Barbiturates are contraindicated in patients with known hypersensitivity to the drugs.
- These drugs are used cautiously in patients with liver or kidney disease, in those with neurological disorders and pulmonary disease, and in hyperactive children.
- When barbiturates are used with other CNS depressants (e.g., alcohol, narcotic analgesics, and antidepressants), an additive CNS depressant effect may occur. See Chapter 7 for additional information on the barbiturates.

Contraindications, Precautions, and Interactions of Benzodiazepines

- Benzodiazepines are contraindicated in patients with known hypersensitivity to the drugs.
- These drugs are used cautiously in patients with psychoses, acute narrow-angle glaucoma, liver or kidney disease, and neurologic disorders; and in elderly or debilitated patients.
- When benzodiazepines are used with other CNS depressants (e.g., alcohol, narcotic analgesics, and antidepressants), an additive CNS depressant effect may occur.
- Increased effects of benzodiazepines are seen when the drugs are administered with cimetidine, disulfiram, and oral contraceptives.
- When a benzodiazepine is given with theophylline, there is a decreased effect of the benzodiazepine. See Chapter 7 for additional information on the benzodiazepines.

Contraindications, Precautions, and Interactions of Hydantoins

- The hydantoins are contraindicated in patients with known hypersensitivity to the drugs.

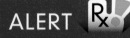

CONSIDERATIONS | Older adults

LIFESPAN

Diazepam

Older or debilitated adults may require a reduced dosage of diazepam to reduce ataxia and oversedation. These patients must be observed carefully. Apnea and cardiac arrest have occurred when diazepam is administered to older adults, very ill patients, and individuals with limited pulmonary reserve.

- Phenytoin is contraindicated in patients with sinus bradycardia, sinoatrial block, second- and third-degree atrioventricular block, and Adams–Stokes syndrome; it also is contraindicated during lactation.
- Ethotoin is contraindicated in patients with hepatic abnormalities.
- When the hydantoins are used with other CNS depressants (e.g., alcohol, narcotic analgesics, and antidepressants), an additive CNS depressant effect may occur.
- The hydantoins are used cautiously in patients with liver or kidney disease and neurologic disorders.
- Phenytoin is used cautiously in patients with hypotension, severe myocardial insufficiency, and hepatic impairment. Phenytoin interacts with many different drugs. For example, isoniazid, chloramphenicol, sulfonamides, benzodiazepines, succinimides, and cimetidine all increase phenytoin blood levels.
- The barbiturates, rifampin, theophylline, and warfarin decrease phenytoin blood levels.
- When a hydantoin is given with meperidine, the analgesic effect of meperidine is decreased.

Contraindications, Precautions, and Interactions of Succinimides

- Succinimides are contraindicated in patients with known hypersensitivity to the drugs and in patients with bone marrow depression or hepatic or renal impairment and during lactation.
- When the succinimides are used with other CNS depressants (e.g., alcohol, narcotic analgesics, and antidepressants), an additive CNS depressant effect may occur.
- When the hydantoins are administered with the succinimides, there may be an increase in the hydantoin blood levels.
- Concurrent administration of valproic acid and the succinimides may result in either a decrease or an increase in succinimide blood levels.
- When primidone is administered with the succinimides, lower primidone levels may occur.

Contraindications, Precautions, and Interactions of Miscellaneous Anticonvulsants

- The miscellaneous anticonvulsants are contraindicated in patients with known hypersensitivity to any of the drugs.
- Carbamazepine is contraindicated in patients with bone marrow depression or hepatic or renal impairment.

- Valproic acid is not administered to patients with renal impairment.
- Oxcarbazepine (Trileptal) may exacerbate dementia.
- The miscellaneous anticonvulsants are used cautiously in patients with glaucoma or increased intraocular pressure; a history of cardiac, renal, or liver dysfunction; or psychiatric disorders.
- When the miscellaneous anticonvulsants are used with other CNS depressants (e.g., alcohol, narcotic analgesics, and antidepressants), an additive CNS depressant effect may occur.
- When carbamazepine is administered with primidone, decreased primidone levels and higher carbamazepine serum levels may result.
- Cimetidine administered with carbamazepine may result in an increase in plasma levels of carbamazepine that can lead to toxicity.
- Blood levels of lamotrigine increase when the agent is administered with valproic acid, requiring a lower dosage of lamotrigine.

FACT CHECK

5-5 Many of the anticonvulsants cause drowsiness or sedation, and as a result, they should be used with caution when combined with what other medications? (List the drug class and give examples).

5-6 Why should these drugs be used with caution when combined?

Patient Management Issues with Anticonvulsants

Seizures that occur in the outpatient setting are almost always seen first by family members or friends, rather than by a member of the medical profession. The occurrence of abnormal behavior patterns or convulsive movements usually prompts the patient to visit a health care provider's office or a neurologic clinic. A family history of seizures (if any) and recent drug therapy (all drugs currently being used) are also important considerations, because either or both could contribute to seizure activity. Depending on the type of seizure disorder, other information may be needed, such as a history of a head injury or a thorough medical history.

Anticonvulsants control, but do not cure, epilepsy. An accurate ongoing assessment is important to obtain the desired effect of the anticonvulsant. The dosage of the anticonvulsant may require frequent adjustments during the initial treatment period. Dosage adjustments are based on the patient's response to therapy (e.g., the control of the seizures), as well as the occurrence of adverse reactions. Depending on the patient's response to therapy, a second anticonvulsant may be added to the therapeutic regimen, or one anticonvulsant may be changed to another. Regular serum plasma levels of the anticonvulsant are taken to monitor for toxicity.

A patient's seizures, as well as response to drug therapy, must be observed when a patient is receiving an anticonvulsant. Most seizures occur without warning, and a health care provider may not see a patient until after the seizure begins or after the seizure is over. However, any observations made during and after the seizure are important and may aid in the diagnosis of the type of seizure, as well as assist the health care provider in evaluating the effectiveness of drug therapy.

A patient must not omit or miss a dose (except by order of the health care provider). An abrupt interruption in therapy by omitting a dose may result in a recurrence of the seizures. In some instances, abrupt withdrawal of an anticonvulsant can result in status epilepticus. If the health care provider discontinues the anticonvulsant therapy, then the dosage is gradually withdrawn or another drug is gradually substituted.

Educating the Patient and Family about Anticonvulsants

When the patient receives a diagnosis of epilepsy, the health care provider must assist the patient and the family to adjust to the diagnosis. The health care provider should instruct family members in the care of a patient before, during, and after a seizure. The health care provider explains the importance of restricting some activities until the seizures are controlled by drugs. Restriction of activities often depends on the age, sex, and occupation of the patient. For example, the health care provider should advise a mother with a seizure disorder who has a newborn infant to have help when caring for her child. The health care provider would also warn a carpenter about climbing ladders or using power tools. For some patients, the restriction of activities may create problems with employment, management of the home environment, or child care. If a problem is recognized, then a referral may be needed to a social worker, discharge planning coordinator, or public health nurse.

The health care provider reviews adverse drug reactions associated with the prescribed anticonvulsant with a patient and family members. The patient and family members are instructed to contact the health care provider if any adverse reactions occur. A patient must not stop taking the drug until the problem is discussed with the health care provider.

Some patients, once their seizures are under control (e.g., stop occurring or occur less frequently), may have a tendency to stop the drug abruptly or begin to omit a dose occasionally. The drug must never be abruptly discontinued or doses omitted. If a patient experiences drowsiness during initial therapy, then a family member should be responsible for administration of the drug.

Following are key points about anticonvulsants a patient or family should know.

- Do not omit, increase, or decrease the prescribed dose.
- Anticonvulsant blood levels must be monitored at regular intervals, even if the seizures are well controlled.
- This drug should never be abruptly discontinued, except when recommended by your health care provider.
- If your health care provider finds it necessary to stop the drug, another drug usually is prescribed. Start taking this drug immediately (at the time the next dose of the previously used drug was due).
- These drugs may cause drowsiness or dizziness. Be careful when performing hazardous tasks. Do not drive unless the adverse reactions of drowsiness, dizziness, or blurred vision are not significant. Driving privileges will

be given by your health care provider based on seizure control.
- Avoid the use of alcohol unless use has been approved by your health care provider.
- Carry identification, such as a Medic-Alert tag, indicating drug use and the type of seizure disorder.
- Do not use any nonprescription drug unless use of a specific drug has been approved by your health care provider.
- Keep a record of all seizures (date, time, length), as well as any minor problems (e.g., drowsiness, dizziness, lethargy), and bring this information to each clinic or office visit.
- Contact the local branches of agencies, such as the Epilepsy Foundation of America, for information and assistance with problems such as legal matters, insurance, driver's license, low-cost prescription services, and job training or retraining.

Hydantoins

- Inform your dentist and other health care providers of use of this drug.
- Brush and floss your teeth after each meal, and make periodic dental appointments for oral examination and care.
- Take the medication with food to reduce gastrointestinal upset.
- Shake the phenytoin suspension thoroughly immediately before use.
- Do not use capsules that are discolored.
- Notify your health care provider if you experience any of the following: skin rash, bleeding, swollen or tender gums, yellow discoloration of the skin or eyes, unexplained fever, sore throat, unusual bleeding or bruising, persistent headache, malaise, or pregnancy.

Succinimides

- If you have gastrointestinal upsets, take the drug with food or milk.
- Notify your health care provider if you experience any of the following: skin rash, joint pain, unexplained fever, sore throat, unusual bleeding or bruising, drowsiness, dizziness, blurred vision, or pregnancy.

FACT CHECK

5-7 A patient's activities may need to be restricted when he or she is initially diagnosed with a seizure while drug therapy is being initiated and adjusted. What is an example of an activity that might need to be restricted?

Antiparkinsonism Drugs

Parkinson disease, also called paralysis agitans, is a degenerative disorder of the CNS. The disease is thought to be caused by a deficiency of dopamine and an excess of acetylcholine within the CNS. Parkinson disease affects the part of the brain that controls muscle movement, causing such symptoms as trembling, rigidity, difficulty walking, and problems in balance. It is characterized by fine tremors and rigidity of some muscle groups and weakness of others. Parkinson disease is progressive, with the symptoms becoming worse over time. As the disease progresses, speech becomes slurred, the face has a mask-like and emotionless expression, and the patient may have difficulty chewing and swallowing. The patient may have a shuffling and unsteady gait, and the upper part of the body bends forward. Fine tremors begin in the fingers with a pill-rolling movement, increase with stress, and decrease with purposeful movement. Depression or dementia may occur, causing memory impairment and alterations in thinking.

Parkinson disease has no cure, but the antiparkinsonism drugs are used to relieve the symptoms and assist in maintaining the patient's mobility and functioning capability as long as possible. For years, levodopa was the drug that provided the mainstay of treatment. Now, there are new drugs that are used either alone or in combination with levodopa. Entacapone (Comtan), pramipexole (Mirapex), and ropinirole (Requip) are newer drugs used in the treatment of Parkinson disease. Drug-induced parkinsonism is treated with the anticholinergics benztropine (Cogentin) and trihexyphenidyl (Artane).

Parkinsonism is a term that refers to the symptoms of Parkinson disease, as well as the Parkinson-like symptoms that may be seen with the use of certain drugs, head injuries, and encephalitis. Drugs used to treat the symptoms associated with parkinsonism are called antiparkinsonism drugs. As with some other types of drugs, it may be necessary to change from one antiparkinsonism drug to another or to increase or decrease the dosage until maximum response is obtained. The Summary Drug Table: Antiparkinsonism Drugs lists the drugs used to treat Parkinson disease. Antiparkinsonism drugs discussed in the chapter are classified as dopaminergic agents, anticholinergic drugs, COMT inhibitors, and dopamine receptor agonists (nonergot).

DOPAMINERGIC DRUGS

Actions of Dopaminergic Drugs

Dopaminergic drugs are drugs that affect the dopamine content of the brain. These drugs include levodopa/carbidopa (Sinement), carbidopa (Lodosyn), amantadine (Symmetrel), and pergolide mesylate (Permax) (see Summary Drug Table: Antiparkinsonism Drugs).

The symptoms of parkinsonism are caused by a depletion of dopamine in the CNS. Dopamine, when given orally, does not cross the blood–brain barrier and therefore is ineffective. The body's **blood–brain barrier** is a meshwork of tightly packed cells in the walls of the brain's capillaries that screen out certain substances. This unique meshwork of cells in the CNS prohibits large and potentially harmful molecules from crossing into the brain. This ability to screen out certain substances has important implications for drug therapy because some drugs are able to pass through the blood–brain barrier more easily than others.

Levodopa is a chemical formulation found in plants and animals that is converted into dopamine by nerve cells in the brain. Levodopa does cross the blood–brain barrier, and a small amount is then converted to dopamine. This allows the drug to have a pharmacologic effect in patients with Parkinson disease (Fig. 5-1). Combining levodopa with another drug (carbidopa) causes more levodopa to reach the brain. When more levodopa is available, the dosage of levodopa may be reduced. Carbidopa has no effect when given alone. Sinemet is a combination of carbidopa and levodopa and is available in several combinations (e.g., Sinemet 10/100 has 10 mg of carbidopa and 100 mg of levodopa; Sinemet CR is a time-released version of the combined drugs).

The mechanism of action of amantadine (Symmetrel) and selegiline (Eldepryl) in the treatment of parkinsonism is not fully understood.

Uses of Dopaminergic Drugs

The dopaminergic drugs are used to treat the signs and symptoms of parkinsonism. As with some other types of drugs, it may be necessary to change from one antiparkinsonism

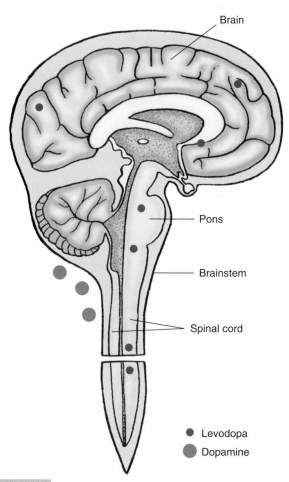

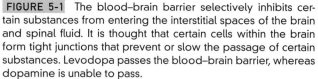

FIGURE 5-1 The blood–brain barrier selectively inhibits certain substances from entering the interstitial spaces of the brain and spinal fluid. It is thought that certain cells within the brain form tight junctions that prevent or slow the passage of certain substances. Levodopa passes the blood–brain barrier, whereas dopamine is unable to pass.

drug to another or to increase or decrease the dosage until maximum response is obtained.

Levodopa has been considered the gold standard drug therapy for Parkinson disease since it was first used in the 1960s. Carbidopa is always given with levodopa, combined together into a single dosage form. When it is necessary to titrate the dose of carbidopa, it may be given at the same time as the carbidopa/levodopa combination dosage form. Sometimes the response with these two drugs can be enhanced by the addition of another drug. For example, selegiline or pergolide may be added to the drug regimen of those being treated with carbidopa and levodopa but who have had a decreased response to therapy with these two drugs.

Amantadine is less effective than levodopa in the treatment of Parkinson disease but more effective than the anticholinergics. Amantadine may be given alone or in combination with an antiparkinsonism drug with anticholinergic activity. Amantadine is also used as an antiviral drug (see Chapter 37).

FACT CHECK

5-8   What are the classic symptoms that characterize Parkinson disease?

5-9   Do any of the current therapies on the market cure Parkinson disease?

5-10 What is the gold standard drug therapy for Parkinson disease?

Adverse Reactions of Dopaminergic Drugs

During early treatment with levodopa and carbidopa, adverse reactions are usually not a problem. But as the disease progresses, the response to the drug may become less, and the period of time that each dose is effective begins to decrease, leading to more frequent doses, and more adverse reactions.

The most serious and frequent adverse reactions seen with levodopa include **choreiform movements** (involuntary muscular twitching of the limbs or facial muscles) and **dystonic movements** (muscular spasms most often affecting the tongue, jaw, eyes, and neck). Less common but serious reactions include mental changes, such as depression, psychotic episodes, paranoia, and suicidal tendencies. Carbidopa is used with levodopa and has no effect when given alone.

In addition to adverse reactions, the **on–off phenomenon** may occur in patients taking levodopa. In this condition, a patient may suddenly alternate between improved clinical status and loss of therapeutic effect. This effect is associated with long-term levodopa treatment. Low doses of the drug, reserving the drug for severe cases, or the use of a "drug holiday" may be prescribed. Should symptoms occur, the health care provider may order a drug holiday that includes complete withdrawal of levodopa for 5 to 14 days, followed by gradually restarting use of the drug at a lower dose.

The most common serious adverse reactions to amantadine are orthostatic hypotension, depression, congestive heart failure, psychosis, urinary retention, convulsions, leukopenia, and neutropenia. Adverse reactions with selegiline include nausea, hallucinations, confusion, depression, loss of balance, and dizziness.

Contraindications, Precautions, and Interactions of Dopaminergic Drugs

- The dopaminergic drugs are contraindicated in patients with known hypersensitivity to the drugs.
- Levodopa is contraindicated in patients with narrow-angle glaucoma, those receiving a monoamine oxidase inhibitor (see Chapter 7), and during lactation.
- Levodopa is used cautiously in patients with cardiovascular disease, bronchial asthma, emphysema, peptic ulcer disease, renal or hepatic disease, and psychosis.
- Levodopa and combination antiparkinsonism drugs (e.g., carbidopa/levodopa) are used with caution during lactation.
- Levodopa interacts with many different drugs. When levodopa is used with phenytoin, reserpine, and papaverine, there is a decrease in response to levodopa.
- The risk of a hypertensive crisis increases when levodopa is used with the monoamine oxidase inhibitors (see Chapter 7).
- Selegiline is used cautiously in patients with psychosis, dementia, or excessive tremor.
- When selegiline is administered with levodopa, the effectiveness of levodopa increases. This effect allows for a decrease in the dosage of levodopa.
- If selegiline is given in higher doses, then there is an increased risk of hypertension, particularly if tyramine-containing foods (e.g., beer, wine, aged cheese, yeast products, chicken livers, and pickled herring) are ingested.
- A potentially serious reaction (confusion, agitation, hypertension, and seizures) can occur when fluoxetine is administered with selegiline. Fluoxetine therapy is discontinued for at least 1 week before treatment with selegiline is initiated.
- Amantadine is used cautiously in patients with seizure disorders, hepatic disease, psychosis, cardiac disease, and renal disease.
- The antihistamines, phenothiazines, disopyramide, and alcohol increase the risk of adverse reactions when administered with amantadine.

FACT CHECK

5-11 What are the most common adverse effects of levodopa?

5-12 What is the "on–off phenomenon"?

ANTICHOLINERGIC DRUGS

Actions of Anticholinergic Drugs

Drugs with anticholinergic activity inhibit acetylcholine (a neurohormone produced in excess in Parkinson disease) in the CNS. Drugs with anticholinergic activity are generally less effective than levodopa.

Uses of Anticholinergic Drugs

Drugs with anticholinergic activity are used as adjunctive therapy in all forms of parkinsonism and in the control of drug-induced extrapyramidal disorders. Examples of drugs with anticholinergic activity include benztropine mesylate (Cogentin), biperiden (Akineton), diphenhydramine, procyclidine (Kemadrin), and trihexyphenidyl (Artane).

Adverse Reactions of Anticholinergic Drugs

Frequently seen adverse reactions to drugs with anticholinergic activity include dry mouth, blurred vision, dizziness, mild nausea, and nervousness. These may become less pronounced as therapy progresses. If any of the adverse reactions are severe, the drug may be discontinued for several days and restarted at a lower dosage, or a different antiparkinsonism drug may be prescribed.

Contraindications, Precautions, and Interactions of Anticholinergic Drugs

- These drugs are contraindicated in those with a hypersensitivity to the anticholinergic drugs, those with glaucoma (angle-closure), pyloric or duodenal obstruction, peptic ulcers, prostatic hypertrophy, achalasia (failure of the muscles of the lower esophagus to relax causing difficulty swallowing), myasthenia gravis, and megacolon.
- These drugs are used with caution in older adults and in patients with tachycardia, cardiac arrhythmias, hypertension, hypotension, those with a tendency toward urinary retention, those with decreased liver or kidney function, or those with obstructive disease of the urinary system or gastrointestinal tract.
- When the anticholinergic drugs are administered with amantadine, there is an increased anticholinergic effect.
- When digoxin is administered with an anticholinergic drug, digoxin blood levels may be increased, leading to an increased risk for digitalis toxicity.
- Haloperidol and anticholinergic coadministration may result in worsening of schizophrenic symptoms, decreased haloperidol blood levels, and development of tardive dyskinesia (see Chapter 7).
- When the anticholinergic drugs are administered with the phenothiazines, there is a decrease in the therapeutic effects of the phenothiazines and an increase in anticholinergic adverse reactions.

FACT CHECK

5-13 Why are anticholinergics used in patients with Parkinson disease?

5-14 Why should anticholinergics be used with caution in the elderly?

COMT INHIBITORS

Actions of COMT Inhibitors

A newer classification of antiparkinsonism drugs is the catechol-O-methyltransferase (COMT) inhibitors. Examples of the COMT inhibitors are entacapone (Comtan) and tolcapone (Tasmar).

These drugs are thought to prolong the effect of levodopa by blocking an enzyme, catechol-O-methyltransferase (COMT), which eliminates dopamine. When given with levodopa, the COMT inhibitors increase the plasma concentrations and duration of action of levodopa.

Uses of COMT Inhibitors

The COMT inhibitors are used as adjuncts to levodopa/carbidopa in Parkinson disease. Tolcapone is a potent COMT inhibitor that easily crosses the blood–brain barrier. However, the drug is associated with liver damage and liver failure. Because of the danger to the liver, tolcapone is reserved for people who are not responding to other therapies. Entacapone is a milder COMT inhibitor and is used to help manage fluctuations in the response to levodopa in individuals with Parkinson disease.

Adverse Reactions of COMT Inhibitors

The adverse reactions most often associated with the administration of the COMT inhibitors include disorientation, confusion, light-headedness, dizziness, dyskinesias, hyperkinesias, nausea, vomiting, hallucinations, and fever. A serious and possibly fatal adverse reaction that can occur with the administration of tolcapone is liver failure.

Contraindications, Precautions, and Interactions of COMT Inhibitors

- These drugs are contraindicated in patients with a hypersensitivity to the drugs and during lactation.

CONSIDERATIONS | Older adults

LIFESPAN

Anticholinergic Drugs

Individuals older than 60 years frequently have increased sensitivity to anticholinergic drugs. Confusion and disorientation may occur, requiring lower doses. Patients experiencing any of these effects should be referred to their physician.

ALERT ℞

Tolcapone

A serious and potentially fatal adverse reaction to tolcapone is hepatic injury. Regular blood testing to monitor liver function is usually prescribed. The health care provider may order testing of serum transaminase levels at frequent intervals (e.g., every 2 weeks for the first year and every 8 weeks thereafter). Treatment is discontinued if the ALT (SGPT) exceeds the upper normal limit or signs or symptoms of liver failure develop.

- Tolcapone is contraindicated in patients with liver dysfunction.
- The COMT inhibitors are used with caution in patients with hypertension, hypotension, and decreased hepatic or renal function. The COMT inhibitors should not be administered with the monoamine oxidase inhibitors (see Chapter 7) because there is an increased risk of toxicity.
- If the COMT inhibitors are administered with norepinephrine, dopamine, dobutamine, methyldopa, or epinephrine, then there is a risk of increased heart rate, arrhythmias, and excessive blood pressure changes.

FACT CHECK

5-15　How do the COMT inhibitors work with levodopa?

5-16　What adverse reaction is a concern for patients taking tolcapone?

DOPAMINE RECEPTOR AGONISTS

Actions of Dopamine Receptor Agonists

The exact mechanism of action of these drugs is not understood. It is thought that these drugs act directly on postsynaptic dopamine receptors of nerve cells in the brain, mimicking the effects of dopamine in the brain.

Uses of Dopamine Receptor Agonists

The dopamine receptor agonists, such as pramipexole (Mirapex) and ropinirole (Requip), are used for the treatment of the signs and symptoms of Parkinson disease.

Adverse Reactions of Dopamine Receptor Agonists

The most common adverse reactions seen with pramipexole and ropinirole include nausea, dizziness, postural hypotension, hallucinations, somnolence, vomiting, confusion, visual disturbances, abnormal involuntary movements, and headache.

Contraindications, Precautions, and Interactions of Dopamine Receptor Agonists

- Dopamine receptor agonists are contraindicated in patients with known hypersensitivity to the drugs, severe ischemic heart disease, or peripheral vascular disease.
- These drugs are used with caution in patients with dyskinesia, orthostatic hypotension, hepatic or renal impairment, and cardiovascular disease, and in patients with a history of hallucinations or psychosis.
- There is an increased risk of CNS depression when the dopamine receptor agonists are administered with other CNS depressants.

- When administered with levodopa, the dopamine receptor agonists increase the effects of levodopa (a lower dosage of levodopa may be required); in addition, there is an increased risk of hallucinations.
- When administered with ciprofloxacin, there is an increased effect of the dopamine receptor agonist.
- The phenothiazines may decrease the effectiveness of the dopamine receptor agonists.
- When pramipexole is administered concurrently with cimetidine, ranitidine, verapamil, and quinidine, there is an increased effect of pramipexole.
- When ropinirole is administered with the estrogens, particularly estradiol, there may be an increased effect of ropinirole.

FACT CHECK

5-17　How do the dopamine receptor agonists work?

Patient Management Issues with Antiparkinsonism Drugs

Because of memory impairment and alterations in thinking in some patients with parkinsonism, a history obtained from the patient may be unreliable. It may be necessary for the health care provider to rely on a family member for information about the symptoms of the disorder, the length of time the symptoms have been present, the ability of the patient to perform on activities of daily living, and the patient's current mental condition (e.g., impairment in memory, signs of depression, or withdrawal).

Before starting the drug therapy, a physical assessment of a patient provides a baseline for future evaluations of drug therapy. It also is important that the patient's neurologic status be evaluated.

A patient's response to drug therapy by neurologic observations can be compared with the data obtained during the initial physical assessment. For example, a patient is assessed for clinical improvement of the symptoms of the disease, such as improvement of tremor of head or hands at rest, muscular rigidity, mask-like facial expression, and ambulation stability. Although the drug response may occur slowly in some patients, these observations aid the health care provider in adjusting the dosage of the drug upward or downward to obtain the desired therapeutic results. The patient is evaluated for imbalanced nutrition related to adverse drug effects (nausea, vomiting); the risk for injury related to parkinsonism or adverse drug reactions (dizziness, light-headedness, orthostatic hypotension, loss of balance); impaired physical mobility related to alterations in balance, unsteady gait, and dizziness; and constipation related to adverse drug reactions.

Effective management of a patient with parkinsonism requires that the health care provider carefully monitor the drug therapy, provide psychological support, and place a strong emphasis on patient and family teaching, as detailed later in the chapter.

The drugs used to treat parkinsonism also may be used to treat the symptoms of parkinsonism that occur with the administration of some of the psychotherapeutic drugs

ALERT Rx

Levodopa

Patients receiving levodopa or carbidopa and levodopa must be monitored for the occurrence of choreiform and dystonic movements, such as facial grimacing, protruding tongue, exaggerated chewing motions and head movements, and jerking movements of the arms and legs. If these occur, then the health care provider should be notified immediately because it may be necessary to reduce the dosage of levodopa or discontinue use of the drug.

ALERT Rx

Dry Mouth

Some adverse reactions, although not serious, may be uncomfortable. An example of a less serious but uncomfortable adverse reaction is dryness of the mouth. Dry mouth can be relieved by offering frequent sips of water, ice chips, or hard candy (if allowed). If dry mouth is so severe that the patient has difficulty swallowing or speaking, or if loss of appetite and weight loss occurs, then the dosage of the antiparkinsonism drug may be reduced.

(see Chapter 7). When used for this purpose, the antiparkinsonism drugs may exacerbate mental symptoms and precipitate a psychosis. A health care provider must observe the patient's behavior at frequent intervals. If sudden behavioral changes are noted, the next dose of the drug is withheld and the health care provider is notified immediately.

Some patients with parkinsonism communicate poorly and do not tell the health care provider that problems are occurring. A patient with parkinsonism must be observed for outward changes that may indicate one or more adverse reactions. For example, a sudden change in the facial expression or changes in posture may indicate abdominal pain or discomfort, which may be caused by urinary retention, paralytic ileus, or constipation. Sudden changes in behavior may be signs of hallucinations, depression, or other psychotic episodes.

Educating the Patient and Family about Antiparkinsonism Drugs

The health care provider evaluates a patient's ability to understand the therapeutic drug regimen, to care for himself or herself at home, and to comply with the prescribed drug therapy. If any type of assistance is needed, then the health care provider arranges for a referral to the discharge planning coordinator or social worker.

If a patient requires supervision or help with daily activities and the drug regimen, the family is encouraged to create a home environment that is least likely to result in accidents or falls. Changes such as removing throw rugs, installing a handrail next to the toilet, and moving obstacles that can result in tripping or falling can be made at little or no expense to the family.

Following are key points about antiparkinsonism drugs the patient or family should know.

- Take this drug as prescribed. Do not increase, decrease, or omit a dose or stop taking the drug unless advised to do so by your health care provider. If you have gastrointestinal upset, take the drug with food.
- If you experience dizziness, drowsiness, or blurred vision, avoid driving or performing other tasks that require alertness.
- Do not use alcohol unless approved by your health care provider.
- Relieve dry mouth by sucking on hard candy (preferably sugar free) or frequent sips of water. Consult your dentist if dryness of the mouth interferes with wearing, inserting, or removing dentures or causes other dental problems.
- Orthostatic hypotension may develop with or without symptoms of dizziness, nausea, fainting, and sweating. Do not rise rapidly after sitting or lying down.
- Notify your health care provider if you experience any of these problems: severe dry mouth, inability to chew or swallow food, inability to urinate, feelings of depression, severe dizziness or drowsiness, rapid or irregular

CONSIDERATIONS | Older adults

LIFESPAN

Hallucinations occur more often in older adults receiving the antiparkinsonism drugs, especially when taking the dopamine receptor agonists. Older adults should be assessed for signs of visual, auditory, or tactile hallucinations. The incidence of hallucinations appears to increase with age.

ALERT Rx

Difficulty Walking

Minimizing the risk for injury is an important aspect in the care of a patient with parkinsonism. These patients may have difficulty walking. Adverse reactions may further increase difficulty with walking. These individuals are especially prone to falls and other accidents because of their disease process and possible adverse drug reactions. A patient should be helped out of the bed or a chair and with walking and other self-care activities. In addition, assistive devices such as a cane or walker may be helpful. It may be suggested to a patient to wear shoes with rubber soles to minimize the possibility of slipping. Patients are prone to orthostatic hypotension as a result of the drug regimen. These patients are instructed to arise slowly from a sitting or lying position, especially after sitting or lying for a prolonged time.

heartbeat, abdominal pain, mood changes, and unusual movements of the head, eyes, neck, arms, legs, feet, mouth, or tongue.

- Keep all appointments with your health care provider or clinic personnel because close monitoring of therapy is necessary.
- If you have diabetes, levodopa may interfere with your urine tests for glucose or ketones. Report any abnormal result to your health care provider before adjusting the dosage of the antidiabetic medication.
- If you are taking tolcapone, keep all appointments with your health care provider. Liver function tests are performed periodically and are an important part of therapy. Report any signs of liver failure, such as persistent

nausea, fatigue, lethargy, anorexia, jaundice, dark urine, pruritus, and right upper quadrant tenderness.

FACT CHECK

5-18   If a family member informs you that the patient is experiencing dry mouth, what could you recommend?

5-19   If a family member notices that the patient seems to be having difficulty walking, what could you recommend?

Chapter Review

KEY POINTS

- Generally, anticonvulsants reduce the excitability of the neurons (nerve cells) of the brain. When neuron excitability is decreased, seizures are theoretically reduced in intensity and frequency of occurrence or, in some instances, are virtually eliminated.
- For some patients, only partial control of the seizure disorder may be obtained with anticonvulsant drug therapy.
- Parkinsonism is a term that refers to the symptoms of Parkinson disease, as well as the Parkinson-like symptoms that may occur with the use of certain drugs, head injuries, and encephalitis.
- Drugs used to treat the symptoms associated with parkinsonism are called antiparkinsonism drugs. As with some other types of drugs, it may be necessary to change from one antiparkinsonism drug to another or to increase or decrease the dosage until maximum response is obtained. The drugs will relieve symptoms and assist in maintaining the patient's mobility and functioning capability as long as possible. Patient management and teaching for all of these drugs focus on the need for strict dosage control and the management of adverse reactions, many of which are severe.

CRITICAL THINKING CASE STUDIES

Epilepsy

Donny is 14 years old and has just been diagnosed with epilepsy. He has been prescribed phenytoin, which is a hydantoin.

1. Which of the following are common adverse reactions associated with the hydantoins?
   a. Nystagmus
   b. Ataxia
   c. Slurred speech
   d. All of the above
2. In addition to the physician Donny sees for treatment of his epilepsy, which other health care provider should he see regularly?

Parkinson Disease

Ms. Chang has Parkinson disease. Her personal assistant is responsible for Ms. Chang's home care and needs guidance about the drug therapy that has been prescribed for Ms. Chang.

3. Ms. Chang has been prescribed amantadine. The personal assistant needs to be aware of adverse reactions, including
   a. none when given alone; in combination with levodopa, levodopa side effects
   b. light-headedness, dizziness, and confusion
   c. blurred vision, increase in hand tremor, and abdominal pain
   d. potential loss of hair and dry skin
4. Ms. Chang's personal assistant phones the health care provider 1 month into treatment to report that Ms. Chang seems to be stumbling more frequently, especially when rising. The assistant is instructed to
   a. contact the health care provider
   b. caution Ms. Chang to rise more slowly, and assist her if necessary
   c. recall whether any dose of the medication was accidentally increased or missed
   d. all of the above
5. What dopaminergic drug would you expect Ms. Chang to be taking in place of amantadine? Why?

Review Questions

MULTIPLE CHOICE

1. A patient is prescribed phenytoin for a recurrent convulsive disorder. The health care provider informs the patient that the most common adverse reactions are
   a. related to the gastrointestinal system
   b. associated with the reproductive system
   c. associated with kidney function
   d. related to the central nervous system

2. Which of the following adverse reactions, if observed in a patient prescribed phenytoin, would indicate that the patient may be developing phenytoin toxicity?
    a. Severe occipital headache
    b. Ataxia
    c. Hyperactivity
    d. Somnolence

3. The most serious adverse reactions seen with levodopa include
    a. choreiform and dystonic movements
    b. depression
    c. suicidal tendencies
    d. paranoia

4. Elderly patients prescribed one of the dopamine receptor agonists are monitored closely for which of the following adverse reactions?
    a. Occipital headache
    b. Hallucinations
    c. Paralytic ileus
    d. Cardiac arrhythmias

MATCHING

_____ 5. lamotrigine   a. Requip
_____ 6. entacapone   b. Lamictal
_____ 7. ropinirole   c. Dilantin
_____ 8. phenytoin   d. Comtan

TRUE OR FALSE

_____ 9. For some patients, only partial control of the seizure disorder may be obtained with anticonvulsant drug therapy.

_____ 10. Anticonvulsant blood levels must be monitored at regular intervals, even if the seizures are well controlled.

_____ 11. Parkinson disease is progressive, with the symptoms becoming worse over time.

_____ 12. Levodopa does not cross the blood–brain barrier when given alone; however, combining levodopa and carbidopa prevents the levodopa from crossing the blood–brain barrier.

FILL IN THE BLANKS

13. The _____ is an adverse reaction that occurs with levodopa in which a patient suddenly alternates between improved clinical status and loss of therapeutic effect.

14. _____ is a permanent, recurrent seizure disorder.

15. _____ is a degenerative disorder of the central nervous system and is caused by a deficiency of _____ and an excess of _____ within the CNS.

16. The most common adverse reaction of most anticonvulsants is _____.

SHORT ANSWERS

17. Why is it necessary for a patient who suffers from epilepsy or another seizure disorder to carry identification, such as a Medic-Alert tag?

18. The most serious and frequent adverse reactions of levodopa are choreiform movements and dystonic movements. What are examples of each of these?

19. How are seizure disorders characterized?

20. What are the four types of drugs used to treat Parkinson disease?

Web Activities

1. Go to the Web site for the Epilepsy Foundation of America (http://www.efa.org) and conduct a search on the ketogenic diet. Write a brief description of the diet and its use in treating epilepsy in children.

2. Does the Epilepsy Foundation of America Web site suggest a way for patients and their families to connect with other epilepsy-impacted households? If so, what are they?

3. Go to the Web site for the National Parkinson Foundation (www.parkinson.org) and find Caregiving 101. What are the 10 early warning signs of Parkinson disease?

SUMMARY DRUG TABLE: Anticonvulsants
(left, generic; right, trade)

Comprehensive Summary Drug Tables, including uses, adverse effects, dosages, and pregnancy classifications, are provided on the companion website, http:// thePoint.lww.com/PharmacologyHP2e

Barbiturates	
phenobarbital *fee-noe-bar'-bi-tal*	*generic* (CIV)
phenobarbital sodium *fee-noe-bar'-bi-tal*	Luminal Sodium (CIV), *generic*

Hydantoins	
ethotoin *eth'-i-toe-in*	Peganone
phenytoin sodium, parenteral *fen'-i-toe-in*	*generic*
phenytoin, phenytoin sodium, oral *fen'-i-toe-in*	Dilantin, *generic*
fosphenytoin sodium *fos'-fen-i-toyn*	*generic*

Succinimides	
ethosuximide *eth-oh-sux'-i-mide*	Zarontin, *generic*
methsuximide *meth-sux'-i-mide*	Celontin

Benzodiazepines	
clonazepam *clo-nay'-zeh-pam*	Klonopin (CIV), *generic*
clorazepate dipotassium *klor-az'-e-pate*	Tranxene-T (CIV), *generic*
diazepam *dye-az'-e-pam*	Valium (CIV), Diastat AcuDial (rectal gel), *generic*

Miscellaneous Preparations	
carbamazepine *kar-ba-maz'-e-peen*	Tegretol, Tegretol-XR, *generic*
felbamate *fell'-ba-mate*	Felbatol
gabapentin *gab-ah-pen'-tin*	Neurontin
lacosamide *la-koe'-sa-mide*	Vimpat
lamotrigine *l* *a mo' tri geen*	Lamictal, Lamictal Chewable, Lamictal ODT, Lamictal XR
levetiracetam *lee-va-tye-ra'-se-tam*	Keppra, Keppra XR
magnesium sulfate *mag-nee'-zhum*	*generic*
oxcarbazepine *ox-car-baz'-e-peen*	Trileptal
pregabalin *Pre-gab'-a-lin*	Lyrica (C-V)
primidone *pri'-mi-done*	Mysoline
rufinamide *Roo-fin'-a-mide*	Banzel
tiagabine hydrochloride *Tye-ag'-a-been*	Gabitril
topiramate *Toe-pyre'-a-mate*	Topamax, *generic*
valproic acid *val-proe'-ik*	Depakene, Depakote, *generic*
vigabatrin *Vye-ga'-ba-trin*	Sabril
zonisamide *Zoh-niss'-ah-mide*	Zonegran

SUMMARY DRUG TABLE: Antiparkinsonism Drugs
(left, generic; right, trade)

Comprehensive Summary Drug Tables, including uses, adverse effects, dosages, and pregnancy classifications, are provided on the companion website, http:// thePoint.lww.com/PharmacologyHP2e

Dopaminergic Agents	
amantadine *a-man'-ta-deen*	*generic*
bromocriptine *broe-moe-krip'-tine*	Parlodel
carbidopa *kar'-bi-doe-pa*	Lodosyn
carbidopa/levodopa *kar'-bi-doe-pa/lee'-voe-doe-pa*	Sinemet CR, Sinemet 10/100, Sinemet 25/100, Sinemet 25/250, *generic*
carbidopa/levodopa/entacapone *kar'-bi-doe-pa/ lee'-voe-doe-pa/ en-ta'-ka-pone*	Stalevo
rasagiline *ra-sa'-ji-leen*	Azilect
selegiline *sell-eh'-geh-leen*	Emsam, Eldepryl, Zelapar, *generic*

Anticholinergic Agents	
benztropine mesylate *benz'-tro-peen*	Cogentin, *generic*
diphenhydramine *dye-fen-hye'-dra-meen*	Benadryl, *generic*
trihexyphenidyl *trye-hex-ee-fen'-i-dill*	*generic*

COMT Inhibitors	
entacapone *en-tah-kap'-own*	Comtan
tolcapone *toll-kap'-own*	Tasmar

Dopamine Receptor Agonists	
apomorphine *a-poe-mor'-feen*	Apokyn
pramipexole *pram-ah-pex'-ole*	Mirapex, Mirapex ER
ropinirole HCL *roe-pin'-o-role*	Requip, Requip XL

6

Cholinesterase Inhibitors

CHAPTER OBJECTIVES

On completion of this chapter, students will be able to:

1. Define the chapter's key terms.
2. Describe the manifestations of Alzheimer disease.
3. Identify the medications that are used to treat Alzheimer disease.
4. Identify common adverse reactions of the cholinesterase inhibitors.
5. Discuss important points that patients and family members should know about the use of cholinesterase inhibitors.

KEY TERMS

acetylcholine—a natural chemical in the brain that is required for memory and thinking

Alzheimer disease—a disease of the elderly causing progressive deterioration of mental and physical abilities

alanine aminotransferase (ALT)—an enzyme found predominately in the liver; high levels may indicate liver damage

anorexia—a diminished appetite

dementia—decrease in cognitive functioning (memory, decision making, speech, etc.)

hepatotoxic—capable of producing liver damage

CHAPTER OVERVIEW

Drug classes covered in this chapter are:

- Cholinesterase inhibitors

Drugs by classification are listed on page 72.

---

thePOINT RESOURCES

- Comprehensive Summary Drug Tables
- Lippincott's Interactive Tutorials: Drugs Affecting the Central Nervous System
- Interactive Practice and Review
- Monographs of Most Commonly Prescribed Drugs

Alzheimer disease is a progressive deterioration of a person's mental and physical abilities from which there is no recovery. Specific pathologic changes occur in the cortex of the brain that are thought to be associated with deficiencies of one or more of the neurohormones, such as acetylcholine or norepinephrine (Fig. 6-1). Alzheimer disease generally occurs in three progressive phases (see Signs and Symptoms box).

While this chapter focuses on cholinesterase inhibitors, an NMDA receptor antagonist has also been approved for Alzheimer treatment. Box 6-1 provides additional information on this drug.

Cholinesterase Inhibitors

Cholinesterase inhibitors are drugs used to treat Alzheimer disease. They do not cure the disease but help slow its progression. These drugs are used to treat mild to moderate **dementia** (a decrease in cognitive functioning) caused by Alzheimer disease. Donepezil has been shown to be effective in patients with both mild to moderate and moderate to severe Alzheimer disease. These patients may also be taking other drugs for symptomatic relief. For example, wandering, irritability, and aggression in people with Alzheimer disease are treated with antipsychotic drugs, such as risperidone and olanzapine (see Chapter 7). Other drugs, such as antidepressants or antianxiety drugs, may be helpful for patients with Alzheimer disease who are experiencing symptoms of depression and anxiety.

Actions of Cholinesterase Inhibitors

Acetylcholine, a natural chemical in the brain, is required for memory and thinking (Fig. 6-2). Individuals with Alzheimer disease slowly lose this chemical. As their levels of the chemical decrease, these patients experience problems with memory and thinking. The cholinesterase inhibitors act to increase the level of acetylcholine in the central nervous system by inhibiting its breakdown and slowing the destruction of neurons. However, the disease is progressive, and although these drugs alter the progress of the disease, they do not cure the disease.

Uses of Cholinesterase Inhibitors

Cholinesterase inhibitors are used to treat the dementia associated with Alzheimer disease. The effectiveness of these drugs varies from individual to individual. The drugs may noticeably diminish the symptoms of Alzheimer disease, the symptoms may improve only slightly, or the symptoms may continue to progress (only at a slower rate).

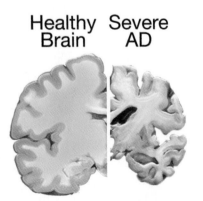

FIGURE 6-1 A. Normal brain. B. Brain with Alzheimer disease.

SIGNS & SYMPTOMS

Manifestations of Alzheimer Disease

Early Phase—Mild Cognitive Decline

- Increased forgetfulness
- Decreased social performance
- Some memory deficit
- Mild to moderate anxiety

Early Dementia Phase—Moderately Severe Cognitive Decline

- Needs assistance in activities of daily living
- Unable to recall important aspects of current life
- Difficulty making choices (e.g., what clothes to wear, what to eat)
- Able to recall major facts (e.g., their name and family members' names)

Late Dementia Phase—Severe Cognitive Decline

- Incontinent of urine
- No verbal ability
- No basic psychomotor skills
- Needs help bathing, toileting, and feeding

FACT CHECK

6-1 What classification of drugs is used to treat Alzheimer disease?

6-2 What natural chemical in the brain is lower in patients with Alzheimer disease?

6-3 Are all of the medications used to treat Alzheimer disease equally effective for all individuals?

ALERT Rx

NMDA Receptor Antagonist

The drug memantine (trade name Namenda) is an NMDA receptor antagonist that is used for moderate to severe Alzheimer disease. Memantine blocks NMDA (N-methyl D-aspartate) receptors that are activated by the amino acid glutamate and that are thought to be a factor in Alzheimer symptoms. There is no evidence that memantine prevents or slows neurodegeneration in patients with Alzheimer disease. Many of the drug's adverse reactions are similar to those of cholinesterase inhibitors and include confusion, dizziness, headache, constipation, agitation, diarrhea, nausea, urinary incontinence, insomnia, abnormal gait, depression, and anorexia. Dosage: Immediate-release tablets and oral solution: 5 to 20 mg daily; extended-release capsules: 7 to 28 mg once daily. This drug is pregnancy category B.

FACTS ABOUT . . .

Alzheimer Disease

- Over 5 million Americans have Alzheimer disease.
- One in eight people over the age of 65 have Alzheimer disease, and those over 85 make up almost half of the Alzheimer patient population.
- Alzheimer disease is the seventh leading cause of death in the United States. It is the fifth leading cause of death for adults over the age of 65.
- The annual cost of Alzheimer disease is $172 billion.
- Approximately 11 million unpaid caregivers are taking care of family members or friends with Alzheimer disease.
- The life span of a patient with Alzheimer disease is usually decreased, although a patient may live 3 to 20 years after the diagnosis.
- Alzheimer is the most common cause of dementia.

Source: Alzheimer's Association

ALERT Rx

Tacrine and Hepatotoxicity

A patient taking tacrine must be monitored for liver damage. This is usually performed by monitoring alanine aminotransferase (ALT) levels. ALT is an enzyme found predominately in the liver. Disease or injury to the liver causes a release of this enzyme into the bloodstream, resulting in elevated ALT levels.

Adverse Reactions of Cholinesterase Inhibitors

Adverse reactions of cholinesterase inhibitors include **anorexia** (a diminished appetite), nausea, vomiting, diarrhea, weight loss, abdominal pain, dizziness, and headache. In most situations, these adverse reactions are mild and are usually experienced only early in treatment. However, two major problems in the late stage of Alzheimer disease are weight loss and eating problems related to the inability to swallow. If the patient is still experiencing anorexia, vomiting, diarrhea, weight loss, and other adverse reactions that could affect the weight, then the patient's health could deteriorate more quickly. Patients taking rivastigmine appear to have more problems with nausea and severe vomiting. In addition, physical decline and the adverse reaction of dizziness place the patient at risk for injury. On the positive side, when adverse reactions occur, they tend to disappear gradually as the body gets used to the treatment and generally do not last for more than several days.

Tacrine, however, is particularly **hepatotoxic** (capable of producing liver damage). Because tacrine is more likely to cause adverse reactions and drug interactions, it is administered in smaller doses given more frequently; tacrine is rarely used today. Donepezil has fewer and milder side effects and is considered the agent of first choice, although some patients may have a better response with one drug than another.

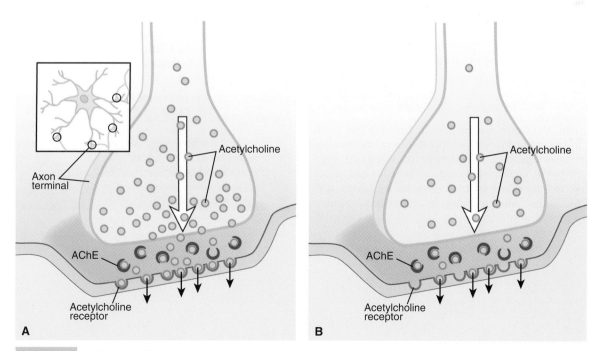

FIGURE 6-2 A. Normal ACh levels. B. Decreased ACh levels with Alzheimer disease.

Contraindications, Precautions, and Interactions of Cholinesterase Inhibitors

- Cholinesterase inhibitors are contraindicated in patients with hypersensitivity to the drugs and during lactation.
- These drugs are used cautiously in patients with renal or hepatic disease, bladder obstruction, seizure disorders, sick sinus syndrome, gastrointestinal bleeding, and asthma. Individuals with a history of ulcer disease may have a recurrence of bleeding.
- When the cholinesterase inhibitors are given to patients using an anticholinergic drug, there is a potential decrease in the activity of the anticholinergic drug.
- There is a greater risk of theophylline toxicity when tacrine is administered. There is a synergistic effect when tacrine is administered with succinylcholine, other cholinesterase inhibitors, or cholinergic agonists (e.g., bethanechol).

FACT CHECK

6-4 Which of the cholinesterase inhibitors is considered the drug of first choice? Why?

6-5 What are the common adverse reactions of cholinesterase inhibitors?

6-6 Which of the cholinesterase inhibitors may cause liver damage?

Patient Management Issues with Cholinesterase Inhibitors

A patient receiving a cholinesterase inhibitor may be treated in a hospital or nursing home or as an outpatient. The patient's cognitive ability and physical ability are assessed before and during therapy. Confusion, agitation, impulsive behavior, speech, ability to perform the activities of daily living, and self-care abilities also are assessed. These assessments will be used to monitor the patient's improvement (if any) after taking a cholinesterase inhibitor (Key Concepts 6-1). These drugs may slow the progression of the disease but are not a cure for Alzheimer disease.

Educating the Patient and Family

Patients with Alzheimer disease may understand and comprehend the extent and severity of this disease while they are early in the disease process. As their cognitive abilities decrease, however, it is the family who needs to be educated about the disease and the effects of drugs given for treatment. It is often important for family members to assume responsibility

KEY CONCEPTS

6-1 Patient Response to Cholinesterase Inhibitors

Patients with poor response to drug therapy with a cholinesterase inhibitor may require dosage changes, discontinuation of the drug therapy, or the addition of other therapies to the treatment regimen. However, response to these drugs may take several weeks. The symptoms that the patient is experiencing may get better or remain the same, or the patient may experience only a small response to therapy. Any treatment that slows the progression of symptoms in Alzheimer disease is considered successful.

for giving drugs to patients at home if they appear unable to manage their own drug therapy. Following are key points about cholinesterase inhibitors the patient or family members should know.

- Keep all appointments with health care providers because close monitoring of the drug therapy is essential. Dose changes may be needed to achieve the best results.
- Take the drug exactly as directed. Do not increase, decrease, or omit a dose or discontinue use of this drug unless directed to do so by your primary health care provider.
- Keep track of when the drug is taken. Patients in the early stages of forgetfulness can mark their calendar each time they take the medicine or use a pill counter that holds the medicine for each day of the week; such methods can help patients remember to take their medication or know if they have already taken the medication for the day.
- Be aware that the patient may need help when walking. The use of assistive devices such as walkers or canes may reduce the risk of falls. To minimize the risk of injury, the patient's environment should be controlled and safe.

FACT CHECK

6-7 What are some of the items that will be assessed after diagnosis and during treatment for a patient with Alzheimer disease?

6-8 When is drug therapy for Alzheimer disease considered successful?

Chapter Review

KEY POINTS

- Alzheimer disease is a common progressive deterioration of mental and physical abilities caused by changes in the brain.
- Medications for Alzheimer disease do not cure the disease but may lessen or delay its symptoms.
- Cholinesterase inhibitors increase the level of acetylcholine in the central nervous system by inhibiting its breakdown and slowing the destruction of neurons.
- Cholinesterase inhibitors may cause anorexia, nausea, vomiting, diarrhea, weight loss, dizziness, and headache. They are contraindicated during pregnancy and lactation and in patients with a known hypersensitivity, and are used with caution in patients with renal or hepatic disease, bladder obstruction, seizure disorders, sick sinus syndrome, gastrointestinal bleeding, and asthma.
- Patient management issues include physical and cognitive assessments to determine the patient's improvement while on the medication and to monitor and care for adverse reactions.
- Patient and family education issues include monitoring the patient's status for adverse effects and to determine a need for dosage changes.

CRITICAL THINKING CASE STUDY

Alzheimer Disease

Mr. Alvarez had mild Alzheimer disease diagnosed, and the doctor has prescribed donepezil. Two weeks later, Mr. Alvarez's family is concerned because he does not seem "better" and is experiencing some nausea.

1. His family members need to know that
   a. it may take a full year before the drug has an effect
   b. even if he does not seem to be getting "better," the drug may be helping to keep his symptoms from worsening
   c. the doctor will double the dosage every week until a positive effect occurs
   d. he does not need to take the drug on days when he does not feel like taking it
2. Mr. Alvarez's symptom of nausea
   a. is a common adverse effect of donepezil and will likely diminish over time
   b. is probably caused by his Alzheimer disease, not the drug
   c. will become worse the longer he continues to use the drug
   d. is a sign that the drug is improving his cognitive performance
3. What are other adverse effects that Mr. Alvarez may experience?

Review Questions

MULTIPLE CHOICE

1. Cholinesterase inhibitors are used to treat which of the following conditions associated with Alzheimer disease?
   a. Urinary incontinence
   b. Dementia
   c. Peripheral paralysis
   d. Depression
2. Cholinesterase inhibitors act by helping maintain or increase the level of what chemical in the brain?
   a. Erythrocytes
   b. Gastric acid
   c. Cerebrospinal fluid
   d. Acetylcholine
3. An adverse reaction that may occur in a patient taking rivastigmine (Exelon) include
   a. occipital headache
   b. vomiting
   c. hyperactivity
   d. hypoactivity
4. When a patient with Alzheimer disease is given tacrine (Cognex), which laboratory examination would most likely be prescribed?
   a. A complete blood count
   b. Cholesterol levels
   c. Alanine aminotransferase (ALT) levels
   d. Electrolytes

MATCHING

_____ 5. donepezil   a. Exelon
_____ 6. galantamine   b. Cognex
_____ 7. rivastigmine   c. Aricept
_____ 8. tacrine   d. Razadyne

TRUE OR FALSE

_____ 9. Alzheimer disease is a progressive deterioration of a person's mental and physical abilities from which there is no recovery.
_____ 10. A patient taking a cholinesterase inhibitor may still need other medications for symptomatic relief, such as an antipsychotic for aggression.
_____ 11. Alzheimer disease is the most common cause of death in adults over the age of 85.
_____ 12. When adverse reactions appear after beginning cholinesterase inhibitor therapy, the patient should switch drugs because the adverse reactions will only worsen over time.

FILL IN THE BLANKS

13. Cholinesterase inhibitors are drugs used to treat mild to moderate or moderate to severe _____.

14. Cholinesterase inhibitors increase the level of _____ in the central nervous system by inhibiting its breakdown and slowing the destruction of neurons.

15. Patient management issues include _____ and _____ assessments to determine the patient's improvement while on the medication.

16. Once medication is begun, it may take several _____ for the patient to have a response.

SHORT ANSWERS

17. What are the three progressive phases of Alzheimer disease? Provide at least two symptoms that are present during each of the phases.

18. Physical decline and the adverse reaction of dizziness can place the patient at risk for injury. If asked by a family member how to best help the patient, what could you recommend?

19. Why is it important that the family and caregivers of a patient with Alzheimer disease be educated about the disease and the effects of the drugs given for treatment?

20. What ideas could you share with the patient and/or caregivers to help keep track of when the patient has taken his or her medication?

Web Activities

1. Go to the Web site of the Alzheimer's Association (http://www.alz.org). What are the 10 warning signs of Alzheimer disease?

2. Go to the Web site of the Alzheimer Disease Education & Referral Center (http://www.nia.nih.gov/alzheimers). Write a summary of the differences between mild, moderate, and severe Alzheimer disease.

SUMMARY DRUG TABLE: Cholinesterase Inhibitors (left, generic; right, trade).

Comprehensive Summary Drug Tables, including uses, adverses effects, dosages, and pregnancy classifications, are provided on the companion website, http://thePoint.lww.com/PharmacologyHP2e

donepezil HCL *doe-nep'-ah-zill*	Aricept, Aricept ODT
galantamine hydrobromide *ga-lan'-ta-meen*	Razadyne, Razadyne ER
rivastigmine tartrate *riv-ah-stig'-meen*	Exelon
tacrine HCL *tay'-krin*	Cognex

7

Psychiatric Drugs

CHAPTER OBJECTIVES

On completion of this chapter, students will be able to:

1. Define the chapter's key terms.
2. Describe the difference between a sedative and a hypnotic.
3. List and discuss the uses, actions, contraindications, precautions, interactions, and adverse reactions associated with the administration of sedatives and hypnotics.
4. Discuss important points to keep in mind when educating patients and family members about the use of sedatives and hypnotics.
5. List and discuss the uses, actions, contraindications, precautions, interactions, and adverse reactions associated with the administration of antianxiety drugs.
6. Discuss important points to keep in mind when educating patients and family members about the use of antianxiety drugs.
7. Discuss the symptoms of depression.
8. Identify the different types of antidepressants.
9. For each category of antidepressants, list and discuss the uses, actions, contraindications, precautions, interactions, and adverse reactions associated with their administration.
10. Discuss important points to keep in mind when educating patients and family members about the use of antidepressants.
11. List and discuss the uses, actions, contraindications, precautions, interactions, and adverse reactions associated with the administration of antipsychotic drugs and lithium.
12. Discuss common adverse reactions and signs of toxicity for lithium.
13. Discuss important points to keep in mind when educating patients and family members about the use of antipsychotic drugs and lithium.

CHAPTER OVERVIEW

Drug classes covered in this chapter are:

- Sedatives and hypnotics
- Antianxiety drugs
- Antidepressants
- Antipsychotic drugs

Drugs by classification are listed on pages 89-90.

thePOINT RESOURCES

- Comprehensive Summary Drug Tables
- Lippincott's Interactive Tutorials: Drugs Affecting the Central Nervous System
- Interactive Practice and Review
- Monographs of Most Commonly Prescribed Drugs

KEY TERMS

addiction—physical drug dependence

akathisia—extreme restlessness and increased motor activity

antianxiety drugs—drugs used to treat anxiety

antidepressant drugs—used to treat depression

antipsychotic drugs—drugs used to treat psychotic disorders

anxiety—a feeling of apprehension, worry, or uneasiness that may or may not be based on reality

anxiolytics—another term that refers to antianxiety drugs

ataxia—a loss of control of voluntary movements, especially producing an unsteady gait

bipolar disorder—a psychiatric disorder characterized by severe mood swings from extreme hyperactivity to depression (manic–depressive disease)

depression—a common psychiatric disorder characterized by feelings of intense sadness, helplessness, and worthlessness and by impaired functioning

dysphoric—extreme or exaggerated sadness, anxiety, or unhappiness

dystonia—facial grimacing and twisting of the neck into unnatural positions

endogenous—made within the body

extrapyramidal effects—a group of adverse reactions occurring in the extrapyramidal portion of the nervous system, causing abnormal muscle movements

hypnotic—a drug that induces sleep

neuroleptic drugs—another term for antipsychotic drugs

neuroleptic malignant syndrome—a rare reaction to antipsychotic drugs characterized by a combination of extrapyramidal effects, hyperthermia, and autonomic disturbance

orthostatic hypotension—a feeling of light-headedness and dizziness after suddenly changing position after sitting or lying down in one place for a long period, caused by a drop in blood pressure when a person sits or stands up

photophobia—an intolerance to light

photosensitivity—abnormally heightened reactivity of the skin to sunlight

psychotherapeutic drug—used to treat disorders of the mind

psychotic disorder—a disorder, such as schizophrenia, characterized by extreme personality disorganization and a loss of contact with reality

psychotropic drug—another term for psychotherapeutic drugs

sedative—a drug that produces a relaxing, calming effect

tardive dyskinesia—a syndrome consisting of potentially irreversible, involuntary dyskinetic movements

tolerance—patient condition in which increasingly larger dosages are required to obtain the desired effect

withdrawal—a syndrome of physical and psychological symptoms caused by abruptly stopping use of a drug in a dependent patient

A wide range of drugs are used to treat patients with mental symptoms or disorders. These include **psychotherapeutic drugs**, also called **psychotropic drugs**, which are used to treat disorders of the mind. The types of psychotherapeutic drugs used to treat mental illness include

- Antianxiety drugs (tranquilizers)
- Antidepressant drugs
- Antipsychotic drugs

Sedatives and hypnotics are also discussed in this chapter because they may also be used for patients experiencing anxiety, although they are used for other medical purposes, also, such as to induce sleep the night before surgery.

Sedatives and Hypnotics

A **sedative** is a drug that produces a relaxing, calming effect. Sedatives are usually given during daytime hours, and although they may make the patient drowsy, they usually do not produce sleep. A **hypnotic** is a drug that induces sleep; that is, it allows the patient to fall asleep and stay asleep. Hypnotics are also called soporifics. Hypnotics are given at night or when the patient needs to go to sleep.

Sedatives and hypnotics can be divided into two classes: barbiturates and miscellaneous sedatives and hypnotics. The barbiturates are divided into several groups, depending on their duration of action.

- Ultrashort acting. The ultrashort-acting barbiturates are used as anesthetics (see Chapter 9). Single doses have a duration of 20 minutes or less.
- Short acting. The average duration of action of short-acting barbiturates is 3 to 4 hours.
- Intermediate acting. The average duration of action of intermediate-acting barbiturates is 6 to 8 hours.
- Long acting. The average duration of action of the long-acting barbiturates is 10 to 16 hours.

The Summary Drug Table: Sedatives and Hypnotics gives examples of the barbiturate sedatives and hypnotics.

The miscellaneous sedatives and hypnotics are a group of unrelated drugs and a second group called the benzodiazepines. The benzodiazepines are also called antianxiety drugs (see later section). The miscellaneous sedatives and hypnotics are listed in the Summary Drug Table: Sedatives and Hypnotics.

Actions of Sedatives and Hypnotics

All barbiturates have essentially the same mode of action. Depending on the dose given, these drugs produce central nervous system depression and mood alteration ranging from mild excitation to mild sedation, hypnosis (sleep), or deep coma. These drugs also are respiratory depressants, with the degree of depression usually depending on the dose given. When these drugs are used as hypnotics, their respiratory depressant effect is usually similar to that normally occurring during sleep. The sedative or hypnotic effects of the barbiturates diminish after approximately 2 weeks. Outpatients taking these drugs for periods longer than 2 weeks may increase the dose to produce the desired effects (e.g., sleep, sedation). Physical and psychological dependence may occur, especially after prolonged use of high doses. Discontinuing use of a barbiturate after prolonged use may result in severe, and sometimes fatal, withdrawal symptoms. **Withdrawal** is a syndrome of physical and psychological symptoms caused by abruptly stopping use of a drug in a dependent patient, as discussed later in this chapter.

Miscellaneous or nonbarbiturate sedatives and hypnotics have essentially the same mode of action as the barbiturates; that is, they depress the central nervous system. However, the miscellaneous sedatives and hypnotics have a lesser effect on the respiratory rate.

Effect of Barbiturates on Sleep

Sleep occurs in four stages. People experience varying degrees of wakefulness followed by deeper sleep throughout the sleep cycle. These stages fall into two areas: rapid eye movement (REM) sleep and nonrapid eye movement sleep. Nonrapid eye movement sleep occurs mostly in the early hours of sleep; REM sleep tends to lengthen progressively during the later sleep period.

Dreaming occurs mostly during REM sleep. Dreams appear to be a necessary part of sleep, and when an individual is deprived of dreaming for a prolonged period, a psychosis can develop. Sleep induced by a barbiturate involves reduced time in the REM stage (the dreaming stage) of sleep. Abrupt discontinuation of a barbiturate can cause increased dreaming, nightmares, or insomnia.

FACT CHECK

7-1   What is the difference between a sedative and a hypnotic?
7-2   What groups are the barbiturates divided into and what is the duration of action for each of the groups?
7-3   What is the mode of action for the barbiturates?

FACTS ABOUT . . .

Insomnia

- Insomnia affects 1 in 3 adults occasionally and 1 in 10 adults chronically.
- Insomnia's main symptom—trouble falling and/or staying asleep—leads to a lack of sleep that can cause other symptoms, such as trouble focusing, anxiety, depression, and irritability.
- Insomnia may affect an individual's daily activities and cause serious problems. For example, driving while drowsy leads to more than 100,000 car crashes annually, and insomnia raises the risk of falling for older women.
- The lifestyle changes listed below may help:
  - Avoid substances that worsen insomnia— for example, caffeine, tobacco, and other stimulants taken too close to bedtime; over-the-counter and prescription drugs that can disrupt sleep; and alcohol.
  - Avoid heavy meals and don't drink a lot before bedtime.
  - Exercise at least 5 to 6 hours before going to bed.
  - Establish a bedtime routine that helps you relax, making it easier to fall asleep.
  - Make your bedroom sleep-friendly—for example, avoid bright lighting, limit use of TV or computers, and keep the temperature cool and the room dark and quiet.
  - Go to sleep around the same time each night and wake up the same time each morning.
  - If possible, avoid night shifts, alternating schedules, or other things that may disrupt your sleep schedule.

Source: National Heart Lung and Blood Institute of the National Institutes of Health

Uses of Sedatives and Hypnotics

Sedatives and hypnotics are primarily used to treat insomnia.

Helping hospitalized patients sleep is an important part of the management of illness. Hospitalized patients are in unfamiliar surroundings unlike their home situation. Noises and lights at night often interfere with or interrupt their sleep. Because sleep deprivation can interfere with the healing process, a hypnotic may be given. These drugs also may be prescribed for short-term use after discharge from the hospital.

Zaleplon, a miscellaneous sedative, is a prescription sleep preparation a patient can take later in the night if at least 4 hours remain before the patient will become active again. With zaleplon, the patient will fall asleep quickly and wake up with little or no aftereffects of the drug.

A hypnotic may be given the night before an operation to prepare the patient for surgery. On the day of surgery, a barbiturate or miscellaneous sedative and hypnotic may be used either alone or with other drugs as part of the preoperative regimen. The anesthesiologist or surgeon selects a drug tailored to the patient's needs. When a barbiturate or miscellaneous sedative and hypnotic are used as a hypnotic, a dose larger than that required to produce sedation is given.

Adverse Reactions of Sedatives and Hypnotics

Adverse reactions associated with the use of barbiturates include

- Central nervous system symptoms: somnolence, agitation, confusion, central nervous system depression, **ataxia** (unsteady gait), nightmares, lethargy, residual sedation (drug hangover), hallucinations, paradoxical excitement

CONSIDERATIONS | Older adults

LIFESPAN

Sedatives and Hypnotics

Elderly patients may require a smaller hypnotic dose. In some instances, a sedative dose produces sleep.

Although barbiturates and miscellaneous sedatives and hypnotics used for sedation have largely been replaced by the antianxiety drugs (see following section), they occasionally may be used to provide sedation before certain types of procedures, such as cardiac catheterization or the administration of a local or general anesthesia. Sedative doses, usually given during daytime hours, may be used to treat anxiety and apprehension. Patients with chronic disease may require sedation to reduce anxiety and as an adjunct in the treatment of their disease.

In addition, some barbiturates are used as anticonvulsants (see Chapter 5).

CONSIDERATIONS | Older adults

LIFESPAN

Adverse Effects of Sedatives and Hypnotics

Older adults are at greater risk for oversedation, dizziness, confusion, or ataxia (unsteady gait) when taking a sedative or hypnotic. If oversedation, extreme dizziness, or ataxia occurs, then the health care provider is notified.

Contraindications, Precautions, and Interactions of Sedatives and Hypnotics

- These drugs are contraindicated in patients with known hypersensitivity to sedatives or hypnotics.
- They are not administered to comatose patients, those with severe respiratory problems, those with a history of drug and alcohol abuse, or lactating women.
- These drugs are given with great caution to patients with liver or kidney disease because their diseased organs will not be able to detoxify or eliminate the drug, and a drug buildup will occur.
- Barbiturates should be administered only with extreme caution to patients with a history of drug abuse (e.g., alcoholics and opiate abusers) or mental illness. If the drugs are prescribed to an outpatient, then the amount dispensed is limited to the amount needed until the next appointment.
- These drugs should be used with great caution during lactation. Drowsiness in infants of breast-feeding mothers who have taken the barbiturates has been reported.
- Sedatives and hypnotics have an additive effect when administered with alcohol, antidepressants, narcotic analgesics, antihistamines, or phenothiazines.

- Respiratory symptoms: hypoventilation, apnea, respiratory depression, bronchospasm, laryngospasm
- Gastrointestinal symptoms: nausea, vomiting, constipation, diarrhea, epigastric pain
- Cardiovascular symptoms: bradycardia, hypotension, syncope
- Hypersensitivity symptoms: rash, angioneurotic edema, fever, urticaria (skin rash)
- Other: headache and liver damage.

Adverse reactions associated with the use of the miscellaneous sedatives and hypnotics vary depending on the drug used. Common adverse reactions include dizziness, drowsiness, headache, and nausea.

FACT CHECK

7-4 What are the parameters for dosing zaleplon?
7-5 Older adults are at a greater risk to experience which adverse effects when taking a sedative or hypnotic?

ALERT Rx

Hypnotics and Drug Hangover

Excessive drowsiness and headache the morning after a hypnotic has been given (drug hangover) may occur in some patients. This problem should be reported to the health care provider because a smaller dose or a different drug may be necessary. The patient should be assisted when walking if necessary. When getting out of bed, the patient is encouraged to rise to a sitting position first, wait a few minutes, and then rise to a standing position.

ALERT Rx

Barbiturate Toxicity

The onset of symptoms of barbiturate toxicity may occur several hours after the drug is administered. Symptoms of acute toxicity include central nervous system and respiratory depression, constriction or paralytic dilation of the pupils, tachycardia, hypotension, lowered body temperature, oliguria (scanty urine production), circulatory collapse, and coma. Any symptoms of toxicity should be reported to the health care provider immediately. The treatment of barbiturate toxicity is mainly supportive and involves maintaining a patent airway, giving oxygen if needed, and monitoring the patient's vital signs and fluid balance. The patient may require treatment for shock, respiratory assistance, administration of activated charcoal, and, in severe cases of toxicity, hemodialysis.

Patient Management Issues with Sedatives and Hypnotics

Before a barbiturate or miscellaneous sedative and hypnotic are given, the patient's blood pressure, pulse, and respiratory rate are checked and recorded. In addition, the following patient needs are assessed:

- Is the patient uncomfortable? If the reason for discomfort is pain, then an analgesic, rather than a hypnotic, may be required.
- Is it too early for the patient to receive the drug? Is a later hour preferred?
- Does the patient receive a narcotic analgesic every 4 to 6 hours? A hypnotic may not be necessary because a narcotic analgesic can also cause drowsiness and sleep.
- Are there disturbances in the environment that may keep the patient awake and decrease the effectiveness of the drug?

Barbiturates have little or no analgesic action and are not used if the patient cannot sleep because of pain. Barbiturates given to a patient with pain may cause restlessness, excitement, and delirium.

After the drug is first used, the patient is checked for response. Did it help the patient sleep? If not, then a different drug or dose may be needed, and the health care provider should be informed about the drug's ineffectiveness. In addition, it is important to determine if any factors such as noise, lights, pain, or discomfort are interfering with the patient's sleep and whether these can be controlled or eliminated.

If the patient has an order for a PRN (as needed) narcotic analgesic or other central nervous system depressant and a hypnotic, then the health care provider must specify the time interval between administration of these drugs. Usually, at least 2 hours should elapse between administration of a hypnotic and any other central nervous system, but this interval may vary, depending on factors such as the patient's age and diagnosis.

Enhancing Sleep Patterns

To promote the effects of the sedative or hypnotic, the patient should be given supportive care, such as back rubs, night lights or a darkened room, and a quiet atmosphere. The patient is discouraged from drinking beverages containing caffeine, such as coffee, tea, or cola drinks, which can contribute to wakefulness.

Managing Drug Dependency

Sedatives and hypnotics are not usually given longer than 2 weeks and are given preferably for a shorter time. Barbiturates and miscellaneous sedatives and hypnotics can cause drug dependency. The drug should not be suddenly discontinued when there is a question of possible dependency. Patients who have been taking a sedative or hypnotic for several weeks are gradually withdrawn from the drug to prevent withdrawal symptoms. Symptoms of withdrawal include restlessness, excitement, euphoria, and confusion. Withdrawal can have serious consequences, especially in those with existing diseases or disorders.

Educating the Patient and Family about Sedatives and Hypnotics

Sedatives and hypnotics are subject to abuse by outpatients. The most common abuses are increasing the dose of the drug and drinking an alcohol beverage soon before, with, or soon after taking the sedative or hypnotic.

Because sedatives and hypnotics can become less effective after they are taken for a period of time, patients may be tempted to increase the dose without consulting their health care provider. The importance of not increasing or decreasing the dose unless a change in dosage is recommended by the health care provider should be emphasized. In addition, the dose should not be repeated during the night if sleep is interrupted or sleep only lasts a few hours, unless the health care provider has approved taking the drug more than once per night.

Alcohol is a central nervous system depressant, as are sedatives and hypnotics. When alcohol and a sedative or hypnotic are taken together, because of the additive effect there is an increase in central nervous system depression, which has sometimes resulted in death. Patients must understand the importance of not drinking alcohol while taking this drug because of the serious effects.

Following are key points that the patient or family members should know about sedatives and hypnotics.

- Do not drink any alcoholic beverage 2 hours before, with, or 8 hours after taking the drug.
- If the drug seems ineffective, contact your health care provider. Do not increase the dose unless advised to do so by your health care provider.
- Notify your health care provider if any adverse drug reactions occur.
- When taking the drug as a sedative, be aware that the drug can impair your mental and physical abilities required for performing potentially dangerous tasks, such as driving a car or operating machinery.
- Be careful when getting out of bed at night after taking a drug for sleep. Keep the room dimly lit and remove any obstacles that may result in injury when getting out of bed. Never attempt to drive or perform any hazardous task after taking a drug intended to produce sleep.
- Do not use these drugs if you are pregnant, considering becoming pregnant, or breast-feeding.
- Do not use over-the-counter cold, cough, or allergy drugs while taking this drug unless your health care provider approves their use. Some of these products contain antihistamines or other drugs that may also cause mild to extreme drowsiness. Others may contain an adrenergic drug, which is a mild stimulant and will therefore defeat the purpose of the prescribed drug.

Zaleplon

- Zaleplon may be taken at bedtime or later in the night if you have at least 4 hours of bedtime left. You will still wake up naturally without excessive drowsiness in the morning.
- Do not take zaleplon with a high-fat meal or snack because fat interferes with absorption of the drug.

FACT CHECK

7-6   A patient taking a sedative or hypnotic should be warned to avoid combining the drug with which other drugs?

7-7   What are the dosing parameters for a patient taking a sedative or hypnotic and a narcotic analgesic or other CNS depressant?

7-8   What complementary and alternative medication is available over the counter as a sedative?

Antianxiety Drugs

Anxiety is a feeling of apprehension, worry, or uneasiness that may or may not be based on reality. Anxiety may occur in many types of situations, ranging from chronic anxiety related to one's job to acute anxiety that may occur during withdrawal from alcohol. Although it is normal for most people to feel some anxiety, excess anxiety interferes with day-to-day functioning and can cause undue stress. Drugs used to treat anxiety are called **antianxiety drugs**, or **anxiolytics**.

Antianxiety drugs include the benzodiazepines and the nonbenzodiazepines. Examples of the benzodiazepines are alprazolam (Xanax), chlordiazepoxide (Librium), diazepam (Valium), and lorazepam (Ativan). All benzodiazepines are classified as schedule IV controlled substances (see Chapter 1). Nonbenzodiazepines that are useful as antianxiety drugs are buspirone (BuSpar), hydroxyzine (Vistaril), and zolpidem (Ambien).

Actions of Antianxiety Drugs

The exact mechanism of action of antianxiety drugs is not fully understood. The benzodiazepines are thought to exert their tranquilizing effect by potentiating the effects of γ-aminobutyric acid, an inhibitory transmitter, by binding to the specific benzodiazepine receptor sites. Nonbenzodiazepines exert their action in various other ways. For example, buspirone is thought to act on the brain's dopamine and serotonin receptors. Hydroxyzine produces its antianxiety effect by acting on the hypothalamus and brain stem reticular formation.

Uses of Antianxiety Drugs

Antianxiety drugs are used in the management of anxiety disorders and for short-term treatment of the symptoms of anxiety. Long-term use of these drugs is usually not recommended because prolonged therapy can result in drug dependence and serious withdrawal symptoms.

Some of these drugs have additional uses as sedatives, muscle relaxants, or anticonvulsants and in the treatment of alcohol withdrawal. For example, clorazepate (Tranxene) and diazepam (Valium) are used as anticonvulsants (see Chapter 5).

Lorazepam and oxazepam are relatively safe for older adults when given in normal dosages. Buspirone (BuSpar) also is a safe choice for older adults with anxiety because it does not cause excessive sedation, and there is less risk of falling. Buspirone, unlike most of the benzodiazepines, must be taken regularly and is not effective on an as-needed basis.

Adverse Reactions of Antianxiety Drugs

Transient, mild drowsiness commonly occurs during the first few days of treatment with antianxiety drugs. It is rare to have to discontinue therapy, however, because of the undesirable effects of the antianxiety agent. Depending on the severity of the patient's anxiety or other circumstances, it may be desirable to allow some degree of sedation to occur during early therapy. Other adverse reactions include lethargy, apathy, fatigue, disorientation, anger, restlessness, constipation, diarrhea, dry mouth, nausea, visual disturbances, and incontinence. Some adverse reactions occur only when higher dosages are used.

The long-term use of antianxiety drugs may result in **addiction** (physical drug dependence) and **tolerance** (increasingly larger dosages required to obtain the desired effect). The withdrawal syndrome may occur after as little as 4 to 6 weeks of therapy with a benzodiazepine. The withdrawal syndrome is more likely to occur when the benzodiazepine is taken for 3 months or more and is abruptly discontinued. Antianxiety drugs must never be discontinued abruptly because withdrawal symptoms, which can be extremely severe, may occur. Withdrawal symptoms usually begin within 1 to 10 days after discontinuing the drug, and last from 5 days to 1 month. Symptoms of withdrawal are listed in the Signs and Symptoms box.

When discontinuing the use of an antianxiety drug in patients who have used the drug for a prolonged period, the health care provider prescribes a decreasing dosage gradually for a period of 4 to 8 weeks to prevent withdrawal symptoms.

Some antianxiety drugs, such as buspirone (BuSpar), seem to have less abuse potential and less effect on motor ability and cognition than do other antianxiety drugs.

Contraindications, Precautions, and Interactions of Antianxiety Drugs

- Antianxiety drugs are contraindicated in patients with a known hypersensitivity, psychoses, acute narrow-angle glaucoma, or shock, as well as in patients in a coma or with acute alcoholic intoxication and depressed vital signs.
- The benzodiazepines are contraindicated during labor because of reports of floppy infant syndrome manifested by sucking difficulties, lethargy, and hypotonia. Lactating women should also avoid the benzodiazepines because of the effect on the infant, who becomes lethargic and loses weight.
- Antianxiety drugs are used cautiously in patients with impaired liver or kidney function and in elderly and debilitated patients. The metabolism of the benzodiazepines is slowed in the liver, increasing the risk of benzodiazepine toxicity. Lorazepam and oxazepam are the only benzodiazepines whose elimination is not significantly affected by liver metabolism.
- Central nervous system depressants, such as alcohol, narcotic analgesics, tricyclic antidepressants (see next section), and antipsychotic drugs (see later section), increase the sedative effects of antianxiety drugs. Combining any of these drugs with an antianxiety drug is dangerous and can cause serious respiratory depression and profound sedation.
- Drinking alcohol with an antianxiety drug can cause convulsions and coma.

ALERT Rx

Benzodiazepine Toxicity

Although rare, benzodiazepine toxicity may occur with an overdose of the drug. Benzodiazepine toxicity causes sedation, respiratory depression, and coma. Flumazenil (Romazicon) is an antidote (antagonist) for benzodiazepine toxicity and acts to reverse the sedation, respiratory depression, and coma within 6 to 10 minutes after intravenous administration. The adverse reactions of flumazenil include agitation, confusion, seizures, and, in some cases, symptoms of benzodiazepine withdrawal. The adverse reactions of flumazenil related to the symptoms of benzodiazepine withdrawal are relieved by the administration of the benzodiazepine.

- Buspirone causes less additive central nervous system depression than other antianxiety drugs but should still be avoided with concurrent of a central nervous system depressant. Buspirone may increase serum digoxin levels, increasing the risk of digitalis toxicity.

Patient Management Issues with Antianxiety Drugs

Both outpatients and hospitalized patients may receive antianxiety drugs. Before starting therapy, a complete medical history is obtained, including the patient's mental status and anxiety level. When severe anxiety is present, the history should be obtained from a family member or friend. The patient is observed for behavioral symptoms indicating anxiety, such as extreme restlessness, facial grimaces, and a tense posture. The physiologic manifestations of anxiety include increased blood pressure and pulse rate, increased rate and depth of respiration, and increased muscle tension. An anxious patient generally has cool, pale skin.

In addition, if possible, a history of any past drug or alcohol abuse should be obtained. Individuals with a history of previous abuse are more likely to abuse other drugs such as an antianxiety drug.

The patient's mental status and anxiety level should be periodically monitored during therapy to check for improvement or worsening of the behavioral and physical symptoms identified before the drug therapy was begun.

The patient is also monitored for adverse reactions. The sedation and drowsiness that sometimes occur with an antianxiety drug may decrease as therapy continues. Prolonged therapy (more than 3–4 months) may lead to dependence.

Antianxiety drugs are not recommended for long-term use. When the antianxiety drugs are used for short periods (1–2 weeks), tolerance, dependence, or withdrawal symptoms usually do not develop. Any signs of tolerance or dependence must be reported, such as the patient requesting larger doses of drug or increased anxiety and agitation (see Signs and Symptoms box).

Oral antianxiety drugs may be taken with food or meals to decrease the possibility of gastrointestinal upset. Some patients have difficulty swallowing the drug (because of a dry mouth, a common adverse effect, or other causes). The patient

SIGNS SYMPTOMS

Symptoms of Withdrawal from Antianxiety Drugs

Increased anxiety	Numbness in the extremities
Fatigue	Nausea
Hypersomnia	Sweating
Metallic taste	Muscle tension and cramps
Concentration difficulties	Psychoses
Fatigue	Hallucinations
Headache	Memory impairment
Tremors	Convulsions (possible)

may chew sugarless gum, suck on hard candy, or take frequent sips of water to reduce the discomfort of dry mouth.

Educating the Patient and Family about Antianxiety Drugs

Adverse reactions that may occur with a specific antianxiety drug should be explained to the patient, who should be encouraged to contact the health care provider immediately if a serious drug reaction occurs. Following are key points the patient or family members should know about antianxiety drugs.

- Take the drug exactly as directed. Do not increase, decrease, or omit a dose or stop taking this drug unless directed to do so by your health care provider.
- Do not stop using the drug abruptly because withdrawal symptoms may occur.
- Do not drive or perform other hazardous tasks if you feel drowsy.
- Do not take any nonprescription drug unless it has been approved by your health care provider.
- Inform physicians, dentists, and other health care providers of your therapy with this drug.
- Do not drink alcoholic beverages unless your health care provider approves.
- If you feel dizzy when changing position, rise slowly when getting out of bed or a chair. For severe dizziness, always ask for help when changing positions.
- If you experience dry mouth, take frequent sips of water, suck on hard candy, or chew gum (preferably sugarless).
- If you experience constipation, eat foods high in fiber, increase your fluid intake, and exercise if your condition permits.
- Keep all appointments with your health care provider because close monitoring of therapy is essential.
- Report any unusual changes or physical effects to your health care provider.

FACT CHECK

7-9   Why is long-term therapy with the benzodiazepines not recommended?

7-10   What are some other uses of antianxiety drugs?

7-11   Which of the antianxiety drugs is the least addictive?

7-12   How is buspirone different from most of the benzodiazepines?

Antidepressants

Depression is one of the most common psychiatric disorders. It is characterized by feelings of intense sadness, helplessness, worthlessness, and impaired functioning. Those experiencing a major depressive episode exhibit physical and psychological symptoms, such as appetite disturbances, sleep disturbances, and diminished interest in their job, family, and other activities they usually enjoy. A major depressive episode is a depressed or **dysphoric** (extreme or exaggerated sadness, anxiety, or unhappiness) mood that interferes with daily functioning and includes five or more of the following symptoms:

- Depressed mood
- Diminished interest in life activities
- Significant weight loss or gain (without dieting)
- Insomnia (inability to sleep) or hypersomnia (excessive sleeping)
- Fatigue or loss of energy
- Feelings of worthlessness
- Excessive or inappropriate guilt feelings
- Diminished ability to think or concentrate or indecisiveness
- Recurrent thoughts on death or suicide (or suicide attempt)

A patient is said to have major depression if his or her symptoms occur daily or nearly every day for a period of 2 weeks or more. A normal bereavement over the loss of a loved one or the effects of a disease such as hypothyroidism are not classified as major depression.

Depression is treated with the use of **antidepressant drugs**. Psychotherapy is often also used with antidepressant drugs to treat major depressive episodes. The four types of antidepressants are

- Tricyclic antidepressants (TCAs)
- Monoamine oxidase inhibitors (MAOIs)
- Selective serotonin reuptake inhibitors (SSRIs)
- Miscellaneous, unrelated drugs

Actions of Antidepressants

It was previously thought that antidepressants blocked the reuptake of the neurohormones, norepinephrine and serotonin,

FACTS ABOUT . . .

Major Depressive Disorder

- Major depressive disorder is the leading cause of disability in the United States for individuals aged 15 to 44.
- It affects approximately 14.8 million American adults, or about 6.7% of the U.S. population aged 18 and older in a given year.
- While this disorder can develop at any age, the median age at onset is 32.
- Major depressive disorder is more prevalent in women than in men.

Source: National Institute of Mental Health

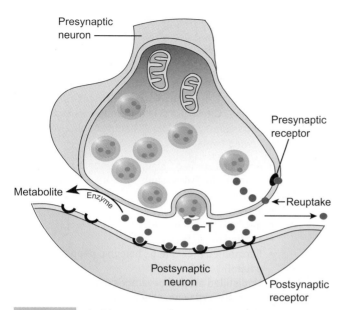

FIGURE 7-1 Antidepressant drugs inhibit the reuptake of the neutotransmitter (T), thus making it available to the postsynaptic neuron.

thereby stimulating the central nervous system. Although their exact action is unknown, this theory is now being questioned. New research indicates that the antidepressants cause changes in the brain's receptors for norepinephrine and serotonin and normalize neurotransmission activity (Fig. 7-1).

The TCAs, for example, amitriptyline (Elavil) and doxepin, inhibit reuptake of norepinephrine or serotonin at the presynaptic neuron. Drugs classified as MAOIs inhibit the activity of monoamine oxidase, resulting in an increase in the **endogenous** (made within the body) neurohormones epinephrine, norepinephrine, and serotonin in the nervous system. This increase stimulates the central nervous system. The action of the SSRIs is linked to their inhibition of neuronal uptake of the central nervous system neurotransmitter serotonin. The increase in serotonin levels is thought to act as a stimulant to reverse depression.

The mechanism of action of most of the miscellaneous antidepressants is not clearly understood.

FACT CHECK

7-13 What are the characteristics of depression?
7-14 What are the four types of antidepressants?

Uses of Antidepressants

Antidepressants are used to manage major depression or depression accompanied by anxiety. The SSRIs also are used to treat obsessive–compulsive disorders. Treatment is usually continued for 9 months after recovery from the first major depressive episode. If the patient later has another major depressive episode, then treatment is continued up to 5 years. If a third episode occurs, then treatment is continued indefinitely.

Adverse Reactions of Antidepressants

Adverse Reactions of Tricyclic Antidepressants

The tricyclics cause anticholinergic effects (see Chapter 14) such as dry mouth, blurred vision, postural hypotension, urinary retention, and constipation. Sedation and dry mouth are the most common adverse reactions. With continued use, the patient develops tolerance to these effects. Orthostatic hypotension can result from the TCAs. **Orthostatic hypotension** is a decrease in blood pressure of 20 to 30 points when a person changes position, such as going from a lying position to a standing position, and may cause sudden dizziness. Mental confusion, lethargy, disorientation, rash, nausea, vomiting, visual disturbances, **photosensitivity** (abnormally heightened reactivity of the skin to sunlight), and nasal congestion also may occur. Sexual dysfunction may result from clomipramine.

Adverse Reactions of Monoamine Oxidase Inhibitors

Orthostatic hypotension is a common adverse reaction of MAOIs. Other common adverse reactions include dizziness, vertigo, nausea, constipation, dry mouth, diarrhea, headache, and overactivity.

Adverse Reactions of Selective Serotonin Reuptake Inhibitors

Common adverse reactions associated with SSRIs include headache, nervousness, dizziness, insomnia, nausea, vomiting, weight loss, sweating, rash, pharyngitis, and painful menstruation. Fluoxetine may cause headache, activation of mania or hypomania, insomnia, anxiety, nervousness, nausea, vomiting, and sexual dysfunction.

Adverse Reactions of Miscellaneous Antidepressants

Adverse reactions of bupropion include agitation, dry mouth, insomnia, headache, nausea, constipation, anorexia, weight loss, and seizures. Trazodone may cause drowsiness, skin disorders, anger, hostility, anemia, priapism, nausea, and vomiting.

FACT CHECK

7-15 What are antidepressants used to treat?
7-16 What adverse reaction is of concern in older men with prostatic enlargement?

Contraindications, Precautions, and Interactions of Antidepressants

Contraindications, Precautions, and Interactions of Tricyclic Antidepressants

- The TCAs are contraindicated in patients with known hypersensitivity to the drugs.
- Doxepin is contraindicated in patients with glaucoma or a tendency for urinary retention.
- The TCAs are not given within 14 days of using a MAOI, in patients with a recent myocardial infarction, or during pregnancy or lactation.
- Tricyclic antidepressants are contraindicated in patients scheduled to have a myelogram (x-ray of the spinal cord and associated nerves) in the next 48 hours or within 24 hours of having a myelogram.
- Tricyclic antidepressants are used cautiously in patients with hepatic or renal impairment, heart disease, angina, paroxysmal tachycardia, increased intraocular pressure, prostatic hypertrophy, or a history of seizures.
- Adverse drug interactions may occur with TCAs if the patient is also taking a MAOI, many antihypertensive drugs, dicumarol, the adrenergic drugs, or clonidine.

Contraindications, Precautions, and Interactions of MAOIs

- Monoamine oxidase inhibitor drugs are contraindicated in patients with known hypersensitivity to the drugs; in patients with liver and kidney disease, cerebrovascular disease, hypertension, and congestive heart failure; and in the elderly.
- These drugs are given cautiously to patients with impaired liver function, history of seizures, parkinsonian symptoms, diabetes, or hyperthyroidism.
- A serious hypertensive crisis (extremely high blood pressure) can occur if a patient taking a MAOI eats a food containing tyramine (an amino acid present in some foods) (see Key Concepts 7-1).
- Adverse drug interactions may occur with MAOIs if the patient is also taking an opiate drug, a thiazide diuretic, or adrenergic drug.
- Monoamine oxidase inhibitors should be discontinued several weeks before surgery because they can cause unpredictable reactions.

Contraindications, Precautions, and Interactions of SSRIs

- Selective serotonin reuptake inhibitors are contraindicated in patients with hypersensitivity to the drugs.
- Selective serotonin reuptake inhibitors are used cautiously in patients with diabetes mellitus, with impaired liver or kidney function, and during lactation.
- Adverse drug interactions may occur with SSRIs if the patient is also taking a MAOI, TCA, or St. John's wort.
- If sertraline is taken with a MAOI, then a potentially fatal reaction can occur.
- Sertraline blood levels are increased when administered with cimetidine.
- Fluoxetine is less effective in patients who smoke cigarettes.
- Fluoxetine is not given with lithium.

KEY CONCEPTS

7-1 Avoiding Drug–Food Interactions with MAOIs

Patients taking MAOIs must avoid foods containing tyramine. Otherwise a life-threatening hypertensive crisis may develop. Patients should avoid the following foods:

- Aged cheese (e.g., bleu, Camembert, cheddar, mozzarella, Parmesan)
- Sour cream
- Yogurt
- Beef or chicken livers
- Pickled herring
- Fermented meats (e.g., bologna, pepperoni, salami)
- Undistilled alcohol beverages (e.g., imported beer, ale, red wine, especially Chianti)
- Coffee
- Tea
- Colas containing caffeine
- Chocolate drinks
- Fruits and vegetables (avocado, dried beans, fava beans, figs, raisins and other dried fruit, raspberries, bananas)
- Sauerkraut
- Yeast extracts
- Soy sauce
- Chocolate

Contraindications, Precautions, and Interactions of Miscellaneous Antidepressants

- The miscellaneous antidepressant drugs are contraindicated in patients with known hypersensitivity to the drugs.
- These drugs are used cautiously in patients with liver or kidney impairment, taking alcohol or other central nervous system depressants, and during lactation.
- Adverse drug interactions may occur with buspirone if the patient is also taking fluoxetine, erythromycin, or itraconazole.
- Venlafaxine adversely reacts with MAOIs or cimetidine.
- Trazadone adversely reacts with the phenothiazines, carbamazepine, digoxin, or phenytoin.

Patient Management Issues with Antidepressants

Health care workers should be alert for any signs of suicidal thoughts in depressed patients. Any expressions of guilt, hopelessness, helplessness, insomnia, weight loss, and direct or indirect threats of suicide should be reported to the primary health care provider. It is also important for the patient's vital signs to be monitored and any changes reported. Some antidepressants cause excessive drowsiness initially, and patients may need help walking or caring for themselves.

The patient or a family member may mention an adverse drug reaction or other problem occurring during antidepressant therapy. These reactions or problems should be reported to the primary health care provider.

Patient Management Issues with Specific Antidepressants

- Tricyclic antidepressants may be administered in a single daily dose at night because sedative effects promote sleep and adverse reactions are less troublesome. Because protriptyline may produce a mild stimulation, it is usually not taken at bedtime.
- Monoamine oxidase inhibitors are not widely used because of their potential for serious adverse reactions. Patients receiving MAOIs require strict dietary control.
- Selective serotonin reuptake inhibitors can cause weight loss. The patient's dietary intake may need to be monitored.
- High doses of bupropion may cause seizure.
- Because trazodone may cause drowsiness or sedation, most of the dose is usually taken at bedtime. An uncommon but potentially serious adverse reaction of trazodone is priapism (a persistent erection of the penis); if not treated immediately, priapism can result in impotence.

Educating the Patient and Family about Antidepressants

Some outpatients may not take their antidepressant drug as prescribed. Family members may need to assist. Family members also need to know to report any adverse reaction that occurs. Following are key points about antidepressants the patient or family members should know.

- Take the drug exactly as directed. Do *not* increase, decrease, or omit a dose or discontinue this drug unless your health care provider directs.
- Do not drive or perform other hazardous tasks if you feel drowsy.
- Do not take any nonprescription drug unless your health care provider approves it.
- Inform other health care providers, your dentist, and other medical personnel that you are taking this drug.

- Do not drink alcoholic beverages without approval from your health care provider.
- If you feel dizzy when changing position, rise slowly when getting out of bed or a chair. If you feel very dizzy, get help when changing positions.
- Relieve dry mouth by taking frequent sips of water, sucking on hard candy, or chewing gum (preferably sugarless).
- Do not take the antidepressants during pregnancy. Notify your health care provider if you are pregnant or you wish to become pregnant.
- Report any unusual changes or physical effects to your health care provider.

FACT CHECK
7-17 Why are TCAs dosed at bedtime?
7-18 Why are MAOIs not widely used?
7-19 What is a natural remedy for depression?

Antipsychotic Drugs

Antipsychotic drugs, also called **neuroleptic drugs**, are given to patients with a psychotic disorder, such as schizophrenia. A **psychotic disorder** is characterized by extreme personality disorganization and the loss of contact with reality. The patient usually has hallucinations (a false perception having no basis in reality) or delusions (false beliefs that cannot be changed with reason). Other symptoms include disorganized speech, behavior disturbances, social withdrawal, flattened affect (reduced or absent emotional response to any situation or condition), and anhedonia (finding no pleasure in activities that are normally pleasurable).

Although lithium is not a true antipsychotic drug, it is considered here with the antipsychotics because of its use in regulating the severe fluctuations of the manic phase of **bipolar disorder** (a psychiatric disorder characterized by severe mood swings of extreme hyperactivity to depression). During the manic phase, the person experiences altered thought processes, which can lead to bizarre delusions. The drug diminishes the frequency and intensity of hyperactive (manic) episodes.

Actions of Antipsychotic Drugs

The exact mechanism of action of antipsychotic drugs is not well understood. These drugs are thought to act by inhibiting or blocking the release of the neurohormone dopamine in the brain and possibly increasing the firing of nerve cells in certain areas of the brain. These effects may suppress the symptoms of certain psychotic disorders. Examples of antipsychotic drugs include chlorpromazine, haloperidol (Haldol), and lithium. Lithium is an antimanic drug. Although its exact mechanism is unknown, it appears to alter sodium transport in nerve and muscle cells and inhibit the release of norepinephrine and dopamine. The Summary Drug Table: Antipsychotic Drugs gives a more complete listing of the antipsychotic drugs.

Uses of Antipsychotic Drugs

Antipsychotic drugs are used to manage acute and chronic psychoses. In addition to its antipsychotic properties, chlorpromazine is used to treat uncontrollable hiccoughs. Clozapine (Clozaril) is used only in patients with schizophrenia that is unresponsive to other antipsychotic drugs. Lithium is effective in the management of bipolar (manic–depressive) illness. Some of these drugs, such as chlorpromazine and prochlorperazine (Compazine), are also used as antiemetics (see Chapter 8). When given in small doses, neuroleptics effectively control acute agitation in the elderly.

Adverse Reactions of Antipsychotic Drugs

These drugs may result in a wide variety of adverse reactions, including sedation, hypotension, postural hypotension, dry mouth, nasal congestion, **photophobia** (an intolerance to light), urticaria, photosensitivity, behavioral changes, and headache. Photosensitivity can result in severe sunburn when patients taking antipsychotic drugs are exposed to the sun or ultraviolet light.

Behavioral changes may also occur with the use of antipsychotic drugs. These changes include an increase in the intensity of the psychotic symptoms, lethargy, hyperactivity, paranoid reactions, agitation, and confusion. A decreased dosage may eliminate some of these symptoms, but it also may be necessary to try another drug.

Three significant adverse reactions, extrapyramidal effects, tardive dyskinesia, and neuroleptic malignant syndrome, are described in the following sections.

Extrapyramidal Effects

Among the most significant adverse reactions of antipsychotic drugs are extrapyramidal effects. The term **extrapyramidal effects** refers to a group of adverse reactions occurring in the extrapyramidal portion of the nervous system. This part of the nervous system affects body posture and coordinates smooth and uninterrupted movement of various muscle groups. Antipsychotics disturb the function of the extrapyramidal portion of the nervous system, causing abnormal muscle movements. Extrapyramidal effects include three main sets of effects:

- Parkinson-like symptoms: fine tremors, muscle rigidity, a mask-like appearance of the face, slowness of movement, slurred speech, and unsteady gait
- **Akathisia**: extreme restlessness and increased motor activity
- **Dystonia**: facial grimacing and twisting of the neck into unnatural positions

Extrapyramidal effects usually diminish with a reduced dosage of the antipsychotic drug. The health care provider may also prescribe an antiparkinsonism drug, such as benztropine (see Chapter 6) to reduce the Parkinson-like symptoms.

Tardive Dyskinesia

Tardive dyskinesia is a syndrome consisting of potentially irreversible, involuntary dyskinetic movements. Tardive dyskinesia is characterized by rhythmic, involuntary movements of the tongue, face, mouth, or jaw, and sometimes the extremities. The patient's tongue may protrude, and the patient may make chewing movements, pucker the mouth, and grimace (Fig. 7-2). Tardive dyskinesia may occur in patients receiving an antipsychotic drug or after discontinuation of antipsychotic drug therapy. When symptoms of tardive dyskinesia occur during the course of therapy, the drug must be discontinued. Depending on the severity of the condition being treated, the health care provider may slowly taper the drug dose because abrupt discontinuation may result in a return of the psychotic symptoms. There is no known treatment for tardive dyskinesia, although partial or complete remission may occur if the antipsychotic drug is withdrawn. The risk of tardive dyskinesia and the likelihood that it will become irreversible increase as the duration of treatment and total cumulative dosage administered increase. The highest incidence of tardive

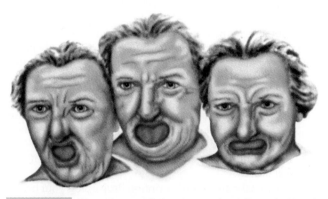

FIGURE 7-2 The characteristic signs of tardive dyskinesia include a protruding tongue, puckered mouth, and facial grimace.

ALERT Rx

Extrapyramidal Effects

The patient is observed for extrapyramidal effects, which include muscular spasms of the face and neck, an inability to sleep or sit still, tremors, rigidity, or involuntary rhythmic movements. The health care provider is notified of any of these symptoms because they may indicate a need for dosage adjustment.

ALERT Rx

Tardive Dyskinesia

Because there is no known treatment for tardive dyskinesia and because it is irreversible in some patients, its symptoms occurring in a patient must be immediately reported. These include rhythmic, involuntary movements of the tongue, face, mouth, jaw, or the extremities.

dyskinesia occurs in patients receiving an antiparkinson drug for extrapyramidal effects along with an antipsychotic drug. Although any patient taking an antipsychotic can experience tardive dyskinesia, elderly women are at highest risk.

Neuroleptic Malignant Syndrome

Neuroleptic malignant syndrome is a rare reaction characterized by a combination of extrapyramidal effects, hyperthermia, and autonomic disturbance. It may occur hours to months after the antipsychotic drug regimen is begun. Once neuroleptic malignant syndrome begins, it progresses rapidly during the next 24 to 72 hours. The syndrome most often occurs in patients taking haloperidol but has occurred also with thiothixene, thioridazine, and clozapine. Neuroleptic malignant syndrome is potentially fatal and requires intensive symptomatic treatment and immediate discontinuation of the causative drug.

Adverse Reactions of Lithium

Lithium carbonate is rapidly absorbed after oral administration. The most common adverse reactions include tremors, nausea, vomiting, thirst, and polyuria (frequent urination). Because some toxic reactions are potentially serious, the patient's lithium blood levels are usually measured during therapy, and the dosage adjusted accordingly.

Lithium toxicity can occur even when the drug is administered at therapeutic doses. Patients taking lithium are observed for signs of toxicity, such as diarrhea, vomiting, nausea, drowsiness, muscular weakness, and lack of coordination. For early symptoms, the health care provider may reduce the patient's dosage or discontinue the drug for 24 to 48 hours and then gradually restart the drug therapy at a lower dosage. Patients

receiving lithium often need more fluids. Fluids should be readily available to the patient, and extra fluids should be offered throughout waking hours.

Adverse Effects of Clozapine

This drug is available only through the Clozaril Patient Management System, a program involving white blood cell (WBC) testing, patient monitoring, and other services. Only 1 week of this drug is dispensed at a time. Patients taking clozapine have a higher risk of bone marrow suppression. A weekly WBC count is made throughout the period of therapy and for 4 weeks after its end. In addition, the patient is monitored for the symptoms of bone marrow suppression: lethargy, weakness, fever, sore throat, malaise, mucous membrane ulceration, or flu-like symptoms.

Contraindications, Precautions, and Interactions of Antipsychotic Drugs

- Antipsychotics are contraindicated in patients with a known hypersensitivity, in comatose patients, and in those who are severely depressed or have bone marrow depression, blood dyscrasias, Parkinson disease (haloperidol), liver impairment, coronary artery disease, or severe hypotension or hypertension.
- Lithium is contraindicated in patients who have hypersensitivity to tartrazine, renal or cardiovascular disease, sodium depletion, or dehydration, and in patients receiving diuretics. Lithium is contraindicated during lactation. Women of childbearing age may choose to use contraceptives while taking lithium.
- Antipsychotic drugs are used cautiously in patients exposed to extreme heat or phosphorous insecticides

ALERT Rx

Extreme Drowsiness

Antipsychotic drugs may cause extreme drowsiness and sedation, especially during the first or second weeks of therapy. This reaction may impair the patient's mental or physical abilities. Drowsiness usually diminishes after 2 to 3 weeks of therapy. However, if the patient continues to be troubled by drowsiness and sedation, a lower dosage may be used.

CONSIDERATIONS | Older adults

LIFESPAN

Lithium Toxicity

Older adults have an increased risk for toxicity because of a decreased rate of excretion. Lower dosages may be necessary to decrease the risk of toxicity.

and in those with respiratory disorders, glaucoma, prostatic hypertrophy, epilepsy, decreased renal function, lactation, or peptic ulcer.

- Antipsychotic drugs are used cautiously in elderly and debilitated patients because these patients are more sensitive to their effects.
- Lithium is used cautiously in patients in situations in which they may sweat profusely and in those who are suicidal, have diarrhea, or who have an infection or fever.
- Taking an antipsychotic drug with alcohol may result in additive central nervous system depression.
- Anticholinergics (see Chapter 14) may reduce the therapeutic effects of the antipsychotic, causing worsening of the psychotic symptoms and an increased risk of tardive dyskinesia.
- Clozapine acts synergistically with other drugs that suppress bone marrow, resulting in increased severity of bone marrow suppression.
- When lithium is administered with another antipsychotic drug, lithium renal clearance may be reduced, making a decreased dosage necessary to prevent lithium toxicity.
- Lithium may have decreased effectiveness when taken with antacids.
- When thiazide or loop diuretics are administered with lithium, serum lithium levels increase, resulting in a greater risk for lithium toxicity.

Patient Management Issues with Antipsychotic Drugs

A patient receiving an antipsychotic drug may be treated in the hospital or as an outpatient. The patient's mental status is assessed before and periodically throughout therapy. Any hallucinations or delusions are documented in the patient's record. Patients with psychosis often are unable to give a reliable history of their illness, and the psychiatric history is obtained from a family member or friend. The patient is observed for any behavior patterns that appear to be deviations from normal, such as poor eye contact, a failure to answer questions completely, inappropriate answers to questions, a monotone speech pattern, and inappropriate laughter, sadness, or crying.

Because antipsychotic drugs are often given for a long time, ongoing assessment is an important part of determining therapeutic drug effects and monitoring for adverse reactions, particularly extrapyramidal effects and tardive dyskinesia. Frequent assessments are necessary because dosage adjustments may be necessary during therapy. It is important to watch for the appearance of adverse drug effects because the patient may not be able to communicate physical changes to the health care provider.

Antipsychotic drugs may be given orally as a single daily dose or in divided doses several times per day. Divided daily doses are recommended when beginning drug therapy, but once-daily doses may be used with continued therapy. Taking the drug at bedtime helps to minimize the effects of postural hypotension and sedation.

Oral administration requires great care because some patients have difficulty swallowing (because of a dry mouth

or other causes). Other patients may refuse to take the drug. The patient should never be forced to take an oral drug. If the patient refuses the drug, then the health care provider is notified because parenteral administration of the drug may be necessary.

After giving an oral drug, the patient's mouth is checked to be sure the drug was swallowed.

Oral liquid concentrates are available for patients who can more easily swallow a liquid. These concentrates are light-sensitive and dispensed in amber or opaque bottles to help protect the concentrate. They are administered mixed in liquids such as fruit juices, tomato juice, milk, or carbonated beverages. Semisolid foods, such as soups or puddings, may also be used. Perphenazine (Trilafon) concentrate should not be mixed with beverages containing caffeine (coffee, cola), tea, or apple juice because of the risk of incompatibility.

When these drugs are given parenterally, the patient should remain lying down for approximately 30 minutes after the drug is given.

With outpatients, at each visit to the health care provider, the patient is observed for a response to therapy. Questions asked depend on the patient and the diagnosis and may include questions such as:

- How are you feeling?
- Do you seem to be less nervous?
- Would you like to tell me how everything is going?

The patient or a family member is asked about adverse drug reactions or any other problems occurring during therapy, which are reported to the health care provider.

Educating the Patient and Family about Antipsychotics

Noncompliance with the drug therapy is a problem with some patients after discharge. The administration of antipsychotic drugs becomes a family responsibility if the outpatient appears to be unable to manage his or her own drug therapy. Patients may need to tolerate some adverse reactions, such as dry mouth, episodes of orthostatic hypotension (feeling dizzy when standing), and drowsiness, because their drug therapy must continue. A patient experiencing extreme sedation may need help with eating, dressing, and walking. Extremely hyperactive patients may need protection from injury to themselves or others.

Any adverse reactions that may occur with a specific antipsychotic drug are explained to the patient and family, who are encouraged to contact the health care provider immediately if a serious drug reaction occurs. Following are key points the patient or family members should know about antipsychotic drugs.

- Keep all appointments with your health care provider because close monitoring of therapy is essential.
- Report any unusual changes or physical effects to your health care provider.
- Take the drug exactly as directed. Do not increase, decrease, or omit a dose or stop using this drug unless directed to do so by your health care provider.
- Do not drive or perform other hazardous tasks if you feel drowsy.

- Do not take any nonprescription drug unless the health care provider approves it.
- Inform physicians, dentists, and other medical personnel about your therapy with this drug.
- Do not drink alcoholic beverages without approval from your health care provider.
- If you become dizzy when changing position, rise slowly when getting out of bed or a chair. If the dizziness is severe, get help when changing positions.
- If you are bothered by dry mouth, relieve it by taking frequent sips of water, sucking on hard candy, or chewing gum (preferably sugarless).
- Notify your health care provider if you become pregnant or intend to become pregnant during therapy.
- Immediately report any of the following adverse reactions: restlessness, inability to sit still, muscle spasms, mask-like expression, rigidity, tremors, drooling, or involuntary rhythmic movements of the mouth, face, or extremities. Avoid exposure to the sun. If exposure is unavoidable, wear sunblock, keep your arms and legs covered, and wear a sun hat.
- Note that only a 1-week supply of clozapine is dispensed at a time. The drug is obtained through a special program designed to ensure the required blood monitoring. Weekly blood tests are required. Immediately report any signs of weakness, fever, sore throat, malaise, or flu-like symptoms to your health care provider.

- Note that olanzapine is available either as a tablet to swallow or in a form to be dissolved in the mouth. When using the dissolving tablet, peel back the foil on the blister. With dry hands, remove the tablet and place the entire tablet in your mouth. The tablet will disintegrate with or without liquid.
- Remember to take lithium with food or immediately after meals to avoid stomach upset. Drink at least 10 large glasses of fluid each day and add extra salt to food. Prolonged exposure to the sun may lead to dehydration. If any of the following symptoms occur, do not take the next dose but immediately notify your health care provider: diarrhea, vomiting, fever, tremors, drowsiness, lack of muscle coordination, or muscle weakness.

FACT CHECK

7-20 What are the characteristics of a psychotic disorder?

7-21 What is lithium used to treat?

7-22 What are three significant adverse reactions that patients and family members should be informed about before antipsychotic therapy is started?

Chapter Review

KEY POINTS

- Sedatives and hypnotics act on the central nervous system and are used primarily to treat insomnia. Common adverse reactions include drowsiness, dizziness, lethargy, headache, and nausea.
- Antianxiety drugs exert tranquilizing effects through various actions in the brain. They are used primarily to treat anxiety disorders and secondarily for specific purposes such as treatment of acute alcohol withdrawal. Common adverse reactions include drowsiness, sedation, confusion, dry mouth, depression, and nausea.
- Antidepressants act on the central nervous system and are used to treat depression. Common adverse reactions include sedation, dry mouth, nausea, orthostatic hypotension, and constipation.
- Antipsychotics have actions that are not perfectly known. Different antipsychotics are used to treat various psychotic disorders ranging from schizophrenia to manic–depressive disorder and other specific disorders, as well as some medical conditions. Common adverse effects include extrapyramidal symptoms, tardive dyskinesia, headache, and photosensitivity.
- Patient management and teaching for all these drugs focus on the need for strict dosage control and the management of common adverse reactions.

CRITICAL THINKING CASE STUDY

Depression

Mr. Hopkins has been severely depressed for several months. Two weeks ago, his physician prescribed amitriptyline 30 mg orally four times per day. His family is concerned because he is still depressed and wants to use some other medication. The physician decides to prescribe a higher dose of amitriptyline.

1. Mr. Hopkins will be more likely to experience which side effect?
   a. Tinnitus
   b. Dry mouth
   c. Insomnia
   d. Diarrhea
2. The family needs to be aware that Mr. Hopkins may experience sudden dizziness
   a. after eating
   b. if he misses a dose
   c. when getting out of bed
   d. from drinking too much water
3. What other adverse reactions should Mr. Hopkins and his family be watching for?

Insomnia

Ms. Wright is having trouble sleeping. Because her insomnia is interfering with her ability to work and enjoy life, she sees her physician, and he prescribes zolpidem.

4. Which of the following should Ms. Wright NOT take with her zolpidem?
   a. Oral contraceptive
   b. Blood pressure medication
   c. Narcotic analgesic
   d. Acetaminophen
5. Why not?
6. Unfortunately, Ms. Wright is able to fall asleep but keeps waking up during the night. She asks if you are aware of any medication that she could take during the night to help her go back to sleep. What would you say?

Review Questions

MULTIPLE CHOICE

1. Ms. Brown has arthritis in her lower back, and the pain keeps her awake at night. She asks if she can have a "sleeping pill." In considering her request, what must be taken into account?
   a. Barbiturates, if given in the presence of pain, may cause excitement or delirium.
   b. A hypnotic may be given instead of an analgesic to relieve her pain.
   c. Hypnotics often increase the pain threshold.
   d. A hypnotic plus an analgesic is best given in this situation.
2. When a hypnotic is given to Ms. Green, aged 82 years, it is important to know that
   a. elderly patients usually require larger doses of a hypnotic
   b. smaller doses of the drug are usually given to older patients
   c. older adults excrete the drug faster than do younger adults
   d. dosages of the hypnotic may be increased each night until the desired effect is achieved
3. Which adverse effects are common with antianxiety drugs?
   a. Skin rash, blurry vision
   b. Tinnitus, hypertension
   c. Anger, combativeness
   d. Sedation, lethargy
4. Which statement is true about long-term use of anti-anxiety drugs?
   a. Long-term use may result in dependence but not tolerance.
   b. Long-term use may result in tolerance but not dependence.
   c. Long-term use may result in both dependence and tolerance.
   d. Long-term use may result in neither dependence nor tolerance.
5. Antidepressant drugs are thought to work by changing the brain's receptor sites for
   a. histamine
   b. glucose
   c. leukocytes
   d. serotonin
6. A patient taking a monoamine oxidase inhibitor should not eat foods containing
   a. glutamine
   b. sugar
   c. tyramine
   d. large amounts of iron
7. Patient education related to taking antidepressant medications includes which of the following?
   a. Slowly increase your dose until all symptoms of depression are relieved.
   b. Avoid drinking too much water.
   c. Do not drink alcoholic beverages without approval from the health care provider.
   d. Avoid exercise during the first hour after taking any medication.
8. Which of the following reactions would be expected in a patient experiencing tardive dyskinesia?
   a. Muscle rigidity, dry mouth, insomnia
   b. Arrhythmic, involuntary movements of the tongue, face, mouth, or jaw
   c. Muscle weakness, paralysis of the eyelids, diarrhea
   d. Dyspnea, somnolence, muscle spasms
9. Which of the following symptoms would indicate that a patient taking lithium is experiencing toxicity?
   a. Constipation, abdominal cramps, rash
   b. Stupor, oliguria, hypertension
   c. Nausea, vomiting, diarrhea
   d. Dry mouth, blurred vision, difficulty swallowing
10. Antipsychotic drugs are likely to cause drug interactions with
    a. alcohol
    b. caffeine
    c. sugar
    d. tyramine

MATCHING

_____	11. alprazolam	a.	Ambien
_____	12. diazepam	b.	Halcion
_____	13. eszopiclone	c.	Lunesta
_____	14. hydroxyzine	d.	Sonata
_____	15. olanzapine	e.	Valium
_____	16. triazolam	f.	Vistaril
_____	17. zaleplon	g.	Xanax
_____	18. zolpidem	h.	Zyprexa

TRUE OR FALSE

_____ 19. The barbiturates are respiratory depressants, with the degree of depression usually depending on the dose given.

_____ 20. St. John's wort can be combined with a prescribed antidepressant to improve depression.

_____ 21. MAOIs are not widely used as antidepressants because of their potential for serious adverse reactions and numerous drug interactions.

_____ 22. When a patient is taking an antipsychotic, the person administering the medication should check the patient's mouth to make sure the drug was actually swallowed.

FILL IN THE BLANKS

23. Sedatives and hypnotics are typically not given for longer than 2 weeks because they can cause

    _____.

24. _____ is a feeling of apprehension, worry, or uneasiness that may or may not be based on reality.

25. _____ is characterized by feelings of intense sadness, helplessness, worthlessness, and impaired functioning.

26. A _____ _____ is characterized by extreme personality disorganization and the loss of contact with reality.

SHORT ANSWERS

27. What foods should be avoided in patients taking an MAOI?

28. Why should sedatives and hypnotics be used with caution in the elderly?

29. Which anxiolytic is a safe choice for older adults? Why?

30. The antipsychotics have some very disruptive adverse reactions. List the three significant adverse reactions. For each reaction, include the signs to watch for that would indicate the patient is experiencing the adverse reaction.

Web Activities

1. Go to the CDC Web site (*http://www.cdc.gov*) and research sleep hygiene tips.
   a. What are the sleep hygiene tips for adults?
   b. What are the sleep hygiene tips for adolescents?
2. Go to the National Institute of Mental Health Web site (*http://www.nimh.nih.gov*). Research depression. How are depressions experienced differently between men, women, elderly, and adolescents?

SUMMARY DRUG TABLE: Antianxiety Drugs (left, generic; right, trade)

Comprehensive Summary Drug Tables, including uses, adverses effects, dosages, and pregnancy classifications, are provided on the companion website, http://thePoint.lww.com/PharmacologyHP2e

Benzodiazepines	
alprazolam *al-prah-zoe-lam*	Xanax (CIV), Xanax XR, *generic*
chlordiazepoxide *klor-dye-az-e-pox'-ide*	Librium (CIV), *generic*
clorazepate *klor-az'-eh-pate*	Tranxene-SD (CIV), Tranxene-T, *generic*
diazepam *dye-az'-e-pam*	Valium (CIV), *generic*
lorazepam *lor-a'-ze-pam*	Ativan (CIV), *generic*
oxazepam *ox-a'-ze-pam*	*generic* (CIV)
Nonbenzodiazepine	
buspirone hydrochloride *byoo-spye-rone*	*generic*
hydroxyzine *high-drox'-ih-zeen*	Vistaril, *generic*
meprobamate *me-pro-ba'-mate*	*generic* (CIV)

SUMMARY DRUG TABLE: Antipsychotic Drugs (left, generic; right, trade)

Comprehensive Summary Drug Tables, including uses, adverses effects, dosages, and pregnancy classifications, are provided on the companion website, http://thePoint.lww.com/PharmacologyHP2e

asenapine *a-sen'-a-peen*	Saphris
chlorpromazine HCL *klor-proe'-ma-zeen*	*generic*
clozapine *kloe'-za-peen*	Clozaril, FazaClo, *generic*
fluphenazine *floo-fen'-a-zeen*	*generic*
haloperidol *ha-loe-per'-i-dole*	Haldol, *generic*
lithium *lith'-ee-um*	Lithobid, *generic*
loxapine *lox'-a-peen*	Loxitane, *generic*
olanzapine *oh-lan'-za-peen*	Zyprexa
perphenazine *per-fen'-a-zeen*	*generic*
pimozide *pi'-moe-zide*	Orap
prochlorperazine *proe-klor-per'-a-zeen*	*generic*
quetiapine fumarate *kwe-tie'-ah-pine*	Seroquel, Seroquel XR
risperidone *ris-per'-i-done*	Risperdal, *generic*
thioridazine *thye-oh-rid'-a-zeen*	*generic*
trifluoperazine HCL *try-floo-oh-per'-a-zeen*	*generic*
ziprasidone HCL *zih-pray'-sih-dohn*	Geodon

SUMMARY DRUG TABLE: Sedatives and Hypnotics
(left, generic; right, trade)

Comprehensive Summary Drug Tables, including uses, adverses effects, dosages, and pregnancy classifications, are provided on the companion website, http:// thePoint.lww.com/PharmacologyHP2e

Barbiturates	
amobarbital sodium *am-oh-bar'-bi-tal*	Amytal sodium (CII)
butabarbital *byoo-ta-bar'-bi-tal*	Butisol sodium (CIII)
mephobarbital *me-foe-bar'-bi-tal*	Mebaral (CIV), *generic*
pentobarbital sodium *pen-toe-bar'-bi-tal*	Nembutal (CII)
phenobarbital *fee-noe-bar'-bi-tal*	Luminal (CIV), *generic*
secobarbital sodium *see-koe-bar'-bi-tal*	*Seconal* (CII)

Miscellaneous Sedatives and Hypnotics	
chloral hydrate *klor-al hye'-drate*	Somnote (CIV), *generic*
dexmedetomidine HCL *dex-meh-dih- toe'- mih-deen*	Precedex
eszopiclone *es-zoe-pik'-lone*	Lunesta (CIV)
zaleplon	Sonata (CIV)
zolpidem tartrate *zol'-pih-dem*	Ambien (CIV), Ambien CR, *generic*

Benzodiazepines	
estazolam *es-taz'-e-lam*	*generic* (CIV)
flurazepam *flur-az'-e-pam*	Dalmane (CIV), *generic*
quazepam *kwa'-ze-pam*	Doral (CIV)
temazepam *te-maz'-e-pam*	Restoril (CIV), *generic*
triazolam *trye-ay'-zoe-lam*	Halcion (CIV), *generic*

SUMMARY DRUG TABLE: Antidepressants
(left, generic; right, trade)

Comprehensive Summary Drug Tables, including uses, adverses effects, dosages, and pregnancy classifications, are provided on the companion website, http:// thePoint.lww.com/PharmacologyHP2e

Tricyclics	
amitriptyline *am-ee-trip'-ti-leen*	*generic*
amoxapine *a-mox'-a-peen*	*generic*
clomipramine *kloe-mi'-pra-meen*	Anafranil, *generic*
desipramine *dess-ip'-ra-meen*	Norpramin, *generic*
doxepin *dox'-e-pin*	Silenor, *generic*
imipramine *im-ip'-ra-meen*	Tofranil, Tofranil-PM, *generic*
nortriptyline *nor-trip'-ti-leen*	Pamelor, *generic*
protriptyline *proe-trip'-ti-leen*	Vivactil, *generic*
trimipramine *trye-mi'-pra-meen*	Surmontil

Monoamine Oxidase Inhibitors	
isocarboxazid *eye-soe-kar-boks'-a-zid*	Marplan
phenelzine *fen'-el-zeen*	Nardil
tranylcypromine *tran-ill-sip'-roe meen*	Parnate, *generic*

Selective Serotonin Reuptake Inhibitors	
citalopram *si-tal'-oh-pram*	Celexa, *generic*
escitalopram *es-sye-tal'-oh-pram*	Lexapro
fluoxetine *floo-ox'-e-teen*	Prozac, Prozac Weekly, Sarafem, Selfemra, *generic*
fluvoxamine *floo-voks'-a-meen*	Luvox CR, *generic*
paroxetine *par-ox'-e-teen*	Paxil, Paxil CR, *generic*
sertraline *sir'-trah-leen*	Zoloft, *generic*

Miscellaneous Antidepressants	
bupropion HCL *byoo-proe'-pee-on*	Wellbutrin, Wellbutrin SR, Wellbutrin XL, *generic* Zyban (smoking cessation), *generic*
Maprotiline *map-roe'-ti-leen*	*generic*
mirtazapine *mer-tah'-zah-peen*	Remeron, *generic*
nefazodone *ne-faz'-oh-done*	*generic*
trazodone *traz'-oh-done*	*generic*
venlafaxine *ven-la-fax'-een*	Effexor XR, *generic*

8

Analgesics and Antagonists

thePOINT RESOURCES

- Comprehensive Summary Drug Tables
- Lippincott's Interactive Tutorials: Drugs Affecting the Central Nervous System
- Interactive Practice and Review
- Monographs of Most Commonly Prescribed Drugs

KEY TERMS

acute pain—pain that is of short duration and lasts less than 3 to 6 months and can be from mild to severe

agonist–antagonist—a narcotic analgesic that has properties of both the agonist and antagonist

analgesic—a drug that alleviates pain

antipyretic—a drug that reduces elevated body temperature

chronic pain—pain that lasts longer than 6 months and ranges in intensity from mild to severe

epidural—drug administration is performed when a catheter is placed into the epidural space outside of the dura mater of the brain and spinal cord

miosis—pinpoint pupils

opioids—narcotic analgesics obtained from the opium plant

pain—an unpleasant sensory and emotional experience associated with actual or potential tissue damage

partial agonist—a category of narcotic analgesic that binds to a receptor, but the response is limited (i.e., is not as great as with the agonist)

patient-controlled analgesia—a method of pain relief that allows patients to administer their own analgesic by means of an intravenous pump system

Reye syndrome—a rare, life-threatening condition that occurs in children and is characterized by vomiting and lethargy, progressing to coma

salicylates—drugs that have analgesic, antipyretic, and anti-inflammatory effects

salicylism—a condition produced by salicylate toxicity

tinnitus—ringing sound in the ear

Pain is an unpleasant sensory and emotional experience that is associated with actual or potential tissue damage. Pain is subjective, and the patient's report of pain should always be taken seriously. Pain management in acute and chronic illness is an important responsibility of health care providers. Many practitioners consider pain as the fifth vital sign and the assessment of pain to be just as important as the assessment of temperature, pulse, respirations, and blood pressure. Accurate assessment of pain is necessary if pain management is to be effective. Patients with pain are often undertreated.

Basically there are three types of pain: acute pain, chronic pain associated with malignant disease, and chronic pain not associated with malignant disease. **Acute pain** is of short duration and lasts less than 3 to 6 months. The intensity of acute pain is from mild to severe. Causes of acute pain include postoperative pain, procedural pain, and traumatic pain. Acute pain usually subsides when the injury heals.

Chronic pain lasts longer than 6 months and ranges in intensity from mild to severe. Chronic pain associated with a malignancy includes the pain of cancer, acquired immunodeficiency syndrome (AIDS), multiple sclerosis, sickle cell disease, and end-stage organ system failure.

A patient's exact cause of chronic pain of a nonmalignant nature may or may not be known. This type of pain includes the pain associated with various neuropathic and musculoskeletal disorders such as headaches, fibromyalgia, rheumatoid arthritis, and osteoarthritis.

This chapter deals with drugs used in the management of pain: nonnarcotic analgesics (salicylates, nonsalicylates, and the nonsteroidal anti-inflammatory drugs [NSAIDs]) and narcotic analgesics. **Analgesics** are drugs that relieve pain. This chapter also includes narcotic antagonists, which are used to counteract the effects of narcotics.

Nonnarcotic analgesics are a group of drugs used to relieve pain without the possibility of causing physical dependency, which can occur with the use of the narcotic analgesics. Nonnarcotic analgesics include salicylates, nonsalicylates (such as acetaminophen), and the NSAIDs. A number of combination nonnarcotic analgesics are available over the counter and by prescription. Nonsteroidal anti-inflammatory drugs have emerged as important drugs in the treatment of the chronic

pain and inflammation associated with disorders such as rheumatoid arthritis and osteoarthritis. Examples of NSAIDs include celecoxib (Celebrex) and naproxen (Naprosyn, Aleve).

FACT CHECK

8-1 What are the three types of pain and what are the differences between them?

8-2 What types of medications are used to treat pain?

Salicylates

Actions of Salicylates

The **salicylates** include aspirin (acetylsalicylic acid) and related drugs, such as magnesium salicylate. The salicylates have analgesic (relieves pain), **antipyretic** (reduces elevated body temperature), and anti-inflammatory effects. All the salicylates are similar in pharmacologic activity, but aspirin has a greater anti-inflammatory effect than the other salicylates. Specific salicylates are listed in the Summary Drug Table: Nonnarcotic Analgesics: Salicylates and Nonsalicylates.

The manner in which salicylates relieve pain and reduce inflammation is not fully understood. It is thought that the analgesic action of the salicylates is caused by the inhibition of prostaglandins. Prostaglandins are fatty acid derivatives found in almost every tissue of the body and body fluid. Release of prostaglandin is thought to increase the sensitivity of peripheral pain receptors. The inhibitory action of salicylates on the prostaglandins is also thought to account for the anti-inflammatory activity. Salicylates lower an elevated body temperature by dilating peripheral blood vessels, which in turn cools the body.

Aspirin more potently inhibits prostaglandin synthesis and has greater anti-inflammatory effects than other salicylates. In addition, aspirin also prolongs bleeding time by inhibiting the aggregation (clumping) of platelets. It takes a longer time for the blood to clot after a cut, surgery, or other injury to the skin or mucous membranes. Other salicylates do not have as great an effect on platelets as aspirin. This effect of aspirin on platelets is irreversible and lasts for the life of the platelet (7–10 days).

Uses of Salicylates

The salicylate nonnarcotic analgesics are used for the following purposes:

- Relief of mild to moderate pain
- Reduction of elevated body temperature (except for diflunisal, which is not used as an antipyretic)
- Treatment of inflammatory conditions, such as rheumatoid arthritis, osteoarthritis, and rheumatic fever
- Reduction of the risk of myocardial infarction in those with unstable angina or previous myocardial infarction (aspirin only)
- Reduction of the risk of transient ischemic attacks or strokes in men who have had transient ischemia of the brain caused by fibrin platelet emboli (aspirin only), although this use has not been found effective in women

Adverse Reactions of Salicylates

Gastric upset, heartburn, nausea, vomiting, anorexia, and gastrointestinal (GI) bleeding may occur with salicylate use. (See Key Concepts 8-1 for details on detecting GI bleeding.) Although

KEY CONCEPTS

8-1   Detecting Gastrointestinal Bleeding

Patients with a musculoskeletal disorder commonly receive salicylates or NSAIDs to help control inflammation and pain. In addition, these drugs are readily available over-the-counter. A patient who is prescribed one drug, such as an NSAID, may also take an OTC salicylate, such as an aspirin, for headaches or additional pain relief. When taken alone, these drugs may cause GI irritation, possibly leading to GI bleeding. If taken in combination or in high doses, or for long periods of time, the patient's risk for GI bleeding increases dramatically. Therefore, the patient may be taught how to look for signs and symptoms of GI bleeding. Patients should be instructed to report any of the following:

- Abdominal pain or distention, especially any sudden increases
- Vomiting that appears bright red or blood streaked (indicates fresh or recent bleeding) dark red, brown, or black, similar to the consistency of coffee grounds (indicates partial digestion of retained blood)
- Stools that appear black, loose and tarry, or bright red, red streaked, maroon, or dark mahogany

Patients should check their stools for occult blood (guaiac) by using an over-the-counter fecal occult blood test.

SIGNS & SYMPTOMS

Salicylism

When high doses of salicylates are administered (such as for severe arthritic disorders), the patient should be observed for signs of salicylism. If signs of salicylism occur, then the health care provider should be notified before the next dose is given because a reduction in dose or determination of the plasma salicylate level may be necessary.

The patient also should be assessed for tinnitus or impaired hearing. Tinnitus or impaired hearing probably indicates high blood salicylate levels. If this is suspected, then the drug should be withheld and any sensory alterations reported immediately. It should be explained to the patient that any hearing loss will disappear after the drug therapy is discontinued

Symptoms of Salicylism

- Dizziness
- **Tinnitus** (a ringing sound in the ear)
- Impaired hearing
- Nausea
- Vomiting
- Flushing
- Sweating
- Rapid deep breathing
- Tachycardia
- Diarrhea
- Mental confusion
- Lassitude
- Drowsiness
- Respiratory depression and coma (large doses)

these drugs are relatively safe when taken as recommended, their use can occasionally result in more serious reactions. Some individuals are allergic to aspirin and other salicylates. Salicylate allergy causes hives, rash, angioedema, bronchospasm with asthma-like symptoms, and anaphylactoid reactions.

Loss of blood through the GI tract occurs with salicylate use. The amount of blood lost is insignificant with one normal dose. However, use of these drugs over a long period, even in normal doses, can result in a significant blood loss.

Salicylate toxicity produces a condition called **salicylism**. The symptoms of this condition are listed in Signs and Symptoms box. Mild salicylism usually occurs with repeated administration of large doses of a salicylate. This condition is reversible with reduction of the drug dosage.

FACT CHECK

8-3   What three types of effects do salicylates have?
8-4   How is aspirin different from other salicylates?
8-5   What are salicylate nonnarcotic analgesics used to treat?

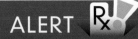

ALERT

Salicylate Gastrointestinal Toxicity

Serious GI toxicity can cause bleeding, ulceration, and perforation that may occur at any time during therapy, with or without symptoms. Although minor GI problems are common, patients receiving long-term therapy may experience ulceration and bleeding, even if they experienced no previous gastric symptoms. The color of the patient's stools must be checked. Black or dark stools (often described as "tarry") or bright red blood in the stool may indicate GI bleeding. Any changes should be reported to the health care provider.

Contraindications, Precautions, and Interactions of Salicylates

- The salicylates are contraindicated in patients with known hypersensitivity.
- Because the salicylates prolong bleeding time, they are contraindicated in those with bleeding disorders or bleeding tendencies. These include patients with GI bleeding (attributed to any cause), blood dyscrasias, and those receiving anticoagulant or antineoplastic drugs.
- Children or teenagers with influenza or chickenpox should not take the salicylates, particularly aspirin.
- The salicylates are used cautiously in patients with hepatic or renal disease, preexisting hypoprothrombinemia, or vitamin K deficiency and during lactation. The drugs are also used with caution in patients with GI irritation such as peptic ulcers, mild diabetes, or gout.
- Food containing salicylate (curry powder, paprika, licorice, prunes, raisins, and tea) may increase the risk of adverse reactions.
- Coadministration of a salicylate with activated charcoal decreases the absorption of the salicylate.
- Antacids may decrease the effects of the salicylate.
- Coadministration with a carbonic anhydrase inhibitor increases the risk of salicylism.
- Aspirin may increase the risk of bleeding during heparin administration.
- Coadministration with a NSAID may increase the blood levels.

CONSIDERATIONS   Older adults

LIFESPAN

Salicylates

Salicylates are often prescribed for the pain and inflammation of arthritis. Because older adults have a higher incidence of both rheumatoid arthritis and osteoarthritis and may use nonnarcotic analgesics on a long-term basis, they are particularly vulnerable to GI bleeding. Patients should be encouraged to take the drug with a full glass of water or with food because this may decrease the GI effects.

CONSIDERATIONS   Infants & Children

LIFESPAN

Salicylates in Children

Studies suggest that the use of salicylates (especially aspirin) may be involved in the development of **Reye syndrome** in children with chickenpox or influenza. This rare but life-threatening disorder is characterized by vomiting and lethargy, progressing to coma. Therefore, use of salicylates is not recommended for children with chickenpox, fever, or flu-like symptoms. Acetaminophen is recommended instead.

Patient Management Issues with Salicylates

The patient should be monitored for relief of pain. If pain recurs, then its severity, location, and intensity should be assessed.

Any adverse reactions, such as unusual or prolonged bleeding or dark stools, must be reported to the health care provider.

Some health care providers may not prescribe an antipyretic for patients with an elevated temperature because of evidence suggesting that fever activates the immune system to produce disease-fighting antibodies. The decision to treat an elevated temperature with an antipyretic (whether a salicylate or nonsalicylate) depends in part on the cause of the fever and the patient's physical condition.

A patient receiving these drugs may have an acute or chronic disorder with varying degrees of mobility. The patient may be in acute pain or have long-standing mild to moderate pain. These patients may need help walking or with other activities.

Salicylates are given with food, milk, or a full glass of water to prevent gastric upset. If gastric distress occurs, then the health care provider is notified because other drug therapy may be necessary. An antacid may be prescribed to minimize GI distress.

Patients should not take salicylates for at least 1 week before any type of major or minor surgery, including dental surgery, because of the possibility of postoperative bleeding. In addition, patients should not use salicylates after any type of surgery until complete healing has occurred. A patient may use acetaminophen or an NSAID after surgery or a dental procedure when relief of mild pain is necessary.

Educating the Patient and Family About Salicylates

Following are key points about salicylates that the patient and family members should know.

- Notify your health care provider if you have any of the following symptoms: ringing in the ears, GI pain, nausea, vomiting, flushing, sweating, thirst, headache, diarrhea, episodes of unusual bleeding or bruising, or dark stools.
- All drugs deteriorate with age. Salicylates often deteriorate more rapidly than many other drugs. If there is a vinegar odor to the salicylate, then discard the entire contents of the container. Purchase salicylates in small amounts when used only occasionally. Keep the container tightly

closed at all times because salicylates deteriorate rapidly when exposed to air, moisture, or heat.

- The ingredients of some over-the-counter (OTC) drugs contain aspirin. The name of the salicylate may not appear in the name of the drug but is listed on the label. Do not use these products while taking a salicylate, especially during high-dose or long-term salicylate therapy. Consult the pharmacist about the product's ingredients if you are in doubt.
- If you are to have surgery or a dental procedure, such as tooth extraction or gum surgery, then notify your health care provider or dentist. Salicylates may be discontinued 1 week before the procedure because of the possibility of postoperative bleeding.

FACT CHECK

8-6   Why should salicylates be taken with food?
8-7   Why are salicylates not recommended for children with chickenpox or influenza?
8-8   A patient who routinely takes a salicylate is having surgery. Should the patient continue taking the salicylate?

Nonsalicylate Analgesics

The major drug classified as a nonsalicylate analgesic is acetaminophen (Tylenol). Acetaminophen is the only drug of this kind available in the United States at this time. It is often abbreviated "APAP." It is the most widely used aspirin substitute for patients who are allergic to aspirin or who experience extreme gastric upset when taking aspirin. Acetaminophen is also the drug of choice for treating children with fever and flu-like symptoms.

Actions of Nonsalicylate Analgesics

The mechanism of action of acetaminophen is unknown. Like the salicylates, acetaminophen has both analgesic and antipyretic activity. However, acetaminophen does not have an anti-inflammatory action and is of no value in the treatment of inflammation or inflammatory disorders.

Uses of Nonsalicylate Analgesics

Acetaminophen is used to relieve mild to moderate pain and to reduce elevated body temperature (fever). This drug is particularly useful for those with aspirin allergy and bleeding disorders, such as bleeding ulcer or hemophilia, those receiving anticoagulant therapy, and those who have recently had minor surgical procedures. Although acetaminophen has no anti-inflammatory action, it may be used to relieve the pain and discomfort associated with arthritic disorders.

Adverse Reactions of Nonsalicylate Analgesics

Acetaminophen causes few adverse reactions when used as recommended. Adverse reactions associated with the use of acetaminophen usually occur with long-term use or when the

COMPLEMENTARY & ALTERNATIVE MEDICINE

Willow Bark

Willow bark has long been used to reduce fever or inflammation and to relieve pain. Salicylate was originally isolated from willow bark and identified as the most likely source of the bark's anti-inflammatory effects. Its chemical structure was replicated in the laboratory and mass-produced as synthetic salicylic acid. While synthetic anti-inflammatory drugs work quickly and have a higher potency than willow bark, willow bark has fewer adverse reactions than salicylates. However, it should be used with caution in patients with peptic ulcers and medical conditions in which aspirin is contraindicated and should not be used at all in patients taking anticoagulant or antiplatelet medications.

recommended dosage is exceeded. Adverse reactions are rare when used as directed but may include skin eruptions, urticaria (hives), hemolytic anemia, pancytopenia (a reduction in all cellular components of the blood), hypoglycemia, jaundice (yellow discoloration of the skin), hepatotoxicity (damage to the liver), and hepatic failure (seen in chronic alcoholics taking the drug).

Acute acetaminophen poisoning or toxicity can occur after a single 10- to 15-g dose of acetaminophen. Dosages of 20 to 25 g may be fatal. The daily dose of acetaminophen should not exceed 4 g. In an effort to combat acetaminophen toxicity, prescription medications are limited to no more than 325 mg of acetaminophen per dosage form. With excessive dosages, the liver cells necrose (die). Death can occur because of liver failure. The risk of liver failure is higher in chronic alcoholics. If a patient is an alcoholic or chronic user of alcohol, then acetaminophen intake is limited to no more than 2 g/day. If a patient is an alcoholic or chronic user of alcohol, then acetaminophen intake is limited to no more than 2 g/day.

Signs of acute acetaminophen toxicity include the following:

- Nausea
- Vomiting
- Confusion
- Liver tenderness
- Hypotension
- Arrhythmias
- Jaundice
- Acute hepatic and renal failure

FACT CHECK

8-9   What is acetaminophen used to treat? For which conditions is it considered the drug of choice?
8-10   What is the maximum daily dose of acetaminophen?

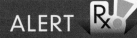

ALERT

Acetaminophen Toxicity

Any signs of acetaminophen toxicity, such as nausea, vomiting, anorexia, malaise, diaphoresis, abdominal pain, confusion, liver tenderness, hypotension, arrhythmias, jaundice, and acute hepatic and renal failure, must be reported immediately to the health care provider. Early diagnosis is important because liver failure may be reversible. Acetylcysteine (Mucomyst) is an antidote to acetaminophen toxicity, protecting liver cells and destroying acetaminophen metabolites.

Contraindications, Precautions, and Interactions of Nonsalicylate Analgesics

- Hypersensitivity to acetaminophen is a contraindication.
- Hepatotoxicity has occurred in chronic alcoholics after therapeutic dosages.
- Patients taking acetaminophen should avoid alcohol if taking more than an occasional dose of acetaminophen and should avoid taking acetaminophen concurrently with a salicylate or NSAID.
- The drug is used cautiously in patients with severe or recurrent pain or high or continued fever, which may indicate the presence of a serious illness.
- If pain persists for more than 5 days or if redness or swelling is present, then the health care provider should be consulted.
- Acetaminophen may alter blood glucose test results, causing falsely lower blood glucose values.
- Use with barbiturates, hydantoins, isoniazid, or rifampin may increase the toxic effects and possibly decrease the therapeutic effects of acetaminophen.
- The effects of loop diuretics may be decreased when administered with acetaminophen.
- Hepatotoxicity has occurred in chronic alcoholics taking moderate doses of acetaminophen.

Patient Management Issues with Nonsalicylate Analgesics

As with salicylates, patients taking nonsalicylate analgesics should be monitored for pain relief or recurrence, and those with disorders that may affect mobility should receive assistance with walking or other activities, as needed. Any adverse reactions must be reported to the health care provider.

Acetaminophen is taken with a full glass of water. A patient may take this drug with meals or on an empty stomach.

Educating the Patient and Family about Nonsalicylate Analgesics

Following are key points the patient and family members should know about nonsalicylate analgesics.

If you have arthritis, then do not change from aspirin to acetaminophen without consulting your health care provider.

ALERT

Acetaminophen Use

The patient's overall health and alcohol usage must be assessed before acetaminophen is prescribed. Patients who are malnourished or abuse alcohol are at risk for hepatotoxicity (damage to the liver) with the use of acetaminophen.

Acetaminophen lacks the anti-inflammatory properties of aspirin.

- Notify your health care provider if you have any of the following adverse reactions: dyspnea, weakness, dizziness, blue discoloration of the nail beds, unexplained bleeding, bruising, or sore throat.
- Do not drink alcoholic beverages.

FACT CHECK

8-11 What are the signs of acute acetaminophen toxicity?
8-12 What patients are specifically at risk for developing hepatotoxicity with acetaminophen use?

Nonsteroidal Anti-inflammatory Drugs

The nonsteroidal anti-inflammatory drug group contains more than 70 drugs, with new drugs frequently becoming available. The chemical and physiologic effects of NSAIDs are similar to the salicylates. The NSAIDs are also nonnarcotic analgesics. This section covers the NSAID group generally and describes three commonly used NSAIDs in more specifics: celecoxib (Celebrex), ibuprofen (Advil/Motrin), and naproxen (Naprosyn/Aleve). Other NSAIDs are listed in the Summary Drug Table: Nonsteroidal Anti-inflammatory Drugs. Like salicylates, NSAIDs have anti-inflammatory, antipyretic, and analgesic effects.

Actions of NSAIDs

NSAIDs are so named because they are not steroids and thus do not cause the adverse reactions associated with steroids (see Chapter 31), yet they have anti-inflammatory effects along with their analgesic and antipyretic properties. Although their exact mechanisms of actions are not known, NSAIDs are thought to act by inhibiting prostaglandin synthesis by inhibiting the action of the enzyme cyclooxygenase, which is responsible for prostaglandin synthesis. The anti-inflammatory effects of the NSAIDs result from inhibition of cyclooxygenase-2 (COX-2). The GI adverse reactions are caused by inhibition of cyclooxygenase-1 (COX-1).

The newer NSAID, celecoxib, appears to work by specifically inhibiting the COX-2 enzyme without inhibiting the COX-1 enzyme. Celecoxib relieves pain and inflammation with less potential for GI adverse reactions. Traditional

NSAIDs, such as ibuprofen and naproxen, are thought to reduce pain and inflammation by blocking COX-2. Unlike celecoxib, these drugs also inhibit COX-1, the enzyme that helps maintain the lining of the stomach. This inhibition of COX-1 causes the unwanted GI reactions, such as stomach irritation and ulcers.

Uses of NSAIDs

The NSAIDs have a variety of uses, including relief of the following conditions:

- Signs and symptoms of osteoarthritis, rheumatoid arthritis, and other musculoskeletal disorders
- Mild to moderate pain
- Primary dysmenorrhea (painful menstruation)
- Fever

Adverse Reactions of NSAIDs

Many adverse reactions are associated with the use of NSAIDs, although many patients take these drugs and experience few, if any, of these effects. The most common adverse reaction associated with most NSAIDs is GI upset and includes nausea, epigastric pain, heartburn, and abdominal pain.

Adverse Reactions of Celecoxib

Celecoxib is different from the other NSAIDs in that it causes less GI upset. However, it does have other adverse reactions that patients should be aware of. The most common adverse reactions of celecoxib include abdominal pain, cough, diarrhea, dizziness, fever, headache, nausea, upper abdominal pain, and vomiting. Like other NSAIDs, celecoxib may compromise renal function. Aminotransferase levels may be elevated.

FACT CHECK

8-13 What are NSAIDs used to treat?
8-14 How is celecoxib different from the other NSAIDs?

Contraindications, Precautions, and Interactions of NSAIDs

- Nonsteroidal anti-inflammatory drugs are contraindicated in patients with known hypersensitivity to any NSAID, because these drugs have a cross-sensitivity.
- Hypersensitivity to aspirin is a contraindication for all NSAIDs.

ALERT Rx

NSAIDs
The health care provider should be notified immediately if any gastric symptoms occur, especially nausea, vomiting, diarrhea, evidence of bleeding (blood in stool, tarry stools), or abdominal pain.

- Nonsteroidal anti-inflammatory drugs are used cautiously in the elderly and in patients with bleeding disorders, renal disease, cardiovascular disease, or hepatic impairment. Patients older than 65 years taking NSAIDs have an increased risk of ulcer formation.
- Nonsteroidal anti-inflammatory drugs prolong bleeding time and increase the effects of anticoagulants, lithium, cyclosporine, and the hydantoins.
- These drugs may decrease the effects of diuretics or antihypertensive drugs.
- Long-term use of NSAIDs with acetaminophen may increase the risk of renal impairment.

Contraindications, Precautions, and Interactions of Specific NSAIDs

Celecoxib

- Celecoxib is contraindicated in patients who are allergic to the drug or to sulfonamides, other NSAIDs, or aspirin.
- The drug is used cautiously in patients with a history of peptic ulcer, patients older than 60 years, and patients taking an anticoagulant or steroids. In rare instances, serious stomach problems such as bleeding can occur without warning.
- When celecoxib is given with an anticoagulant, the patient has an increased risk for bleeding.

Ibuprofen

- Ibuprofen is contraindicated in patients with hypertension, peptic ulceration, or GI bleeding.
- The drug is used cautiously in patients with renal or liver dysfunction.
- When ibuprofen is taken with lithium, the patient has an increased risk of lithium toxicity.
- Ibuprofen may cause a diuretic to have a decreased effect when they are taken together.
- Ibuprofen may cause a decreased antihypertensive effect of β-adrenergic blocking drugs.

Naproxen

- The drug is used cautiously in patients with asthma, hypertension, cardiac problems, peptic ulcer disease, or impaired liver or kidney function.
- Like ibuprofen, naproxen increases the risk of lithium toxicity when a patient is taking both drugs.
- When naproxen is administered with an anticoagulant, the patient has an increased risk for bleeding.
- When naproxen is administered with an antihypertensive, the antihypertensive's effect is diminished.
- Naproxen decreases the diuretic effect of diuretics.

Patient Management Issues with Nonsteroidal Anti-inflammatory Drugs

The patient is monitored for relief of pain. If pain recurs, then its severity, location, and intensity are assessed. Hot, dry, flushed skin and decreased urinary output may develop with prolonged fever and dehydration. The patient's joints are assessed for reduced inflammation and greater mobility. Any adverse reactions, such as unusual or prolonged bleeding or dark stools, should be reported to the health care provider. Patients who do not experience a therapeutic response to one

NSAID may respond to another NSAID. However, several weeks of treatment may be necessary for a full therapeutic response to develop.

NSAIDs are prescribed for the pain and inflammation of arthritis. Because older adults more commonly have rheumatoid arthritis and osteoarthritis and may use the NSAID for a long term, they are particularly vulnerable to GI bleeding. The patient should take the drug with a full glass of water or with food because this may decrease the GI effects.

Patients with pain in their limbs or joints may need additional comfort measures. Therapy may include the use of heat or cold along with joint rest. Various orthodontic devices, such as splints and braces, may be used to support inflamed joints. Braces, splints, and assistive mobility devices such as canes, crutches, and walkers help ease pain.

Educating the Patient and Family about Nonsteroidal Anti-inflammatory Drugs

An NSAID may be prescribed for a patient for a prolonged period, such as for arthritis. Some patients may discontinue their use of the drug, fail to take the drug at the prescribed or recommended intervals, increase their dose, or decrease the time interval between doses, especially if their symptoms change. The patient and family must understand that the drug should be taken even when symptoms are relieved.

Many NSAIDs are available as OTC products. Over-the-counter formulations such as ibuprofen (Advil, Motrin) and naproxen (Aleve) are available to any consumer. The potential for misuse and abuse is high, especially because frequent advertisements on television and in print herald the wonderful benefits of these products. Therefore, patients need to be educated about these products, emphasizing the following points:

- Indications for using the drug (the reason the patient might take it)
- Dosage information, including frequency and maximum daily amounts
- Possible drug–drug and drug–food interactions
- Possible adverse effects, including life-threatening ones such as bleeding
- The need to read and heed all manufacturer's instructions, including the maximum number of days one should use the drug and when to notify the health care provider (e.g., if fever is not resolved within 3 days or pain persists)

Following are key points about NSAIDs that the patient or family members should know.

- Take the drug exactly as prescribed by your health care provider. Do not increase or decrease the dosage, and do not take any OTC drugs without first consulting your health care provider. Notify your health care provider or dentist if the pain is not relieved.
- Take the drug with food or a full glass of water unless indicated otherwise by your health care provider. If you experience gastric upset, then take the drug with food or milk. If the problem persists, then contact your health care provider.
- Inform all health care providers, including dentists, if you take these drugs regularly or occasionally.
- If you use the drug to reduce fever, then contact your health care provider if your temperature continues elevated for more than 24 hours.
- Do not consistently use an NSAID to treat chronic pain without first consulting your health care provider.
- Severe or recurrent pain or high or continued fever may indicate a serious illness. If your pain persists more than 10 days (in an adult), or if your fever persists more than 3 days, then consult your health care provider.
- Do not use aspirin or other salicylates when taking an NSAID.
- The drug may take several days to take effect (relief of pain and tenderness). If some or all of your symptoms are not relieved after 2 weeks of therapy, then continue taking the drug, but notify your health care provider.
- These drugs may cause drowsiness, dizziness, or blurred vision. Use caution while driving or performing tasks that require alertness.
- Notify your health care provider if you have any of the following adverse reactions: skin rash, itching, visual disturbances, weight gain, edema, diarrhea, black stools, nausea, vomiting, or persistent headache.

For general teaching points that apply to all of the nonnarcotic analgesics addressed above, see Box 8-1.

FACT CHECK

8-15 Before taking an OTC NSAID, a patient should receive counseling on what points?

8-16 If a patient is experiencing GI upset when taking an NSAID, what could he or she do to prevent future GI upset?

Narcotic Analgesics

Narcotic analgesics are controlled substances (see Chapter 1) used to treat moderate to severe pain. Narcotic antagonists, which are drugs that counteract the effects of narcotic analgesics by competing with narcotic at receptor sites, are used to reverse the depressant effects of narcotic analgesics.

Actions of Narcotic Analgesics

Opioid analgesics are narcotic drugs derived from the opium plant. The analgesic properties of opium have been known for hundreds of years. Narcotics obtained from raw opium (also called opiates, opioids, or opiate narcotics) include morphine, codeine, hydrochlorides of opium alkaloids, and tincture of opium.

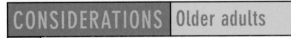

CONSIDERATIONS   Older adults

LIFESPAN

Adverse Reactions to NSAIDs

Age appears to increase the possibility of adverse reactions to NSAIDs. The risk of serious ulcer disease in adults older than 65 years is increased with higher doses of NSAIDs. Therapy often begins with reduced dosages, which are increased slowly.

Morphine is extracted from raw opium and treated chemically to produce the semisynthetic narcotics hydromorphone, oxymorphone, oxycodone, and heroin. Heroin is an illegal narcotic in the United States and is not used in medicine. Synthetic narcotics are laboratory-made analgesics with properties and actions similar to the natural opioids. Examples of synthetic narcotic analgesics are methadone, levorphanol, remifentanil, and meperidine. Additional narcotics are listed in the Summary Drug Table: Narcotic Analgesics.

Narcotic analgesics are classified as agonists, partial agonists, and mixed agonists–antagonists. An agonist binds to a receptor and causes a response (Fig. 8-1). A **partial agonist** binds to a receptor but has only a limited response. Antagonists bind to a receptor and cause no response of their own, but an antagonist can reverse the effects of an agonist. This reversal occurs possibly because the antagonist competes with the agonist for the receptor site. (Narcotic antagonists are discussed later in this chapter.) An **agonist–antagonist** drug has properties of both the agonist and antagonist.

Narcotic analgesics are categorized based on the opioid receptor sites where they are active. Five categories of opioid receptors have been identified, three of which are involved in the actions of narcotic analgesics; these are called the mu, kappa, and delta receptors. Table 8-1 identifies the responses in the body associated with each of these receptors.

Remifentanil is a very short-acting agonist with potent analgesic activity. It is a mu opioid agonist with rapid onset and peak effect, and short duration of action. The mixed agonist–antagonist drugs act on the mu receptors by competing with other substances at the mu receptor (antagonist activity) and are agonists at other receptors. Partial agonists have limited agonist activity at the mu receptor.

Uses of Narcotic Analgesics

The major use of narcotic analgesics is to manage moderate to severe acute and chronic pain. The ability of a narcotic analgesic to relieve pain depends on several factors, such as the drug, the dose, the route of administration, the type of pain, the

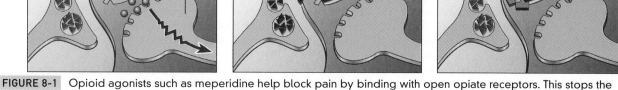

FIGURE 8-1 Opioid agonists such as meperidine help block pain by binding with open opiate receptors. This stops the release of substance P (a pain neurotransmitter) and slows the transmission of the pain impulse.

TABLE 8-1   Activities within the Body Associated With Receptor Sites

Receptor	Bodily Response
Mu	Morphine-like supraspinal analgesia, respiratory and physical depression, miosis, reduced G motility
Delta	Dysphoria, psychotomimetic effects (e.g., hallucinations), respiratory and vasomotor stimulations caused by drugs with antagonist activity
Kappa	Sedation and miosis

patient, and the length of time the drug has been administered. Morphine is the most widely used opioid and is an effective drug for moderately severe to severe pain. Morphine is considered the prototype or "model narcotic." Morphine's actions, uses, and ability to relieve pain are standards to which other narcotic analgesics are often compared. Other narcotics, such as meperidine and levorphanol, are effective for the treatment of moderate to severe pain. For mild to moderate pain, the health care provider may order a narcotic such as codeine or pentazocine.

In addition to the management of moderate to severe acute and chronic pain, narcotic analgesics may be used for the following reasons:

- To lessen anxiety and sedate a patient before surgery. Patients who are relaxed and sedated when anesthesia is given are easier to anesthetize (requiring a smaller dose of an induction anesthetic), as well as easier to maintain under anesthesia.
- To support anesthesia (as an adjunct during anesthesia)
- For obstetrical analgesia
- To relieve anxiety in patients with dyspnea associated with pulmonary edema
- Intrathecally or epidurally to relieve pain for extended periods without apparent loss of motor, sensory, or sympathetic function
- To relieve pain associated with heart attack (morphine)
- For detoxification of and temporary maintenance of narcotic addiction (methadone)
- To induce conscious sedation before a diagnostic or therapeutic procedure
- To treat severe diarrhea and intestinal cramping (tincture of opium)
- To relieve severe, persistent cough (codeine, although the drug's use has declined)

Narcotic Analgesic Use in Management of Opioid Dependence

The opioid that is used in the treatment and management of opiate dependence is methadone. Methadone, a synthetic narcotic, may be used for the relief of pain, but it also is used in the detoxification and maintenance treatment of those addicted to narcotics. Detoxification involves withdrawing the patient from the narcotic while preventing withdrawal symptoms.

Maintenance therapy is designed to reduce the patient's desire to return to the drug that caused addiction and to prevent withdrawal symptoms. The dosages used vary with the patient, the length of time the individual has been addicted, and the average daily amount of the addictive drug that had been used. Patients enrolled in an outpatient methadone program for detoxification or maintenance therapy on methadone must continue to receive methadone when hospitalized.

FACT CHECK

8-17   What type of pain is treated with narcotic analgesics?

8-18   What are other uses of narcotic analgesics?

8-19   Which opioid is used in the treatment and management of opiate dependence?

Adverse Reactions of Narcotic Analgesics

The adverse reactions differ according to whether the narcotic analgesic acts as an agonist or as an agonist–antagonist.

Adverse Reactions of Agonists

One of the major hazards of narcotic administration is respiratory depression, in which the respiratory rate and depth decrease. The most common adverse reactions include light-headedness, dizziness, sedation, constipation, anorexia, nausea, vomiting, and sweating. When these effects occur, the health care provider may lower the dose in an effort to eliminate or decrease their intensity. Other adverse reactions that may occur with the administration of an agonist narcotic analgesic include the following:

- Central nervous system: euphoria, weakness, headache, **miosis** (pinpoint pupils), insomnia agitation, tremor, and impairment of mental and physical tasks
- Gastrointestinal: dry mouth and biliary tract spasms
- Cardiovascular: flushing of the face, peripheral circulatory collapse, tachycardia, bradycardia, and palpitations
- Genitourinary: spasms of the ureters and bladder sphincter, urinary retention or hesitancy
- Allergic: pruritus, rash, and urticaria
- Other: physical dependence, pain at injection site, and local tissue irritation

Adverse Reactions of Agonist–Antagonists

Administration of a narcotic agonist–antagonist may result in symptoms of narcotic withdrawal in those addicted to narcotics. Other adverse reactions include sedation, nausea, vomiting, sweating, headache, vertigo, dry mouth, euphoria, and dizziness.

Narcotic Drug Dependence

Most patients receiving a narcotic analgesic for medical purposes do not develop dependence. However, drug dependence can occur when a narcotic is administered over a long period. For some patients, such as those who are terminally ill and in severe pain, drug dependence is not considered a problem because the most important task is to keep patients

Narcotic Analgesics

The narcotic analgesic should be withheld and the health care provider contacted immediately if any of the following are present:

1. A significant decrease in the respiratory rate or a respiratory rate of 10/min or below
2. A significant increase or decrease in the pulse rate or a change in the pulse quality
3. A significant decrease in blood pressure (systolic or diastolic) or a systolic pressure below 100 mm Hg

Constipation

Constipation can occur with repeated doses of a narcotic. A daily record of bowel movements is kept, and the health care provider is informed if constipation appears to be a problem. Most patients should begin taking a stool softener or laxative with the initial dose of a narcotic analgesic. Many patients need to continue taking a laxative as long as they take the narcotic analgesic. If a patient is constipated despite the use of a stool softener, then the health care provider may prescribe an enema or another means of relieving constipation.

as comfortable as possible for the time they have remaining (see the section on "Relieving Chronic Severe Pain" below).

When a patient does not have a painful terminal illness, drug dependence must be avoided. Signs of drug dependence include the appearance of withdrawal symptoms (acute abstinence syndrome) when the narcotic is discontinued, requests for the narcotic at frequent intervals around the clock, personality changes if the narcotic is not given immediately, and constant reports of pain and failure of the narcotic to relieve pain. Although these behaviors can have other causes, drug dependence should be considered. Specific symptoms of the abstinence syndrome are listed in the Signs and Symptoms box.

Contraindications, Precautions, and Interactions of Narcotic Analgesics

- All narcotic analgesics are contraindicated in patients with known hypersensitivity.
- These drugs are contraindicated in patients with acute bronchial asthma, emphysema, or upper airway obstruction; in patients with head injury or increased intracranial pressure; and in patients with convulsive disorders, severe renal or hepatic dysfunction, or acute ulcerative colitis.
- These drugs are used cautiously in the elderly and in patients with undiagnosed abdominal pain, liver disease, a history of addiction to the opioids, hypoxia, supraventricular tachycardia, prostatic hypertrophy, or renal or hepatic impairment.

- Narcotics are used cautiously during lactation, and the mother is advised to wait at least 4 to 6 hours after taking the drug before breast-feeding the infant. These drugs also are used cautiously in patients undergoing biliary

SIGNS SYMPTOMS

Symptoms of the Abstinence Syndrome

Early Symptoms

Yawning
Lacrimation
Rhinorrhea
Sweating

Intermediate Symptoms

Mydriasis
Tachycardia
Twitching
Tremor
Restlessness
Irritability
Anxiety
Anorexia

Late Symptoms

Muscle spasm
Fever
Nausea
Vomiting
Kicking movements
Weakness
Depression
Body aches
Weight loss
Severe backache
Abdominal and leg pains
Hot and cold flashes
Insomnia
Repetitive sneezing
Increased blood pressure, respiratory rate, and heart rate

CONSIDERATIONS | Older adults

LIFESPAN

Narcotic Analgesics

Older adults are especially prone to adverse reactions of narcotic analgesics, particularly respiratory depression, somnolence (sedation), and confusion. The health care provider may order a lower dosage of the narcotic for an older adult.

surgery because these drugs may cause spasm of the sphincter of Oddi.

- Narcotic analgesics potentiate the central nervous system depressant properties of other central nervous system depressants, such as alcohol, antihistamines, antidepressants, sedatives, phenothiazines, and monoamine oxidase inhibitors.
- Use of a narcotic analgesic within 14 days of a MAO inhibitor (see Chapter 7) may potentiate the effect of either drug.
- Patients taking an agonist–antagonist narcotic analgesic may experience withdrawal symptoms if they have been abusing or using narcotics. The agonist–antagonists drugs can cause opioid withdrawal symptoms in those who are physically dependent on an opioid.
- The patient has an increased risk of respiratory depression, hypotension, and sedation when narcotic analgesics are administered too soon after barbiturate general anesthesia.

Patient Management Issues with Narcotic Analgesics

The health care provider may request that a patient evaluate the pain using a standardized pain scale measurement tool. The pain is usually rated on a scale of 1 to 10, with 10 being the most severe pain and 1 being the least discomfort. Failure to adequately assess pain is a major factor in the common undertreatment of pain.

When these drugs are administered, the health care provider should regularly ask about the pain and believe the patient's and family's reports of pain. The exact location of the pain, a description of the pain (e.g., sharp, dull, or stabbing), and an estimate of when the pain began are assessed each time the patient requests a narcotic analgesic. Further questioning and more detailed information about the pain are necessary if the pain is different from that experienced previously or if it is in a different area. Not all instances of a change in pain type, location, or intensity require notifying the health care provider. For example, if a patient recovering from recent abdominal surgery experiences pain in the leg, then the health care provider should be notified immediately. However, it may not be necessary to contact the health care provider for pain that is slightly worse because the patient has been moving in bed.

In addition, if any controllable factors (e.g., uncomfortable position, cold room, drafts, bright lights, noise, thirst) may decrease the patient's tolerance to pain, then the adjustment should be made as soon as possible.

Narcotic analgesics can produce serious or potentially fatal respiratory depression if given too frequently or in excessive doses. Respiratory depression may occur in patients receiving a normal dose if the patient is vulnerable, such as in weakened state or debilitated state.

Relieving Acute Pain

The health care provider should be notified if the analgesic is ineffective because a higher dose or a different narcotic analgesic may be required.

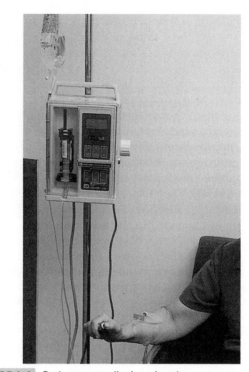

FIGURE 8-2 Patient-controlled analgesia.

During the time when the drug is producing its greatest analgesic effect, usually 1 to 2 hours after being administered, the patient may need help getting out of bed and performing therapeutic activities, such as deep breathing, coughing, and leg exercises (when ordered).

Patient-controlled analgesia (PCA) allows patients to administer their own analgesic by means of an intravenous pump system (Fig. 8-2). The dose and the time interval permitted between doses is programmed into the device to prevent accidental overdosage.

Many postoperative patients require narcotics less often when they are able to self-administer a narcotic for pain. Because the self-administration system is under the control of a nurse or health care provider, who adds the drug to the infusion pump and sets the time interval (or lockout interval) between doses, the patient cannot receive an overdose of the drug.

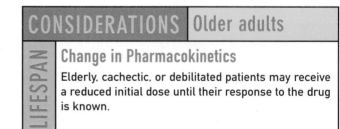

CONSIDERATIONS | Older adults

LIFESPAN

Change in Pharmacokinetics
Elderly, cachectic, or debilitated patients may receive a reduced initial dose until their response to the drug is known.

Relieving Chronic Severe Pain

Morphine is the most widely used drug for chronic severe pain, such as pain associated with cancer. The fact that this drug can be given orally, subcutaneously, intramuscularly, intravenous, and rectally in the form of a suppository allows tremendous versatility. Medication for chronic pain should be scheduled around the clock and not given on a PRN (as needed) basis. Most patients with cancer can be treated with oral morphine. The oral route is preferred as long as a patient is able to swallow or can tolerate sublingual administration. Respiratory depression is less likely to occur when the drug is given orally.

OxyContin is a controlled-release form of oxycodone for moderate to severe pain when a continuous, around-the-clock analgesic is needed for an extended period of time. OxyContin is not intended for use as a PRN analgesic. A patient may experience fewer adverse reactions with oxycodone than morphine, and the drug is effective and generally considered safe for the elderly. The tablets are to be swallowed whole and should not be broken, chewed, or crushed.

Fentanyl transdermal is a transdermal system that is effective for the severe pain associated with cancer. The transdermal system allows for a timed-release patch containing the drug fentanyl used over a 72-hour period. A small number of patients may require systems applied every 48 hours. Adverse effects are monitored in the same manner as for other narcotic analgesics (e.g., the health care provider is notified if the respiratory rate is 10/minute or less).

When narcotics are administered for severe pain, the goal is to prevent or control the patient's pain, not to prevent addiction. Patients taking a narcotic for severe pain rarely become addicted. Although some dependence may occur in rare instances, a patient who recovers from the illness may be gradually weaned from the drug.

When long-acting forms of a narcotic are used, a fast-acting form may be given for breakthrough pain. Patients should be given the drug as ordered and on time. Oral transmucosal fentanyl (Actiq) is used to treat breakthrough pain. Making a patient wait for the effect of a long-acting drug may result in withdrawal symptoms, which will only add to the pain of the illness.

Tolerance results over a period of time in the patient taking a narcotic analgesic. The rate at which a patient develops tolerance varies according to the dosage, the route or administration, and the individual. Patients taking oral or transdermal morphine develop tolerance more slowly than those taking the drug parenterally. Some patients develop tolerance

quickly and need larger doses every few weeks, whereas others are maintained on the same dosage schedule throughout the course of their illness.

The risk of respiratory depression is a concern for health care professionals who administer narcotics and may cause some to hesitate to administer the drug. However, respiratory depression rarely occurs in patients using a narcotic for pain because these patients usually very quickly develop tolerance to the respiratory depressant effects of the drug. Naloxone can be administered to reverse the narcotic effects if absolutely necessary.

Epidural Pain Management

Epidural administration of certain narcotic analgesics, specifically morphine and fentanyl, is an alternative to the intramuscular or oral route. **Epidural** administration is performed when a catheter is placed into the epidural space outside the dura mater of the brain and spinal cord. The analgesic effect is produced by the direct effect on the opiate receptors in the dorsal horn of the spinal cord. Epidural administration offers several advantages over other routes. Lower total dosages of the drug are used, fewer adverse reactions occur, and the patient has greater comfort with epidural administration.

Access to the epidural route is made through the use of a percutaneous epidural catheter. The epidural catheter is placed into the space between the dura mater and the vertebral column. The drug injected through the catheter spreads freely throughout all the tissues in the space, interrupting pain conduction at the points where sensory fibers exit from the spinal cord. The narcotic is administered either by bolus or by continuous infusion pump.

This type of pain management is used for postoperative pain, labor pain, and cancer pain. The most serious adverse reaction associated with the administration of narcotics by the epidural route is respiratory depression. A patient may also experience sedation, confusion, nausea, pruritus, or urinary retention. Fentanyl is increasingly used as an alternative to morphine sulfate because patients experience fewer adverse reactions.

Educating the Patient and Family about Narcotic Analgesics

The health care provider explains to the patient that the drug he or she is receiving is for pain. Additional information is also often included, such as how often the drug can be taken. Box 8-2 explains the process of receiving drugs through a PCA infusion pump.

Narcotics for outpatient use may be prescribed in the oral form or as a timed-release transdermal patch. In certain cases, such as when terminally ill patients are being cared for at home, the health care provider may instruct the family in the parenteral administration of the drug or use of PCA. Following are key points the patient or family member needs to know about narcotics.

- This drug may cause drowsiness, dizziness, and blurring of vision. Be cautious when driving or performing tasks requiring alertness.

ALERT ℞

Naloxone

Naloxone should be administered with great caution and only when necessary in patients receiving a narcotic for severe pain. Naloxone cancels out all of the pain-relieving effects of the narcotic and may lead to withdrawal symptoms or the return of pain.

BOX 8.2

Key Points for Receiving Drugs through a PCA Infusion Pump

Patients using a PCA system need to be taught and/or shown the following:

- The location of the control button that activates the administration of the drug
- The difference between the control button and the button to call the health care provider (when both are similar in appearance and feel)
- The machine regulates the dose of the drug as well as the time interval between doses
- If the control button is used too soon after the last dose, then the machine will not deliver the drug until the correct time
- Pain relief should occur soon after pushing the button
- Call the health care provider if pain relief does not occur after two successive doses

In some situations, narcotic analgesics may be ordered for pain relief using PCA. If the patient will be receiving PCA at home, then the following steps are reviewed with the patient and the caregiver:

- How the pump works
- What drug is being given
- When to administer a dose
- What the power source is (battery or electricity)
- What to do if the battery fails or a power failure occurs
- How to check the insertion site
- How to change the cartridge or syringe

- Do not drink alcoholic beverages unless your health care provider approves. Alcohol may intensify the action of the drug and cause extreme drowsiness or dizziness. In some instances, drinking while taking a narcotic can have extremely serious and even life-threatening consequences that may require emergency medical treatment.
- Take the drug as directed by the container label and do not exceed the prescribed dose. Contact your health care provider if the drug is not effective.
- If you experience GI upset, take the drug with food.
- Notify your health care provider if you experience severe nausea, vomiting, or/and constipation.
- To put on a transdermal patch, remove the patch from the package and immediately apply it to the nonhairy skin of your upper torso. To ensure complete contact with the skin, press on it for 10 to 20 seconds with your palm. After 72 hours, remove the patch. Put on a new one if prescribed. Use only water to cleanse the site before putting it on because soaps, oils, and other substances may irritate the skin. Rotate your sites of application. Fold the

used patch carefully so that it adheres to itself, and dispose of it appropriately.

FACT CHECK

8-20   What is one of the major hazards of narcotic administration?
8-21   Why is a lower dosage of a narcotic often needed for older adults?
8-22   What is patient-controlled analgesia (PCA)?

Narcotic Antagonists

An antagonist is a substance that counteracts the action of something else. An antagonist drug has an affinity for a cell receptor and by binding to it prevents the cell from responding to another drug. Thus, a narcotic antagonist reverses the actions of a narcotic. Specific antagonists have been developed to reverse the respiratory depression associated with the opiates. Two narcotic antagonists in use today are naloxone (Narcan) and naltrexone (ReVia); see the Summary Drug Table: Narcotic Antagonists. Naloxone can restore respiratory function within 1 to 2 minutes after administration. Naltrexone is used primarily for the treatment of narcotic dependence to block the effects of the opiates, especially the euphoric effects experienced in opiate dependence.

Actions of Narcotic Antagonists

Administration of naloxone prevents or reverses the effects of the opiates. The exact mechanism of action is not fully understood, but it is believed that naloxone reverses opioid effects by competing for opiate receptor sites. If the individual has taken or received an opiate, then the effects of the opiate are reversed. If the individual has not taken or received an opiate, then naloxone has no drug activity.

Naltrexone completely blocks the effects of intravenous opiates, as well as drugs with agonist–antagonist actions (butorphanol, nalbuphine, and pentazocine). The mechanism of action appears to be the same as that for naloxone.

Uses of Narcotic Antagonists

Naloxone is used for complete or partial reversal of narcotic depression, including respiratory depression. Narcotic depression may be caused by intentional or accidental overdose (self-administration by an individual), accidental overdose by medical personnel, or a drug idiosyncratic reaction. Naloxone also may be used to diagnose a suspected acute opioid overdosage.

Naltrexone is used to treat persons dependent on opioids. Patients receiving naltrexone have been detoxified and are enrolled in a program for treatment of narcotic addiction. Naltrexone, along with other methods of treatment, such as counseling or psychotherapy, is used to maintain an opioid-free state. Patients taking naltrexone on a scheduled basis will not experience any narcotic effects if they use an opioid.

Adverse Reactions of Narcotic Antagonists

Although not a true adverse reaction of naloxone, the abrupt reversal of narcotic depression may result in nausea, vomiting, sweating, tachycardia, increased blood pressure, and tremors.

Administration of naltrexone may result in anxiety, difficulty sleeping, abdominal cramps, nasal congestion, joint and muscle pain, nausea, vomiting, dizziness, irritability, depression, fatigue, and drowsiness.

Contraindications, Precautions, and Interactions of Narcotic Antagonists

Naloxone

- Naloxone is contraindicated in those with a hypersensitivity to narcotic antagonists.
- Naloxone is used cautiously in those with a narcotic addiction. Naloxone is used cautiously in patients with cardiovascular disease, lactating women, and infants of opioid-dependent mothers.
- These drugs may produce withdrawal symptoms in those physically dependent on a narcotic drug. These patients must not have taken any opiate for the last 7 to 10 days.
- Naloxone may prevent the action of opioid antidiarrheals, antitussives, and analgesics.

Naltrexone

- Naltrexone is contraindicated in those with a hypersensitivity to narcotic antagonists.
- Naltrexone is used cautiously in those with a narcotic addiction; in patients with cardiovascular disease, acute hepatitis, liver failure, or depression; in patients who are suicidal; and during lactation.
- Naltrexone may produce withdrawal symptoms in those physically dependent on narcotics. These patients must not have taken any opiate for the last 7 to 10 days.
- Concurrent use of naltrexone with thioridazine may cause increased drowsiness and lethargy.
- Naltrexone may prevent the action of opioid antidiarrheals, antitussives, and analgesics.

Patient Management Issues with Narcotic Antagonists

Narcotic Antagonists for Respiratory Depression

As part of the ongoing assessment during the administration of naloxone, the patient's blood pressure, pulse, and respiratory rate are monitored frequently, usually every 5 minutes, until the patient responds. After the patient has shown response to the drug, vital signs are monitored every 5 to 15 minutes. The health care provider should be notified if any adverse drug reactions occur because additional medical treatment may be needed. The patient's respiratory rate, rhythm, and depth; pulse; blood pressure; and level of consciousness are monitored until the effects of the narcotic wear off.

Narcotic Antagonists for Treatment of Opioid Dependency

Each time a patient visits the outpatient clinic, the patient's response to therapy is evaluated and the health care provider

looks for any signs that drug dependency might again be a problem. These signs might include ineffective coping related to difficulty staying drug free, anxiety, or other factors, including an indifference to the requirements of the treatment program.

Entering a program for drug dependency may cause great anxiety. Possible causes of anxiety include the socioeconomic impact of drug dependency, questions about the effectiveness of the treatment program, and concern over remaining drug free. Individuals vary in their ability to communicate their fears and concerns. At times, the health care provider may be able to identify situations causing anxiety and explore possible solutions to the many problems faced by these patients.

One of the greatest problems experienced by those with former drug dependency is remaining drug free. Some people find it difficult to break away from situations, individuals, or pressures that promote drug use. Because of this, some opioid users entering a drug rehabilitation program may eventually not report to the program or agency to receive their drug and thus become more likely to return to using an opiate.

All staff members in a rehabilitation program should work to encourage the patient to stick with the regimen and to identify situations in which the patient is encouraged to return to drug use.

Educating the Patient and Family about Narcotic Antagonists

Patients under treatment for narcotic addiction should be instructed to wear or carry identification indicating that they are receiving naltrexone. If a patient taking naltrexone requires hospitalization, then medical personnel must be aware of therapy with this drug. Narcotics administered to these patients have no effect and cannot relieve pain. The health care provider must decide what methods must be used to control pain in patients receiving naltrexone.

Patients taking naltrexone should be made aware of the impact of therapy. While they are taking the drug, any use of heroin or another opiate generally will have no effect. Large doses of heroin or other opiates, however, can overcome the drug's effect and result in coma or death.

FACT CHECK

8-23 What is naltrexone used to treat?
8-24 What is naloxone used to treat?

Chapter Review

KEY POINTS

- Nonnarcotic analgesics are drugs used to relieve pain without the possibility of causing physical dependency, such as can occur with the use of the narcotic analgesics. Nonnarcotic analgesics include the salicylates, nonsalicylates (acetaminophen), and NSAIDs.
- Adverse reactions of salicylate drugs include gastric upset, heartburn, nausea, vomiting, anorexia, and GI bleeding. Adverse reactions of acetaminophen usually occur with chronic use or when the recommended dosage is exceeded, and are otherwise uncommon.
- Adverse reactions of aceteminophen are rare, but it is hepatotoxic.
- Many adverse reactions may occur with NSAIDs. However, many patients take these drugs and experience few, if any, side effects. Taking an NSAID with food will help prevent GI upset.
- Narcotic analgesics are controlled substances used to treat moderate to severe pain. Narcotic analgesics are classified as agonists, partial agonists, and mixed agonists–antagonists. Drugs that counteract the effects of the narcotic analgesics are narcotic antagonists.
- One of the major hazards of agonist narcotic administration is respiratory depression. The most common adverse reactions to agonists include light-headedness, dizziness, sedation, constipation, anorexia, nausea, vomiting, and sweating. Administration of a narcotic agonist–antagonist may result in symptoms of narcotic withdrawal in those addicted to narcotics.
- Morphine is the most widely used drug in the management of chronic severe pain, such as pain associated with cancer. This drug can be given orally, subcutaneously, intramuscularly, intravenously, and rectally in the form of a suppository and has tremendous versatility.
- Narcotic antagonists are available to reverse the respiratory depression associated with opiates in the event of overdose and to treat opioid dependence.

CRITICAL THINKING CASE STUDY

Understanding NSAIDs

Mr. Nunn, aged 68 years, has been diagnosed with arthritis and has been prescribed an NSAID.

1. What should Mr. Nunn know before taking his medication?
   a. It should be taken with food to prevent GI upset.
   b. It can cause GI bleeding. He should watch for any signs of blood in his stool.
   c. Because of his age, he is at an increased risk of ulcer formation.
   d. All of the above
2. Mr. Nunn's right knee is really bothering him. What might you recommend to help him with his knee pain?
   a. Heating pad
   b. Resting his knee
   c. A cane to help him walk more easily
   d. All of the above
3. The next time you see him, Mr. Nunn is running a fever of 100.5 °F. You know that he is still taking an NSAID. What should he take for his fever? Why?
4. Mr. Nunn goes to the hospital for heart surgery. Can he continue to take his NSAID? Why or why not?

Review Questions

MULTIPLE CHOICE

1. Which of the following symptoms would you expect in a patient experiencing salicylism?
   a. Dizziness, tinnitus, mental confusion
   b. Diarrhea, nausea, weight loss
   c. Constipation, anorexia, rash
   d. Weight gain, hyperglycemia, urinary frequency
2. The health care provider observes a patient for which of these common adverse reactions when administering naproxen?
   a. Headache, dyspepsia
   b. Drowsiness, heartburn
   c. Anorexia, tinnitus
   d. Stomatitis, confusion
3. It is explained to patients that some narcotics may be used as part of the preoperative medication regimen to
   a. increase their intestinal motility
   b. facilitate passage of an endotracheal tube
   c. enhance the effects of a skeletal muscle relaxant
   d. lessen their anxiety and provide sedation
4. Which narcotic antagonist is most likely prescribed for treatment of a patient experiencing an overdose of a narcotic?
   a. naltrexone
   b. naloxone
   c. naproxen
   d. nifedipine

MATCHING

_____ 5. naproxen	a.	Dilaudid
_____ 6. oxycodone	b.	Stadol
_____ 7. aspirin	c.	ReVia
_____ 8. acetaminophen	d.	Celebrex
_____ 9. celecoxib	e.	OxyContin
_____ 10. hydromorphone	f.	Tylenol
_____ 11. butorphanol	g.	Aleve
_____ 12. naltrexone	h.	Bayer

TRUE OR FALSE

_____ 13. Aspirin more potently inhibits prostaglandin synthesis and has greater anti-inflammatory effects than other salicylates.

_____ 14. The inhibition of COX-1 by NSAIDs causes the unwanted gastrointestinal reactions, such as stomach irritation and ulcers.

_____ 15. Elderly, cachectic, or debilitated patients may receive a reduced initial dose of narcotic analgesic until their response to the drug is known.

_____ 16. The salicylates act at the mu receptor.

FILL IN THE BLANKS

17. It is thought that the analgesic action of the salicylates is caused by the inhibition of _____.

18. Aspirin prolongs bleeding time by inhibiting the aggregation (clumping) of _____.

19. NSAIDs have _____, _____ and _____ properties.

20. One of the major hazards of narcotic administration is _____ _____.

SHORT ANSWERS

21. What is acetaminophen used to treat? What advantage does it offer over salicylates and NSAIDs?

22. One of your patients, Mrs. Downey, is going into the hospital for a surgical procedure. She will be discharged on a narcotic analgesic for pain. She will likely take the medication for several days and is worried about the adverse effects and dependence. What should you tell her?

23. Mr. Jones has pancreatic cancer and has been prescribed a Duragesic patch. How should the patch be used?

24. Compare and contrast the uses of the salicylates, acetaminophen, NSAIDs, and the narcotic analgesics.

Web Activities

1. Go to the Mayo Clinic Web site (www.mayoclinic.org) and search for information about the use of an epidural for labor pain management. Write a brief statement about what an expectant mother might learn from the site.

2. Go to Hospice Web site (http://www.hospicenet.org) and conduct a search for "Pain Control: Dispelling the Myths". Write a brief description about the different myths.

SUMMARY DRUG TABLE: Nonnarcotic Analgesics: Salicylates and Nonsalicylates (left, generic; right, trade)

Comprehensive Summary Drug Tables, including uses, adverses effects, dosages, and pregnancy classifications, are provided on the companion website, http://thePoint.lww.com/PharmacologyHP2e

Salicylates	
aspirin (acetylsalicylic acid) *ass'-purr-in*	Bayer (OTC), Ecotrin (OTC), Easprin (Rx), Zorprin (Rx), miscellaneous (OTC), *generic*
buffered aspirin *ass'-purr-in*	Bufferin (OTC)
diflunisal *dye-floo-'ni-sal*	*generic* (Rx)
magnesium salicylate *mag-nee'-see-um-sal-ih'-sah-late*	DeWitts Pain Reliever (OTC), Extra Strength Doan's (OTC), Momentum Muscular Backache (OTC), MST 600 (Rx)
salsalate *sal-sa'-late*	*generic*
Nonsalicylate	
acetaminophen *a-sea-tah-min'-oh-fen*	Tylenol (OTC), miscellaneous, *generic*

SUMMARY DRUG TABLE: Narcotic Antagonists (left, generic; right, trade)

Comprehensive Summary Drug Tables, including uses, adverses effects, dosages, and pregnancy classifications, are provided on the companion website, http://thePoint.lww.com/PharmacologyHP2e

naloxone hydrochloride *nal-ox'-ohn*	*generic*
naltrexone hydrochloride *nal-trex'-ohn*	ReVia, Depade, Vivitrol

SUMMARY DRUG TABLE: Nonsteroidal Anti-Inflammatory Drugs (left, generic; right, trade)

Comprehensive Summary Drug Tables, including uses, adverses effects, dosages, and pregnancy classifications, are provided on the companion website, http://thePoint.lww.com/PharmacologyHP2e

celecoxib *sell-ah-cocx'-ib*	Celebrex
diclofenac sodium *dye-kloe'-fen-ak*	Voltaren, *generic*
diclofenac potassium *dye-kloe'-fen-ak*	Cataflam, *generic*
etodolac *ee-toe-doe'-lak*	*generic*
fenoprofen calcium *fen-oh-proe'-fen*	Nalfon, *generic*
flurbiprofen	*generic*
ibuprofen *eye-byoo-proe'-fen*	Advil (OTC), Motrin (OTC), *generic* (OTC), *generic* (Rx)
indomethacin *in-doe-meth'-a-sin*	Indocin, *generic*
ketoprofen *kee-toe-proe'-fen*	*generic*
ketorolac *kee'-toe-role-ak*	*generic*
meclofenamate *me-kloe-fen-am'-ate*	*generic*
mefenamic acid *me-fe-nam'-ik*	Ponstel
meloxicam *mel-ox'-i-kam*	Mobic
nabumetone *nah-byew'-meh-tone*	*generic*
naproxen *na-prox'-en*	Aleve (OTC), Pamprin All Day Relief Max Str (OTC), Anaprox DS (Rx), EC-Naprosyn (Rx), Naprelan (Rx), Naprosyn (Rx), *generic*
oxaprozin *oks-a-pro'-zin*	Daypro, *generic*
piroxicam *peer-ox'-i-kam*	Feldene, *generic*
sulindac *sul-in'-dak*	Clinoril, *generic*
tolmetin sodium *tole'-met-in*	*generic*

SUMMARY DRUG TABLE: Narcotic Analgesics (left, generic; right, trade)

Comprehensive Summary Drug Tables, including uses, adverses effects, dosages, and pregnancy classifications, are provided on the companion website, http://thePoint.lww.com/PharmacologyHP2e

Agonist	
alfentanil HCL *al-fen'-ta-nil*	Alfenta (CII), *generic*
codeine *koe'-deen*	*generic* (CII)
fentanyl *fen'-ta-nil*	Sublimaze, *generic*
fentanyl *fen'-ta-nil* transmucosal system	Actiq (CII), Fentora, Onsolis, *generic*
fentanyl *fen'-ta-nil* transdermal system	Duragesic (CII)
hydromorphone *hy-droe-mor'-fone*	Dilaudid (CII), *generic*
levorphanol tartrate *lee-vor'-fa nole*	*generic* (CII)
meperidine *me-per'-i-deen*	Demerol (CII), *generic*
methadone *meth'-a-doan*	Dolophine (CII), *generic*
morphine sulfate *mor'-feen*	MS Contin (CII), *generic*
opium *oh'-pee-um*	Paregoric (CIII), opium tincture (CII)
oxycodone *ox-ee-koe'-done*	OxyContin (CII), Roxicodone, *generic*
oxymorphone *ox-ee-mor'-fone*	Opana (CII), Opana ER, *generic*
remifentanil HCL *reh-mih-fen'-tah-nill*	Ultiva (CII)
sufentanil citrate *soo-fen'-ta-nil*	Sufenta (CII), *generic*
tapentadol *ta-pen'-ta-dol*	Nucynta (CII)
tramadol *tra'-ma-dole*	Ultram, Ultram ER, *generic*
Partial Agonist	
buprenorphine *byoo-pre-nor'-feen*	Buprenex (CIII), Subutex, *generic*
butorphanol *byoo-tor'fa-nole*	Stadol (CIV), *generic*
Agonist Antagonist	
nalbuphine *nal'-byoo-feen*	*generic*
pentazocine *pen-taz'-oh-seen*	Talwin (CIV)
pentazocine combination *pen-taz'-oh-seen*	Pentazocine and acetaminophen (CIV), pentazocine and naloxone (CIV), pentazocine and aspirin (CIV)

9

Anesthetic Drugs

KEY TERMS

analgesia—absence of pain
anesthesia—a loss of feeling or sensation
anesthesiologist—a physician with special training in administering anesthetics
anesthetist—a nurse with special training who is qualified to administer anesthetics
atelectasis—reduction of air in the lung
brachial plexus block—type of regional anesthesia produced by injection of a local anesthetic into the brachial plexus
conduction block—type of regional anesthesia produced by injection of a local anesthetic into or near a nerve trunk
epidural block—type of regional anesthesia produced by injection of a local anesthetic into the space surrounding the dura of the spinal cord
general anesthesia—provision of a pain-free state for the entire body
induction drug—drug given at the beginning of an anesthesia process that results in a general anesthesia state
local anesthesia—provision of a pain-free state in a specific area
local infiltration anesthesia—anesthesia produced by injecting a local anesthetic drug into tissues

thePOINT RESOURCES

- Comprehensive Summary Drug Tables
- Lippincott's Interactive Tutorials: Drugs Affecting the Central Nervous System
- Interactive Practice and Review
- Monographs of Most Commonly Prescribed Drugs

neuroleptanalgesia—a state of general quietness achieved through a combination of analgesic and neuroleptic drugs

patency—being open or exposed

preanesthetic drug—a drug given before the administration of anesthesia

regional anesthesia—anesthesia produced by injecting a local anesthetic around nerves to limit the pain signals sent to the brain

spinal anesthesia—a type of regional anesthesia produced by injecting a local anesthetic drug into the subarachnoid space of the spinal cord

transsacral block—type of regional anesthesia produced by injection of a local anesthetic into the epidural space at the level of the sacrococcygeal notch

volatile liquid—a liquid that evaporates on exposure to the air

This chapter focuses on anesthetic drugs. Because either an anesthesiologist or a nurse anesthetist is responsible for administering this drug group, this chapter's information on dosages, adverse reactions, contraindications, precautions, and interactions will be kept to a minimum.

Anesthesia is a loss of feeling or sensation. Anesthesia may be induced by various drugs that are able to bring about partial or complete loss of sensation. The two types of anesthesia are local anesthesia and general anesthesia.

Local Anesthetics

Local anesthesia, as the term implies, is the condition of a pain-free state in a specific area (or region) of the body. This condition is achieved by inhibiting the transmission of pain signals from the pain receptors where the anesthetic has been administered to the brain. With a local anesthetic, a patient is fully awake but does not feel pain in the area that has been anesthetized. However, some procedures performed under local anesthesia may require a patient to be sedated. Although

not fully awake, sedated patients may still hear what is going on around them. A physician or dentist administers a local injectable anesthetic. Table 9-1 lists commonly used local anesthetics.

Uses of Local Anesthetics

Topical Anesthetics

Topical anesthesia involves the application of the anesthetic to the surface of the skin, open area, or mucous membrane. The anesthetic may be applied with a cotton swab or sprayed on the area. This type of anesthesia may be used to desensitize the skin or mucous membrane before the injection of a deeper local anesthetic. In some instances, a topical anesthetic may be applied by a health care provider other than a physician.

Some topical anesthetics are available over-the-counter. For example, benzocaine is a common topical anesthetic found in medications for toothaches, teething, or other mouth pains. It is also found in topical medications used to treat burns and

TABLE 9-1 Examples of Local Anesthetics

Generic Name	Trade Name	Pregnancy Category
Injectables		
Amide		
bupivacaine HCl	Marcaine, Sensorcaine	C
lidocaine HCl	Xylocaine, *generic*	B
lidocaine and epinephrine	Xylocaine, *generic*	B
mepivacaine HCl	Carbocaine, Polocaine, *generic*	C
prilocaine HCl	Citanest	B
ropivacaine HCl	Naropin	B
Ester		
chloroprocaine HCl	Nesacaine, *generic*	C
procaine HCl	Novocain	C
tetracaine HCl	Pontocaine,	
	generic	C
Topicals		
Amide		
dibucaine	Nupercainal, *generic*	Undetermined
lidocaine HCl	Xylocaine, miscellaneous	B
Ester		
benzocaine	Lanacane, Orajel, Orabase, miscellaneous	C
Miscellaneous		
pramoxine	Sarna, Itch-X, Vagisil, miscellaneous	C

insect bites. Lidocaine is a topical anesthetic that is available both over the counter and by prescription.

Local Infiltration Anesthetics

Local infiltration anesthesia is produced by the injection of a local anesthetic drug into tissues. This type of anesthesia may be used for dental procedures, suturing small wounds, or making an incision into a small area such as that required for removing a superficial tissue sample for biopsy.

Regional Anesthetics

Regional anesthesia is produced by the injection of a local anesthetic around nerves so that the area supplied by these nerves will not send pain signals to the brain. The anesthetized area is usually larger than the area affected by local infiltration anesthesia. Spinal anesthesia and conduction blocks are two types of regional anesthesia.

Spinal Anesthetics. Spinal anesthesia is a type of regional anesthesia resulting from the injection of a local anesthetic drug into the subarachnoid space of the spinal cord, usually at the level of the second lumbar vertebra. There is a loss of feeling (anesthesia) and movement in the lower extremities, lower abdomen, and perineum. Any drug that is injected into the spinal cord must be preservative free.

Conduction Block Anesthetics. A **conduction block** is a type of regional anesthesia produced by injection of a local anesthetic drug into or near a nerve trunk. Examples of a conduction block include an **epidural block** (injection of a local anesthetic into the space surrounding the dura of the spinal cord), a **transsacral** (caudal) **block** (injection of a local anesthetic into the epidural space at the level of the sacrococcygeal notch), and **brachial plexus block** (injection of a local anesthetic into the brachial plexus). Epidural and transsacral blocks are often used in obstetrics. A brachial plexus block may be used for surgery of the arm or hand.

Patient Management Issues with Local Anesthetics

Depending on the procedure performed, preparing a patient for local anesthesia may or may not be similar to preparing the patient for general anesthesia. For example, administering a local anesthetic for dental surgery or for suturing a small wound may require the health care provider to explain to the patient how the anesthetic will be administered. The patient's allergy history may be taken. When applicable, the area of the patient's body to be anesthetized may require preparation, such as cleaning the area with an antiseptic or shaving the area. Other local anesthetic procedures may require the patient to be in a fasting state because a sedative may also be administered. An intravenous sedative such as the antianxiety drug diazepam (Valium) (see Chapter 7) may also be given during some local anesthetic procedures, such as cataract surgery or surgery performed under spinal anesthesia.

Educating the Patient and Family about Local Anesthetics

When a local anesthetic is being administered, the patient is usually in a medical office or facility under the care of health care professionals who will determine when the patient is fit to return home. However, a patient who is using an over-the-counter topical anesthetic at home needs to be aware of the following points:

- The effects of the anesthetic will last for a relatively short period of time, between 15 and 45 minutes.
- The anesthetic should only be applied to a small area. Overuse could result in hypersensitivity and/or systemic toxicity of some anesthetics.
- Using the anesthetic more than three or four times a day could result in systemic toxicity.
- Benzocaine can cause a hypersensitivity reaction. If the patient seems to be developing an allergic reaction (e.g., rash, itching), then the medication should be discontinued. The patient and family member should document this reaction, inform the health care provider of the hypersensitivity, and avoid benzocaine in the future.

FACT CHECK

9-1   What are the three uses of local anesthetics?
9-2   Which topical local anesthetic may cause a hypersensitivity reaction?

Preanesthetic Drugs

A **preanesthetic drug** is one given before the administration of anesthesia. It is usually used before the administration of general anesthesia but also on occasion before injection of a local anesthetic. The preanesthetic may consist of one drug or a combination of drugs.

Uses of Preanesthetic Drugs

The general purpose of the preanesthetic drug is to prepare the patient for anesthesia.

Narcotic or antianxiety drugs are used to decrease anxiety and apprehension immediately before surgery. The patient who is calm and relaxed can be anesthetized more quickly, usually requires a smaller dose of an **induction drug** (drug given at the beginning of anesthesia), may require less anesthesia during surgery, and may have a smoother anesthesia recovery period (awakening from anesthesia). Preanesthetic drugs are usually given 30 minutes before surgery.

Cholinergic blocking drugs are used to decrease secretions of the upper respiratory tract. Some anesthetic gases and volatile liquids are irritating to the lining of the respiratory tract and increase mucus secretions. The cough and swallowing reflexes are lost during general anesthesia, and excessive secretions can pool in the lungs, resulting in pneumonia or **atelectasis** (a reduction of air in the lung) after surgery. The cholinergic blocking drug, such as glycopyrrolate (Robinul), dries up secretions of the upper respiratory tract and lessens the possibility of excessive mucus production.

Antiemetics are used to prevent nausea and vomiting during the immediate postoperative recovery period.

The preanesthetic drug is usually selected by the anesthesiologist and may consist of one or more drugs (Table 9-2). A narcotic (see Chapter 8), antianxiety drug (see Chapter 7), or barbiturate (see Chapter 7) may be given to relax or sedate a patient. Barbiturates are used only occasionally; narcotics

LIFESPAN

Preanesthetic Drugs

Preanesthetic drugs are often not used in patients 60 years or older because many of the medical disorders for which these drugs are contraindicated occur in older individuals. For example, atropine and glycopyrrolate, drugs that can be used to decrease secretions of the upper respiratory tract, are contraindicated in patients with certain medical disorders, such as prostatic hypertrophy, glaucoma, and myocardial ischemia. Other preanesthetic drugs that depress the central nervous system, such as narcotics, barbiturates, and antianxiety drugs with or without antiemetic properties, may also be contraindicated in older individuals.

are usually preferred for sedation. A cholinergic blocking drug (see Chapter 14) is given to dry secretions in the upper respiratory tract. Scopolamine and glycopyrrolate also have mild sedative properties, and atropine may or may not produce some sedation. Antianxiety drugs have sedative action; when combined with a narcotic, they allow for a lowering of the narcotic dosage because they potentiate the sedative action of the narcotic. Diazepam (Valium), an antianxiety drug, is one of the more commonly used drugs for preoperative sedation.

Contraindications, Precautions, and Interactions of Preanesthetic Drugs

Preanesthetic drugs must be administered on time to produce their intended effects. Failure to give the preanesthetic drug on time may result in events such as increased respiratory secretions caused by the irritating effect of anesthetic gases and the need for a greater dose of the induction drug because the preanesthetic drug has not had time to sedate a patient.

Patient Management Issues with Preanesthetic Drugs

A health care provider, usually a nurse, evaluates the patient's physical status and explains the anesthesia to the patient. In some situations, an anesthesiologist examines the patient the day or evening before surgery. In some hospitals, members of the operating room or postanesthesia recovery room staff visit a patient the night before or the morning of surgery to explain certain facts, such as the time of surgery, the effects of the preanesthetic drug, preparations for surgery, and the postanesthesia recovery room. Proper explanation of anesthesia, the surgery itself, and the events that may occur in preparation for surgery, as well as care after surgery, require a team approach.

Examples of preoperative preparations include fasting from midnight (or the time specified by a health care provider), enemas, shaving of the operative site, use of a hypnotic for sleep the night before, and a preoperative injection approximately 30 minutes before going to surgery.

FACT CHECK

9-3   Why would a patient need a preanesthetic drug?
9-4   Why is there concern over using preanesthetic drugs in the elderly?

TABLE 9-2   Examples of Preanesthetic Drugs

Generic Name	Trade Name	Pregnancy Category
Narcotics		
droperidol	Inapsine	C
fentanyl	Actiq, Duragesic, Fentora, Onsolis, Sublimaze (CII), *generic*	C
meperidine hydrochloride	Demerol (CII), *generic*	B
morphine sulfate	Astramorph (CII), DepoDur, Infumorph, miscellaneous, *generic*	C
Barbiturates		
pentobarbital	Nembutal (CII)	D
secobarbital	*Seconal (CII)*	D
Cholinergic-Blocking Drugs		
atropine sulfate	*AtroPen, Sal-Tropine, generic*	C
glycopyrrolate	Robinul, *generic*	B
scopolamine	*Maldemar, Scopace, generic*	C
Antianxiety Drugs with Antiemetic Properties		
hydroxyzine	Vistaril, *generic*	C
Antianxiety Drugs		
chlordiazepoxide	Librium (CIV), *generic*	D
diazepam	Valium (CIV), *generic*	D
midazolam	*Generic* (CIV)	D

General Anesthetics

Uses of General Anesthetics

General anesthesia is a condition of a pain-free state for the entire body. When a general anesthetic is given, a patient loses consciousness and feels no pain. Reflexes, such as the swallowing and gag reflexes, are lost during deep general anesthesia (Fig. 9-1). An **anesthesiologist** is a physician with special training in administering anesthesia. A nurse **anesthetist** is a nurse with special training who is qualified to administer anesthetics.

General anesthesia results from the use of one or more drugs. The choice of anesthetic drug depends on many factors, including the patient's general physical condition; the area, organ, or body system undergoing surgery; and the anticipated length of the surgical procedure. An anesthesiologist selects the anesthetic drugs that will produce safe anesthesia, **analgesia** (absence of pain), and, for some surgeries, skeletal muscle relaxation.

General surgical anesthesia usually has four stages:

- Stage I: analgesia
- Stage II: delirium
- Stage III: surgical analgesia
- Stage IV: respiratory paralysis

Key Concepts 9-1 describes the stages of general anesthesia more completely. With newer drugs and techniques, the stages of anesthesia may not be as prominent as those described in Key Concepts 9-1. In addition, most patients' movement through the first two stages is very rapid.

Anesthesia begins with a loss of consciousness. This occurs at the end of the induction stage (stage I). The patient relaxes and after becoming unconscious cannot see or hear what is going on. Additional anesthetic drugs are usually administered once the patient is unconscious for deepening anesthesia. Depending on the type of surgery, an endotracheal tube may be inserted into the patient's trachea to ensure an adequate airway and assist in the administration of oxygen and anesthetic drugs. The endotracheal tube is removed during the postanesthesia period when the gag and swallowing reflexes return.

Administration of General Anesthetics

General anesthetics are most commonly administered by inhalation or intravenously. Volatile liquid anesthetics produce anesthesia when their vapors are inhaled. **Volatile liquids** are liquids that evaporate when exposed to air. Examples of volatile liquids include desflurane, isoflurane, sevoflurane, and enflurane. Gas anesthetics are combined with oxygen and administered by inhalation. Examples of

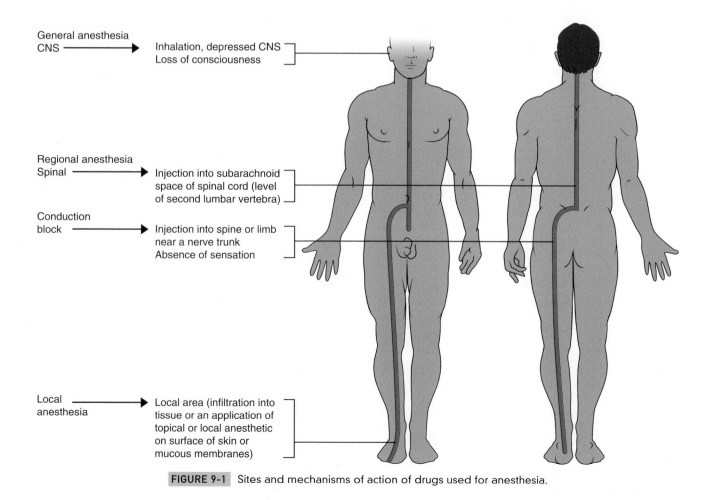

General anesthesia CNS → Inhalation, depressed CNS — Loss of consciousness

Regional anesthesia Spinal → Injection into subarachnoid space of spinal cord (level of second lumbar vertebra)

Conduction block → Injection into spine or limb near a nerve trunk — Absence of sensation

Local anesthesia → Local area (infiltration into tissue or an application of topical or local anesthetic on surface of skin or mucous membranes)

FIGURE 9-1 Sites and mechanisms of action of drugs used for anesthesia.

KEY CONCEPTS

9-1   Stages of General Anesthesia

Stage I

Induction is a part of stage I anesthesia. It begins with the administration of an anesthetic drug and lasts until the patient loses consciousness. With some induction drugs, such as short-acting barbiturates, this stage may last only 5 to 10 seconds.

Stage II

Stage II is a brief stage of delirium and excitement. During this stage, the patient may move about and mumble incoherently, although the patient is unconscious and cannot feel pain. The muscles are somewhat rigid. The patient would have a physical reaction to painful stimuli yet not remember sensing pain. During the first two stages of anesthesia, health care professionals avoid any unnecessary noise or motion around the patient.

Stage III

Stage III is the stage of surgical analgesia, which is usually divided into four planes or substages. The anesthesiologist differentiates these planes by the character of the patient's respirations, eye movements, reflexes, pupil size, and other factors. The level of anesthesia ranges from plane 1 (light) to plane 4 (deep). At plane 2 or 3, the patient is ready for the surgical procedure.

Stage IV

Stage IV is the stage of respiratory paralysis, a rare and dangerous stage of anesthesia. Respiratory arrest may occur.

gas anesthetics are ethylene, nitrous oxide, and cyclopropane. Other general anesthetics are administered intravenously. Examples of intravenous anesthetics are droperidol, etomidate, propofol, and ketamine. Commonly used general anesthetics are listed in the Summary Drug Table at the end of the chapter.

Drugs Used for General Anesthesia

Methohexital and Thiopental. Methohexital (Brevital) and thiopental (Pentothal), which are ultrashort-acting barbiturates, are used for

- Induction of anesthesia
- Short surgical procedures with minimal painful stimuli
- In conjunction with or as a supplement to other anesthetics
- Control of convulsive states (thiopental)

These drugs have a rapid onset and a short duration of action. They depress the central nervous system to produce hypnosis

and anesthesia but do not produce analgesia. Recovery after a small dose is rapid.

Etomidate. Etomidate (Amidate), a nonbarbiturate, is used for induction of anesthesia. Etomidate also may be used to supplement other anesthetics, such as nitrous oxide, for short surgical procedures. It is a hypnotic without analgesic activity.

Propofol. Propofol (Diprivan) is used for induction and maintenance of anesthesia. It also may be used for sedation during diagnostic procedures and procedures that use a local anesthetic. This drug also is used for continuous sedation of intubated or respiratory-controlled patients in intensive care units.

Fospropofol (Lusedra) is used for monitored anesthesia care sedation. It is a prodrug of propofol, which means it is converted to propofol in the body.

Midazolam. Midazolam (Versed), a short-acting benzodiazepine central nervous system depressant, is used as a preanesthetic drug to relieve anxiety, for induction of anesthesia, for conscious sedation before minor procedures such as endoscopic procedures, and to supplement nitrous oxide and oxygen for short surgical procedures.

Sevoflurane. Sevoflurane (Ultane) is an inhaled analgesic. It is used for induction and maintenance of general anesthesia in adult and pediatric patients for inpatient and outpatient surgical procedures.

Ketamine. Ketamine (Ketalar) is a rapid-acting general anesthetic. It produces an anesthetic state characterized by profound analgesia, cardiovascular and respiratory stimulation, normal or enhanced skeletal muscle tone, and occasionally mild respiratory depression. Ketamine is used for diagnostic and surgical procedures that do not require relaxation of skeletal muscles, for induction of anesthesia before the administration of other anesthetic drugs, and as a supplement to other anesthetic drugs.

Cyclopropane. An anesthetic gas, cyclopropane has a rapid onset of action and may be used for induction and maintenance of anesthesia. Skeletal muscle relaxation is produced with full anesthetic doses.

Ethylene. Ethylene is an anesthetic gas with a rapid onset of action and a rapid recovery from its anesthetic effects. It provides adequate analgesia but has poor muscle relaxant properties.

Nitrous Oxide. Nitrous oxide is the most commonly used anesthetic gas. It is a weak anesthetic and is usually used in combination with other anesthetic drugs. It does not cause skeletal muscle relaxation.

Enflurane. Enflurane (Ethrane) is a volatile liquid anesthetic that is delivered by inhalation. Induction and recovery from anesthesia are rapid. Muscle relaxation for abdominal surgery is adequate, but greater muscle relaxation may be necessary for other surgeries and may require the use of a skeletal muscle relaxant.

Isoflurane. Isoflurane (Forane) is a volatile liquid given by inhalation. It is used for induction and maintenance of anesthesia.

Desflurane. Desflurane (Suprane), a volatile liquid, is used for induction and maintenance of anesthesia. A special vaporizer is used to deliver this anesthetic because delivery by mask results in irritation of the respiratory tract.

Fentanyl and Droperidol. The narcotic analgesic fentanyl (Sublimaze) and the neuroleptic (major tranquilizer) droperidol (Inapsine) may be used together as a single drug called Innovar. The combination of these two drugs results in **neuroleptanalgesia**, which is characterized by general quietness, reduced motor activity, and profound analgesia. Complete loss of consciousness may not occur unless other anesthetic drugs are used. A combination of fentanyl and droperidol may be used for the tranquilizing effect and analgesia for surgical and diagnostic procedures. It may also be used as a preanesthetic for the induction of anesthesia and in the maintenance of general anesthesia.

Droperidol may be used alone as a tranquilizer, as an antiemetic to prevent nausea and vomiting during the immediate postanesthesia period, as an induction drug, and as an adjunct to general anesthesia. Fentanyl may be used alone as a supplement to general or regional anesthesia. It may also be administered alone or with other drugs as a preoperative drug and as an analgesic during the immediate postoperative (recovery room) period.

Remifentanil Hydrochloride. Remifentanil (Ultiva) is used for induction and maintenance of general anesthesia and for continued analgesia during the immediate postoperative period. This drug is used cautiously in patients with a history of hypersensitivity to fentanyl.

Skeletal Muscle Relaxants

Various skeletal muscle relaxants may be used during general anesthesia (Table 9-3). These drugs are given to produce relaxation of the skeletal muscles during certain types of surgeries, such as those involving the chest or abdomen. They may also be used to facilitate the insertion of an endotracheal tube. Their onset of action is usually rapid (45 seconds to a few minutes), and the duration of action is 30 minutes or more.

Adverse Reactions of General Anesthetics

The most common adverse reactions that patients experience after administration of a general anesthetic are paresthesia (stinging, tingling, burning) and pruritis (itching). The patient will experience these fairly soon after administration. Again, the patient and family members need to document these adverse reactions and inform the health care providers at the time of the occurrence and prior to any future anesthesia.

Patient Management Issues with General Anesthetics

After surgery, a number of patient management issues must be monitored. These include checking the patient's airway for **patency** (being open and clear), assessing the patient's respiratory status and giving oxygen as needed, positioning the patient to prevent aspiration of vomitus and secretions, and checking the patient's blood pressure, pulse, intravenous lines, catheters, drainage tubes, surgical dressings, and casts. The patient's blood pressure, pulse, and respiratory rate may be monitored every 5 to 15 minutes. The

TABLE 9-3   Examples of Muscle Relaxants Used during General Anesthesia

Generic Name	Trade Name	Pregnancy Category
Depolarizing Neuromuscular Blockers		
succinylcholine chloride	Anectine, Quelicin	C
Nondepolarizing Neuromuscular Blockers		
atracurium besylate	*Generic*	C
cisatracurium besylate	Nimbex	B
pancuronium bromide	*Generic*	C
rocuronium bromide	Zemuron	C
vecuronium bromide	*Generic*	C

patient is checked every 5 to 15 minutes for emergence from anesthesia.

FACT CHECK

9-5   What is general anesthesia?
9-6   How is general anesthesia administered?

Educating the Patient and Family about General Anesthetics

Before surgery, the immediate postoperative care is explained to the patient, such as the postanesthesia recovery room or postoperative surgical unit and the activities of physicians, nurses, and other health care workers during this period. The patient is told that his or her vital signs will be monitored frequently and that other equipment, such as intravenous fluids and monitors, may be used.

Postoperative patient activities, such as deep breathing, coughing, and leg exercises, are also explained and demonstrated, as appropriate.

ALERT ℞

Postsurgical Narcotic Administration
Caution is needed when narcotics are administered after surgery. A patient's respiratory rate, blood pressure, and pulse are taken before these drugs are given and 20 to 30 minutes afterwards (see Chapter 8). The health care provider is contacted if the patient's respiratory rate is below 10 before the drug is given or falls below 10 after the drug is given.

Chapter Review

KEY POINTS

- With a local anesthetic, a patient is fully awake but does not feel pain in the area that has been anesthetized. In some cases, the patient may also be sedated.
- Local anesthetics may be administered by topical application, local infiltration, or methods to result in regional anesthesia.
- Narcotic or antianxiety drugs are used to decrease the patient's anxiety and apprehension immediately before surgery and are referred to as preanesthetic drugs. Cholinergic blocking drugs are used to decrease secretions of the upper respiratory tract. Some anesthetic gases and volatile liquids are irritating to the lining of the respiratory tract and increase mucus secretions. Antiemetics are used to prevent nausea and vomiting during the immediate postoperative recovery period.
- Preanesthetic drugs may not be used in patients 60 years or older because many of the medical disorders for which these drugs are contraindicated occur in older individuals.
- When a general anesthetic is given, a patient loses consciousness and feels no pain. Reflexes, such as the swallowing and gag reflexes, are lost during deep general anesthesia.
- The choice of anesthetic drug depends on many factors, including the patient's general physical condition; the area, organ, or body system being operated on; and the anticipated length of the surgical procedure.
- Careful monitoring of a patient is essential after surgery. This usually includes respiratory observation, and checking the patient's pulse, blood pressure, intravenous lines, catheters, drainage tubes, surgical dressings, and casts.

CRITICAL THINKING CASE STUDY

Local vs. General Anesthesia

Sally Smithers is visiting her dentist to discuss having her wisdom teeth removed. She is nervous about the procedure and is hoping it can be done in the dentist's office.

1. If Sally is able to have her wisdom teeth removed in the office, what type of anesthesia may be used?
   a. Topical local to numb the gum
   b. Local infiltration to numb the area
   c. General anesthesia
   d. A and b only
2. After reviewing Sally's x-rays, the dentist determines that the procedure is more involved and will require general anesthesia. What might you tell Sally about the advantages of general anesthesia versus local anesthesia?

Review Questions

MULTIPLE CHOICE

1. Which of the following is/are commonly used in obstetrics?
   a. Transsacral block
   b. Brachial plexus block
   c. Epidural block
   d. a and c
2. What is the purpose of cholinergic blocking drugs (anticholinergics) as preanesthetic drugs?
   a. To decrease secretions of the upper respiratory tract
   b. To decrease anxiety
   c. To prevent postoperative nausea
   d. All of the above
3. Which population is particularly at risk for problems with preanesthetic drugs?
   a. Children
   b. Patients 60 years or older
   c. Pregnant women
   d. Anyone weighing less than 100 lb

MATCHING

_____ 4. Preanesthetic drug   a. lidocaine
_____ 5. General anesthetic   b. atropine
_____ 6. Local anesthetic   c. succinylcholine
_____ 7. Muscle relaxant   d. propofol

TRUE OR FALSE

_____ 8. Benzocaine is a topical anesthetic that is available over the counter.
_____ 9. Local anesthetics have a long duration of action.
_____ 10. Spinal anesthesia and conduction blocks are two types of regional anesthesia.

FILL IN THE BLANKS

11. Preanesthesia drugs are usually given _____ minutes before surgery.
12. Common adverse reactions of general anesthetics are _____ and _____.
13. General anesthesia should be administered by either a(n) _____ or a(n) _____.

SHORT ANSWERS

14. Name and describe the four stages of general anesthesia.

15. Name at least two types of drugs that may be used as preanesthetics.
16. What are some examples or preoperative preparations that the patient and family should know about?

Web Activities

1. Go to the American Academy of Pediatric Dentistry Web site (http://www.aapd.org) and conduct a search of the site for nitrous oxide.
   a. What is nitrous oxide often called?
   b. How does it make the patient feel?

2. Go to the Institute for Safe Medication Practices Web site (www.ismp.org) and conduct a search for propofol.
   a. What are the advantages of propofol over other drugs used for sedation?
   b. Who should administer propofol?

SUMMARY DRUG TABLE: General Anesthetics (left, generic; right, trade)

Comprehensive Summary Drug Tables, including uses, adverses effects, dosages, and pregnancy classifications, are provided on the companion website, http://thePoint.lww.com/PharmacologyHP2e

Barbiturates	
methohexital sodium *meth-oh-heks′-i-tal*	Brevital sodium (CIV)
thiopental sodium *thye-oh-pen′-tal*	Pentothal (CIII)
Benzodiazepines	
midazolam *mid′-aye-zoe-lam*	Midazolam (CIV)
Gases	
cyclopropane*	
ethylene*	
nitrous oxide *nye′-trus-oks′-ide*	Nitrous Oxide
Volatile Liquids	
desflurane *des′-flure-ane*	Suprane

enflurane *en′-floo-rane*	Compound 347, Ethrane
isoflurane *eye-soe-flure′-ane*	Forane, Terrell, *generic*
sevoflurane *see-voe-floo′-rane*	Sojourn, Ultane, *generic*
Others	
etomidate *e-tom′-i-date*	Amidate, *generic*
fospropofol *fos-proe′-po-fole*	Lusedra
ketamine *keet′-a-meen*	Ketalar (CIII), *generic*
propofol *proe′-po-fole*	Diprivan, *generic*
remifentanil *rem-i-fen′-ta-nil*	Ultiva

*Rarely used because they are flammable and explosive when mixed with oxygen.

10

Antiemetic and Antivertigo Drugs

CHAPTER OBJECTIVES

On completion of this chapter, students will be able to:

1. Define the chapter's key terms.
2. Identify the actions of antiemetics and antivertigo drugs.
3. Describe the uses of antiemetics and antivertigo drugs.
4. Explain the similarities between the uses of antiemetic and antivertigo drugs and the differences.
5. Identify common adverse reactions of antiemetic and antivertigo drugs.
6. Discuss important points that patients and family members should know about the use of an antiemetic or antivertigo drug.

KEY TERMS

antiemetic—a drug used to treat or prevent nausea or vomiting

antivertigo—a drug used to treat or prevent vertigo

chemoreceptor trigger zone—a group of nerve fibers in the brain that when stimulated by chemicals, such as drugs or toxic substances, sends impulses to the vomiting center of the brain

emesis—the expelled gastric contents; vomitus

nausea—an unpleasant gastric sensation usually preceding vomiting

prophylaxis—a drug or treatment designed for prevention of a condition or symptom

vertigo—an abnormal feeling of spinning or rotation-type motion that may occur with motion sickness and other disorders

vestibular neuritis—inflammation of the vestibular nerve to the inner ear

vomiting—forceful expulsion of gastric contents through the mouth

CHAPTER OVERVIEW

Drug classes covered in this chapter are:

- Antiemetic drugs
- Antivertigo drugs

Drugs by classification are listed on page 124.

thePOINT RESOURCES

- Comprehensive Summary Drug Tables
- Lippincott's Interactive Tutorials: Drugs Affecting the Central Nervous System
- Interactive Practice and Review
- Monographs of Most Commonly Prescribed Drugs

An **antiemetic** drug is used to treat or prevent **nausea** (unpleasant gastric sensation usually preceding vomiting) or **vomiting** (forceful expulsion of gastric contents through the mouth). An **antivertigo** drug is used to treat or prevent **vertigo** (a feeling of a spinning or rotation-type motion), which may occur with motion sickness, Ménière disease of the ear, middle or inner ear surgery, and other disorders.

Vomiting caused by drugs, radiation, and metabolic disorders usually occurs because of stimulation of the **chemoreceptor trigger zone**, a group of nerve fibers in the brain. When these fibers are stimulated by chemicals, such as drugs or toxic substances, impulses are sent to the vomiting center located in the medulla (Fig. 10-1). The vomiting center may also be directly stimulated by disorders such as gastrointestinal irritation, motion sickness, and **vestibular neuritis** (inflammation of the vestibular nerve in the inner ear).

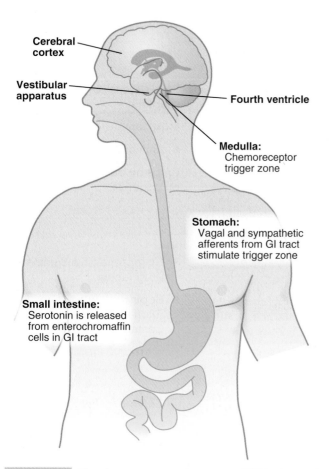

Cerebral cortex

Vestibular apparatus

Fourth ventricle

Medulla: Chemoreceptor trigger zone

Stomach: Vagal and sympathetic afferents from GI tract stimulate trigger zone

Small intestine: Serotonin is released from enterochromaffin cells in GI tract

FIGURE 10-1 The chemoreceptor trigger zone (CTZ) is located in the brain. When stimulated, the CTZ sends impulses to the vomiting center located in the medulla, which then triggers a series of motor activities in the chest and abdomen. The end result is emesis (vomiting).

Antiemetic and Antivertigo Drugs

Actions of Antiemetics and Antivertigo Drugs

These drugs appear to act primarily by inhibiting the chemoreceptor trigger zone or by depressing the sensitivity of the vestibular apparatus of the inner ear. Drugs that act on the chemoreceptor trigger zone are more effective for vomiting caused by stimulation of the chemoreceptor trigger zone, whereas those that act on the vestibular apparatus of the inner ear are more effective for vertigo associated with motion sickness or middle or inner ear surgery.

Uses of Antiemetics and Antivertigo Drugs

Uses of Antiemetic Drugs

An antiemetic is used for **prophylaxis** (prevention) or treatment of nausea and vomiting. An example of prophylactic use is giving an antiemetic before surgery to prevent vomiting during the immediate postoperative period when the patient is recovering from anesthesia. Another example is giving an antiemetic before administration of antineoplastic drugs (drugs used in the treatment of cancer; see Chapter 41), which are likely to cause vomiting.

Antiemetics are also used for other causes of nausea and vomiting such as radiation therapy for a malignancy, bacterial and viral infections, nausea and vomiting caused by drugs, Ménière disease and other ear disorders, and some neurological diseases and disorders. Some of these drugs also are used to treat the nausea and vomiting that occur with motion sickness.

Severe nausea and vomiting should not be treated only with antiemetic drugs. The cause of the vomiting must be investigated. Antiemetic drugs may hamper the diagnosis of disorders such as brain tumors, appendicitis, intestinal obstruction, or drug toxicity (e.g., digitalis toxicity). A delayed diagnosis of any of these disorders could have serious consequences for the patient.

Nausea and vomiting can occur during pregnancy as well; this condition is often referred to as morning sickness. Most cases of nausea and vomiting during pregnancy occur during the first trimester and usually improve or go away entirely by the 16th week of pregnancy. However, some cases can last for the entire pregnancy. Medications are typically avoided during the first trimester, with a few exceptions.

Some antiemetics also are antivertigo drugs (see the Summary Drug Table: Antiemetic and Antivertigo Drugs).

Uses of Antivertigo Drugs

An antivertigo drug is used to treat vertigo, which is usually accompanied by light-headedness, dizziness, and weakness. A person experiencing vertigo often has difficulty walking. Some of the causes of vertigo include inebriation with alcohol, certain drugs, inner ear disease, and postural hypotension. Motion sickness (seasickness, carsickness) has similar symptoms but is caused by repetitive motion (e.g., riding in an airplane, boat, or car). Both vertigo and motion sickness may result in nausea and vomiting. An antivertigo drug may also be used to treat Ménière disease of the ear, middle or inner ear surgery, and other disorders.

Antivertigo drugs are essentially antiemetics because many of these drugs, whether used for motion sickness or vertigo, also have direct or indirect antiemetic properties. They prevent the nausea and vomiting that occur because of stimulation of the vestibular apparatus in the ear. Stimulation of this apparatus results in vertigo, which is often followed by nausea and vomiting.

FACT CHECK

10-1 What is an antiemetic drug used to prevent or treat?
10-2 What is an antivertigo drug used to treat?
10-3 Where do the antiemetics and antivertigo drugs act?

Adverse Reactions of Antiemetics and Antivertigo Drugs

The most common adverse reactions of these drugs are varying degrees of drowsiness. The 5-HT$_3$ receptor antagonists are the one class of drugs that do not typically cause drowsiness, and are generally well tolerated. Several of the medications for motion sickness are classified as anticholinergics and will cause anticholinergic side effects such as dry mouth. (See Chapter 14 for more detailed information about anticholinergics.)

Contraindications, Precautions, and Interactions of Antiemetics and Antivertigo Drugs

- Antiemetic and antivertigo drugs are contraindicated in patients with known hypersensitivity to these drugs, those in a coma, or those with severe central nervous system depression.
- In general, these drugs are not recommended during lactation or for uncomplicated vomiting in young children.
- Prochlorperazine is contraindicated in patients with bone marrow depression, blood dyscrasia, Parkinson disease, or severe liver or cardiovascular disease.
- Antiemetics and antivertigo drugs are used cautiously in patients with glaucoma or obstructive disease of the

ALERT ℞

Drowsiness
Many antiemetic and antivertigo drugs cause variable degrees of drowsiness. The patient should avoid activities requiring alertness and may need help when getting out of bed if drowsiness occurs. If the medication is being taken for motion sickness, then the patient should not be the one driving.

gastrointestinal or genitourinary system, in patients with renal or hepatic dysfunction, and in older men with possible prostatic hypertrophy.

- Promethazine is used cautiously in patients with hypertension, sleep apnea, or epilepsy.
- Trimethobenzamide is used cautiously in children with a viral illness because it may increase the risk of Reye syndrome.
- Many of the antiemetics and antivertigo drugs cause drowsiness and may have additive effects when used with alcohol and other central nervous system depressants such as sedatives, hypnotics, antianxiety drugs, opiates, and antidepressants.
- The anticholinergics will cause dry mouth and other anticholinergic effects.
- These drugs may cause additive anticholinergic effects (see Chapter 14) when administered with drugs that have anticholinergic activity, such as the antihistamines, antidepressants, phenothiazines, and disopyramide.
- Antacids decrease the absorption of the antiemetics.
- When ondansetron is administered with rifampin, blood levels of ondansetron may be reduced, decreasing the antiemetic effect.
- Dimenhydrinate may mask the signs and symptoms of ototoxicity when administered with ototoxic drugs, such as the aminoglycosides (see Chapter 35), causing irreversible hearing damage.
- When lithium is administered with prochlorperazine, the risk of extrapyramidal reactions increases (see Chapter 7).

FACT CHECK

10-4 What is the most common adverse reaction of the antiemetic and antivertigo drugs?
10-5 A patient who is taking an antiemetic or antivertigo drug that causes drowsiness should avoid what other medications?

Patient Management Issues with Antiemetics and Antivertigo Drugs

Patients who have vomited repeatedly are at risk for fluid and electrolyte imbalances. It may be necessary to document the number of times the patient has vomited and the approximate amount of fluid lost. The health care provider should be notified if there is blood in the patient's **emesis** (vomitus) or if the vomiting suddenly becomes more severe.

If the patient continues vomiting after being given the oral form of an antiemetic drug, then the drug may need to be administered parenterally or as a rectal suppository (if available in these forms) until the risk of vomiting has passed.

A number of different antiemetics are used to prevent nausea in patients being treated for cancer. Most are administered before the chemotherapy is given and for some time afterwards to prevent or relieve nausea and vomiting.

KEY CONCEPTS

10-1   Dehydration

An elderly or chronically ill patient who is experiencing vomiting may have severe dehydration develop in a short time, leading to fluid and electrolyte disturbances. Health care workers should be alert for and immediately report symptoms of dehydration, such as poor skin turgor, dry mucous membranes, decreased urinary output, concentrated urine, increased respiratory rate, irritability, restlessness, or confusion in older adults. Likewise, infants and small children need to be watched for signs of dehydration if they are experiencing recurrent or prolonged vomiting.

Dehydration is a serious concern in patients experiencing vomiting (Key Concepts 10-1). If the patient can retain small amounts of oral fluids, then sips of water should be offered at frequent intervals. In addition, the patient is observed for signs of an electrolyte imbalance, particularly sodium and potassium deficits (see Chapter 45); in such cases, parenteral administration of fluids or fluids with electrolytes may be necessary.

FACT CHECK

10-6   What is the most serious concern for patients who are vomiting and unable to keep anything down? Which patient populations are most frequently at risk?

Educating the Patient and Family about Antiemetic and Antivertigo Drugs

Following are key points about antiemetic and antivertigo drugs that the patient or family members should know.

- Avoid driving or performing other hazardous tasks when taking these drugs because drowsiness may occur with use.
- Contact the health care provider if nausea, vomiting, or vertigo persists or worsens.

COMPLEMENTARY & ALTERNATIVE MEDICINE

Ginger

Ginger, a medicinal herb, is usually taken to reduce nausea, vomiting, and indigestion. Research suggests that it can be effective in preventing the nausea associated with motion sickness, seasickness, and anesthesia. Ginger is not recommended for morning sickness associated with pregnancy and is not advised for patients with gallstones or hypertension. Small amounts present in food preparation are generally regarded as safe. The medicinal use of ginger should cease 2 to 3 weeks before surgery to reduce the risk of bleeding.

- Use these drugs only as directed. Do not increase the dose or frequency of use unless advised by the health care provider.
- Do not use alcohol and other drugs with sedative effects except as advised by the health care provider.
- Follow the directions for application of transdermal scopolamine that are supplied with the drug.
- Patients taking the medication for motion sickness might find acupressure or acustimulation devices to be beneficial with or in place of an antiemetic.

COMPLEMENTARY & ALTERNATIVE MEDICINE

Pyridoxine (Vitamin B6)

The American College of Obstetrics and Gynecology supports the off-label use of pyridoxine as a first-line treatment for nausea and vomiting in pregnancy. The usual dose is 10 to 25 mg three to four times a day. Pyridoxine is a water-soluble vitamin that is generally well tolerated. Pyridoxine can also be found in a combination prescription product for nausea during pregnancy that is taken once daily with a meal. This product contains 75 mg of sustained-release pyridoxine, 12 mcg cyanocobalamin (Vitamin B12), 1 mg folic acid and 200 mg calcium carbonate.

Chapter Review

KEY POINTS

- An antiemetic drug is used to treat or prevent nausea or vomiting. An antivertigo drug is used to treat or prevent vertigo, which may occur with motion sickness.
- Antiemetics and antivertigo drugs appear to act primarily by inhibiting the chemoreceptor trigger zone, a group of nerve fibers in the brain, or by depressing the sensitivity of the vestibular apparatus of the inner ear.
- The most common adverse reactions of both antiemetics and antivertigo drugs are varying degrees of drowsiness. The patient should avoid activities requiring alertness.
- The antiemetic and antivertigo drugs are contraindicated in patients with known hypersensitivity to these drugs, those in a coma, or those with severe central nervous system depression. In general, these drugs are not recommended during pregnancy or lactation or for uncomplicated vomiting in young children. Specific agents also have specific contraindications and precautions.
- Patients who have vomited repeatedly are at risk for fluid and electrolyte imbalances, especially dehydration. Patients especially at risk for dehydration include the elderly or chronically ill, infants, and children.

CRITICAL THINKING CASE STUDY

Motion Sickness

Ms. Davis was prescribed meclizine (Antivert-50) 50 mg for motion sickness. After returning from a long car trip, she tells you that the medicine did not help.

1. When should she have taken the medication to prevent experiencing motion sickness?
   a. The day before the car trip
   b. One hour before the car trip began
   c. At the beginning of the car trip
   d. When she first began to feel nauseous
2. Which of the following is *not* a common adverse reaction to meclizine and should therefore be reported to Ms. Davis's health care provider?
   a. Bleeding
   b. Dry mouth
   c. Drowsiness
   d. All of the above are common adverse reactions.
3. Before Ms. Davis's next trip, which happens to be a 7-day cruise, her health care provider prescribes a transdermal scopolamine patch. What advantage(s) does the patch have over the meclizine?

Review Questions

MULTIPLE CHOICE

1. What is the most common adverse reaction in patients receiving an antiemetic?
   a. Occipital headache
   b. Drowsiness
   c. Edema
   d. Nausea

2. When an antivertigo drug is prescribed for a patient experiencing motion sickness, the patient should be advised to
   a. take the drug with food immediately before traveling
   b. administer the drug at least 6 hours before travel
   c. avoid driving or performing hazardous tasks
   d. take the drug at the first sign of motion sickness
3. Repeated vomiting may lead to what potentially serious condition?
   a. Dehydration
   b. Stomach ulcers
   c. Migraine headache
   d. Anaphylaxis
4. Which of the following is NOT a group of drugs used as an antiemetic or antivertigo treatment?
   a. Antidopaminergic
   b. Anticholinergic
   c. 5-HT3 Receptor agonist
   d. Antidepressant

MATCHING

_____ 5. Zofran   a. meclizine
_____ 6. Antivert   b. dronabinol
_____ 7. Phenergan   c. ondansetron
_____ 8. Marinol   d. promethazine

TRUE OR FALSE

_____ 9. Taking an antiemetic and an antacid at the same time may cause the antiemetic to not work as well.
_____ 10. If a patient who has been experiencing vomiting can retain small amounts of oral fluids, then sips of water should be offered at frequent intervals.
_____ 11. Ginger is a medicinal herb that has been proven effective for treating nausea and vomiting associated with pregnancy.
_____ 12. If a patient is vomiting and unable to keep anything down, an antiemetic could be administered rectally as a suppository.

FILL IN THE BLANKS

13. An antiemetic is used to treat or prevent _____ or _____.
14. Vomiting occurs because of stimulation of the _____ _____ _____, a group of nerve fibers in the brain.
15. Vitamin _____ is recommended as a first-line treatment for women suffering from nausea and vomiting associated with pregnancy.
16. The antiemetics and antivertigo drugs cause drowsiness and may have _____ effects when used with alcohol and other central nervous system depressants

SHORT ANSWERS

17. What are some causes of vertigo?
18. When would an antiemetic be used prophylactically?
19. Why should severe nausea and vomiting not be treated only with antiemetic drugs?
20. Why is an antiemetic needed for patients who are undergoing chemotherapy, and why is it administered before the chemotherapy?

Web Activities

1. Go to the Mayo Clinic's public health information Web site (http://www.mayoclinic. com) and navigate to the "diseases and conditions A–Z" section. Read the information on the treatment of vertigo and write brief answers to these questions:
   a. What is the procedure called BPPV?
   b. What conditions can a physical therapist help with?
   c. When might counseling help a patient?
   d. What other types of drugs might help a patient with Ménière disease?
2. Go to the National Cancer Institute Web site (www. cancer.gov). Conduct a search on nausea and vomiting.
   a. What are some foods that are easy on the stomach that you could recommend for a patient suffering from nausea and vomiting?
   b. What are some other tips that you could recommend the patient try to help settle his or her stomach?

SUMMARY DRUG TABLE: Antiemetics and Antivertigo Drugs (left, generic; right, trade)

Comprehensive Summary Drug Tables, including uses, adverses effects, dosages, and pregnancy classifications, are provided on the companion website, http://thePoint.lww. com/PharmacologyHP2e

5-HT₃ Receptor Antagonists	
dolasetron mesylate *dol-a'-se-tron*	Anzemet
granisetron *gra-ni'-se-tron*	Granisol, Kytril, Sancuso
ondansetron *on-dan'-se-tron*	Zofran
palonosetron *pal-oh-noe'-se-tron*	Aloxi
Anticholinergics	
cyclizine	Bonine for Kids (OTC), Marezine (OTC)
dimenhydrinate *dye-men-hye'-dri-nate*	Dramamine (OTC), Triptone (OTC)
diphenhydramine injection	*generic* (Rx)
meclizine	Antivert (Rx), Bonine (OTC), Dramamine Less Drowsy (OTC), *generic*
scopolamine	Transderm-Scop (Rx)
trimethobenzamide hydrochloride	Tigan (Rx)

Antidopaminergics	
chlorpromazine hydrochloride	*generic* (Rx)
perphenazine	*generic* (Rx)
prochlorperazine	Compro (Rx), *generic*
promethazine *proe-meth'-a-zeen*	Phenadoz (Rx), Phenergan (Rx), *generic*
Miscellaneous	
aprepitant *ap-re'-pt-tant*	Emend (Rx)
dronabinol *droe-nab'-i'-nol*	Marinol (CIII), *generic*
fosaprepitant *fos-a-pre'-pi-tant*	Emend (Rx)
nabilone	Cesamet (CII)
phosphorated carbohydrate solution	Emetrol (OTC)

11

Adrenergic Drugs

CHAPTER OBJECTIVES

On completion of this chapter, students will be able to:

1. Define the chapter's key terms.
2. Discuss the anatomy of the central nervous system, the peripheral nervous system, and the sympathetic and parasympathetic nervous systems.
3. Identify common uses of adrenergic drugs.
4. Describe the different types of shock.
5. Identify common adverse reactions of adrenergic drugs.
6. Describe how to manage the adverse reactions of adrenergic drugs.
7. Discuss the management of shock.
8. Identify the key points about caring for a patient taking an adrenergic drug.

KEY TERMS

acetylcholine—a neurotransmitter in the parasympathetic nervous system

acetylcholinesterase—a neurotransmitter that inactivates acetylcholine

adrenergic drugs—drugs with effects similar to those that occur in the body when the adrenergic nerves are stimulated

autonomic nervous system—the branch of the peripheral nervous system that controls functions essential for survival

cardiac arrhythmia—irregular heartbeat

central nervous system—consists of the brain and the spinal cord

neurotransmitter—a chemical substance, also called a neurohormone, released at nerve endings to help transmit nerve impulses

orthostatic hypotension—a feeling of light-headedness and dizziness after suddenly changing position, caused by a decrease in blood pressure when a person sits or stands; also referred to as postural hypotension

parasympathetic nervous system—a branch of the autonomic nervous system partly responsible for activities such as slowing the heart rate, digesting food, and eliminating body wastes

CHAPTER OVERVIEW

Drug classes covered in this chapter are:

- Adrenergic drugs

Drugs by classification are listed on page 133.

thePOINT RESOURCES

- Comprehensive Summary Drug Tables
- Lippincott's Interactive Tutorials: Drugs Affecting the Autonomic Nervous System
- Interactive Practice and Review
- Monographs of Most Commonly Prescribed Drugs

peripheral nervous system—all nerves outside of the brain and spinal cord, connecting all parts of the body with the central nervous system

receptor sites—specific protein-like macromolecules required for a drug's action at the cellular level

shock—a life-threatening condition occurring when the supply of arterial blood flow and oxygen to the cells and tissues is inadequate

somatic nervous system—branch of the peripheral nervous system that controls sensation and voluntary movement

sympathetic nervous system—branch of the autonomic nervous system that regulates the expenditure of energy and has key effects in stressful situations

vasopressor—a drug that raises the blood pressure because it constricts blood vessels

A basic knowledge of the anatomy and physiology of the nervous system is necessary to understand how drugs affect this body system. Therefore, we will begin with an introduction to the nervous system before discussing the adrenergic drugs in detail.

The Nervous System

The nervous system is a complex part of the human body that regulates and coordinates body activities such as movement, digestion of food, sleep, and elimination of waste products. The nervous system has two main divisions: the central nervous system and the peripheral nervous system. Figure 11-1 illustrates the divisions of the nervous system.

The **central nervous system** consists of the brain and the spinal cord, which receive, integrate, and interpret nerve impulses from the body. The **peripheral nervous system** encompasses all nerves outside of the brain and spinal cord. The peripheral nervous system connects all parts of the body with the central nervous system.

Peripheral Nervous System

The peripheral nervous system is further divided into the **somatic nervous system** and the **autonomic nervous system.** The somatic branch of the peripheral nervous system controls sensation and voluntary movement. The sensory part of the somatic nervous system sends messages to the brain about the internal and external environment, such as sensations of heat, pain, cold, and pressure. The voluntary part of the somatic nervous system controls the voluntary movement of skeletal muscles, such as walking, chewing food, or writing a letter.

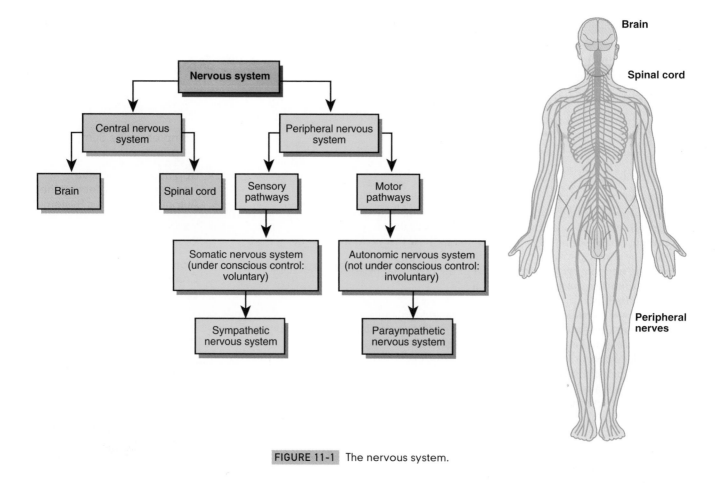

FIGURE 11-1 The nervous system.

Autonomic Branch of the Peripheral Nervous System

The autonomic branch of the peripheral nervous system controls functions essential for survival. Functional activity of the autonomic nervous system is not consciously controlled (i.e., the activity is automatic). This system controls blood pressure, heart rate, gastrointestinal activity, and glandular secretions. Table 11-1 describes the main actions of the autonomic nervous system in the body. Figure 11-2 shows sympathetic (adrenergic) effects on the body's organs and structures.

The autonomic nervous system is divided into the sympathetic and parasympathetic nervous systems. The **sympathetic nervous system** generally regulates the expenditure of energy and has key effects when one is confronted with stressful situations, such as danger, intense emotion, or severe illness.

The **parasympathetic nervous system** helps conserve body energy and is partly responsible for activities such as slowing the heart rate, digesting food, and eliminating body wastes.

Neurotransmitters

Neurotransmitters are chemical substances called neurohormones. The two neurohormones (neurotransmitters) of the sympathetic nervous system are epinephrine and norepinephrine. Epinephrine is secreted by the adrenal medulla. Norepinephrine is secreted mainly at nerve endings of sympathetic (also called adrenergic) nerve fibers (Fig. 11-3).

The parasympathetic nervous system has two different neurotransmitters: **acetylcholine** (ACh) and **acetylcholinesterase** (AChE). These two neurohormones are released at nerve endings of parasympathetic nerve fibers, at some nerve endings in the sympathetic nervous system, and at nerve endings of skeletal muscles. The neurohormone then acts at the **receptor site** and exerts a response. When a parasympathetic nerve fiber is stimulated, the nerve fiber releases ACh, and the nerve impulse travels from the nerve fiber to the

TABLE 11-1   Action of the Autonomic Nervous System on Body Organs and Structures

Organs or Structures	Sympathetic (Adrenergic) Effects	Types of Sympathetic (Adrenergic) Receptor	Parasympathetic (Cholinergic) Effects
Heart	Increase in heart rate, heart muscle contractility, increase in speed of atrioventricular conduction	β	Decrease in heart rate, decrease in heart muscle contractility
Blood Vessels Skin, mucous membranes Skeletal muscle	Constriction Usually dilatation	α Cholinergic, *β	
Bronchial Muscles	Relaxation	β	Contraction
Gastrointestinal Muscle motility, tone decrease Sphincters Gallbladder	Usually contraction Relaxation	β α	Increase Usually relaxation Contraction
Urinary Bladder Detrusor muscle Trigone, sphincter muscles	Relaxation Contraction	β α	Contraction Relaxation
Eye Radial muscle of iris Sphincter muscle of iris Ciliary muscle	Contraction (pupil dilates)	α	Contraction (pupil constricts) Contraction
Skin Sweat glands Pilomotor muscles	Increased activity in localized areas Contraction (gooseflesh)	Cholinergic* α	
Uterus	Relaxation	β	
Salivary Glands	Thickened secretions	α	Copious, watery secretions
Liver	Glycogenolysis	β	
Lacrimal and Nasopharyngeal Glands		α	Increased secretion
Male Sex Organs	Emission	α	Erection

*Cholinergic transmission, but nerve cell chain originates in the thoracolumbar part of the spinal cord and is therefore sympathetic. alpha, α; beta, β.

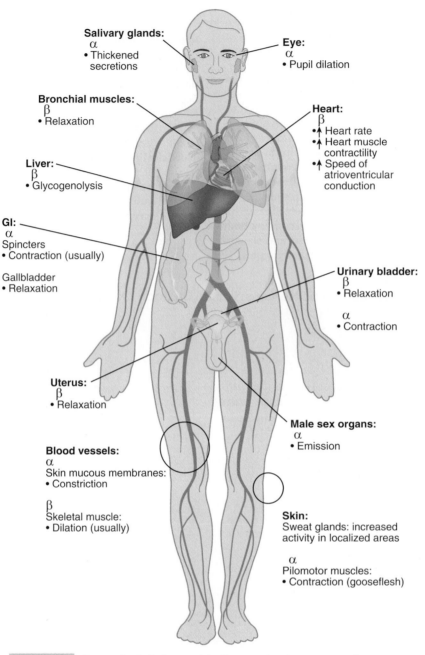

Salivary glands:
α
• Thickened secretions

Eye:
α
• Pupil dilation

Bronchial muscles:
β
• Relaxation

Heart:
β
•↑ Heart rate
•↑ Heart muscle contractility
•↑ Speed of atrioventricular conduction

Liver:
β
• Glycogenolysis

GI:
α
Spincters
• Contraction (usually)

Gallbladder
• Relaxation

Urinary bladder:
β
• Relaxation

α
• Contraction

Uterus:
β
• Relaxation

Male sex organs:
α
• Emission

Blood vessels:
α
Skin mucous membranes:
• Constriction

β
Skeletal muscle:
• Dilation (usually)

Skin:
Sweat glands: increased activity in localized areas

α
Pilomotor muscles:
• Contraction (gooseflesh)

FIGURE 11-2 Sympathetic (adrenergic) effects on body organs and structures.

effector organ or structure (Fig. 11-4). After the impulse has crossed over to the effector organ or structure, ACh is inactivated (destroyed) by AChE. When the next nerve impulse is ready to travel along the nerve fiber, ACh is again released and then inactivated by AChE.

FACT CHECK

11-1   The autonomic nervous system is divided into what two divisions?
11-2   What are the neurotransmitters of the sympathetic nervous system?

Adrenergic Drugs

Actions of Adrenergic Drugs

Adrenergic drugs have effects similar to those that occur in the body when the adrenergic nerves are stimulated. Adrenergic nerves are nerves in the autonomic nervous system that use norepinephrine as a neurotransmitter. The primary effects of these drugs occur in the heart, the blood vessels, and the smooth muscles, such as the bronchi. Adrenergic drugs mimic the activity of the sympathetic nervous system and therefore are also called sympathomimetic drugs. Epinephrine and norepinephrine are neurohormones produced naturally by the body. Synthetic preparations of these two neurohormones, which are identical

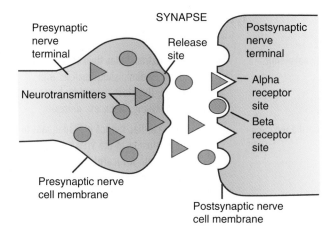

FIGURE 11-3 Neurotransmission in the central nervous system. Neurotransmitter molecules (e.g., norepinephrine), released by the presynaptic nerve, cross the synapse and bind with receptors in the cell membrane of the postsynaptic nerve, resulting in the transmission of the nerve impulse.

to those naturally produced by the body, are used in medicine. Adrenergic drugs such as metaraminol (Aramine), isoproterenol (Isuprel), and ephedrine are synthetic adrenergic drugs.

Generally, adrenergic drugs produce one or more of the following responses:

- In the central nervous system: wakefulness, quickened reaction to stimuli, and quickened reflexes

- In the parasympathetic nervous system: relaxation of the smooth muscles of the bronchi, constriction of blood vessels and the sphincters of the stomach, decrease in gastric motility, and dilation of coronary blood vessels
- Heart: increase in the heart rate
- Metabolism: increased use of glucose (sugar) and liberation of fatty acids from adipose tissue

See Table 11-1 for additional information.

Adrenergic nerve fibers have either alpha (α) or beta (β) receptors. Adrenergic drugs may act on α receptors only, on β receptors only, or on both α and β receptors. For example, phenylephrine (Neo-Synephrine) acts chiefly on α receptors, isoproterenol acts chiefly on β receptors, and epinephrine acts on both α and β receptors. Whether an adrenergic drug acts on α, β, or α and β receptors accounts for variations in the effects of adrenergic drugs.

When a drug binds at a receptor, it will produce a receptor-specific effect depending on the site of the receptor. An adrenergic drug that binds at an α receptor will produce a response specific to that receptor. For example, an α receptor in the blood vessels will cause vasoconstriction when a drug or norepinephrine binds to it. An adrenergic blocking drug that binds at an α receptor will block a response from occurring. For example, an α receptor in the blood vessels will remain dilated when a drug blocks the α receptor from being activated by norepinephrine or an α-adrenergic drug (Fig. 11-5). The same things occurs at the β receptors (see Table 11-1).

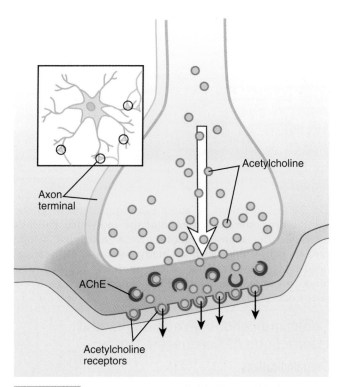

FIGURE 11-4 How ACh works. Acetylcholine is released from the nerve and enters the space between the two nerves. The acetylcholine either attaches to the receptor site to continue the nerve transmission or it is inactivated by acetylcholinesterase.

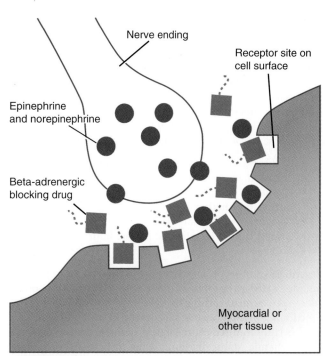

FIGURE 11-5 β-Adrenergic blocking drugs prevent epinephrine and norepinephrine from occupying receptor sites on cell membranes. This action alters cell functions normally stimulated by epinephrine and norepinephrine, according to the number of receptor sites occupied by the β-blocking drugs.

Uses of Adrenergic Drugs

Adrenergic drugs have a wide variety of uses. They may be used to treat

- Hypovolemic and septic shock
- Moderately severe to severe episodes of hypotension
- Control of superficial bleeding during surgical and dental procedures of the mouth, nose, throat, and skin
- Bronchial asthma
- Cardiac decompensation and arrest
- Allergic reactions (anaphylactic shock, angioneurotic edema)
- Temporary treatment of heart block
- Ventricular arrhythmias (under certain conditions)
- Nasal congestion (applied topically)
- Along with local anesthetics to prolong anesthetic action

Other adrenergic drugs have specific uses. Isoproterenol may be used in the treatment of some **cardiac arrhythmias** (irregular heartbeat), cardiac arrest, Adams–Stokes syndrome, or as a systemic bronchodilator (see Chapter 15). Midodrine is used to treat **orthostatic hypotension** (a feeling of light-headedness and dizziness after suddenly changing position after sitting or standing in one place for a long period). (Because adrenergic drugs affect various body systems, the list of drugs in this chapter is not comprehensive. Additional adrenergic drugs will be covered in their respective body system chapters.)

The adrenergic drugs are an important treatment for patients in shock. **Shock** is a life-threatening condition of inadequate perfusion. In shock, the supply of arterial blood flow and oxygen to the cells and tissues is inadequate. The body uses compensatory mechanisms to counteract the symptoms of shock, including the release of epinephrine and norepinephrine. In some situations, the body can compensate and maintain blood pressure. However, if shock is untreated and the body's compensatory mechanisms fail, then death will occur. There are five types of shock: hypovolemic shock, cardiogenic shock, septic shock, obstructive shock, and neurogenic shock. Table 11-2 describes the various types of shock.

Shock causes a number of clinical manifestations:

- Pallor, cyanosis, cold and clammy skin, sweating
- Agitation, confusion, disorientation, coma
- Hypotension, tachycardia, arrhythmias, wide pulse pressure, gallop rhythm
- Tachypnea, pulmonary edema
- Urinary output less than 20 mL per hour
- Acidosis

Regardless of the type, shock results in decreased cardiac output, decreased arterial blood pressure (hypotension), hypoxia (decreased oxygen reaching the cells), and other problems. The functioning of vital organs, such as the heart, brain, and kidneys, is compromised. Adrenergic drugs improve the patient's hemodynamic status by improving myocardial contractility and increasing heart rate, which increase cardiac output. Peripheral resistance is increased by vasoconstriction, making more blood available for vital organs. In cardiogenic shock or advanced shock associated with low cardiac output, an adrenergic drug may be used with a vasodilating drug. A vasodilator

TABLE 11-2 Types of Shock

Type*	Description
Hypovolemic	Occurs when extracellular fluid volume is significantly diminished, such as with hemorrhage, fluid loss caused by burns, diarrhea, vomiting, or excess diuresis
Cardiogenic	Occurs when cardiac output is inadequate to maintain perfusion to the vital organs, such as with an acute myocardial infarction, ventricular arrhythmias, congestive heart failure, or severe cardiomyopathy
Septic	Occurs as a result of circulatory insufficiency associated with overwhelming infection
Obstructive	Occurs when obstruction of blood flow results in inadequate tissue perfusion, such as with a massive pulmonary embolism, pericardial tamponade, restrictive pericarditis, or severe cardiac valve dysfunction
Neurogenic (rare)	Occurs as a result of blockade of neurohumoral outflow such as caused by spinal anesthesia or direct injury to the spinal cord

*Other causes of shock include anaphylaxis, hypoglycemia, hypothyroidism, or Addison disease.

such as nitroprusside (Chapter 21) or nitroglycerin (Chapter 20) improves myocardial performance as the adrenergic drug maintains blood pressure.

FACT CHECK

11-3 What are the clinical manifestations of shock?
11-4 How does an adrenergic drug improve a patient's hemodynamic status?

Adverse Reactions of Adrenergic Drugs

The adverse reactions of adrenergic drugs depend on the specific drug, the dose used, and the individual patient's response. The more common adverse reactions include cardiac arrhythmias, such as bradycardia and tachycardia, headache, insomnia, nervousness, anorexia, and increased blood pressure, which may reach dangerously high levels (Key Concepts 11-1).

Contraindications, Precautions, and Interactions of Adrenergic Drugs

Contraindications

- Known hypersensitivity
- Isoproterenol: tachyarrhythmias, tachycardia, or heart block caused by digitalis toxicity, ventricular arrhythmias, and angina pectoris

KEY CONCEPTS

11-1 Flight or Fight

To remember the adverse reactions of adrenergic drugs, keep in mind that they are similar to reactions experienced during the "flight or fight" response.

* Dopamine: pheochromocytoma (tumor of adrenal gland), unmanaged arrhythmias, and ventricular fibrillation
* Epinephrine: narrow-angle glaucoma, cerebral arteriosclerosis, or cardiac insufficiency
* Norepinephrine and ephedrine: hypotension caused by a loss of blood volume
* Midodrine: severe organic heart disease, acute renal disease, pheochromocytoma, or supine hypertension

Precautions

* Used cautiously for patients with coronary insufficiency, cardiac arrhythmias, angina pectoris, diabetes, hyperthyroidism, occlusive vascular disease, or prostatic hypertrophy, and for those taking digoxin. Patients with diabetes may require a higher dosage of insulin. Used with extreme caution during pregnancy.
* Epinephrine: Parkinson disease or ventricular fibrillation, and in the elderly
* Ephedrine: acute-closure glaucoma
* Midodrine: urinary problems or hepatic disease, and during lactation

Interactions

* Dobutamine: Increased risk of hypertension when given along with a β-adrenergic blocking drug
* Dopamine: When given with a monoamine oxidase inhibitor (see Chapter 7) or tricyclic antidepressant (see Chapter 7), effects may be increased. Increased risk of seizures, hypotension, and bradycardia when administered with phenytoin.
* Epinephrine: When administered with a tricyclic antidepressant, the patient has an increased risk of sympathomimetic effects. Excessive hypertension can occur when administered with propranolol. A decreased

bronchodilating effect occurs when administered with the β-adrenergic drugs.
* Midodrine: When administered with cardiac glycosides, psychotropic drugs, or β blockers, bradycardia, heart block, or arrhythmias can occur.

Patient Management Issues with Adrenergic Drugs

Because adrenergic drugs are powerful and potentially dangerous, proper supervision and patient management before, during, and after administration of the drug is needed to minimize any serious problems.

Caring for a Patient in Shock

When an adrenergic drug is to be given for shock, the patient's blood pressure, pulse rate and quality, and respiratory rate and rhythm are first assessed. This information is important for treatment.

Management of shock is aimed at providing basic life support (airway, breathing, and circulation) while attempting to correct the underlying cause. The initial pharmacologic intervention is aimed at supporting the circulation with a **vasopressor** (a drug that raises the blood pressure because it constricts blood vessels). Some hypotensive episodes require the use of a less potent vasopressor, such as metaraminol, whereas at other times a more potent vasopressor, such as dobutamine (Dobutrex), dopamine (Intropin), or norepinephrine (Levophed), is necessary. The patient's heart rate, blood pressure, and ECG are monitored continuously.

The less potent vasopressors, such as metaraminol, also require close patient supervision during use. Blood pressure and pulse assessments are also made.

Caring for Patients Taking Midodrine

When midodrine is prescribed for orthostatic hypotension, the patient's blood pressure should be checked before therapy with the patient both lying down and sitting. This is important because midodrine is contraindicated in patients with supine hypertension.

This drug is given only when the patient is out of bed. Bedridden patients should not receive the drug. Patients taking midodrine need frequent monitoring of blood pressure and heart rate. Bradycardia is common at the beginning of therapy. Persistent bradycardia should be reported to the health care provider. Because the drug can cause dysuria, the patient is asked to urinate before being given the drug.

Managing Anorexia

Adrenergic drugs may cause anorexia (lack of appetite). The patient's food preferences should be considered and modifications made in the diet. An easily digested diet high in carbohydrates and protein and low in fat is usually well tolerated. Several small meals may be better tolerated than three large meals. The patient should be monitored for weight loss.

Managing Sleep Disturbances

Patients taking an adrenergic drug may experience insomnia and nervousness, which can cause considerable stress. The care of hospitalized patients may have to be modified to prevent disturbing their sleep. Caffeinated beverages should be avoided,

CONSIDERATIONS | Older adults

LIFESPAN

Adverse Reactions of Adrenergic Drugs

Older adults are particularly vulnerable to adverse reactions of adrenergic drugs, particularly epinephrine. Older adults are also more likely to have cardiovascular problems that predispose them to potentially serious cardiac arrhythmias. All elderly patients taking an adrenergic drug should be monitored, and any changes in pulse rate or rhythm must be reported immediately

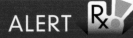

ALERT

Blood Pressure Drops with Adrenergic Drugs

Regardless of the actual numerical reading, any continuing fall of blood pressure is serious. Any progressive fall of the blood pressure, or a fall in systolic blood pressure below 100 mm Hg, should be reported to the health care provider.

especially after late afternoon. Other sleep aids may be used (e.g., warm milk, back rub, progressive relaxation, or a bedtime snack). The patient should be assured that the sleeplessness and nervousness will pass when the drug therapy is over.

Educating the Patient and Family about Adrenergic Drugs

Some adrenergic drugs, such as the vasopressors, are given only by medical personnel. In this case, the drug must be explained to the patient or family, along with what results are expected and what effects may occur. Below are the key points about adrenergic drugs that the patient or family members should know.

Midodrine

- Patients with severe orthostatic hypotension need to take this drug during daytime hours when they are upright.
- Take doses at 3-hour intervals if needed to control symptoms.
- Do not take the drug within 4 hours of bedtime.
- Do not lie down soon after taking the drug.
- It may be necessary to sleep with the head of the bed elevated.
- If urinary retention is a problem, then urinate before taking the drug.
- See the health care provider regularly for medical evaluation.
- Report any changes in vision, pounding in the head when lying down, slow heart rate, or difficulty urinating.

FACT CHECK

11-5 What are the more common adverse reactions associated with adrenergic drugs?

11-6 How does an adrenergic drug help with the management of shock?

Chapter Review

KEY POINTS

- Adrenergic drugs mimic the activity of the sympathetic nervous system and have many effects throughout the body based on cellular receptor activity.
- These drugs have many uses, including the treatment of shock, asthma, and nasal congestion.
- Common adverse effects include insomnia, nervousness, anorexia, dizziness, headache, and cardiac arrhythmias.
- Patient management and teaching for adrenergic drugs focus on the need for strict dosage control and the management of common adverse reactions.

CRITICAL THINKING CASE STUDY

Treating Shock

Samuel Everette is admitted to the hospital for shock and a recent MI.

1. Which of the following symptoms would you NOT expect the patient to exhibit?
   a. Agitation and confusion
   b. Hypertension
   c. Tachycardia
   d. Decreased urine output
2. When looking at the chart, which of the following would you expect to see prescribed for the treatment of shock?
   a. Ephedrine
   b. Isoproterenol
   c. Dopamine
   d. Midodrine

3. The patient is warned that he may experience orthostatic hypotension. The family wants to know what orthostatic hypotension is. How would you explain it?

Review Questions

MULTIPLE CHOICE

1. Which of the following is an adrenergic effect on the heart?
   a. Increase in heart rate
   b. Decrease in speed of atrioventricular conduction
   c. Decrease in heart muscle contractility
   d. All of the above
2. Which of the following is a common adverse reaction of adrenergic drugs?
   a. Bradycardia
   b. Increase in appetite
   c. Decreased blood pressure
   d. Drowsiness
3. When caring for a patient taking an adrenergic drug, which of the following is important for the caregiver to do?
   a. Take the patient's blood pressure when he or she is sitting up.
   b. Take the patient's blood pressure when he or she is lying down.
   c. Have the patient take the medication when he or she is sitting upright.
   d. All of the above

4. Which of the following organs contains b receptors?
   a. Bronchial muscles
   b. Urinary bladder
   c. The uterus and liver
   d. All of the above

MATCHING

_____ 5. dopamine   a. Adrenaline
_____ 6. dobutamine   b. Levophed
_____ 7. epinephrine   c. Intropin
_____ 8. norepinephrine   d. Dobutrex

TRUE OR FALSE

_____ 9. The parasympathetic nervous system has two different neurotransmitters: norepinephrine and acetylcholine.
_____ 10. There are five types of shock: hypovolemic, cardiogenic, septic, obstructive, and neurogenic.
_____ 11. The GI tract contains both α- and β-adrenergic receptors.
_____ 12. Adrenergic drugs are commonly used to treat shock, asthma, and nasal congestion.

FILL IN THE BLANKS

13. _____ is a life-threatening condition of inadequate perfusion.
14. In cardiogenic shock, an adrenergic drug may be used with a vasodilating drug. The vasodilator improves _____ _____ as the adrenergic drug maintains _____.

15. Adrenergic drugs may cause _____ (lack of appetite).
16. Patients taking an adrenergic drug may experience insomnia and nervousness, which can cause considerable _____.

SHORT ANSWERS

17. Where do the primary effects of adrenergic drugs occur?
18. What are adrenergic drugs used to treat?
19. Compare the actions of an adrenergic drug with an adrenergic blocking drug.
20. What are the adverse reactions of adrenergic drugs similar to?

Web Activities

1. Go to the Medline Plus Web site at http://www.nlm.nih.gov and look up "Hypovolemic shock." What are possible complications of hypovolemic shock?
2. On the same Web site, look up "Cardiogenic Shock." What are the symptoms of cardiogenic shock?

SUMMARY DRUG TABLE: Adrenergic Drugs (left, generic; right, trade)

Comprehensive Summary Drug Tables, including uses, adverses effects, dosages, and pregnancy classifications, are provided on the companion website, http://thePoint.lww.com/PharmacologyHP2e

dobutamine HCL *doe'-byoo-ta-meen*	Dobutrex, *generic*	isoproterenol *eye-sew-proe-tear'-e-nall*	Isuprel, Medihaler-Iso
dopamine *doe'-pa-meen*	Intropin, *generic*	midodrine *mid'-oh-dryn*	ProAmatine
ephedrine sulfate *e-fed'-rin*	*generic*	norepinephrine *nor-ep-i-nef'-rin* (levarterenol)	Levophed
epinephrine *ep-i-nef'-rin*	Adrenalin chloride, AsthmaHaler, Bronkaid, *generic*		

12

Adrenergic Blocking Drugs

CHAPTER OBJECTIVES

On completion of this chapter, students will be able to:

1. Define the chapter's key terms.
2. Identify four groups of adrenergic blocking drugs.
3. Discuss the uses, general drug actions, contraindications, precautions, interactions, and adverse reactions associated with the administration of adrenergic blocking drugs, based on their group.
4. Discuss important points to keep in mind when educating patients about the use of adrenergic blocking drugs,.

KEY TERMS

adrenergic blocking drugs—drugs that impede certain sympathetic nervous system functions
first dose effect—an unusually strong therapeutic effect experienced by some patients with the first doses of a medication
glaucoma—an eye condition in which a blockage of drainage channels within the eye results in increased intraocular pressure that may lead to blindness
postural hypotension—a feeling of light-headedness and dizziness after suddenly changing position, caused by a decrease in blood pressure when a person sits or stands; also referred to as orthostatic hypotension

CHAPTER OVERVIEW

Drug classes covered in this chapter are:

- α-Adrenergic blocking drugs
- β-Adrenergic blocking drugs
- Antiadrenergic blocking drugs
- α/β-Adrenergic blocking drugs

Drugs by classification are listed on page 142.

thePOINT RESOURCES

- Comprehensive Summary Drug Tables
- Lippincott's Interactive Tutorials: Drugs Affecting the Autonomic Nervous System
- Interactive Practice and Review
- Monographs of Most Commonly Prescribed Drugs

Adrenergic blocking drugs, also called sympathomimetic blocking drugs, have generally the opposite effects of adrenergic drugs. They impede sympathetic nervous system functions. The four classes of adrenergic blocking drugs block four different sets of nervous system receptors and therefore have four related but different actions in the body.

A basic knowledge of the nervous system is necessary to understand adrenergic blocking drugs and how they work in the body. Please refer to Chapter 11 for a detailed discussion.

Adrenergic Blocking Drugs

Adrenergic blocking drugs may be divided into four groups. Their actions, uses, adverse reactions, and contraindications and precautions vary according to the group.

- Alpha (α)-adrenergic blocking drugs—drugs that block α-adrenergic receptors. These drugs have their greatest effect in the vascular system.
- Beta (β)-adrenergic blocking drugs—drugs that block β-adrenergic receptors. These drugs produce their greatest effect on adrenergic nerves in the heart.
- Antiadrenergic drugs—drugs that block adrenergic nerve fibers. These drugs have effects within the central nervous system and the peripheral nervous system.
- α/β-Adrenergic blocking drugs—drugs that block both α- and β-adrenergic receptors. These drugs have a wider range of effects.

This chapter provides a general overview of the adrenergic blockers. Because these drugs have so many effects, they will be covered in more detail in subsequent chapters.

α-ADRENERGIC BLOCKING DRUGS

Actions of α-Adrenergic Blocking Drugs

Stimulation of α-adrenergic fibers results in vasoconstriction. If stimulation of these α-adrenergic fibers is blocked, then the result instead is vasodilation—the directly opposite effect (Fig. 12-1). Phentolamine (Regitine) is an example of an α-adrenergic blocking drug. A number of other α-adrenergic blockers will be covered in the Unit V: Drugs That Affect the Cardiovascular System.

Uses of α-Adrenergic Blocking Drugs

Phentolamine (Regitine) is used for its vasodilating effect on peripheral blood vessels. It can be beneficial in the treatment of hypertension caused by pheochromocytoma, a tumor of the adrenal gland that produces excessive amounts of epinephrine and norepinephrine. This drug is used to control hypertension before surgical excision of pheochromocytoma.

Some drugs such as norepinephrine or dopamine are particularly damaging to surrounding tissues if extravasation (infiltration) occurs when they are given intravenously. Phentolamine is also used to prevent or treat tissue damage caused by extravasation of these drugs.

Adverse Reactions of α-Adrenergic Blocking Drugs

α-Adrenergic blocking drugs may result in weakness, orthostatic hypotension, cardiac arrhythmias, hypotension, and tachycardia.

Contraindications, Precautions, and Interactions of α-Adrenergic Blocking Drugs

- Contraindicated in patients who are hypersensitive to them and in patients with coronary artery disease
- Used cautiously during pregnancy and lactation, after a recent myocardial infarction, and in patients with renal failure or Raynaud disease
- When phentolamine is given with epinephrine or ephedrine, the vasoconstrictor and hypertensive effects are decreased

FACT CHECK

12-1 What is the effect of blocking an α-adrenergic receptor?
12-2 What are the common adverse reactions of α-adrenergic blockers?

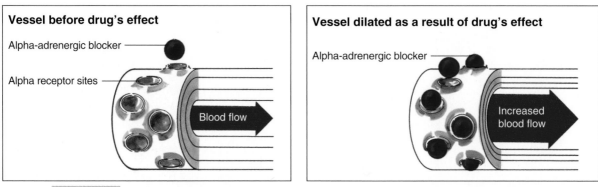

FIGURE 12-1 Graphic representation of α-adrenergic blockers affecting peripheral blood vessels.

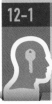
β-ADRENERGIC BLOCKING DRUGS

Actions of β-Adrenergic Blocking Drugs

β-Adrenergic blocking drugs decrease the activity of the sympathetic nervous system in certain tissues. β-Adrenergic receptors are found mainly in the heart. Stimulation of β receptors of the heart results in an increase in the heart rate. If stimulation of these β-adrenergic fibers is blocked, then the heart rate decreases and blood vessels dilate. Examples of β-adrenergic blocking drugs are esmolol (Brevibloc), nadolol (Corgard), and propranolol (Inderal). β-Adrenergic blocking drugs, such as betaxolol (Betoptic) and timolol (Timoptic), when used topically as eye drops, appear to reduce the production of aqueous humor in the anterior chamber of the eye (see Key Concepts 12-1).

Uses of β-Adrenergic Blocking Drugs

These drugs are primarily used in the treatment of hypertension (also see Chapter 21) and certain cardiac arrhythmias. They are used to prevent another heart attack in patients with a recent myocardial infarction (heart attack). Some of these drugs have additional uses, such as the use of propranolol for migraine headaches and nadolol for angina pectoris.

β-Adrenergic blocking drugs also can be used topically as eye drops. For example, betaxolol (Betoptic) and timolol (Timoptic) are used in the treatment of glaucoma. **Glaucoma** is a narrowing or blockage of the drainage channels (canals of Schlemm) between the anterior and posterior chambers of the eye. This results in increased intraocular pressure in the eye. Blindness may occur if glaucoma is left untreated.

CONSIDERATIONS | Older Adults

LIFESPAN

β-Adrenergic Blocking Drugs

Older adults have a greater risk for adverse reactions from β-adrenergic blocking drugs. They should be monitored for confusion, heart failure, worsening of angina, shortness of breath, and peripheral vascular insufficiency (e.g., cold extremities, paresthesia of the hands, weak peripheral pulses). If these adverse reactions occur, alternative therapies should be discussed with their health care provider to improve patients' quality of life.

Adverse Reactions of β-Adrenergic Blocking Drugs

The adverse reactions of β-adrenergic blocking drugs include orthostatic hypotension, bradycardia, dizziness, vertigo, bronchospasm (especially in those with a history of asthma), hyperglycemia, nausea, vomiting, and diarrhea. Many of these reactions are mild and may disappear as therapy continues. More serious adverse reactions include symptoms of congestive heart failure (dyspnea, weight gain, peripheral edema). Adverse reactions of β-adrenergic ophthalmic preparations include headache, depression, cardiac arrhythmias, and bronchospasm.

Contraindications, Precautions, and Interactions of β-Adrenergic Blocking Drugs

- Contraindicated in patients with an allergy to them and patients with sinus bradycardia, second-degree or third-degree heart block, heart failure, asthma, emphysema, or hypotension
- Used cautiously in patients with diabetes, thyrotoxicosis, and peptic ulcer
- When used with verapamil, the effects of the β-blockers are increased.
- When the β-blockers are used with indomethacin, ibuprofen, sulindac, or barbiturates, the effects of the β-blockers may decrease.
- Diuretics may increase the hypotensive effects of the β-adrenergic blocking drugs.
- A paradoxical hypertensive effect may occur when clonidine is given with a β-adrenergic blocking drug.
- When given with lidocaine and cimetidine, β-adrenergic blocking drugs may have increased serum levels and cause toxic effects.

FACT CHECK

12-3   What is the effect of β-adrenergic blocking drugs?
12-4   What are β-adrenergic blocking drugs used to treat?

ANTIADRENERGIC BLOCKING DRUGS

Actions of Antiadrenergic Blocking Drugs

One group of antiadrenergic drugs inhibits the release of norepinephrine from certain adrenergic nerve endings in the peripheral nervous system. This group is composed of antiadrenergic drugs that act on peripheral structures. The other antiadrenergic drugs are called centrally acting antiadrenergic drugs because they act on the central nervous system, rather than on the peripheral nervous system. This group affects specific central nervous system centers and decreases some of the activity of the sympathetic nervous system. Although the actions of these types of antiadrenergic drugs are somewhat different, the results are basically the same. An example of a centrally acting antiadrenergic drug is clonidine (Catapres).

Uses of Antiadrenergic Blocking Drugs

Antiadrenergic drugs are used mainly for the treatment of certain cardiac arrhythmias and hypertension.

Adverse Reactions of Antiadrenergic Blocking Drugs

The adverse reactions of centrally acting antiadrenergic drugs include dry mouth, drowsiness, sedation, anorexia, rash, malaise, and weakness. Adverse reactions of peripherally acting antiadrenergic drugs include hypotension, weakness, light-headedness, and bradycardia.

Contraindications, Precautions, and Interactions of Antiadrenergic Blocking Drugs

Centrally Acting Antiadrenergic Drugs

- Contraindicated in patients with active hepatic disease such as acute hepatitis or active cirrhosis and in patients with a history of hypersensitivity.
- Used cautiously in patients with a history of liver disease or renal function impairment, and during lactation.
- If methyldopa is administered with anesthetics, then the effect of the anesthetic is increased.
- Centrally acting antiadrenergic drugs increase the activity of sympathomimetics, possibly causing hypertension.
- Clonidine decreases the effectiveness of levodopa. When clonidine is given along with a β-adrenergic blocking drug, a potentially life-threatening hypertensive episode may occur.

Peripherally Acting Antiadrenergic Drugs

- Contraindicated in patients with a known hypersensitivity.
- Reserpine is contraindicated in patients with active peptic ulcer or ulcerative colitis or depression.
- Reserpine is used cautiously in patients with renal impairment or cardiovascular disease, and during lactation.
- Guanethidine is contraindicated in patients with pheochromocytoma or congestive heart failure. The drug is used cautiously in patients with bronchial asthma or renal impairment, and during lactation.
- Anorexiants, haloperidol, monoamine oxidase inhibitors, tricyclic antidepressants, and phenothiazines decrease the hypotensive effects of guanethidine.

FACT CHECK

12-5   What are the two types of antiadrenergic drugs?
12-6   Which conditions are antiadrenergic drugs used to treat?

α/β-ADRENERGIC BLOCKING DRUGS

Actions of α/β-Adrenergic Blocking Drugs

α/β-Adrenergic blocking drugs block the stimulation of both α- and β-adrenergic receptors, resulting in peripheral vasodilation. The two drugs in this category are carvedilol (Coreg) and labetalol (Normodyne).

Uses of α/β-Adrenergic Blocking Drugs

Labetalol is used to treat hypertension, either alone or in combination with another drug such as a diuretic. Carvedilol is used to treat essential hypertension and to reduce progression of congestive heart failure.

Adverse Reactions of α/β-Adrenergic Blocking Drugs

The adverse reactions of labetalol include fatigue, drowsiness, insomnia, weakness, hypotension, diarrhea, dyspnea, and skin rash. Most adverse effects are mild and do not require discontinuation of therapy. Adverse reactions of carvedilol include fatigue, hypotension, cardiac insufficiency, chest pain, bradycardia, dizziness, diarrhea, hypotension, and fatigue.

Contraindications, Precautions, and Interactions of α/β-Adrenergic Blocking Drugs

- Contraindicated in patients with hypersensitivity and in patients with bronchial asthma, decompensated heart failure, or severe bradycardia.
- Used cautiously in patients with drug-controlled congestive heart failure, chronic bronchitis, impaired hepatic or cardiac function, or diabetes, and during lactation.
- When either drug is taken along with a diuretic or other hypotensive drug, an increased hypotensive effect may occur.
- When labetalol is given with cimetidine, the effects of labetalol are increased.
- Halothane increases the effects of labetalol.
- When carvedilol is given with an antidiabetic drug, the antidiabetic drug has increased effect.
- Clonidine taken with carvedilol has increased effectiveness.
- Digoxin has an increased serum level when taken with carvedilol.

FACT CHECK

12-7   What are the two α/β–adrenergic blocking drugs?
12-8   What are α/β–adrenergic blocking drugs used to treat?

ALERT ℞

Blood Pressure Drop

If a patient has significant decrease in blood pressure (a drop of 20 mm Hg systolic or a systolic pressure below 90 mm Hg) after a dose of an adrenergic blocking drug, then the health care provider should be notified immediately. A dosage reduction or discontinuation of the drug may be necessary.

Patient Management Issues with Adrenergic Blocking Drugs

An accurate patient database is needed before any adrenergic blocking drug is first given. For example, patients with hypertension have their blood pressure and pulse taken on both arms in sitting, standing, and supine positions. Patients with a cardiac arrhythmia have their pulse taken and their pulse rhythm determined. Once drug therapy is started, the effects of therapy can be evaluated by comparing the patient's current symptoms with the symptoms before therapy started.

Patients receiving adrenergic drug therapy are continually observed for adverse reactions. Some adverse reactions are mild, whereas others, such as diarrhea, may cause a problem, especially if the patient is elderly or debilitated.

Patients receiving adrenergic blocking drugs for cardiac arrhythmias also require monitoring. Some cardiac arrhythmias, such as ventricular fibrillation, are life threatening and require immediate attention. A patient with a life-threatening arrhythmia may receive an adrenergic blocking drug, such as propranolol, by the intravenous route, in which case specialized cardiac monitoring is necessary.

Most adrenergic blocking drugs can be given without regard to food. Propranolol and metoprolol, however, should be given at the same time each day because food may affect their absorption. Sotalol is given on an empty stomach because food may reduce its absorption.

When β-adrenergic blocking eye drops, such as timolol, are administered to patients with glaucoma, they need periodic follow-up examinations by an ophthalmologist. The intraocular pressure should be measured to determine the effectiveness of drug therapy.

Managing Hypotension

Adrenergic blocking drugs may cause hypotension. If the drug is administered for hypertension, then a blood pressure decrease is expected.

Some adrenergic blocking drugs (such as prazosin and terazosin) may cause a "first dose" effect. A **first dose effect** occurs when the patient experiences marked hypotension and syncope (fainting) with the first few doses of the drug. The first dose effect may be minimized if the initial dose is decreased and the drug given at bedtime. The dosage is then slowly increased until a full therapeutic effect is achieved. A patient who experiences syncope should lie down. This effect is self-limiting and in most cases does not recur after the initial period of therapy. Light-headedness and dizziness are more common, however, than fainting.

Decreasing the Patient's Risk for Injury

Some patients receiving an adrenergic blocking drug may experience **postural hypotension**, also known as orthostatic hypotension. This is a feeling of light-headedness and dizziness after suddenly changing from a lying to a sitting or standing position, or from a sitting to a standing position. The following measures help minimize these adverse reactions:

- Instruct patients to rise slowly from a sitting or lying position.
- Help the patients get out of a bed or a chair if symptoms of postural hypotension are severe. Place the call light nearby, and instruct patients to ask for assistance each time they get in and out of a bed or a chair.
- Assist patients in bed to a sitting position, and have the patients sit on the edge of the bed for approximately 1 minute before standing.
- Help seated patients to a standing position, and instruct them to stand in one place for approximately 1 minute before walking.
- Stay with the patients while they are standing in one place and when walking.
- Instruct the patients to avoid standing in one place for prolonged periods.
- Teach the patients to avoid taking hot showers or baths, which may increase these symptoms.

Symptoms of postural or orthostatic hypotension often lessen with time, but patients should be allowed to get out of bed or a chair without assistance only when it is clear they have no danger of falling.

Educating the Patient and Family about Adrenergic Blocking Drugs

Patients need to know why they are taking these drugs and why therapy must be continuous to attain and maintain an optimal state of health and well-being. Below are the key points about adrenergic blocking drugs for specific conditions that the patient or family members should know.

Patients with Hypertension, Cardiac Arrhythmia, or Angina

Some hypertensive patients may be advised to lose weight or eat a special diet, such as a low-salt diet. Patients with angina or a cardiac arrhythmia may also need a special diet. Some patients with hypertension may be taught to monitor their own blood pressure between office visits. If patients are unable to measure their own, then a family member will need be taught how to monitor the patients' blood pressure. In addition

- Do not stop taking the drug abruptly except as advised by your health care provider. Most of these drugs require gradually decreasing the dosage to prevent worsening the adverse effects.
- Notify your health care provider promptly if adverse drug reactions occur.
- Be cautious while driving or performing other hazardous tasks because these drugs (β-adrenergic blockers) may cause drowsiness, dizziness, or light-headedness.
- Immediately report any signs of congestive heart failure (weight gain, difficulty breathing, or edema of the extremities).

- Do not use any nonprescription drug (e.g., cold or flu preparations or nasal decongestants) unless it is approved by the health care provider.
- Inform dentists and other care providers you are taking this drug.
- Keep all health care appointments because close monitoring of therapy is essential with these drugs.

Monitoring Blood Pressure

The patient and family member are taught how to take an accurate blood pressure reading. This involves choosing the correct instrument and the steps to taking a blood pressure reading. The patient and family member are supervised during several trial blood pressure readings to ensure accuracy of the measurements.

- Use the same arm and body position each time to take the blood pressure.
- Blood pressure can vary slightly with emotion, the time of day, and the position of your body.
- Slight changes in readings are normal, but if a drastic change occurs in either or both the systolic or diastolic

readings, then contact your health care provider as soon as possible.

Patients with Glaucoma

When an adrenergic blocking drug is prescribed for glaucoma, the patient needs a demonstration of how to correctly use eye drops. In addition

- Stay on the eye drop instillation schedule, because delaying or discontinuing the drug may result in a marked increase in intraocular pressure, which can lead to blindness.
- Contact your health care provider if you experience eye pain, excessive tearing, or any change in vision.

FACT CHECK

12-9   What is the first dose effect and how can it be minimized?

12-10   Some patients taking adrenergic blocking drugs need to monitor their blood pressure. What should they know to ensure that they are taking it properly?

Chapter Review

KEY POINTS

- Adrenergic blocking drugs inhibit actions in the sympathetic nervous system.
- These drugs are divided into four classes: α-adrenergic blocking drugs, β-adrenergic blocking drugs, antiadrenergic drugs, and α/β-adrenergic blocking drugs.
- Adrenergic blocking drugs have many uses, including the treatment of hypertension, glaucoma, and cardiac arrhythmias.
- Common adverse effects for all adrenergic blockers include bradycardia, dizziness, hypotension, and nausea and vomiting. However, some classes have more adverse effects than others.
- α-Adrenergic blocking drugs may cause a first dose effect. It is very important that the patients understand that they must take the first dose at night and expect to experience adverse effects.
- Patient management and teaching for adrenergic blocking drugs focus on the need for strict dosage control and the management of common adverse reactions.

CRITICAL THINKING CASE STUDY
Treating Hypertension

Ms. Martin has been prescribed propranolol (Inderal) for hypertension. A few days later, she says that she is feeling dizzy and sometimes feels as if she is going to faint.

1. Ms. Martin needs to know that
   a. dizziness is a rare, life-threatening adverse reaction that must be reported immediately to her health care provider
   b. dizziness is a common adverse effect that may disappear with continued therapy
   c. she can stop taking the drug whenever the adverse reactions bother her
   d. taking the drug only with meals will make this adverse effect go away
2. Ms. Martin has a massage scheduled today. Why is it important that she let her massage therapist know about her new medication?
   a. She should not get a massage if she is on propranolol.
   b. She will need to get up slowly after her massage and may need assistance due to postural hypotension.
   c. The massage will likely interfere with the drug effects.
   d. The massage will likely increase her blood pressure.
3. To lower the risk that Ms. Martin may be injured when she feels dizzy, what should she be advised to do?

Review Questions

MULTIPLE CHOICE

1. Which of the following adverse reactions would NOT be expected when taking an α-adrenergic blocking drug?
   a. Orthostatic hypotension
   b. Tachycardia
   c. Hypertension
   d. All of the above would be expected adverse reactions of an α-adrenergic blocking drug.

2. Beta-blockers would NOT be used for which of the following conditions?
   a. Hypertension
   b. Migraines
   c. Glaucoma
   d. Benign prostatic hypertrophy (BPH)

3. When instructing a patient who is taking an adrenergic blocking drug for hypertension, which of the following statements is/are appropriate for patient education?
   a. Do not stop taking the medication abruptly.
   b. Monitor your blood pressure at home on a daily basis.
   c. Do not use any over-the-counter medications for cold or flu without first talking with a health care provider.
   d. All of the above

3. Which of the following adrenergic blocking drugs produce their greatest effect on adrenergic nerves in the heart?
   a. α-Adrenergic blocking drugs
   b. β-Adrenergic blocking drugs
   c. Antiadrenergic drugs
   d. α/β-Adrenergic blocking drugs

MATCHING

_____ 5. clonidine   a. Hytrin
_____ 6. terazosin   b. Inderal
_____ 7. propranolol   c. Regitine
_____ 8. phentolamine   d. Catapres

TRUE OR FALSE

_____ 9. The antiadrenergic drugs inhibit the release of norepinephreine from certain adrenergic nerve endings in the peripheral nervous system.

_____ 10. Most of the adverse effects associated with α/β-adrenergic blocking drugs are mild and do not require discontinuation of the drug.

_____ 11. α-Adrenergic blocking drugs cause vasoconstriction.

_____ 12. Most adrenergic blocking agents must be taken with food.

FILL IN THE BLANKS

13. Most β-adrenergic blockers have a generic name that ends in _____.

14. _____ is a narrowing or blockage of the drainage channels between the anterior and posterior chambers of the eye.

15. The _____ _____ _____ occurs when the patient experiences marked hypotension and syncope with the first few doses of a drug.

16. The α/β-adrenergic blocking drug blocks the stimulation of both α- and β-adrenergic receptors resulting in peripheral _____.

SHORT ANSWERS

17. Adrenergic blocking drugs are used to treat what medication conditions?
18. What are the four adrenergic blocking drugs?
19. What is postural hypotension?
20. Why must a patient taking a β-blocking drug be cautious while driving?

Web Activities

1. Go to the mayo clinic website (http://www.mayoclinic.com). Conduct a search for "orthostatic hypotension" under the Health Information tab. What are five risk factors for orthostatic hypotension?

2. Go to the American heart Association website (http://www.heart.org). Conduct a search on "understanding blood pressure readings." What do the two numbers stand for? What is an optimal blood pressure?

SUMMARY DRUG TABLE Adrenergic Blocking Drugs (left, generic; right, trade)

Comprehensive Summary Drug Tables, including uses, adverses effects, dosages, and pregnancy classifications, are provided on the companion website, http://thePoint.lww. com/PharmacologyHP2e

α-Adrenergic Blocking Agents	
phentolamine *fen-tole-a-meen*	Regitine

β-Adrenergic Blocking Drugs	
betaxolol HCl *beh-tax'-oh-lol*	Kerlone
betaxolol HCl *beh-tax'-oh-lol* (ophthalmic)	Betoptic
esmolol HCl *ess'-moe-lol*	Brevibloc
nadolol *nay-doe'-lol*	Corgard, *generic*
propranolol *pro-pran'-oh-lol*	Inderal, *generic*
timolol maleate *tye-moe'-lole*	Blocadren, *generic*
timolol maleate (ophthalmic) *tye-moe'-lole*	Timoptic

α/β-Adrenergic Blocking Agents	
carvedilol *car-veh'-dih-lol*	Coreg
labetalol *lah-bet'-ah-lol*	Normodyne, Trandate, *generic*

Antiadrenergic Drugs: Peripherally Acting	
reserpine *re-ser'-peen*	*generic*

Antiadrenergic Drugs: Centrally Acting	
clonidine HCl *kloe'-ni-deen*	Catapres, Catapres-TTS, *generic*
prazosin *pray-zoe'-sin*	Minipress, *generic*
terazosin *tear-aye'-zoe-sin*	Hytrin

13

Cholinergic Drugs

CHAPTER OBJECTIVES

On completion of this chapter, students will be able to:

1. Define the chapter's key terms.
2. Discuss the uses, general drug actions, contraindications, precautions, interactions, and adverse reactions associated with the administration of cholinergic drugs.
3. Discuss important points to keep in mind when educating patients about the use of cholinergic drugs.

KEY TERMS

cholinergic drugs—drugs that mimic the activity of the parasympathetic nervous system
cholinergic crisis—cholinergic drug toxicity
myasthenia gravis—a disease that causes fatigue of skeletal muscles because of the lack of acetylcholine released at the nerve endings of parasympathetic nerve fibers

CHAPTER OVERVIEW

Drug classes covered in this chapter are:

- Cholinergic drugs

Drugs by classification are listed on page 148.

thePOINT RESOURCES

- Comprehensive Summary Drug Tables
- Lippincott's Interactive Tutorials: Drugs Affecting the Autonomic Nervous System
- Interactive Practice and Review
- Monographs of Most Commonly Prescribed Drugs

Cholinergic **drugs**—mimic the activity of the parasympathetic nervous system. They also are called parasympathomimetic drugs. Cholinergic drugs have limited usefulness in medicine, partly because of their adverse reactions, but are used for certain diseases or conditions.

A basic knowledge of the nervous system is necessary to understand cholinergic drugs and how they work in the body. Refer to Chapter 11 for an overview of the nervous system. Figure 13-1 shows the effects of the parasympathetic nervous system on body organs and structures .

Cholinergic Drugs

Actions of Cholinergic Drugs

Cholinergic drugs may act like the neurohormone ACh or may inhibit the release of the neurohormone AChE. Cholinergic drugs that act like ACh are called direct-acting cholinergics. A cholinergic drug that inhibits the release of AChE prolongs the activity of the ACh produced naturally by the body. Cholinergic drugs that prolong the activity of ACh by inhibiting the release

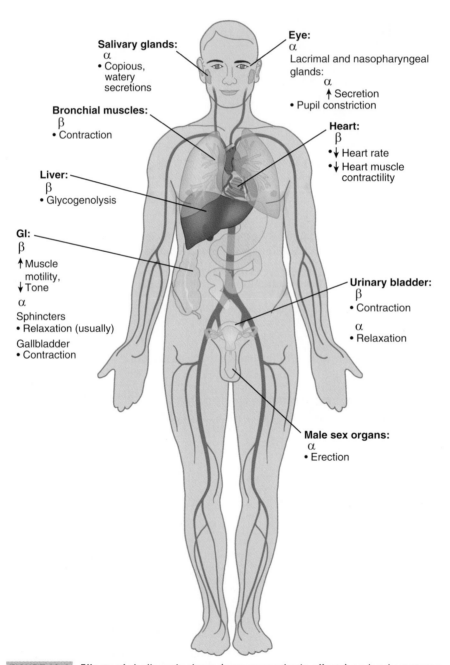

FIGURE 13-1 Effects of cholinergic drugs (parasympathetic effects) on body systems.

of AChE are called indirect-acting cholinergics. The results of these different drug actions, however, are basically the same.

Uses of Cholinergic Drugs

The major uses of cholinergic drugs are for treating glaucoma, myasthenia gravis, and urinary retention.

Glaucoma is a disorder of increased pressure within the eye caused by an obstruction of the outflow of aqueous humor through the canal of Schlemm. The normal flow of aqueous humor keeps the pressure within the eye within normal limits. Glaucoma may be treated by topical application (eye drops) of a cholinergic drug, such as carbachol or pilocarpine (Isopto Carpine). Treating glaucoma with a cholinergic drug produces miosis (constriction of the iris). This opens the blocked channels and allows the normal flow of aqueous humor, thus reducing intraocular pressure.

Myasthenia gravis is a disease that causes fatigue of skeletal muscles because of the lack of ACh released at the nerve endings of parasympathetic nerve fibers. Drugs used to treat this disorder include ambenonium (Mytelase) and pyridostigmine (Mestinon).

Urinary retention results when urination is impaired. Urination is a voluntary and an involuntary act. The parasympathetic nervous system partly controls the process of urination by constricting the detrusor muscle and relaxing the bladder sphincter (see Table 11-1). Treatment of urinary retention with cholinergic drugs, such as ambenonium, bethanechol chloride (Urecholine), or pyridostigmine, results in the spontaneous passage of urine.

> ### FACT CHECK
> 13-1 Cholinergic drugs act like which neurohormone?
> 13-2 What are the major uses of cholinergic drugs?

Adverse Reactions of Cholinergic Drugs

Unless applied topically, as in the treatment of glaucoma, cholinergic drugs are not selective in their action. This means they may affect many different organs and structures in the body and cause a variety of adverse effects. Oral or parenteral administration can result in nausea, diarrhea, abdominal cramping, salivation, flushing of the skin, cardiac arrhythmias, and muscle weakness. Topical administration usually produces few adverse effects, but a temporary reduction of visual acuity (sharpness of vision) and headache may occur.

Contraindications, Precautions, and Interactions of Cholinergic Drugs

Contraindications

- Known hypersensitivity and in patients with asthma, peptic ulcer disease, coronary artery disease, or hyperthyroidism.
- Bethanechol is contraindicated in patients with mechanical obstruction of the gastrointestinal or genitourinary tract.

> ### ALERT ℞
> **Managing Disturbed Visual Perception**
> Because drug-induced myopia (nearsightedness) may occur after cholinergic eye drops are given to treat glaucoma, the patient may need help getting out of bed or walking. Obstacles that might not be seen and might trip a patient, such as slippers, chairs, and tables, should be placed out of the way, especially at night.

- Patients with secondary glaucoma, iritis, corneal abrasion, or any acute inflammatory disease of the eye should not use cholinergic eyedrops.

Precautions

- Use cautiously in patients with hypertension, epilepsy, cardiac arrhythmias, bradycardia, recent coronary occlusion, or megacolon.
- The safety of these drugs has not been established for use during lactation, or in children.

Interactions

- When given along with another cholinergic, the effects of these drugs are increased and the patient has a greater risk for toxicity.
- When used concurrently with an anticholinergic drug, the effects of the cholinergic drug are minimized. Because of this, atropine is used as an antidote for an overdosage of cholinergic drugs.
- Carbachol and pilocarpine have an additive effect when used together.
- Edrophonium, neostigmine, and pyridostigmine have decreased effects, along with possible muscular depression, when given with a corticosteroid.

Patient Management Issues with Cholinergic Drugs

Patients receiving a cholinergic drug should be monitored for drug toxicity or **cholinergic crisis.** Specific patient management issues apply also to patients with glaucoma, myasthenia gravis, or urinary retention.

> ### ALERT ℞
> **Cholinergic Crisis**
> Symptoms of cholinergic crisis (cholinergic drug toxicity) include severe abdominal cramping, diarrhea, excessive salivation, muscle weakness, rigidity and spasm, and clenching of the jaw. Patients with these symptoms require immediate medical treatment, and their condition must be immediately reported to the health care provider. An antidote such as atropine may be given in case of an overdose.

ALERT Rx

Cholinergic Drugs for Myasthenia Gravis

Because dosage adjustments may be frequent, the patient must be observed closely for symptoms of drug overdosage or underdosage. Signs of drug overdosage include muscle rigidity and spasm, salivation, and clenching of the jaw. Signs of drug underdosage are the signs of the disease itself: rapid fatigability of the muscles, drooping of the eyelids, and difficulty breathing. If symptoms of drug overdosage or underdosage develop, the health care provider must be notified immediately.

Patients with urinary retention must be monitored for fluid intake and output. The health care provider should be notified if the patient fails to urinate after taking the drug. Urination usually occurs 5 to 15 minutes after subcutaneous drug administration and 30 to 90 minutes after oral administration. With a hospitalized patient, the call light and any other items the patient might need, such as a urinal or the bedpan, should be within easy reach.

Educating the Patient and Family about Cholinergic Drugs

The purpose of the drug therapy should be explained to the patient and family members, along with the adverse reactions that may occur. Below are the key points about cholinergic drugs the patient or family members should know.

Patients with Glaucoma

When a cholinergic drug is prescribed for glaucoma, the patient and family member are shown how to correctly instill the eye drops.

- The eye drops may sting when put in the eye; this is normal but usually temporary.
- Be cautious while driving or performing any task that requires visual acuity.

- Local irritation and headache may occur at the beginning of therapy.
- Notify your health care provider if you experience abdominal cramping, diarrhea, or excessive salivation.

Instilling Liquid Eye Medication

- It is important to keep the bottle tightly closed.
- Do not wash or touch the tip of the dropper.
- Do not put the dropper down on a table or other surface.
- Support your hand holding the dropper against your forehead.
- Do not let the tip of the dropper touch the eye.
- Put the dropper back in the bottle immediately after use.
- Tilt your head back to instill the prescribed number of drops in the inner lower eyelid.
- If you or a family member cannot instill the eye drops, then contact your health care provider immediately.

Patients with Myasthenia Gravis

Many patients with myasthenia gravis learn to adjust their drug dosage according to their needs because dosages may vary slightly from day to day. The patient and family members are taught to recognize symptoms of overdosage and underdosage and what steps to take if either occurs. The patient should be given a written or printed description of the signs and symptoms of drug overdosage or underdosage. In addition

- Keep a record of your response to drug therapy (e.g., time of day, increased or decreased muscle strength, fatigue), and bring this to each provider or clinic visit until your symptoms are well controlled and the drug dosage is stabilized.
- Wear or carry identification (such as a Medic-Alert tag) indicating that you have myasthenia gravis.

FACT CHECK

13-3   What condition may be caused by cholinergic eyedrops?

13-4   What are the symptoms of a cholinergic crisis?

Chapter Review

KEY POINTS

- Cholinergic drugs mimic the activity of the parasympathetic nervous system.
- These drugs are used primarily for treatment of glaucoma, myasthenia gravis, and urinary retention.
- Common adverse effects include cardiac arrhythmias, abdominal discomfort, temporary reduction in visual acuity, and headache.
- Patient management and teaching for cholinergic drugs focus on the need for strict dosage control and the management of common adverse reactions.

CRITICAL THINKING CASE STUDIES

Pilocarpine Effects

Ms. Windham recently started using pilocarpine for her glaucoma. Her daughter is concerned because Ms. Windham's pupils seem to be constricted, which is not normal.

1. What should you tell Ms. Windham's daughter about the pupil constriction?
   a. She should call the physician.
   b. Ms. Windham is having an adverse reaction to her medication.
   c. This a normal adverse effect of pilocarpine.
   d. Ms. Windham is using too much of the medication, and her daughter should call the physician.

2. What other adverse effects should Ms. Windham's daughter be aware of?
    a. The drops may cause constipation.
    b. The drops may cause myopia, which will interfere with the patient's vision, especially at night.
    c. The drops may cause dry mouth.
    d. The drops should be stopped if they sting when Ms. Windham uses them.

Cholinergic Drug Issues

3. A patient is taking bethanechol for urinary retention. He is experiencing severe abdominal cramping, diarrhea, and muscle weakness. What is wrong with him?

Review Questions

MULTIPLE CHOICE

1. Pilocarpine eye drops may be prescribed to treat
    a. nearsightedness
    b. glaucoma
    c. eye infection
    d. mydriasis of the eyes
2. Cholinergic drugs are used to treat
    a. urinary retention
    b. glaucoma
    c. hypertension
    d. a and b only
3. Patients using a cholinergic drop for glaucoma should know
    a. the eye drops may sting when put in the eye, this is normal but usually temporary
    b. the eye drops will not affect visual acuity
    c. local irritation and headache may occur at the beginning of therapy
    d. a and c only

MATCHING

_____ 4. neostigmine   a. Urecholine
_____ 5. pilocarpine   b. Mestinon
_____ 6. pyridostigmine   c. Prostigmin
_____ 7. bethanechol   d. Isopto Carpine

TRUE OR FALSE

_____ 8. The parasympathetic nervous system partly controls the process of urination by dilating the detrusor muscle and constricting the bladder sphincter.

_____ 9. Cholinergic drugs administered orally or parenterally are not selective in their action like those that are administered topically.
_____ 10. Atropine, which is an anticholinergic, is used as an antidote for an overdosage of cholinergic drugs.
_____ 11. Patients with symptoms of a cholinergic crisis require immediate medical treatment.

FILL IN THE BLANKS

12. Cholinergic drugs treat glaucoma by producing _____ (constriction of the iris), which opens the blocked channels and allows the normal flow of aqueous humor.
13. Myasthenia gravis is a disease that causes fatigue of skeletal muscles because of the lack of _____ released at the nerve endings of parasympathetic nerve fibers.
14. Cholinergic drugs mimic the activity of the _____ nervous system.
15. Patients with severe symptoms of myasthenia gravis require the drug every 2 to 4 hours, even during the night. _____ tablets may be used to allow for less frequent dosing and give the patients longer undisturbed periods at night.

SHORT ANSWERS

16. What are the symptoms of a cholinergic crisis?
17. Why is it necessary for patients to keep a record of their response to drug therapy?

Web Activities

1. Go to the website for the National Institute of Neurologic Disorders and Stroke (http://www.ninds.nih.gov). Under "Disorders A-Z," find myasthenia gravis. What is it?
2. Go to the website for the National Kidney and Urologic Diseases Information Clearinghouse (http://kidney.niddk.nih.gov). Under "Kidney and Urologic Diseases," conduct a search for Urinary Retention. List five causes of urinary retention.

SUMMARY DRUG TABLE Cholinergic Drugs
(left, generic; right, trade)

Comprehensive Summary Drug Tables, including uses, adverses effects, dosages, and pregnancy classifications, are provided on the companion website, http:// thePoint.lww.com/PharmacologyHP2e

ambenonium *am-be-noe'-nee-um*	Mytelase
bethanechol chloride *be-than'-e-kole*	Duvoid, Urecholine, *generic*
carbachol, topical *kar'-ba-kole*	Isopto Carbachol, Miostat
edrophonium *ed-roe-fone'-ee-yum*	Enlon, Tensilon
neostigmine *nee-oh-stig'-meen*	Prostigmin, *generic*
pilocarpine hydrochloride *pye-loe-kar'-peen*	Isopto Carpine, Pilocar, *generic*
pyridostigmine bromide *peer-id-oh-stig'-meen*	Mestinon, Regonol

14

Cholinergic Blocking Drugs (Anticholinergics)

CHAPTER OBJECTIVES

On completion of this chapter, students will be able to:

1. Define the chapter's key terms.
2. Discuss the uses, general drug actions, contraindications, precautions, interactions, and adverse reactions associated with the administration of cholinergic blocking drugs.
3. Discuss important points to keep in mind when educating patients about the use of cholinergic blocking drugs.

KEY TERMS

cholinergic blocking drugs—drugs that impede certain parasympathetic nervous system functions

thePOINT RESOURCES

- Comprehensive Summary Drug Tables

- Lippincott's Interactive Tutorials: Drugs Affecting the Autonomic Nervous System

- Interactive Practice and Review

- Monographs of Most Commonly Prescribed Drugs

Cholinergic blocking drugs, like adrenergic blocking drugs, also have effects on the autonomic nervous system. These drugs block the action of the neurotransmitter acetylcholine in the parasympathetic nervous system. Because parasympathetic nerves control many areas of the body, cholinergic blocking drugs have numerous effects. Cholinergic blocking drugs also are called anticholinergics or parasympathomimetic blocking drugs.

A basic knowledge of the nervous system is necessary to understand cholinergic drugs and how they work in the body. Refer to Chapter 11 for an overview of the nervous system.

Cholinergic Blocking Drugs

Actions of Cholinergic Blocking Drugs

Cholinergic blocking drugs inhibit the activity of acetylcholine in parasympathetic nerve fibers (Fig. 14-1). When the activity of acetylcholine is inhibited, nerve impulses traveling along parasympathetic nerve fibers cannot pass to the effector organ or structure. Because of the wide distribution of parasympathetic nerves, these drugs affect many organs and structures in the body, including the eyes, the respiratory and gastrointestinal tracts, the heart, and the bladder (see Key Concepts 14-1).

Patients' responses to cholinergic blocking drugs vary, often depending on the drug and the dosage. For example, scopolamine may occasionally cause excitement, delirium, and restlessness. This reaction is considered a drug idiosyncrasy (an unexpected or unusual drug effect).

Uses of Cholinergic Blocking Drugs

Because of their widespread effects on many organs and structures, cholinergic blocking drugs have a variety of uses. The

uses of atropine include treatment of pylorospasm, peptic ulcer, ureteral and biliary colic, vagal-induced bradycardia, and parkinsonism; preoperatively, it is given to reduce secretions of the upper respiratory tract before the administration of a general anesthetic. The action of some other cholinergic blocking drugs is more selective, affecting principally one structure of the body.

KEY CONCEPTS
14-1   Effects of Cholinergic Blocking Drugs

Cholinergic blocking drugs produce the following responses:

- *Central nervous system*—dreamless sleep, drowsiness; atropine may produce mild stimulation in some patients
- *Eye*—mydriasis (dilatation of the pupil), cycloplegia (paralysis of accommodation or inability to focus the eye)
- *Respiratory tract*—drying of the secretions of the mouth, nose, throat, bronchi, relaxation of smooth muscles of the bronchi resulting in slight bronchodilatation
- *Gastrointestinal tract*—decrease in secretions of the stomach, decrease in gastric and intestinal movement (motility)
- *Cardiovascular system*—increase in pulse rate (most pronounced with atropine)
- *Urinary tract*—dilatation of smooth muscles of the ureters and kidney pelvis, contraction of the detrusor muscle of the bladder

FACT CHECK

14-1   What is the action of cholinergic blocking drugs?
14-2   Why do cholinergic blocking drugs have a variety of uses?

Adverse Reactions of Cholinergic Blocking Drugs

Dryness of the mouth with difficulty in swallowing, blurred vision, and photophobia (aversion to bright light) commonly occur with cholinergic blocking drugs. These reactions are commonly called "anticholinergic effects." The severity of many adverse reactions often depends on the dose: the larger the dose, the more intense the reaction. Even in normal doses, some degree of dryness of the mouth almost always occurs.

Constipation may occur in patients taking one of these drugs regularly. Drowsiness may occur with these drugs, but sometimes this adverse reaction is desirable, such as when atropine is used preoperatively to reduce respiratory secretions.

Elderly patients may experience confusion or excitement, even at small doses.

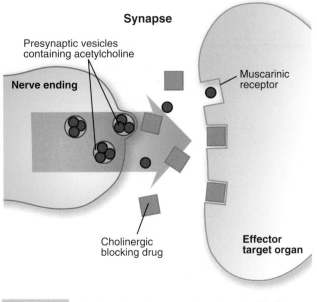

FIGURE 14-1 Mechanism of action of cholinergic blocking drugs.

Other adverse reactions that may occur with cholinergic blocking drugs include

- Central nervous system—headache, flushing, nervousness, drowsiness, weakness, insomnia, nasal congestion, fever
- Eyes—blurred vision, mydriasis (dilated pupils), photophobia, increased ocular tension
- Gastrointestinal tract—nausea, vomiting, difficulty swallowing, heartburn
- Urinary tract—urinary hesitancy and retention, dysuria (difficult or painful urination)
- Cardiovascular system—palpitations, bradycardia (after low doses of atropine), tachycardia (after higher doses of atropine)
- Other—urticaria (skin rash) or other skin manifestations, anaphylactic shock

Contraindications, Precautions, and Interactions of Cholinergic Blocking Drugs

Contraindications

- Glaucoma (may cause an attack of acute glaucoma)
- Tachyarrhythmias, myocardial infarction (heart attack), and congestive heart failure (unless bradycardia is present)

Precautions

- In pregnancy, use only when the benefit to the woman outweighs the risk to the fetus.
- Can cause urinary retention in patients with an enlarged prostate. This caution applies also to some over-the-counter medications for allergy and cold symptoms and for aiding sleep. Some of these products contain atropine, scopolamine, or other cholinergic blocking drugs.
- Used with caution in patients with gastrointestinal infections, benign prostatic hypertrophy, hyperthyroidism, hepatic or renal disease, or hypertension
- Atropine: used with caution in patients with asthma

Interactions

- Decreased effectiveness of haloperidol when that drug is administered with an anticholinergic
- Atropine: When given with meperidine (Demerol), flurazepam (Dalmane), diphenhydramine (Benadryl), phenothiazines, or tricyclic antidepressants, atropine effects may increase.

CONSIDERATIONS | **Older adults**

LIFESPAN

Visual Difficulties

For elderly patients, as well as all patients experiencing visual difficulties, any furniture (e.g., footstools, chairs, stands) that may obstruct walking should be moved out of the way. Throw rugs should be removed.

Patient Management Issues with Cholinergic Blocking Drugs

Patients taking a cholinergic blocking drug should be closely observed. Vital signs are monitored and the patient observed for adverse reactions. Any increase in the severity of symptoms of the condition for which the patient is being treated must be reported to the health care provider immediately.

In hot weather, sweating may be decreased, causing heat prostration. Patients should be observed for signs of heat prostration (fever, tachycardia, flushing, warm dry skin, mental confusion), especially if the patient is elderly or debilitated. The health care provider should be notified immediately if heat prostration is suspected. Elderly patients receiving a cholinergic blocking drug should be observed for agitation, mental confusion, drowsiness, urinary retention, or other adverse effects. If any of these occur, then the health care provider should be informed and the patient's safety ensured.

Caring for Patients with Heart Block

The patient receiving atropine for third-degree heart block is placed on a cardiac monitor during and after administration of the drug to monitor for changes in pulse rate or rhythm. Tachycardia or other arrhythmias must be immediately reported, as well as a failure of the drug to increase the patient's heart rate. Other drugs or medical management may be necessary.

Caring for Patients Receiving a Preoperative Drug

If a cholinergic blocking drug is to be given before surgery, the patient is asked to urinate before the drug is given. Patients are told that their mouth will become very dry but that they cannot drink any fluid before the surgery.

Managing Alterations in Visual Acuity

Blurred vision and photophobia commonly occur with cholinergic blocking drugs. The patient may need help walking. If photophobia is a problem, then the patient may need to wear sunglasses outside, even on cloudy days. The patient's room should be dimly lit and curtains or blinds closed to keep bright sunlight from the room.

Managing Dry Mouth

Patients who take these drugs daily may experience severe and very uncomfortable mouth dryness. Patients may have difficulty swallowing oral drugs and food. The patient should take a few sips of water before and with an oral drug, and sip water at intervals during meals. If allowed, hard candy slowly dissolved in the mouth and frequent sips of water during the day may help relieve a dry mouth.

Minimizing Risk for Injury

Cholinergic blocking drugs may cause drowsiness, dizziness, and blurred vision. Patients (especially the elderly) may need help walking.

Managing Constipation

Constipation can be a problem with cholinergic blocking drugs. The patient may obtain relief by increasing fluid intake up to 2000 mL daily (if health conditions permit), eating a diet high in fiber, and getting adequate exercise. The health care provider may prescribe a stool softener, if necessary, to prevent constipation.

Educating the Patient and Family about Cholinergic Blocking Drugs

A cholinergic blocking drug may be prescribed for a prolonged period. Some patients may discontinue drug use, especially if their original symptoms have been relieved. The patient and family need to understand that the prescribed drug must still be taken even though symptoms have been relieved. Below are the key points about cholinergic blocking drugs the patient or family members should know.

- If you experience drowsiness, dizziness, or blurred vision, then avoid driving or performing other tasks requiring alertness and good vision.
- If you experience photophobia, then wear sunglasses when outside, even on cloudy days, keep rooms dimly lit, and close curtains or blinds to eliminate bright sunlight in the room. Schedule outdoor activities (when necessary) before taking the first dose of the drug, such as early in the morning.
- For constipation, drink plenty of fluids during the day, exercise if approved by your health care provider, and eat foods high in fiber.
- To prevent heat prostration, avoid going outside on hot, sunny days; use fans to stay cool if the day is extremely warm; sponge your skin with cool water if other cooling measures are not available; and wear loose-fitting clothes in warm weather.

For Dry Mouth

- Perform frequent mouth care, including brushing, rinsing, and flossing.
- Keep a glass or sports bottle filled with fluid on hand at all times.
- Sip small amounts of cool water or fluids throughout the day and with meals.
- Take a few sips of water before taking any oral drugs.
- Suck on ice chips or frozen ices, such as popsicles.
- Chew gum.

CONSIDERATIONS | Older adults

LIFESPAN

Cholinergic Blocking Drugs

Family members of an elderly patient should be told about possible visual and mental impairments (blurred vision, confusion, agitation) that may occur during therapy with cholinergic blocking drugs. Objects or situations that may cause falls, such as throw rugs, footstools, and wet or newly waxed floors, should be removed or avoided whenever possible. The patient must be closely observed during the first few days of therapy and the health care provider notified if mental changes occur.

- Suck on sugar-free hard candies.
- Avoid alcohol-based mouthwashes.

Patients Receiving a Preoperative Drug

- Urinate before the preoperative drug is administered.
- Drowsiness and extreme dryness of the mouth and nose will occur approximately 20 to 30 minutes after the drug is given.
- Stay in bed with the side rails raised after the drug is administered.

Patients with Peptic Ulcer

- A special diet may be ordered by the health care provider; following this diet is important.
- Take the drug exactly as prescribed (e.g., 30 minutes before meals or between meals) to obtain the desired results.

FACT CHECK

14-3 What are the most common adverse reactions of cholinergic blocking drugs?

14-4 What can be recommended for a patient who is experiencing dry mouth?

Chapter Review: Anticholinergic Adverse Effects

KEY POINTS

- Cholinergic blocking drugs inhibit actions in the parasympathetic nervous system and have widespread effects throughout the body.
- Common uses are the treatment of pylorospasm, peptic ulcer, and parkinsonism.
- Common adverse effects, often called "anticholinergic effects," include drowsiness, blurred vision, photophobia, dry mouth, and tachycardia.
- Patient management and teaching for cholinergic blocking drugs focus on the need for strict dosage control and the management of common adverse reactions.

CRITICAL THINKING CASE STUDY

Coming in for her weekly massage, Ms. Mock informs you that she has started a new medication. She cannot remember the name of it but recalls the term "anticholinergic" was mentioned when she visited with the pharmacist.

1. What can you tell Ms. Mock to expect when taking an anticholinergic?
   a. It will probably make her mouth dry.
   b. It may cause constipation.
   c. It may cause urinary hesistancy and retention
   d. All of the above

2. Ms. Mock tells you that she is experiencing a dry mouth. What can you recommend to help with this adverse reaction?

3. After finishing the massage, Ms. Mock indicates that lights seem to be bothering her. Is this normal when taking an anticholinergic?

Review Questions

MULTIPLE CHOICE

1. A patient taking clidinium for a peptic ulcer complains of dry mouth. This patient should be told
   a. that this effect is unusual and the health care provider should be notified
   b. to take frequent sips of water
   c. to rinse the mouth with salt water
   d. to ignore this reaction because it is only temporary

2. Because of the effect of cholinergic blocking drugs on intestinal motility, patients taking these drugs should be monitored for the development of
   a. esophageal ulcers
   b. diarrhea
   c. heartburn
   d. constipation

3. How should a patient manage constipation caused by a cholinergic blocking drug?
   a. Drink plenty of fluids.
   b. Eat a diet high in fiber.
   c. Get adequate exercise.
   d. All of the above

MATCHING

_____ 4. dicyclomine   a. Artane
_____ 5. glycopyrrolate   b. Bentyl
_____ 6. trihexyphenidyl c. Pro-Banthine
_____ 7. propantheline   d. Robinul

TRUE OR FALSE

_____ 8. The severity of many adverse reactions associated with cholinergic blocking drugs often depends on the dose.

_____ 9. Elderly patients may experience confusion or excitement, even at small doses.

_____ 10. If a cholinergic blocking drug is to be given before surgery, the patient is asked to urinate before the drug is given.

FILL IN THE BLANKS

11. In hot weather, cholinergic blocking drugs may cause a decrease in sweating, which can cause _____ _____.

12. Cholinergic blocking drugs block the action of _____ in the parasympathetic nervous system.

13. The adverse reactions associated with the cholinergic blocking drugs are commonly called _____ effects.

SHORT ANSWERS

14. Why is atropine used preoperatively?
15. What are the signs of heat prostration?
16. How can photophobia be managed?

Web Activities

1. Go to the merck manual website (http://www.merck manuals.com). Click on the Home Health Handbook tab. Conduct a search on "aging and drugs." Why do older people experience more anticholinergic effects when taking an anticholinergic drug?

2. Go to the National Center for Biotechnology Information website (http://www.ncbi.nlm.nih.gov). Conduct a search for an article titled "Managing Anticholinergic Side Effects" by Dr. Joseph Lieberman, III. How does Dr. Lieberman suggest anticholinergic adverse reactions be handled by the physician prescribing an antipsychotic?

SUMMARY DRUG TABLE Cholinergic Blocking Drugs (left, generic; right, trade)

Comprehensive Summary Drug Tables, including uses, adverses effects, dosages, and pregnancy classifications, are provided on the companion website, http://thePoint.lww.com/PharmacologyHP2e

atropine *a'-troe-peen*	*generic*
dicyclomine HCl *dye-sye'-kloe-meen*	Bentyl, Di-Spasz, *generic*
flavoxate *fla-vox'-ate*	Urispas
glycopyrrolate *glye-koe-pye'-roe-late*	Robinul
l-hyoscyamine sulfate *high-oh-sigh'- ah-meen*	Anaspaz, Donnamar, Levbid
mepenzolate bromide *meh-pen'-zoe-late*	Cantil
methscopolamine *mehth-scoe-pol'-a-meen*	Pamine
propantheline bromide *proe-pan'-the-leen*	Pro-Banthine, *generic*
scopolamine hydrobromide *scoe-pol'-a-meen*	*generic*
trihexyphenidyl *trye-hex-ee-fen'-i-dill*	Artane

15

Bronchodilators and Antiasthma Drugs

CHAPTER OBJECTIVES

On completion of this chapter, students will be able to:

1. Define the chapter's key terms.
2. Describe the actions of the sympathomimetics.
3. Identify common adverse reactions, contraindications, precautions, and interactions of the sympathomimetics.
4. Describe the actions of the xanthine derivatives.
5. Identify common adverse reactions, contraindications, precautions, and interactions of the xanthine derivatives.
6. Discuss important points to keep in mind when speaking to patients and family members about the bronchodilators.
7. Describe the actions of the corticosteroids.
8. Identify common adverse reactions, contraindications, precautions, and interactions of the corticosteroids.
9. Describe the actions of the leukotriene receptor antagonists and leukotriene formation inhibitors.
10. Identify common adverse reactions, contraindications, precautions, and interactions of the leukotriene receptor antagonists and leukotriene formation inhibitors.
11. Describe the actions of the mast cell stabilizer.
12. Identify common adverse reactions, contraindications, precautions, and interactions of the mast cell stabilizer.
13. Discuss important points to keep in mind when speaking to patients and family members about the use of the antiasthma drugs.

KEY TERMS

asthma—a reversible obstructive disease of the lower airway
bronchodilator—a drug used to relieve bronchospasm associated with respiratory disorders
leukotrienes—substances that are released by the body during the inflammatory process and constrict the bronchia

CHAPTER OVERVIEW

Drug classes covered in this chapter are:

- Sympathomimetics
- Xanthine derivatives
- Corticosteroids
- Leukotriene receptor antagonists and leukotriene formation inhibitors
- Mast cell stabilizers

Drugs by classification are listed on page 166.

thePoint RESOURCES

- Comprehensive Summary Drug Tables
- Animations: Asthma; Gas Exchange in Alveoli
- Lippincott's Interactive Tutorials: Drugs Affecting the Respiratory System
- Interactive Practice and Review
- Monographs of Most Commonly Prescribed Drugs

sympathomimetics—drugs that mimic the activities or actions of the sympathetic nervous system

theophyllinization—process of giving the patient a higher initial dose, called a loading dose, of a prescription drug

to bring blood levels of theophylline to a therapeutic range more quickly

xanthine derivatives—drugs that stimulate the central nervous system and result in bronchodilation

The respiratory system consists of the upper and lower airways, the lungs, and the thoracic cavity. The function of the respiratory system is to exchange oxygen and carbon dioxide from the blood in the lungs (Fig. 15-1). Any change in a patient's respiratory status has the potential to affect every other body system because all cells need an adequate supply of oxygen for optimal functioning. The next three chapters focus on drugs used to treat some of the more common disorders affecting the respiratory system.

Within recent years, a number of new drugs have been introduced to treat respiratory disorders such as bronchial **asthma** and disorders that produce chronic airway obstruction. This chapter discusses the **bronchodilators**, drugs that have been around for a long time but are still effective in specific instances, and newer antiasthma drugs that have proven to be highly effective in the prophylaxis (prevention) of breathing difficulty.

Asthma is a respiratory condition characterized by recurrent attacks of dyspnea (difficulty breathing) and wheezing caused by spasmodic constriction of the bronchi. With asthma, the body responds with a massive inflammatory response. During the inflammatory process, large amounts of histamine are released from the mast cells of the respiratory tract, causing symptoms such as increased mucus production and edema of the airway and resulting in bronchospasm and inflammation. With asthma, the airways become narrow, the muscles around the airway tighten, the inner lining of the bronchi swells, and extra mucus clogs the smaller airways.

Asthma is a reversible obstructive disease of the lower airway. Patients with asthma experience airway obstruction caused by bronchospasm and bronchoconstriction, inflammation and edema of the lining of the bronchioles, and the production of thick mucus that can plug the airway (Fig. 15-2).

There are three types of asthma:

- Extrinsic (also referred to as allergic asthma), resulting from response to an allergen such as pollen, dust, and animal dander (see Key Concepts 15-1).
- Intrinsic asthma (also called nonallergic asthma), caused by chronic or recurrent respiratory infections, emotional upset, and exercise
- Mixed asthma, caused by both intrinsic and extrinsic factors

Other disorders of the lower respiratory tract include emphysema (a lung disorder in which the terminal bronchioles or alveoli become enlarged and plugged with mucus) and chronic bronchitis (chronic inflammation and possibly infection of the bronchi). Chronic obstructive pulmonary disease (COPD) is the name given collectively to emphysema and chronic bronchitis because the airflow is limited most of the time. Asthma that is persistent and present most of the time may also be referred to as COPD.

Bronchodilators

A bronchodilator is a drug used to relieve bronchospasm associated with respiratory disorders such as bronchial asthma, chronic bronchitis, and emphysema. These conditions are progressive disorders characterized by a decrease in the inspiratory and expiratory capacity of the lung. Collectively, they are often referred to as COPD. A patient with COPD experiences dyspnea (difficulty breathing) with physical exertion, has difficulty inhaling and exhaling, and may have a chronic cough.

The two major types of bronchodilators are the **sympathomimetics** and the **xanthine derivatives.** The anticholinergic drug ipratropium bromide (Atrovent) is used for bronchospasm associated with COPD, chronic bronchitis, and emphysema. Ipratropium is included in the Summary Drug Table: Bronchodilators. Chapter 4 describes the anticholinergic drugs (cholinergic blocking drugs).

SYMPATHOMIMETICS

Examples of sympathomimetic bronchodilators include albuterol (Ventolin HFA), epinephrine (Adrenalin), salmeterol (Serevent), and terbutaline (Brethine). Many of the

FACTS ABOUT . . .

Asthma

- Asthma is a severe and chronic disease that affects approximately 300 million people worldwide and more than 16 million adults and nearly 7 million children in the United States alone.
- Asthma is one of the leading chronic childhood diseases, a major cause of childhood disability, and places a huge burden on affected children and their families, limiting the child's ability to learn, play, and even sleep. Children miss about 13 million school days each year because of asthma.
- African Americans are diagnosed with asthma at a 28% greater rate than the rate in whites. African American children are hospitalized for asthma at 250% of the rate, and die at 500% of the rate, of white children.

Source: National Institute of Allergy and Infectious Disease

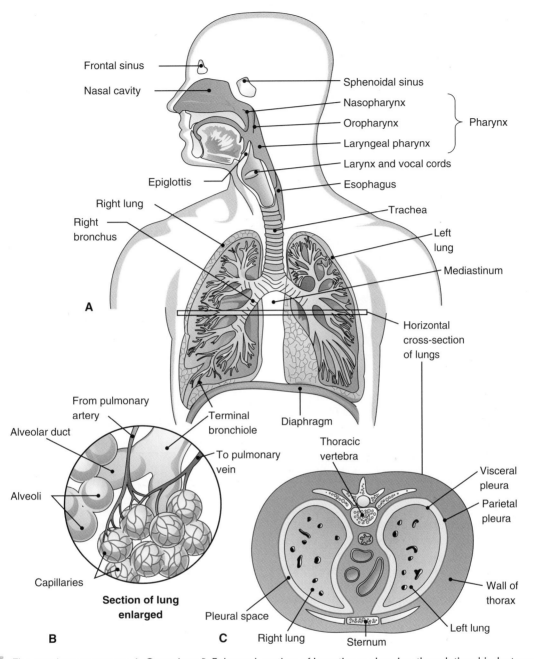

FIGURE 15-1 The respiratory system. A. Overview. B. Enlarged section of lung tissue showing the relationship between the alveoli (air sacs) of the lungs and the blood capillaries. C. A cross section of the chest cavity.

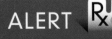 ALERT

Bronchospasm
Acute bronchospasm causes severe respiratory distress and a wheezing sound from the forceful expiration of air. It is considered a medical emergency. It is characterized by severe respiratory distress, dyspnea, forceful expiration, and wheezing. These symptoms should be reported to the health care provider immediately.

sympathomimetics used as bronchodilators are β-2 receptor agonists (e.g., albuterol, salmeterol, and terbutaline).

Actions of Sympathomimetics

When bronchospasm occurs, there is a decrease in the lumen (or inside diameter) of the bronchi, which decreases the amount of air taken into the lungs with each breath. This decreased amount of air taken into the lungs results in respiratory distress. Use of a bronchodilating drug opens the bronchi and allows more air

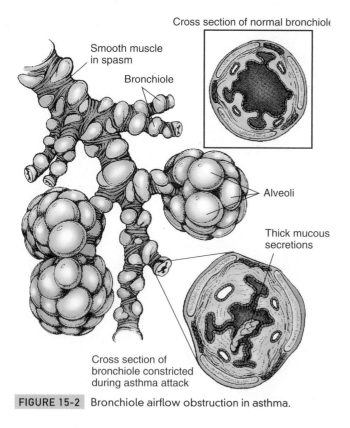

FIGURE 15-2 Bronchiole airflow obstruction in asthma.

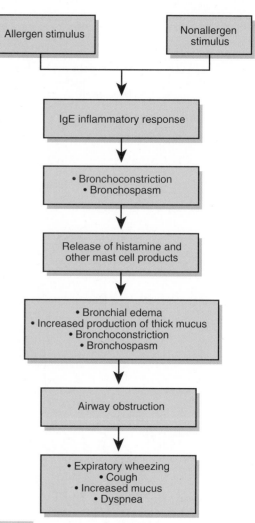

FIGURE 15-3 Asthmatic pathway from intrinsic and extrinsic stimuli.

to enter the lungs, which in turn completely or partially relieves respiratory distress.

Uses of Sympathomimetics

Sympathomimetics (drugs that mimic the sympathetic nervous system) are used primarily to treat reversible airway obstruction caused by bronchospasm associated with acute and chronic bronchial asthma, exercise-induced bronchospasm, bronchitis, emphysema, bronchiectasis (abnormal condition of the bronchial tree), or other obstructive pulmonary diseases.

KEY CONCEPTS

15-1   Extrinsic (Allergic) Asthma

Extrinsic or allergic asthma causes the immunoglobulin (IgE) inflammatory response. With exposure, the IgE antibodies are produced and attach to mast cells in the lungs. Reexposure to the antigen causes them to bind to the IgE antibody, releasing histamine and other mast cell products. The release of these products causes bronchospasm, mucous membrane swelling, and excessive mucus production. Gas exchange is impaired, causing carbon dioxide to be trapped in the alveoli so that oxygen is unable to enter. Figure 15-3 identifies the asthmatic pathway from both the intrinsic and extrinsic stimuli.

There are two types of sympathomimetics: short-acting and long-acting. The short-acting, such as albuterol, are used for an acute attack. The long-acting (i.e., salmeterol, formoterol, arformoterol) are used on a regular basis but are not appropriate for an acute attack.

Adverse Reactions of Sympathomimetics

A sympathomimetic bronchodilator may result in restlessness, anxiety, increased blood pressure, palpitations, cardiac arrhythmias, and insomnia. When these drugs are used by inhalation, excessive use (more often than recommended) may result in paradoxical bronchospasm.

Contraindications, Precautions, and Interactions of Sympathomimetics

- Sympathomimetic bronchodilators are contraindicated in patients with known hypersensitivity, cardiac

ALERT Rx!

Breathing Difficulties

Patients who have difficulty breathing and are receiving a sympathomimetic drug may experience extreme anxiety, nervousness, and restlessness, which may be caused by their breathing difficulty or the action of the sympathomimetic drug. In these patients, it may be difficult to determine if the patient is having an adverse drug reaction or if the problem is related to the respiratory disorder. Health care workers should speak and act in a calm manner, being careful not to increase the patient's anxiety or nervousness caused by the sympathomimetic drug. Explaining the effects of the drug may help the patient to tolerate these uncomfortable adverse reactions.

arrhythmias associated with tachycardia, organic brain damage, cerebral arteriosclerosis, or narrow-angle glaucoma.

- Salmeterol is contraindicated during acute bronchospasm.
- Sympathomimetics are used cautiously in patients with hypertension, cardiac dysfunction, hyperthyroidism, glaucoma, diabetes, prostatic hypertrophy, or a history of seizures.
- Sympathomimetic drugs are used cautiously during lactation.
- When the sympathomimetics are used concurrently with another sympathomimetic drug (see Chapter 11), additive adrenergic effects can occur.
- When used with a monoamine oxidase inhibitor (see Chapter 7), the patient is at increased risk for a hypertensive crisis.
- When a sympathomimetic is administered with a β-adrenergic blocker, the drugs may inhibit the cardiac, bronchodilating, and vasodilating effects of the sympathomimetic.
- When a β-blocker such as propranolol is administered with a sympathomimetic such as epinephrine,

an initial hypertensive episode may occur, followed by bradycardia.
- Concurrent use of a sympathomimetic with an oxytocic drug may result in severe hypotension.
- When a sympathomimetic is administered with theophylline, the patient has an increased risk for cardiotoxicity.
- When epinephrine is administered with insulin or an oral hypoglycemic drug, the patient may require an increased dose of the hypoglycemic drug.

XANTHINE DERIVATIVES

Xanthine derivatives, also called methylxanthines, are drugs that stimulate the central nervous system and result in bronchodilation. Examples are theophylline and aminophylline.

Actions of Xanthine Derivatives

Xanthine derivatives, although a different class of drugs, also have bronchodilating activity by means of their direct relaxation of the smooth muscles of the bronchi.

Uses of Xanthine Derivatives

Xanthine derivatives are used for symptomatic relief or prevention of bronchial asthma and reversible bronchospasm associated with chronic bronchitis and emphysema.

For acute respiratory symptoms, rapid theophyllinization using one of the xanthine derivatives may be required. **Theophyllinization** is accomplished by giving the patient a higher initial dose, called a loading dose, to bring blood levels to therapeutic range more quickly than waiting several days for the drug to exert a therapeutic effect. A patient taking theophylline must be frequently monitored for signs of toxicity. A daily plasma theophylline level is useful in monitoring for toxicity.

Adverse Reactions of Xanthine Derivatives

Adverse reactions of xanthine derivatives include nausea, vomiting, restlessness, nervousness, tachycardia, tremors, headache, palpitations, increased respirations, fever, hyperglycemia, and electrocardiographic changes.

Contraindications, Precautions, and Interactions of Xanthine Derivatives

- Xanthine derivatives are contraindicated in those with known hypersensitivity, peptic ulcers, seizure disorders (unless well controlled with appropriate anticonvulsant medication), serious uncontrolled arrhythmias, or hyperthyroidism.
- Xanthine derivatives are used cautiously in patients older than 60 years and in patients with cardiac disease,

LIFESPAN CONSIDERATIONS Older adults

Sympathomimetic Bronchodilators

Older adults taking sympathomimetic bronchodilators are at increased risk for adverse reactions related to the cardiovascular system (tachycardia, arrhythmias, palpitations, and hypertension) as well as adverse reactions related to the central nervous system (restlessness, agitation, insomnia).

hypoxemia, hypertension, congestive heart failure, or liver disease.
- Xanthines should be used cautiously during lactation.
- When a xanthine bronchodilator is administered with a sympathomimetic drug (see Chapter 11), additive central nervous system and cardiovascular effects may occur.
- If a patient eats large amounts of charcoal-broiled foods while taking a xanthine, then the therapeutic effect of the xanthine may be diminished. Certain foods contain xanthine (e.g., coffee, colas, or chocolate) and may increase the risk of cardiac and central nervous system adverse reactions.
- Cigarettes, nicotine gum and patches, barbiturates, phenytoin, loop diuretics, isoniazid, and rifampin may decrease the effectiveness of the xanthines.
- There is an increased risk of xanthine toxicity when the drugs are administered with influenza vaccination, oral contraceptives, glucocorticoids, β-adrenergic blockers, cimetidine, macrolides, thyroid hormones, or allopurinol.

Patient Management Issues with Bronchodilators

Xanthine derivatives should be taken routinely as prescribed. The short-acting bronchodilators are used either to prevent an asthma attack prior to exercise or to stop an acute bronchospasm. The long-acting bronchodilators should be used on a consistent basis as prescribed and are not to be used for an acute bronchospasm.

Patients taking theophylline may report heartburn because the drug relaxes the lower esophageal sphincter, allowing gastroesophageal reflux. Heartburn is minimized if the patient remains in an upright position and sleeps with the head of the bed elevated.

Educating the Patient and Family about Bronchodilators

Following are key points about bronchodilators that the patient and family members should know:

- Adverse reactions must be reported to the health care provider as soon as possible.

ALERT ℞

Theophylline Toxicity
Notify the health care provider immediately if any of the following signs of theophylline toxicity develop: anorexia, nausea, vomiting, diarrhea, confusion, abdominal cramping, headache, restlessness, insomnia, tachycardia, arrhythmias, or seizures. Toxicity is more likely to occur in patients requiring high doses or during prolonged therapy.

- Patients should be shown how to use inhalers and other devices needed to ensure proper delivery of the bronchodilator.
- Patients using an aerosol inhaler for administration of the bronchodilator should follow these general guidelines:
  - Drink six to eight glasses of water each day to decrease the thickness of secretions.
  - Do not use nonprescription drugs (some may contain sympathomimetic drugs) unless the health care provider approves them.
  - Stop smoking. Smoking may make it difficult to adjust the dosage and may worsen breathing problems.
  - Do not puncture metered dose inhalers or store them near heat or open flame; the contents of such inhalers are under pressure. Never throw the container into a fire or incinerator.
  - If patients notice an unusual smell or taste with use of the inhaler, they should stop using it and contact the health care provider.

For treatment with sympathomimetics, patients should follow these guidelines:
- Do not exceed the recommended dosage.
- These drugs may cause nervousness, insomnia, and restlessness (especially the sympathomimetics). Contact your health care provider if your symptoms become severe.
- Contact your health care provider if you experience palpitations, tachycardia, chest pain, muscle tremors, dizziness, headache, flushing, or difficulty with urination or breathing.
- Salmeterol is not meant to relieve acute asthmatic symptoms. Notify your health care provider immediately if salmeterol becomes less effective for relief of your symptoms, if you need more inhalations than usual, or if you need more than the maximum number of inhalations of short-acting bronchodilators.
- Formoterol fumarate (Foradil Aerolizer) is administered only by oral inhalation using the Aerolizer inhaler. When using the Aerolizer inhaler, do not exhale into the device. Always store formoterol capsules in the blister pack and remove them immediately before use. Always discard the capsule and Aerolizer inhaler by the expiration date included in the manufacturer's instructions. When treatment with formoterol begins, discontinue the regular use of the short-acting β2-agonist and use it only for relief of acute asthma symptoms. Do not substitute formoterol for inhaled oral corticosteroids and do not reduce your use of the corticosteroids.

For treatment with xanthine derivatives, patient should follow these guidelines:
- Avoid foods that contain xanthine, such as colas, coffee, and chocolate, as well as charcoal-grilled foods.
- If you experience gastrointestinal upset, then take the drug with food. Do not chew or crush coated or sustained-release tablets.
- Do not change from one brand to another without consulting your health care provider.

Antiasthma Drugs

CORTICOSTEROIDS

Along with the bronchodilators, several types of drugs are
effective in the treatment of asthma, including corticosteroids.

Actions of Corticosteroids

Corticosteroids, such as beclomethasone (QVAR), flunisolide
(AeroBid), and fluticasone (FloVent Diskus), are given by inhalation and act to decrease the inflammatory process in the airways
of patients with asthma. In addition, corticosteroids increase the
sensitivity of the β2-receptors. With increased sensitivity of the
β2-receptors, the β2-receptor agonist drugs are more effective.

Uses of Corticosteroids

The corticosteroids are used in the management and prophylactic
treatment of the inflammation associated with chronic asthma or
allergic rhinitis. This chapter will focus on those inhaled orally,
but many of them are also available in intranasal sprays.

Adverse Reactions of Corticosteroids

When used to manage chronic asthma, corticosteroids are
most often given by inhalation. Adverse reactions to corticosteroids are less likely to occur when the drugs are given by
inhalation rather than taken orally. Occasionally, patients may
experience throat irritation causing hoarseness, cough, or fungal infection of the mouth and throat. Vertigo or headache
also may occur. See Chapter 31 for adverse reactions after oral
administration of corticosteroids.

Contraindications, Precautions, and Interactions of Corticosteroids

- Corticosteroids are contraindicated in patients with
  hypersensitivity and patients with acute bronchospasm,
  status asthmaticus, or other acute episodes of asthma.
- Corticosteroids are used cautiously in patients with compromised immune systems, glaucoma, kidney or liver
  disease, convulsive disorders, or diabetes; in those taking
  systemic corticosteroids; and during lactation.
- Ketoconazole may increase plasma levels of budesonide
  and fluticasone.

LEUKOTRIENE RECEPTOR ANTAGONISTS AND LEUKOTRIENE FORMATION INHIBITORS

Leukotriene receptor antagonists include montelukast sodium
(Singulair) and zafirlukast (Accolate). Zileuton (Zyflo) is classified as a leukotriene formation inhibitor.

Actions of Leukotriene Receptor Antagonists and Leukotriene Formation Inhibitors

Leukotrienes are bronchoconstrictive substances released by
the body during inflammation. When leukotriene production
is inhibited, bronchodilation is facilitated. Zileuton acts by
decreasing the formation of leukotrienes. Although the result
is the same, montelukast and zafirlukast work in a slightly
different manner. Montelukast and zafirlukast are considered
leukotriene receptor antagonists because they inhibit leukotriene receptor sites in the respiratory tract, preventing airway
edema and facilitating bronchodilation.

Uses of Leukotriene Receptor Antagonists and Leukotriene Formation Inhibitors

Zleuton is used in the prophylaxis and treatment of chronic
asthma in adults and children older than 12 years. Zafirlukast
is used in the prophylaxis and treatment of chronic asthma
in adults and children older than 5 years. Montelukast is
used in the prophylaxis and treatment of chronic asthma in
adults and in children older than 2 years. Leukotriene receptor
antagonists and leukotriene formation inhibitors should never
be administered during an acute asthma attack. These agents
are used for the management of chronic asthma and are not
bronchodilators or fast acting.

Adverse Reactions of Leukotriene Receptor Antagonists and Leukotriene Formation Inhibitors

Adverse reactions of zafirlukast (Accolate) include headache, dizziness, myalgia, pain, nausea, diarrhea, abdominal pain, vomiting, and fever. Montelukast (Singulair) may cause headache, dizziness, dyspepsia, flu-like symptoms, cough, abdominal pain, and fatigue. Adverse reactions of zileuton (Zyflo) include dyspepsia, nausea, abdominal pain, and headache. Liver enzyme elevations may occur with the administration of zileuton; these elevations may continue to rise, remain unchanged, or resolve with continued therapy. Alanine aminotransferase (ALT) is an enzyme produced by the liver that acts as a catalyst in the transamination reaction necessary for amino acid production. Alanine aminotransferase is found in liver cells in high concentrations. When liver damage occurs, ALT levels increase, which makes ALT testing a valuable test for monitoring liver function.

Contraindications, Precautions, and Interactions of Leukotriene Receptor Antagonists and Leukotriene Formation Inhibitors

- These drugs are contraindicated in patients with a known hypersensitivity.
- Montelukast, zafirlukast, and zileuton are not used in the reversal of bronchospasm in acute asthma attacks.
- Zileuton is contraindicated in patients with active liver disease.
- The drugs are used cautiously in patients with hepatic dysfunction and during lactation.
- Administration of zafirlukast and aspirin increases plasma levels of zafirlukast.
- When zafirlukast is administered with warfarin, there is an increased effect of the anticoagulant.
- Administration of zafirlukast and theophylline or erythromycin may result in a decreased level of zafirlukast.
- Administration of montelukast with aspirin or nonsteroidal antiinflammatory drugs (NSAIDs) is avoided in patients with known aspirin sensitivity.

ALERT Rx

Zileuton

The patient is carefully monitored for hepatic transaminase levels at the beginning of treatment and during therapy with zileuton. Alanine aminotransferase levels are measured before treatment begins, once per month for the first 3 months, then every 2 to 3 months for the remainder of the 1st year. After the 1st year, ALT levels are measured periodically. If symptoms of liver impairment (such as right upper quadrant pain, nausea, fatigue, lethargy, pruritus, jaundice, or flu-like symptoms) occur or if the ALT elevation is greater than five times the upper limits of normal, then the drug is discontinued. Transaminase levels are monitored until they return to normal.

- Administration of zileuton with propranolol increases the activity of the propranolol, with theophylline increases serum theophylline levels, and with warfarin may increase prothrombin time. A prothrombin blood test should be performed regularly in the event that dosages of warfarin need to be decreased.

FACT CHECK

15-4 How do the actions of the leukotriene receptor antagonist differ from those of the leukotriene formation inhibitor?

MAST CELL STABILIZER

The only mast cell stabilizer available is cromolyn sodium.

Actions of Mast Cell Stabilizer

Cromolyn sodium inhibits the release of substances that cause bronchoconstriction and inflammation from the mast cells in the respiratory tract.

Uses of Mast Cell Stabilizer

Cromolyn sodium is used in combination with other drugs in the treatment of asthma and other allergic disorders, including allergic rhinitis (using a nasal solution), and in the prevention of exercise-induced bronchospasm. When a mast cell stabilizer is used along with another antiasthma drug, a reduction in dosage of the drugs may be possible after using the mast cell stabilizer for 3 to 4 weeks. Cromolyn sodium may be given by nebulization or as a nasal spray.

When added to an existing treatment regimen, other medications such as corticosteroids are decreased gradually when the patient experiences a therapeutic response to cromolyn in 2 to 4 weeks and the asthma is under good control. The corticosteroid or other antiasthma drug may be reinstituted based on the patient's symptoms. If use of a mast cell stabilizer must be discontinued for any reason, then the dosage is gradually tapered.

Adverse Reactions of Mast Cell Stabilizer

The more common adverse reactions associated with cromolyn sodium include headache, dizziness, nausea, fatigue, hypotension, and an unpleasant taste in the mouth. This drug may cause nasal or throat irritation when given intranasally or by inhalation.

Contraindications, Precautions, and Interactions of Mast Cell Stabilizer

- Cromolyn sodium is contraindicated in patients with a known hypersensitivity and in patients during attacks of acute asthma because it may worsen bronchospasm during the acute asthma attack.
- This drug is used cautiously in patients with impaired renal or hepatic function and during lactation. No significant drug interactions have been reported.

FACT CHECK

15-5 How long may it take for a patient to experience a therapeutic response to cromolyn?

Patient Management Issues with Antiasthma Drugs

Patients who are using corticosteroids should use them on a regular basis. If they are also using a bronchodilator, they should use the bronchodilator first. The bronchodilator will open the airways to allow better action by the corticosteroid. The patient should understand that the corticosteroid is not for relief of an acute bronchospasm.

Patients should take leukotriene receptor agonists and leukotriene formation inhibitors on a routine basis. These drugs should not be used for acute bronchospasm.

Patients who are taking a mast cell stabilizer should use the drug on a regular basis. The full beneficial effects may not be seen immediately and may take up to 2 weeks.

Some antiasthma drugs may cause an unpleasant taste in the mouth. Having the patient take frequent sips of water, suck on sugarless candy, or chew gum helps to alleviate the problem. If dizziness occurs, then the patient may need help walking. For nausea, frequent small meals are recommended rather than three larger meals.

The inhalers may cause throat irritation and infection with *Candida albicans*. The patient is instructed to use strict oral hygiene, cleanse the inhaler as directed in the package directions, and use the proper technique when taking an inhalation. These measures decrease the incidence of candidiasis and help soothe the throat. Occasionally an antifungal drug may be prescribed to manage the candidiasis.

Educating the Patient and Family about Antiasthma Drugs

For treatment with corticosteroid inhalants, patients should follow these guidelines:

- Rinse your mouth with water without swallowing after inhaling the prescribed doses to reduce the risk of oral candidiasis.
- Carry a warning card indicating the need for supplemental systemic steroids in the event of stress or severe asthmatic attack that is unresponsive to bronchodilators.

- Do not stop the drug therapy abruptly.
- These drugs are not bronchodilators and do not contain medication to provide rapid relief of breathing difficulties during an asthma attack.
- If taking bronchodilators by inhalation, then use the bronchodilator several minutes before the corticosteroid to enhance application of the steroid into the bronchial tract.

For treatment with leukotriene receptor agonists and leukotriene formation inhibitors, patients should follow these guidelines:

- Zafirlukast: Take this drug regularly as prescribed, even during symptom-free times. Do not use it to treat acute episodes of asthma.
- Montelukast: Take once daily in the evening, even when free of symptoms. Contact your health care provider if your asthma is not well controlled. This drug is not for the treatment of an acute attack. Avoid taking aspirin and/or NSAIDs while taking montelukast.
- Zileuton: Contact your health care provider if you need a bronchodilator more often than usual or more than the maximum number of inhalations in a 24-hour period. This drug can interact with other drugs; consult your health care provider before starting or stopping any prescription or nonprescription drug. Have liver enzyme tests performed on a regular basis. Immediately report any symptoms of liver dysfunction, such as upper right quadrant pain, nausea, fatigue, lethargy, pruritus, and jaundice.

For treatment with a mast cell stabilizer, patients should follow these guidelines:

- Inform your health care provider if your asthma symptoms do not improve within 4 weeks after starting treatment. Your health care provider may discontinue the drug therapy.
- To prevent exercise-induced asthma, this drug should be taken approximately 15 minutes before activity but no earlier than 1 hour before the expected activity. The oral form should be taken at least 30 minutes before meals and at bedtime. Do not mix the drug with any other food or beverage.

FACT CHECK

15-6 If a patient is using both a bronchodilator and a corticosteroid inhaler, which is used first?

Chapter Review

KEY POINTS

- Asthma is a respiratory condition characterized by recurrent attacks of dyspnea (difficulty breathing) and wheezing caused by spasmodic constriction of the bronchi.
- Asthma is a reversible obstructive disease of the lower airway. Airway obstruction is caused by bronchospasm and bronchoconstriction, inflammation and edema of

the lining of the bronchioles, and the production of thick mucus that can plug the airway.
- Antiasthma drugs are used in various combinations to treat and manage asthma. Using several drugs may be more beneficial than using a single drug.
- A bronchodilator is a drug used to relieve bronchospasm associated with respiratory disorders such as bronchial asthma, chronic bronchitis, and emphysema.

- Patients who have difficulty breathing and are receiving a sympathomimetic drug may experience extreme anxiety, nervousness, and restlessness, which may be caused by their breathing difficulty or the action of the sympathomimetic drug.
- Xanthine derivatives relax the smooth muscles of the bronchia and are used for symptomatic relief or prevention of bronchial asthma and reversible bronchospasm associated with chronic bronchitis and emphysema.
- Adverse reactions of xanthine derivatives include nausea, vomiting, restlessness, nervousness, tachycardia, tremors, headache, palpitations, increased respirations, fever, hyperglycemia, and electrocardiographic changes.
- Corticosteroids are given by inhalation and act to decrease the inflammatory process in the airways of patients with asthma.
- Adverse reactions of corticosteroids are less likely to occur when the drugs are given by inhalation rather than taken orally. Occasionally, patients may experience throat irritation causing hoarseness, cough, or fungal infection of the mouth and throat. Vertigo or headache also may occur.
- Leukotrienes are bronchoconstrictive substances released by the body during the inflammatory process; when leukotriene production is inhibited, bronchodilation is facilitated.
- Adverse reactions of leukotriene receptor antagonists and leukotriene formation inhibitors are specific to each drug. Zafirlukast (Accolate) may cause headache, dizziness, myalgia, pain, nausea, diarrhea, abdominal pain, vomiting, and fever. Montelukast (Singulair) may cause headache, dizziness, dyspepsia, flu-like symptoms, cough, abdominal pain, and fatigue. Zileuton (Zyflo) may cause dyspepsia, nausea, abdominal pain, headache, and liver enzyme elevations.
- The mast cell stabilizer cromolyn sodium inhibits the release of substances that cause bronchoconstriction and inflammation from the mast cells in the respiratory tract.
- The more common adverse reactions associated with cromolyn include headache, dizziness, nausea, fatigue, hypotension, and an unpleasant taste in the mouth. These drugs may cause nasal or throat irritation when given intranasally or by inhalation.

CRITICAL THINKING CASE STUDY
Asthma Drugs

Ms. Sinclair, who lives alone, says that the montelukast (Singulair) her physician prescribed is not having the desired effect. She broke her reading glasses and admits she does not remember how often she is supposed to take it.

1. How often and at what time of day should Ms. Sinclair take montelukast (Singulair)?
   a. Once daily in the evening
   b. Twice daily in the morning and evening
   c. Every 8 hours
   d. Once daily in the morning

2. Ms. Sinclair's 1-year-old granddaughter also has chronic asthma. Ms. Sinclair mentions that the child had an attack while visiting, and Ms. Sinclair wondered whether giving her montelukast (Sinclair) might have helped. The correct response would be
   a. it is not appropriate to give medication to anyone other than the person for whom it was prescribed
   b. the drug is not used in the reversal of bronchospasm in acute asthma attacks
   c. montelukast (Sinclair) is intended to prevent airway edema
   d. all of the above

3. If Ms. Sinclair's asthma is not being controlled with the montelukast, what should you recommend?

Review Questions

MULTIPLE CHOICE

1. When the sympathomimetics are administered to older adults, there is an increased risk of
   a. gastrointestinal effects
   b. nephrotoxic effects
   c. neurotoxic effects
   d. cardiovascular effects

2. Zafirlukast (Accolate) has what primary treatment function?
   a. Anti-inflammatory
   b. Symptomatic relief
   c. Prophylactic
   d. Mast cell stabilizer

3. Which food(s) should be avoided when taking a xanthine derivative?
   a. Shellfish
   b. Products containing nuts
   c. Cola and coffee
   d. Dairy products

4. Which of the following is NOT a common adverse reaction of cromolyn sodium?
   a. Dizziness
   b. Headache
   c. Nausea
   d. Constipation

MATCHING

_____ 5.	albuterol	a.	Atrovent
_____ 6.	ievalbuterol	b.	Proventil HFA
_____ 7.	ipratropium	c.	AeroBid
_____ 8.	flunisolide	d.	Xopenex

TRUE OR FALSE

_____ 9. Extrinsic or allergic asthma causes the immunoglobulin (IgE) inflammatory response.

_____ 10. Older adults who are taking sympathomimetic bronchodilators are at increased risk for adverse reactions related to the cardiovascular and central nervous systems.

_____ 11. Corticosteroids are effective in the acute treatment of bronchospasms.

_____ 12. A patient who is taking both a bronchodilator and a corticosteroid should use the bronchodilator first and the corticosteroid second.

FILL IN THE BLANKS

13. Asthma is a respiratory condition characterized by recurrent attacks of _____ and _____ caused by spasmodic constriction of the bronchi.

14. _____ are bronchoconstrictive substances released by the body during inflammation.

15. _____ is an anticholinergic that is used for the treatment of bronchospasm associated with chronic obstructive pulmonary disease, chronic bronchitis and emphysema, and rhinorrhea.

16. Xanthine derivates have bronchodilating activity by means of their direct relaxation of the _____ _____ of the bronchi.

SHORT ANSWERS

17. Describe the three types of asthma.

18. A patient who is using an orally inhaled corticosteroid complains that it leaves an unpleasant taste in the mouth. What could you suggest?

19. A patient who is taking Zileuton asks about the symptoms of liver impairment. What should you tell the patient to watch for?

20. One of your patients is having an asthma attack and is experiencing a lot of trouble breathing. The patient is using a sympathomimetic inhaler for symptom relief but appears to be having an adverse reaction to the inhaler. What can you do to help the patient?

Web Activities

1. Go to the National Library of Medicine home page (http://www.nlm.nih.gov). Go to "MedlinePlus." Under "Health Topics," select asthma. Under "Related Issues," find the page from the National Institute of Environmental Health Sciences that discusses "Asthma and Its Environmental Triggers." What are common environmental triggers? Write a brief description about The Inner-City Asthma Study.

2. Go to the NIH home page (http://www.nih.gov). Go to "MedlinePlus" and perform a general search for "ipratropium oral inhalation." Read the provided information and write a brief description of how the medication should be used and what special precautions that the patient should know.

SUMMARY DRUG TABLE Bronchodilators
(left, generic; right, trade)

Comprehensive Summary Drug Tables, including uses, adverses effects, dosages, and pregnancy classifications, are provided on the companion website, http://thePoint.lww.com/PharmacologyHP2e

Sympathomimetics	
albuterol sulfate *al-byoo'-ter-ole*	Proventil HFA, Ventolin HFA, ProAir HFA, VoSpire ER, AccuNeb, *generic*
arformoterol *ar-for-moe'-ter-ol*	Brovana
ephedrine sulfate *e-fed'-rin*	*generic*
epinephrine *ep-i-nef'-rin*	Adrenalin (Rx), *generic* (Rx)
formoterol fumarate *for-moh'-te-rol*	Foradil Aerolizer
isoproterenol HCl *eye-soe-proe- ter'-a-nole*	Isuprel
levalbuterol HCl *lev-al-byoo'-ter-ole*	Xopenex
metaproterenol sulfate *met-a-proe- ter'-e-nole*	*generic*
pirbuterol acetate *peer-byoo'-ter-ole*	Maxair Autohaler
salmeterol *sal-mee'-ter-ol*	Serevent
terbutaline sulfate *ter-byoo'-ta-leen*	Brethine, *generic*
Xanthine Derivatives	
aminophylline *am-in-off'-i-lin*	*generic*
dyphylline *dye'-fi-lin*	Lufyllin
theophylline *thee-off'-i-lin*	Theo-24, Theochron, Uniphyl, *generic*
Anticholinergic	
ipratropium bromide *ih-prah-trow'-pea- um*	Atrovent, Atrovent HFA, *generic*

SUMMARY DRUG TABLE Antiasthma Drugs
(left, generic; right, trade)

Comprehensive Summary Drug Tables, including uses, adverses effects, dosages, and pregnancy classifications, are provided on the companion website, http://thePoint.lww.com/PharmacologyHP2e

Corticosteroids	
beclomethasone dipropionate *be-kloe-meth'-a-sone*	Beconase AQ, QVAR
budesonide *bue-des'-oh-nide*	Pulmicort Flexhaler, Rhinicort Aqua, *generic*
ciclesonide *sye-kles'-oh-nide*	Alvesco
flunisolide *floo-niss'-oh-lide*	AeroBid, AeroBid-M, Nasarel, *generic*
fluticasone propionate *flew-tick'-ah-sone pro'-pee-oh-nate*	FloVent Diskus, FloVent HFA, Flonase, Veramyst
mometasone *moe-met'-a-sone*	Asmanex
Leukotriene Receptor Antagonists	
montelukast sodium *mon-tell-oo'-kast*	Singulair
zafirlukast *zah-fir'-luh-kast*	Accolate
Leukotriene Formation Inhibitors	
zileuton *zye-loot'-on*	Zyflo, Zyflo CR
Mast Cell Stabilizers	
cromolyn *kroe'-moe-lin*	Nasalcrom (OTC), *generic*

16

Antihistamines and Decongestants

CHAPTER OBJECTIVES

On completion of this chapter, students will be able to:

1 Define the chapter's key terms.

2 Describe disorders and symptoms that are treated with antihistamines.

3 Identify the difference between first- and second-generation antihistamines.

4 Describe the general adverse reactions, contraindications, precautions, and interactions of antihistamines.

5 Describe disorders and symptoms that are treated with decongestants.

6 Describe the general adverse reactions, contraindications, precautions, and interactions of decongestants.

7 Discuss important points a patient or family member should know about using an antihistamine or decongestant.

KEY TERMS

antihistamine—a drug used to counteract the effects of histamine on body organs and structures

decongestant—a drug that reduces the swelling of nasal passages and relieves congestion

epigastric distress—discomfort in the abdomen

expectoration—the elimination of thick, tenacious mucus from the respiratory tract by spitting it up

histamine—a substance in various body tissues, such as the heart, lungs, gastric mucosa, and skin, that is produced in response to injury

photosensitivity—exaggerated response to brief exposure to the sun, resulting in moderate to severe sunburn

rebound—causing the opposite of the desired effect

rhinitis—nasal congestion, often referred to as a stuffy nose

rhinitis medicamentosa—rebound nasal congestion caused by extended use of topical nasal decongestants

vasoconstriction—a narrowing of the blood vessel

CHAPTER OVERVIEW

Drug classes covered in this chapter are:

- Antihistamines
- Decongestants

Drugs by classification are listed on page 173.

thePOINT RESOURCES

- Comprehensive Summary Drug Tables
- Lippincott's Interactive Tutorials: Drugs Affecting the Respiratory System
- Interactive Practice and Review
- Monographs of Most Commonly Prescribed Drugs

Histamine is a substance present in various tissues of the body, such as the heart, lungs, gastric mucosa, and skin (Fig. 16-1). The highest concentration of histamine is found in basophils (a type of white blood cell) and mast cells that are found near capillaries. Histamine is released in response to injury. It acts on areas such as the vascular system and smooth muscle, producing dilation of arterioles and an increased permeability of capillaries and venules. Dilation of the arterioles results in localized redness. An increase in the permeability of small blood vessels allows fluid to escape from these blood vessels into the surrounding tissues, which produces localized swelling. Thus, the release of histamine produces an inflammatory response. Histamine is also released in allergic reactions or hypersensitivity reactions, such as anaphylactic shock.

Antihistamines

Antihistamines are drugs used to counteract the effects of histamine on body organs and structures.

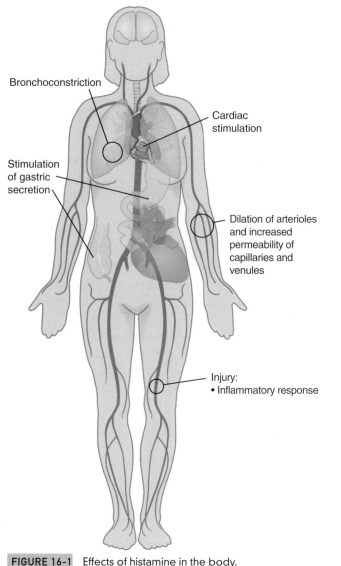

FIGURE 16-1   Effects of histamine in the body.

Actions of Antihistamines

Antihistamines block most, but not all, of the effects of histamine. They do this by competing for histamine at histamine receptor sites, thereby preventing histamine from entering these receptor sites and producing its effect on body tissues. Some antihistamines have additional effects, such as antipruritic (prevents itching), antiemetic (prevents vomiting), and sedative effects.

Uses of Antihistamines

Antihistamines are used whenever there is a histamine response in the body. The most common uses include relief of the symptoms of seasonal and perennial allergies, allergic and vasomotor **rhinitis** (Fig. 16-2), and allergic conjunctivitis. The classic seasonal and perennial allergy symptoms that antihistamines will treat include itchy, watery eyes; sneezing; and a runny nose. They are also used to relieve the symptoms of other types of allergic reactions, such as an insect bite or bee sting. They are used for mild and uncomplicated angioneurotic edema and urticaria and relief of allergic reactions to drugs, blood, or plasma. Some of the antihistamines are indicated for the relief of coughs caused by colds or allergy. In addition, the uses include adjunctive therapy in anaphylactic shock, treatment of parkinsonism, relief of nausea and vomiting, relief of motion sickness, sedation, and as adjuncts to analgesics. Each antihistamine may be used for one or more of these reasons and will be covered in those respective chapters where appropriate.

Two generations of antihistamines are currently available. First-generation antihistamines, the first group of antihistamines on the market, readily cross the blood–brain barrier and have more adverse reactions. Examples of first-generation antihistamines include diphenhydramine (Benadryl) and chlorpheniramine (Chlor-Trimeton). The second-generation antihistamines are newer; they do not readily cross the blood–brain barrier and have fewer adverse reactions (see Key Concepts 16-1). Examples of second-generation antihistamines include loratadine (Claritin), fexofenadine (Allegra), and desloratadine (Clarinex). While there are advantages to the second-generation antihistamines when it comes to adverse reactions, the first-generation antihistamines are usually more potent antihistamines. Additional antihistamines are listed in the Summary Drug Table: Antihistamines.

Rhinitis

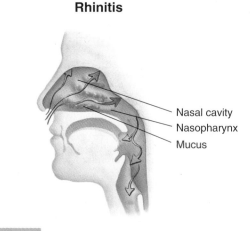

FIGURE 16-2   Rhinitis.

KEY CONCEPTS

16-1 First- and Second-Generation Antihistamines

Not all antihistamines are created equal. The first-generation antihistamines all cause drowsiness, but some are highly sedating and others are less sedating. The second-generation antihistamines have low-sedating and nonsedating options. This makes a difference for a patient when choosing among antihistamines.

First generation
Less sedating: brompheniramine, chlorpheniramine
Highly sedating: clemastine, diphenhydramine, doxylamine
Second generation
Low-sedating: cetirizine
Nonsedating: loratadine, fexofenadine, desloratadine

FACT CHECK

16-1 How does an antihistamine work?
16-2 What is the difference between the first- and second-generation antihistamines?

Adverse Reactions of Antihistamines

Drowsiness and sedation are common adverse reactions of the first-generation antihistamines. Some antihistamines appear to cause more drowsiness and sedation than others. These drugs may also have varying degrees of anticholinergic (cholinergic blocking) effects, which may result in dryness of the mouth, nose, and throat and a thickening of bronchial secretions. The first-generation antihistamines are often referred to as sedating antihistamines. On the other hand, the second-generation antihistamines are referred to as nonsedating antihistamines and cause little, if any, drowsiness and fewer anticholinergic effects than the first-generation antihistamines. Some antihistamines may cause dizziness, disturbed coordination, fatigue, hypotension, headache, **epigastric distress,** and **photosensitivity** (exaggerated response to brief exposure to the sun, resulting in moderate to severe sunburn). Although these drugs are sometimes used to treat allergies, a drug allergy can occur with the use of an antihistamine. Symptoms that may indicate an allergy to these drugs include skin rash, urticaria, and anaphylactic shock.

Contraindications, Precautions, and Interactions of Antihistamines

- Antihistamines are contraindicated in patients with a known hypersensitivity.
- The antihistamines, specifically first generation, are also contraindicated in lactating women; these drugs pass readily into breast milk and may adversely affect newborns.

ALERT R℞

Antihistamines and Lower Respiratory Tract Diseases
Antihistamines should not be taken by patients with lower respiratory tract diseases, including asthma. The drying effect of the antihistamine may cause thickening of respiratory secretions and make expectoration more difficult.

- Antihistamines are used cautiously in patients with bronchial asthma, cardiovascular disease, narrow-angle glaucoma, symptomatic prostatic hypertrophy, hypertension, impaired kidney function, peptic ulcer, urinary retention, pyloroduodenal obstruction, or hyperthyroidism.
- Anticholinergic effects are likely to increase when antihistamines are administered with a monoamine oxidase inhibitor (MAOI), and additive sedative effects occur if they are administered with central nervous system depressants (e.g., narcotic analgesics or alcohol).
- When cimetidine and loratadine are administered together, the patient has a risk of increased loratadine levels.

Patient Management Issues with Antihistamines

Most antihistamines are given orally with food to prevent gastrointestinal upset. The patient's risk of injury is greater when adverse drug reactions such as drowsiness, dizziness, or disturbed coordination are experienced.

Educating the Patient and Family about Antihistamines

Following are key points about antihistamines that the patient or family members should know:
- Do not drive or perform other hazardous tasks if you feel drowsy. This effect may diminish with continued use.
- Do not drink alcohol or use other drugs that cause sleepiness or drowsiness while taking an antihistamine.
- These drugs may cause dryness of the mouth and throat. Frequent sips of water, hard candy, or chewing gum (preferably sugarless) may relieve this problem.
- If you experience gastric upset, then take this drug with food or meals. Loratadine should be taken on an empty

CONSIDERATIONS Older adults

LIFESPAN

Antihistamines
Older adults are more likely to experience anticholinergic effects (e.g., dryness of the mouth, nose, and throat), dizziness, sedation, hypotension, and confusion from antihistamines. First-generation antihistamines should be used with extreme caution. Second-generation antihistamines would be more appropriate, if effective for the patient's symptoms.

stomach, if possible. If your gastric upset is not relieved, then discuss this with your health care provider.

- Avoid ultraviolet light or sunlight because of the possibility of photosensitivity. Wear sunglasses, protective clothing, and a sunscreen when exposed to sunlight.
- Do not crush or chew sustained-release preparations.

FACT CHECK

16-3   What are the most common adverse reactions for first-generation antihistamines?

16-4   Why should first-generation antihistamines be used with caution in the elderly?

Decongestants

A **decongestant** is a drug that reduces swelling of the nasal passages, which in turn opens clogged nasal passages and enhances drainage of the sinuses. These drugs are used for the temporary relief of nasal congestion caused by the common cold, hay fever, sinusitis, and other respiratory allergies.

Actions of Decongestants

Nasal decongestants are sympathomimetic drugs, which produce localized **vasoconstriction** of the small blood vessels of the nasal membranes. Vasoconstriction reduces swelling in nasal passages (decongestive activity). Nasal decongestants may be applied topically by drops or spray, and some are available in oral form. Decongestants are used in other preparations where vasoconstriction is desired, such as ophthalmic drops (for redness) and hemorrhoidal products.

Uses of Decongestants

Decongestants are used to treat the congestion associated with rhinitis, hay fever, allergic rhinitis, sinusitis, and the common cold. In addition, they are an adjunctive therapy for middle ear infections to decrease congestion around the eustachian tube. Nasal inhalers may relieve ear block and pressure pain during air travel. Many have oral as well as topical forms, but topical application is more effective than the oral route.

Examples of oral nasal decongestants include phenylephrine (Sudafed PE) and pseudoephedrine (Sudafed). Examples of topical nasal decongestants include phenylephrine (Neo-Synephrine) and oxymetazoline (Afrin), which are available as nasal sprays or drops. Additional nasal decongestants are listed in the Summary Drug Table: Systemic and Topical Nasal Decongestants.

FACT CHECK

16-5   What nasal symptom does a decongestant relieve?

16-6   How is a decongestant administered for nasal decongestion?

Adverse Reactions of Decongestants

When used topically in prescribed doses, decongestants usually have minimal systemic effects in most individuals. Nasal burning, stinging, and dryness may sometimes occur. Because they are absorbed systemically, oral decongestants have significantly more adverse reactions than topical decongestants. Oral decongestants may cause tachycardia and other cardiac arrhythmias, nervousness, restlessness, insomnia, blurred vision, nausea, and vomiting. When the topical form is used frequently, or if the liquid is swallowed, the same adverse reactions of oral decongestants may occur. In addition, the topical form should be used for no longer than 3 to 5 days to prevent **rhinitis medicamentosa** (rebound congestion).

Contraindications, Precautions, and Interactions of Decongestants

- Decongestants are contraindicated in patients with known hypersensitivity, hypertension, or severe coronary artery disease and in patients taking MAOIs.
- Naphazoline is contraindicated in patients with glaucoma.
- Decongestants are used cautiously in patients with hyperthyroidism, diabetes mellitus, prostatic hypertrophy, ischemic heart disease, and glaucoma.
- Safe use of decongestants during lactation has not been established.
- Additive sympathomimetic effects may develop when decongestants are administered with other sympathomimetic drugs (see Chapter 11).
- Use of a nasal decongestant along with a MAOI may cause hypertensive crisis.
- Use of a decongestant with a β-adrenergic blocking drug may cause hypertension or bradycardia.
- When ephedrine is administered with theophylline, the patient is at increased risk for theophylline toxicity.

Patient Management Issues with Decongestants

Overuse of the topical form of these drugs can cause **rebound** nasal congestion. This means that the congestion becomes worse with continued use of the drug. Although congestion may be relieved for a brief time after the drug is used, it recurs within a short time, which prompts the patient to use the drug at more frequent intervals, perpetuating the rebound congestion. To minimize the occurrence of rebound nasal congestion, drug therapy should be discontinued gradually by initially discontinuing the medication first in one nostril, then in the other.

After using a topical nasal decongestant, some patients may experience a mild, transient stinging sensation. This usually disappears with continued use.

Educating the Patient and Family about Decongestants

Following are key points about decongestants that the patient or family members should know:

- The patient or family member needs to be shown the correct method of using topical nasal decongestants.

- Over-the-counter nasal decongestants, topical or oral, should not be used by patients with high blood pressure.
- Overuse of topical nasal decongestants can actually increase nasal congestion (rebound congestion). To prevent rebound congestion, topical nasal decongestants should be used for no more than 3 to 5 days.
- Some outpatients may not use decongestants as prescribed. Family members may need to monitor the patient's use and report any adverse reactions that occur.
- Remember that overuse of topical nasal decongestants can make the symptoms worse.
- Nasal burning and stinging may occur with the topical decongestants. This effect usually disappears with use. If burning or stinging becomes severe, then stop using the drug and discuss this problem with your health care provider who may prescribe or recommend another drug.
- When using a spray, do not allow the tip of the container to touch the nasal mucosa. Do not share the container with anyone, and wipe it after each use.
- If your symptoms do not improve in 7 days or if you have a high fever, then consult your health care provider before continuing use.

FACT CHECK

16-7 What happens if a patient overuses a topical nasal decongestant?
16-8 What are the most common adverse reactions of oral decongestants?

Combination Antihistamine/ Decongestant Products

Many combination products are available that contain both an antihistamine and a decongestant. Such products are useful if the patient is experiencing symptoms that would be best treated by both an antihistamine and a decongestant. For example, if the patient has nasal congestion as well as symptoms of allergies, then a combination product might be used. Another option would be for the patient to take a single-ingredient antihistamine along with a single-ingredient decongestant.

Combination products allow for convenient dosing because they are of one dosage form instead of two and they often come in sustained-release formulations. However, since the ingredients are in a set strength, there is an increased risk of adverse reactions. If taken as a single ingredient product, a decongestant would not be taken near bedtime because it has a tendency to cause insomnia. In addition, a sedating antihistamine might be welcome at night to help with sleep, but it is not ideal during the day at school or work.

It is very important to read the labels on over-the-counter products to ensure that there is not a duplication of therapy. Many combination products are on the market, and most of them have the same types of ingredients. It is very easy for patients to take two ingredients from the same category of drugs without realizing it.

Chapter Review

KEY POINTS

- Antihistamines are used to counteract the effects of histamine on body organs and structures, a substance present in various tissues of the body produced in response to injury.
- Antihistamines may cause dizziness, disturbed coordination, fatigue, hypotension, headache, epigastric distress, and photosensitivity. Drowsiness and sedation are also common adverse reactions of many of the antihistamines. Symptoms that may indicate an allergy to these drugs include skin rash, urticaria, and anaphylactic shock.
- A decongestant reduces swelling of the nasal passages, which in turn opens clogged nasal passages and enhances drainage of the sinuses.

- Oral decongestants may cause tachycardia and other cardiac arrhythmias, nervousness, restlessness, insomnia, blurred vision, nausea, and vomiting. Decongestants are contraindicated in patients with known hypersensitivity, hypertension, and severe coronary artery disease. These drugs are also contraindicated in patients taking MAOIs. Naphazoline is contraindicated in patients with glaucoma.
- Antihistamine/decongestant combination products have advantages over using either product alone. Combination products are typically available in sustained-release forms that allow for convenient dosing. Patients can, however, take single ingredient products to achieve the same result and have more flexible dosing.

CRITICAL THINKING CASE STUDY
The Common Cold

Mrs. Martin, 76, is visiting her massage therapist for her weekly massage. She complains that her nose is runny and stuffy, and laying with her face down is uncomfortable. She blows her nose and continues with her massage. At the end, Mrs. Martin asks for some advice on how best to treat her nasal stuffiness.

1. What symptoms will a decongestant treat?
   a. Nasal stuffiness
   b. Runny nose
   c. Sneezing
   d. All of the above
2. What symptoms will an antihistamine treat?
   a. Runny nose
   b. Sneezing
   c. Itchy watery eyes
   d. All of the above
3. If Mrs. Martin is experiencing a runny nose that is also stuffy along with sneezing and itchy, watery eyes, which of the following would you suggest she try?
   a. Oral decongestant
   b. Nasal decongestant
   c. Antihistamine
   d. Combination antihistamine–decongestant
4. What rationale did you use to make your recommendation?
5. Does Mrs. Martin's age present any contraindications or warnings?

Review Questions

MULTIPLE CHOICE

1. Which of the following is a common adverse reaction of antihistamines?
   a. Sedation
   b. Blurred vision
   c. Headache
   d. Hypertension
2. When antihistamines are given to patients receiving central nervous system depressants, a potential adverse effect may be
   a. an increase in anticholinergic effects
   b. excessive sedation
   c. seizure activity
   d. loss of hearing
3. Decongestants should not be used in patients with
   a. hyperthyroidism
   b. diabetes mellitus
   c. glaucoma
   d. all of the above
4. An oral decongestant will NOT cause which of the following adverse reactions?
   a. Insomnia
   b. Restlessness
   c. Drowsiness
   d. Nervousness

MATCHING

_____ 5. pseudoephedrine   a. Neo-Synephrine
_____ 6. cetirizine   b. Benadryl
_____ 7. phenylephrine   c. Sudafed
_____ 8. diphenhydramine   d. Zyrtec

TRUE OR FALSE

_____ 9. Oral nasal decongestants cause rebound congestion if taken for more than 3 days.
_____ 10. An antihistamine would help with the histamine response caused by a bee sting.
_____ 11. A patient should be advised to not drive or drink alcohol if they are taking diphenhydramine.
_____ 12. A decongestant should not be used in patients with high blood pressure, unless approved by their health care provider.

FILL IN THE BLANKS

13. _____ is a substance present in various tissues of the body that is released in response to injury and produces an inflammatory response.
14. Decongestants work by producing localized _____ of the small blood vessels of the nasal membranes.
15. Decongestants are _____ drugs.
16. Use of a decongestant with a _____ may cause a hypertensive crisis.

SHORT ANSWERS

17. Why are antihistamines not routinely given to patients with lower respiratory disorders?
18. What are the most common adverse reactions associated with the use of topical nasal decongestants?
19. How do antihistamines work?
20. What are the symptoms that a patient will exhibit if suffering from allergies?

Web Activities

1. Go to the National Guideline Clearinghouse home page (www.guideline.gov). Do a search for guidelines related to cough. Find the guideline titled "Cough and the common cold: ACCP evidence-based clinical practice guidelines." What are the first two major recommendations?
2. On the Web site of the American Academy of Allergy, Asthma, and Immunology is an article about asthma that defines a "second-generation antihistamine." Go to http://www.aaaai.org and select "Patients and Consumers." Conduct a search for "tips to remember: asthma and allergy medications" (www.aaaai.org/patients/seniorsandasthma/medications_and_dosage.stm). Write a brief summary of the discussion about antihistamines and decongestants.

SUMMARY DRUG TABLE Antihistamines (left, generic; right, trade)

Comprehensive Summary Drug Tables, including uses, adverses effects, dosages, and pregnancy classifications, are provided on the companion website, http://thePoint.lww.com/PharmacologyHP2e

brompheniramine maleate *brome-fen-ir'-a-meen*	*generic* (Rx)
carbinoxamine *kar-bi-noks'-a-meen*	Palgic (Rx), *generic*
cetirizine HCl *se-tear'-i-zeen*	Zyrtec (OTC)
chlorpheniramine maleate *klor-fen-eer'-a-meen*	(Chlor-Trimeton Rx), *generic*
clemastine fumarate *klem'-as-teen*	Tavist Allergy (OTC), *generic*
cyproheptadine *si-proe-hep'-ta-deen*	*generic* (Rx)
desloratadine *des-low-rah'-tah-deen*	Clarinex (Rx)
diphenhydramine hydrochloride *edye-fen-hye'-dra- meen*	Benadryl (OTC), miscellaneous, *generic*
doxylamine *dox-il'-a-meen*	Doxytex (Rx), Unisom (OTC), Aldex AN (OTC)
fexofenadine hydrochloride *fecks-oh-fen'-a-deen*	Allegra (Rx), Allegra ODT, *generic*
hydroxyzine *hye-drox'-i-zeen*	Vistaril (Rx), *generic*
levocetirizine *lee'-vo-se-ti'-ra-zeen*	Xyzal (Rx)
loratadine *lor-a'-ta-dine*	Claritin (OTC), Alavert, Triaminic Allerchews, *generic*
promethazine HCl *proe-meth'-a-zeen*	Phenergan (Rx), *generic*
tripelennamine HCl *trip-el-en'-a-meen*	PBZ, PBZ-SR

SUMMARY DRUG TABLE Systemic and Topical Nasal Decongestants (left, generic; right, trade)

Comprehensive Summary Drug Tables, including uses, adverses effects, dosages, and pregnancy classifications, are provided on the companion website, http://thePoint.lww.com/PharmacologyHP2e

epinephrine HCl *ep-i-nef'-rin*	Adrenalin (Rx), Primatene Mist (OTC)
naphazoline HCl *na-faz'-o-line*	Privine (OTC)
oxymetazoline HCl *oxy-met-az'-oh-leen*	Afrin (OTC), Dristan 12-h nasal, miscellaneous, *generic*
phenylephrine HCl *fen-ill-ef'-rin*	Sudafed-PE (OTC), Neo-Synephrine, Miscellaneous
pseudoephedrine HCl *soo-dow-e-fed'-rin*	Sudafed (OTC), *generic*
tetrahydrozoline HCl *tet-rah-hi-draz'-oh-leen*	Tyzine (Rx)

17

Antitussives, Mucolytics, and Expectorants

CHAPTER OBJECTIVES

On completion of this chapter, students will be able to:

1 Define the chapter's key terms.

2 Describe the two types of cough.

3 Identify when to use an antitussive and when to use an expectorant.

4 Describe the common adverse reactions, contraindications, precautions, and interactions of antitussives.

5 Describe the common adverse reactions, contraindications, precautions, and interactions of expectorants and mucolytics.

6 Discuss important points to keep in mind when educating the patient or family members about the use of an antitussive, mucolytic, or expectorant drug.

KEY TERMS

antitussive—a drug used to relieve coughing
auscultating—listening to sounds within the body
coughing—the forceful expulsion of air from the lungs
dyspnea—shortness of breath
expectorant—a drug that aids in raising thick, tenacious mucus from the respiratory passages
mucolytic—a drug that loosens respiratory secretions
nebulization—the dispersing of liquid medication in a mist of extremely fine particles to be inhaled into the deeper parts of the respiratory tract
nonproductive cough—a dry, hacking cough that produces no secretions
productive cough—a cough that expels secretions from the lower respiratory tract

CHAPTER OVERVIEW

Drug classes covered in this chapter are:

- Antitussives
- Mucolytics
- Expectorants

Drugs by classification are listed on page 180.

thePOINT RESOURCES

- Comprehensive Summary Drug Tables
- Lippincott's Interactive Tutorials: Drugs Affecting the Respiratory System
- Interactive Practice and Review
- Monographs of Most Commonly Prescribed Drugs

Upper respiratory infections are among the most common afflictions of humans. The drugs used to treat the discomfort associated with an upper respiratory infection include antitussives, mucolytics, and expectorants. Many of these drugs are available as nonprescription (over-the-counter) drugs, whereas others are available only by prescription.

Antitussives

Actions of Antitussives

Some antitussives depress the cough center located in the medulla and are called centrally acting drugs. Codeine and dextromethorphan are examples of centrally acting antitussives. Other antitussives are peripherally acting drugs, which act by anesthetizing stretch receptors in the respiratory passages, thereby decreasing coughing. An example of a peripherally acting antitussive is benzonatate (Tessalon). If the cough is caused by the common cold, then a first-generation antihistamine, such as diphenhydramine, is considered to be the drug of choice.

Coughing is the forceful expulsion of air from the lungs and is one of the body's natural defense mechanisms. A cough may be productive or nonproductive (Key Concepts 17-1). With a **productive cough**, secretions from the lower respiratory tract are expelled. A **nonproductive cough** is a dry, hacking one that produces no secretions. An **antitussive** is a drug used to relieve coughing. Many antitussive drugs are combined with another drug, such as an antihistamine or expectorant, and sold as nonprescription cough medicine. Other antitussives, either alone or in combination with other drugs, are available by prescription only.

Uses of Antitussives

Antitussives are used to relieve a nonproductive cough. When the cough is productive of sputum, it should be treated by the health care provider who, based on a physical examination, may or may not prescribe or recommend an antitussive.

The color and amount of any sputum present may indicate an infection, particularly in patients with a productive cough.

If the patient's sleep is frequently interrupted by coughing, then the problem should be discussed with the health care provider.

Adverse Reactions of Antitussives

Use of codeine may result in respiratory depression, euphoria, light-headedness, sedation, nausea, vomiting, and hypersensitivity reactions.

Contraindications, Precautions, and Interactions of Antitussives

- Antitussives are contraindicated in patients with a known hypersensitivity.
- All antitussives are given with caution to patients with a persistent or chronic cough or when the cough is accompanied by excessive secretion.
- Individuals with a high fever, rash, persistent headache, nausea, or vomiting should take antitussives only when advised by their health care provider.
- Antitussives containing codeine are used with caution in patients having an acute asthmatic attack, those with congestive obstructive pulmonary disease, and those with preexisting respiratory disorders. Administration of codeine may obscure the diagnosis in patients with acute abdominal conditions.
- Narcotic antitussives are used cautiously in patients with head injury and increased intracranial pressure, acute abdominal disorders, convulsive disorders, hepatic or renal impairment, prostatic hypertrophy, or asthma or other respiratory conditions.
- Other central nervous system depressants and alcohol may cause additive depressant effects when administered with antitussives containing codeine.
- When dextromethorphan is administered with the monoamine oxidase inhibitors (see Chapter 7), patients may experience hypotension, fever, nausea, jerking motions of the leg, and coma.
- Some medications, such as angiotensin-converting enzyme inhibitors, will cause a nonproductive cough as an adverse reaction. If this is the case, the cough should not be treated with an antitussive. The health care provider should be contacted.

KEY CONCEPTS

17-1   Types of Coughs

There are two types of cough: productive and nonproductive.

A productive cough has a purpose. Its job is to help the patient bring mucous up and out of the respiratory tract. A productive cough should be treated with an expectorant, which will help thin the mucus. When the patient coughs, the mucus will then be expectorated from the lungs. It is not appropriate to suppress a productive cough unless under the direction of a health care provider.

A nonproductive cough does not have a purpose. Therefore, it is appropriate to suppress or eliminate the cough. First, however, the cause of the cough should be determined..

ALERT Rx

Extended Use of Nonprescription Cough Medicine

Patients taking nonprescription cough medicine for a cough that has lasted for more than 10 days or is accompanied by fever, chest pain, severe headache, or skin rash should be advised to consult with the health care provider. Indiscriminate use of antitussives by the general public may prevent early diagnosis and treatment of serious disorders, such as lung cancer and emphysema.

ALERT Rx

Drug Action of Antitussives

One problem associated with the use of antitussives is related to its drug action. Although not an adverse reaction, depression of the cough reflex can cause a pooling of secretions in the lungs. A pooling of secretions that are normally removed by coughing may result in more serious problems, such as pneumonia and atelectasis. For this reason, using an antitussive for a productive cough is often contraindicated.

Patient Management Issues with Antitussives

Periodically taking and recording vital signs and **auscultating** the lungs help establish a baseline for patient's condition. When a patient has a cough, the frequency of coughing, whether the cough is productive or nonproductive, and whether the cough interrupts sleep or causes pain in the chest or other parts of the body should be noted.

Educating the Patient and Family about Antitussives

Following are key points about antitussives that the patient and family members should know.

Indiscriminate use of nonprescription cough medicines, especially when coughing produces sputum, is not advised. If an antitussive is prescribed for use at home, then the following information is important:

- Read the label carefully, follow the dosage recommendations, and consult your health care provider if your cough is not relieved, persists for more than 10 days, or if your symptoms worsen.
- Do not exceed the recommended dose.
- If you experience chills, fever, chest pain, or sputum production, contact your health care provider as soon as possible.
- Drink plenty of fluids.
- If taking oral capsules, then do not chew or break open the capsules; swallow them whole and with a full glass of water.
- Avoid irritants such as cigarette smoke, dust, or fumes to decrease throat irritation. Take frequent sips of water, suck on sugarless hard candy, or chew gum to diminish coughing.
- Codeine may impair mental or physical abilities required for potentially hazardous tasks. Be cautious when driving or performing tasks requiring alertness, coordination, or physical dexterity. Do not use with alcohol or other central nervous system depressants (e.g., antidepressants, hypnotics, sedatives, tranquilizers). Codeine may cause orthostatic hypotension (reduced blood pressure and dizziness) when rising too quickly from a sitting or lying position. Do not take it for persistent or chronic cough, such as occurs with smoking, asthma,

or emphysema, or when the cough is accompanied by excessive secretions, except when prescribed by your health care provider.
- Notify your health care provider if you have difficulty breathing because of an inability to raise sputum and clear the respiratory passages.

FACT CHECK

17-1 An antitussive is appropriate for which type of cough?

17-2 What are the three types of antitussives and examples of each?

Mucolytics and Expectorants

Actions of Mucolytics and Expectorants

A **mucolytic** is a drug that loosens respiratory secretions. An **expectorant** is a drug that aids in raising thick, tenacious mucus from the respiratory passages to be coughed out.

A drug with mucolytic activity appears to reduce the viscosity (thickness) of respiratory secretions by direct action on the mucus. An example of a mucolytic drug is acetylcysteine (Mucomyst).

Expectorants increase the production of respiratory secretions, which in turn appears to decrease the viscosity of the mucus. This helps to raise secretions from the respiratory passages. An example of an expectorant is guaifenesin.

Uses of Mucolytics and Expectorants

Uses of Mucolytics

The mucolytic acetylcysteine may be used as part of the treatment of bronchopulmonary diseases such as emphysema. It is primarily given by **nebulization** (liquid medication in a mist form inhaled into respiratory tract) but also may be directly instilled into a tracheostomy to liquefy (thin) secretions. Mucolytic drugs are effective as adjunctive therapy in patients with chronic bronchopulmonary diseases, such as chronic emphysema, emphysema with bronchitis, chronic asthma, tuberculosis, and bronchiectasis, and acute bronchopulmonary diseases, such as pneumonia and tracheobronchitis. It is also used for pulmonary conditions of cystic fibrosis and in tracheostomy care. Acetylcysteine has an additional use in preventing liver damage caused by acetaminophen overdosage.

Uses of Expectorants

Expectorants are used to help raise respiratory secretions. Guaifenesin is the most commonly used expectorant. It may also be included along with one or more additional drugs, such as an antihistamine, decongestant, or antitussive, in some prescription and nonprescription cough medicines.

Adverse Reactions of Mucolytics and Expectorants

Common adverse reactions of mucolytic and expectorant drugs include nausea, vomiting, and drowsiness.

Contraindications, Precautions, and Interactions of Mucolytics and Expectorants

- Expectorants and mucolytics are contraindicated in patients with a known hypersensitivity.
- Expectorants are used cautiously in patients with persistent cough that may be caused by a serious condition needing medical evaluation.
- Acetylcysteine is used cautiously in those with severe respiratory insufficiency or asthma and in older adults or debilitated patients.
- No significant interactions have been reported when guaifenesin is used as directed.
- The iodine products when taken with lithium will potentiate the incidence of hypothyroidism and goiter. When potassium-containing medications and potassium-sparing diuretics are administered with iodine products, the patient may experience hypokalemia, cardiac arrhythmias, or cardiac arrest. Thyroid function tests may also be altered by iodine.

Patient Management Issues with Mucolytics and Expectorants

The respiratory status of the patient is assessed before a drug is administered. Lung sounds, amount of **dyspnea** (if any), and consistency of sputum (if present) are documented. A description of the sputum is important as a baseline for future comparison. Any increase in sputum or change in its consistency is assessed after a drug has been administered as well. Patients with thick, tenacious mucus may have difficulty breathing. The health care provider should be notified if the patient has difficulty breathing because of an inability to raise sputum and clear the respiratory passages.

If any problem occurs during or after treatment, or if the patient is uncooperative, then the problem should be discussed with the health care provider.

Educating the Patient and Family about Mucolytics and Expectorants

Following are key points about mucolytics and expectorants that the patient or family members should know.

- The signs and symptoms of possible adverse reactions should be reported.
- Impaired respiratory function including changes in cough, the color or amount of sputum, shortness of breath, or difficulty breathing should be reported immediately to the health care provider.
- Drink plenty of fluids, especially water, because it will aid the expectorant in thinning the mucus.
- A humidifier or vaporizer might be useful to help thin the mucus. Or, the patient could take a hot, steamy shower.
- If the coughing is making the throat sore, then the patient could suck on sugar-free hard candy. Many patients find hot teas to be soothing to the throat that is raw from coughing.

FACT CHECK
17-3   When a patient is suffering from a productive cough, what needs to be noted about the cough and the patient's condition?
17-4   What is the most commonly used expectorant?

Chapter Review

KEY POINTS

- Drugs used to treat the discomfort associated with an upper respiratory infection include nonprescription and prescription antitussives, mucolytics, and expectorants.
- Some centrally acting antitussives depress the cough center located in the medulla. Peripherally acting antitussives act by anesthetizing stretch receptors in the respiratory passages, thereby decreasing coughing.
- A drug with mucolytic activity appears to reduce the viscosity (thickness) of respiratory secretions by direct action on the mucus.
- Expectorants increase the production of respiratory secretions, which in turn appears to decrease the viscosity of the mucus. This helps to raise secretions from the respiratory passages.
- When used as directed, nonprescription cough medicines containing two or more ingredients have few adverse reactions. However, those that contain an antihistamine may cause drowsiness.

- Narcotic antitussives are used cautiously in patients with head injury and increased intracranial pressure, acute abdominal disorders, convulsive disorders, hepatic or renal impairment, prostatic hypertrophy, asthma, or other respiratory conditions. All antitussives are given with caution to patients with a persistent or chronic cough or when the cough is accompanied by excessive secretion. Individuals with a high fever, rash, persistent headache, nausea, or vomiting should take antitussives only when advised by their health care provider.
- Expectorants are used cautiously in patients with persistent cough that may be caused by a serious condition needing medical evaluation. Acetylcysteine is used cautiously in those with severe respiratory insufficiency or asthma and in older adults or debilitated patients. Expectorants are used cautiously during pregnancy and lactation. Adverse reactions include nausea, vomiting, and drowsiness.

CRITICAL THINKING CASE STUDY

Productive versus Nonproductive Cough

Ms. Tollster, a middle school math teacher, has had a cough for 3 days. She is finding it difficult to teach because of her chest congestion, and she cannot seem to stop coughing. She asks you for some advice.

1. What type of cough does Ms. Tollster have?
   a. Productive
   b. Nonproductive
   c. You do not have enough information to know
   d. None of the above
2. Based on Ms. Tollster's symptoms, which would be the most appropriate product for her to take?
   a. Codeine
   b. Diphenhydramine
   c. Guaifenesin
   d. Dextromethorphan
3. What would be some other things that you could recommend to Ms. Tollster?

Review Questions

MULTIPLE CHOICE

1. What symptom is an antitussive used to relieve?
   a. Productive cough
   b. Nonproductive cough
   c. Lung congestion
   d. Nasal congestion
2. Dextromethorphan has which of the following as a potential adverse reaction?
   a. Constipation
   b. Gastrointestinal upset
   c. Skin eruptions
   d. All of the above
3. Auscultating the lungs is an important diagnostic tool because it
   a. allows a baseline to be determined
   b. determines the color of sputum
   c. helps to determine how the patient's vocal cords are affected by congestion
   d. may indicate whether an allergen is present
4. Narcotic antitussives are used cautiously when the following condition is present:
   a. Head injury
   b. Glaucoma
   c. Arthritis
   d. Gastrointestinal disorders

MATCHING

_____ 5. guaifenesin   a. Tessalon
_____ 6. dextromethorphan   b. Benadryl
_____ 7. benzonatate   c. Mucinex
_____ 8. diphenhydramine   d. Delsym

TRUE OR FALSE

_____ 9. Codeine and dextromethorphan are examples of centrally acting antitussives.
_____ 10. Diphenhydramine is an antihistamine, but it is also used as an antitussive.
_____ 11. Acetylcysteine is a mucolytic that is administered via nebulization.
_____ 12. The most common adverse reaction of guaifenesin is excitation.

FILL IN THE BLANKS

13. Some antitussives depress the cough center located in the _____ and are called centrally acting drugs.
14. A(n) _____ is a drug that aids in raising thick, tenacious mucus from the respiratory passages to be coughed out.
15. Benzonatate is a peripherally acting drug that acts by anesthetizing _____ _____ in the respiratory passages.
16. A(n) _____ is a drug that loosens respiratory secretions.

SHORT ANSWERS

17. Why is an antitussive often contraindicated for a productive cough?
18. Benzonatate is available in a capsule and a "perle" dosage form. How would you instruct the patient to take the medication?

Web Activities

1. Do a web search to find out information on the abuse of dextromethorphan. Write a brief summary of what you have learned.
2. Go to the National Institute of Health Web site MedlinePlus Web site (http://medlineplus.gov) and click on the heading for Drug Information. Use the A to Z drug list to search for guaifenesin. What other classifications of medications is guaifenesin typically combined with in the combination products?

SUMMARY DRUG TABLE Antitussive, Mucolytic, and Expectorant Drugs (left, generic; right, trade)

Comprehensive Summary Drug Tables, including uses, adverses effects, dosages, and pregnancy classifications, are provided on the companion website, http://thePoint.lww.com/PharmacologyHP2e

Antitussives Narcotic	
codeine sulfate *koe'-deen*	Miscellaneous combination products (CV), *generic*
Nonnarcotic	
benzonatate *ben-zoe'-naa-tate*	Tessalon, Tessalon Perles, *generic*
dextromethorphan HBr *dex-troe-meth-or'-fan*	Delsym (OTC), Robitussin Pediatric, Sucrets, Suppress, miscellaneous, *generic*
diphenhydramine HCl *dye-fen-hye'-dra-meen*	Benadryl (OTC), miscellaneous, *generic*
Mucolytic	
acetylcysteine *a-se-teel-sis'-tay-een*	*generic* (Rx)
Expectorants	
guaifenesin (glyceryl guaiacolate) *gwye-fen'-e-sin*	Mucinex (OTC), Organidin NR (Rx), miscellaneous (OTC), *generic*
potassium iodide *poe-tass'-ee-um-eye-o-dide*	SSKI (Rx)

18

Cardiotonics and Miscellaneous Inotropic Drugs

CHAPTER OBJECTIVES

On completion of this chapter, students will be able to:

1. Define the chapter's key terms.
2. Describe heart failure.
3. Describe the uses and general drug actions of cardiotonics and miscellaneous inotropic drugs.
4. Identify common adverse reactions of cardiotonics and miscellaneous inotropic drugs.
5. Describe contraindications, precautions, and interactions of cardiotonics and miscellaneous inotropic drugs.
6. Discuss important points to keep in mind when educating the patient or family members about the use of cardiotonics and miscellaneous inotropic drugs.

KEY TERMS

atrial fibrillation—a cardiac arrhythmia characterized by rapid contractions of the atrial myocardium, resulting in an irregular and often rapid ventricular rate

cardiac output—the amount of blood leaving the left ventricle with each contraction

digitalization—a series of digitalis doses given until the drug begins to exert a full therapeutic effect

ejection fraction—the amount of blood that the ventricle ejects per beat in relationship to the amount of blood available to eject

heart failure—denoted by the area of the initial ventricle dysfunction: left-side (left ventricular) dysfunction and right-side (right ventricular) dysfunction; because both sides work together, both sides are affected in heart failure

ischemic—marked by reduced blood flow caused by arterial narrowing or blockage or other causes

CHAPTER OVERVIEW

Drug classes covered in this chapter are:

- Cardiotonics
- Miscellaneous inotropic drugs

Drugs by classification are listed on page 188.

thePOINT RESOURCES

- Comprehensive Summary Drug Tables
- Animations: Cardiac Cycle; Congestive Heart Failure
- Lippincott's Interactive Tutorials: Drugs Affecting the Cardiovascular System
- Interactive Practice and Review
- Monographs of Most Commonly Prescribed Drugs

left ventricular dysfunction—also called left ventricular systolic dysfunction, the most common form of heart failure

positive inotropic action—the increased force of the contraction of the muscle (myocardium) of the heart through the use of cardiotonic drugs

Cardiotonics are drugs used to improve the efficiency and contraction of the heart muscle (myocardium), leading to improved blood flow to all tissues of the body. These drugs have long been used to treat congestive heart failure (CHF), a condition in which the heart cannot pump enough blood to meet the tissue needs of the body. Although the term "congestive heart failure" continues to be used by some, a more accurate term is simply "heart failure."

Approximately 5 million Americans have heart failure. It is the most common diagnosis upon hospital admission for individuals older than 65 years. With treatment, some patients may lead nearly normal lives, but more than 50% of individuals with heart failure die within 5 years of diagnosis. Heart failure is a complex clinical syndrome that can result from any number of cardiac or metabolic disorders such as **ischemic** heart disease, hypertension, or hyperthyroidism (Fig. 18-1). Any condition that impairs the ability of the ventricles to pump blood can lead to heart failure.

Cardiotonics and Miscellaneous Inotropic Drugs

Heart failure causes a number of neurohormonal changes as the body tries to compensate for the increased workload of the heart. The sympathetic nervous system increases the secretions of catecholamines (the neurohormones epinephrine and norepinephrine), which results in increased heart rate and vasoconstriction. The activation of the renin–angiotensin–aldosterone (RAA) system occurs because of decreased perfusion to the kidneys. As the RAA system is activated, levels of angiotensin II and aldosterone rise, which increases the blood pressure, adding to the workload of the heart. These increases in neurohormonal activity cause a remodeling of cardiac muscle cells, leading to hypertrophy of the heart, an increased need for oxygen, and cardiac necrosis, which worsens the heart failure. Heart tissue changes increase the cellular mass of cardiac tissue, change the shape of the ventricle(s), and reduce the heart's ability to contract effectively.

Heart failure is usually described in terms of the area of initial ventricle dysfunction: left-side (left ventricular) dysfunction or right-side (right ventricular) dysfunction. Left ventricular dysfunction leads to pulmonary symptoms such as dyspnea and moist cough. Right ventricular dysfunction leads to neck vein distention, peripheral edema, weight gain, and hepatic engorgement. Because both sides of the heart work together, ultimately both sides are affected in heart failure. Typically the left side of the heart is affected first, followed by right ventricular involvement. The Signs and Symptoms Box lists the most common symptoms of heart failure.

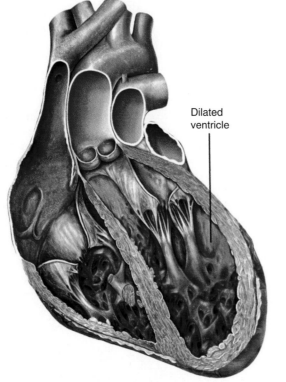

Dilated ventricle

FIGURE 18-1 Congestive heart failure.

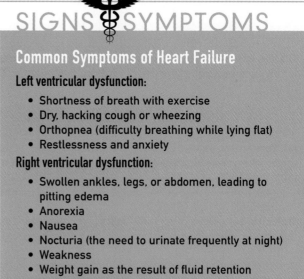

SIGNS ☤ SYMPTOMS

Common Symptoms of Heart Failure

Left ventricular dysfunction:

- Shortness of breath with exercise
- Dry, hacking cough or wheezing
- Orthopnea (difficulty breathing while lying flat)
- Restlessness and anxiety

Right ventricular dysfunction:

- Swollen ankles, legs, or abdomen, leading to pitting edema
- Anorexia
- Nausea
- Nocturia (the need to urinate frequently at night)
- Weakness
- Weight gain as the result of fluid retention

Other symptoms include:

- Palpitations, fatigue, or pain when performing normal activities
- Tachycardia or irregular heart rate
- Dizziness or confusion

Left ventricular dysfunction, also called left ventricular systolic dysfunction, is the most common form of heart failure and results in decreased cardiac output and decreased **ejection fraction** (the amount of blood that the ventricle ejects per beat in relationship to the amount of blood available to eject). Normally the ejection fraction is greater than 60%. With left ventricular systolic dysfunction, the ejection fraction is less than 40%, and the heart is enlarged and dilated.

Until recently, a cardiotonic and a diuretic were the treatment of choice for heart failure. Drugs such as angiotensin-converting enzyme (ACE) inhibitors and β-blockers have now become the treatment of choice. See Chapter 21 for more information on β-blockers and ACE inhibitors. See Chapter 25 for more information on diuretics.

Digoxin (Lanoxin) is the most commonly used cardiotonic drug. Other terms for cardiotonics are cardiac glycosides or digitalis glycosides.

Miscellaneous drugs with positive inotropic action such as inamrinone and milrinone are nonglycosides used in the short-term management of heart failure. Although in the past the cardiotonics were a mainstay of treatment for heart failure, currently they are used as the fourth line of treatment for patients who continue to experience symptoms after using ACE inhibitors, diuretics, and β-blockers.

FACT CHECK

18-1   What are the symptoms of left ventricular dysfunction and right ventricular dysfunction?
18-2   What is the most common form of heart failure?
18-3   What is the most commonly used cardiotonic drug?

Actions of Cardiotonic Drugs

Cardiotonics act in two ways:

- Increase cardiac output through positive inotropic activity
- Decrease the conduction velocity through the atrioventricular (AV) and sinoatrial (SA) nodes in the heart

These are described in the following sections.

Increased Cardiac Output

Cardiotonic drugs increase the force of the contraction of the muscle (myocardium) of the heart. This is called a **positive inotropic action.** When the force of contraction of the myocardium is increased, the amount of blood leaving the left ventricle with each contraction, called **cardiac output**, is increased.

The most profound effect of a cardiotonic drug occurs in patients with heart failure. In heart failure, the heart, weakened by disease or age, cannot pump a sufficient amount of blood to meet the demands of the body. A decreased amount of oxygenated blood leaves the left ventricle during each myocardial contraction (decreased cardiac output). A marked decrease in cardiac output deprives the kidneys, brain, and other vital organs of an adequate blood supply. The weakened heart also cannot pump enough circulated blood back into the heart. The blood accumulates or congests in the body's tissues. With congestion, legs and ankles swell. Fluid collects

in the lungs, and the individual finds it increasingly difficult to breathe, especially when lying down. When the kidneys are deprived of an adequate blood supply, they cannot effectively remove water, electrolytes, and waste products from the bloodstream. Excess fluid (edema) may occur in the lungs or tissues, increasing the congestion. The body attempts to make up for this cardiac output deficit by increasing the heart rate, which in turn circulates more blood through the kidneys, brain, and other vital organs. Often, however, this increased heart rate ultimately fails to deliver an adequate amount of blood to the kidneys and other vital organs. The increased heart rate also places added strain on the heart's muscle, which may further weaken the heart. Untreated, congestion worsens and may prevent the heart from pumping enough blood to keep the individual alive.

When a cardiotonic drug is administered, the positive inotropic action increases the force of the contraction, resulting in an increased cardiac output. When cardiac output is increased, the blood supply to the kidneys and other vital organs is increased. Water, electrolytes, and waste products are removed in adequate amounts, and the symptoms of inadequate heart action or heart failure are relieved. In most instances, the heart rate also decreases. This occurs because vital organs are now receiving an adequate blood supply because of the increased force of myocardial contraction.

Depression of the Sinoatrial and Atrioventricular Nodes

Cardiotonics also affect the transmission of electrical impulses in the conduction system of the heart. The conduction system of the heart involves a group of specialized nerve fibers consisting of the SA node, the AV node, the bundle of His, and the branches of Purkinje (Fig. 18-2). Each heartbeat (contraction of the ventricles) results from an electrical impulse that normally starts in the SA node, is then received by the AV node, and travels down the bundle of His and through the Purkinje fibers. When the electrical impulse reaches the Purkinje fibers, the ventricles contract. Normally, once the ventricles contract, another electrical impulse is generated by the SA node, and the cycle begins again. Cardiotonic drugs depress the SA node and slow conduction of the electrical impulse to and through the AV node. Slowing this part of the transmission of nerve impulses decreases the number of impulses and the number of ventricular contractions per minute, thereby decreasing the heart rate and allowing the heart to function more normally. The therapeutic effects of cardiotonics on atrial arrhythmias are thought to be related to the depressive action on the SA and AV nodes and baroreceptor sensitization.

FACT CHECK

18-4   In what two ways do cardiotonic drugs act?
18-5   What is cardiac output?

Uses of Cardiotonic Drugs

The cardiotonics are used to treat heart failure and atrial fibrillation. **Atrial fibrillation** is a cardiac arrhythmia characterized by

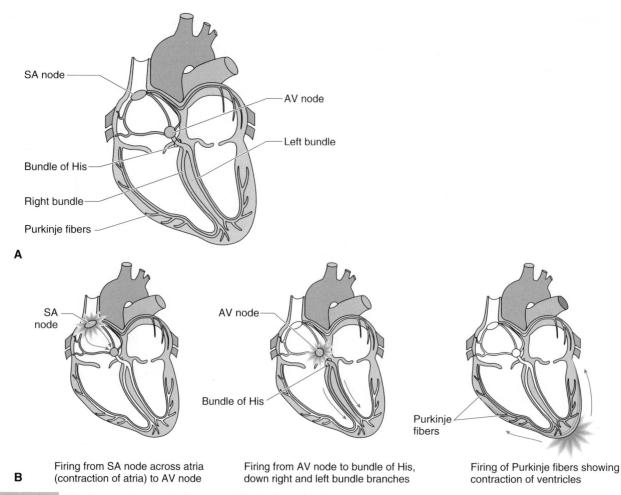

SA node

AV node

Left bundle

Bundle of His

Right bundle

Purkinje fibers

A

SA node

AV node

Bundle of His

Purkinje fibers

B   Firing from SA node across atria   Firing from AV node to bundle of His,   Firing of Purkinje fibers showing
         (contraction of atria) to AV node   down right and left bundle branches   contraction of ventricles

FIGURE 18-2   Cardiac conduction. A. Anatomy. B. Path of conduction.

rapid contractions of the atrial myocardium, resulting in an irregular and often rapid ventricular rate. Arrhythmias are discussed later in this chapter.

Adverse Reactions of Cardiotonic Drugs

Adverse reactions are dose dependent. Dosages are individualized based on several factors, including the following:
- The patient's ideal body weight
- The patient's renal function, evaluated by creatinine clearance
- The patient's age (infants and children require lower dosages, and the elderly may have decreased renal function, requiring a lower dosage)
- The patient's other medications, other medical problems, or other factors affecting the activity of digoxin

Because some patients are more sensitive to the adverse reactions of digoxin, the dosage is selected carefully and adjusted as the clinical condition indicates. Adverse reactions were more common and severe in past years before careful attention was given to weight, renal function, and the concurrent administration of certain medications.

There is a narrow margin of safety between the full therapeutic effects and the toxic effects of cardiotonic drugs. Even normal doses of a cardiotonic drug can cause toxic drug effects. Because substantial individual variations may occur, the dosage must be individualized. The term digitalis toxicity (or digitalis intoxication) is used when toxic drug effects occur when digoxin is administered. The signs of digitalis toxicity are listed in the Signs and Symptoms Box.

Digoxin has a rapid onset and a short duration of action. If the drug is withheld, then the toxic effects of digoxin will disappear rapidly. At times, the health care provider may deem it necessary to administer digoxin immune fab if a life-threatening digoxin overdosage occurs. Digoxin immune fab, composed of digoxin-specific antigen-binding fragments (fab), is used as an antidote in the treatment of digoxin overdosage. The dosage depends on the amount of digoxin the patient was given. Digoxin immune fab is administered by the intravenous (IV) route during a 30-minute period. Few adverse reactions have been observed with the use of immune fab, but there is a possibility of a worsening of the heart failure, low cardiac output, hypokalemia, or atrial fibrillation. Hypokalemia is of particular concern in patients taking

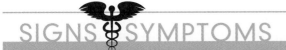

SIGNS & SYMPTOMS

Signs of Digitalis Toxicity

- Gastrointestinal: anorexia (usually the first sign), nausea, vomiting, diarrhea
- Muscular: weakness
- Central nervous system: headache, apathy, drowsiness, visual disturbances (blurred vision, disturbance in yellow/green vision, halo effect around dark objects), mental depression, confusion, disorientation, delirium
- Cardiac: changes in pulse rate or rhythm; electrocardiographic changes, such as bradycardia, tachycardia, premature ventricular contractions, bigeminal (2 beats followed by a pause) or trigeminal (3 beats followed by a pause) pulse. Other arrhythmias (abnormal heart rhythms) also may be seen.

digoxin immune fab, particularly because hypokalemia usually coexists with toxicity.

Contraindications, Precautions, and Interactions of Cardiotonics

- Cardiotonics are contraindicated in patients with known hypersensitivity, ventricular failure, ventricular tachycardia, or AV block, and in the presence of digitalis toxicity.
- Cardiotonics are given cautiously in patients with an electrolyte imbalance (especially hypokalemia, hypocalcemia, and hypomagnesemia), severe carditis, heart block, myocardial infarction, severe pulmonary disease, acute glomerulonephritis, or impaired renal or hepatic function.
- When a cardiotonic is taken with food, absorption is slowed, but the amount absorbed is the same. However, if taken with high-fiber meals, absorption of the cardiotonic may be decreased.

ALERT ℞

Digitalis Toxicity
The drug should be withheld and the health care provider informed immediately if the patient shows any signs of digitalis toxicity, if the patient has any change in pulse rhythm or a marked increase or decrease in the pulse rate since the last time it was taken, or if the patient's general condition appears to have worsened.

CONSIDERATIONS | Older adults

LIFESPAN

Digitalis Toxicity
Older adults are particularly prone to digitalis toxicity. All older adults must be carefully monitored for signs of digitalis toxicity.

- Cardiotonics react with many different drugs. Drugs that may increase plasma digitalis levels leading to toxicity include amiodarone, benzodiazepines, cyclosporine, diphenoxylate, indomethacin, itraconazole, macrolides (erythromycin, clarithromycin), propafenone, quinidine, quinine, spironolactone, tetracyclines, and verapamil.
- Drugs that may decrease plasma digitalis levels include the oral aminoglycosides, antacids, antineoplastics (bleomycin, carmustine, cyclophosphamide, methotrexate, and vincristine), activated charcoal, cholestyramine, colestipol, kaolin/pectin, neomycin, penicillamine, rifampin, St. John's wort, and sulfasalazine.
- Thyroid hormones may decrease the effectiveness of digoxin, requiring a larger dosage of digoxin.
- Thiazide and loop diuretics may increase diuretic-induced electrolyte disturbances, predisposing the patient to digitalis-induced arrhythmias. Patients taking a diuretic and a digitalis glycoside must be monitored closely. Thiazide and loop diuretics (see Chapter 25) may increase the risk and effects of toxicity.

FACT CHECK
18-6 What are the signs of digitalis toxicity?
18-7 When are cardiotonics contraindicated?

Miscellaneous Inotropic Drugs

Inamrinone and milrinone have inotropic actions and are used in the short-term management of severe heart failure that is not controlled by digitalis. Milrinone is used more often than inamrinone, appears to be more effective, and has fewer adverse reactions. Both drugs are given IV, and close monitoring is required during therapy. The patient's heart rate and blood pressure must be continuously monitored with either drug. If hypotension occurs, then the drug is discontinued or the rate of administration reduced. Continuous cardiac monitoring is necessary because life-threatening arrhythmias may occur. These drugs do not cure, but rather control, the signs and symptoms of heart failure.

FACT CHECK
18-8   What is the main use of inamrinone?

Patient Management Issues with Cardiotonic and Miscellaneous Inotropic Drugs

Cardiotonics are potentially toxic drugs. Therefore, the patient must be observed closely, especially during initial therapy. Before therapy is started, the patient is assessed to establish a database for comparison during therapy. The physical assessment should include, among other things:

- Taking blood pressure, apical–radial pulse rate, respiratory rate
- Auscultating the lungs, noting any unusual sounds during inspiration and expiration
- Examining the extremities for edema
- Checking the jugular veins for distention
- Measuring weight

The health care provider also may order laboratory and diagnostic tests. These tests are reviewed before the first dose of the drug is given. Renal function is particularly important because diminished renal function could affect the dosage of digoxin. Because digoxin reacts with many medications, a careful drug history must also be taken.

Patients being started on therapy with a cardiotonic are said to be "digitalized." Digitalization may be accomplished by two general methods:

- Rapid digitalization (accomplished by administering a loading dose)
- Gradual digitalization (giving a maintenance dose allowing the body to gradually accumulate therapeutic blood levels)

Digitalization involves a series of doses given until the drug begins to exert a full therapeutic effect. The digitalizing, or loading, dose is administered in several doses, with approximately half the total digitalization dose administered in the first dose. Additional fractions of the digitalis dose are administered at 6- to 8-hour intervals. Once a full therapeutic effect is achieved, a patient is usually prescribed a maintenance dose schedule. Digoxin injections are usually used for rapid digitalization; digoxin tablets are used for maintenance therapy.

Digitalizing doses vary, and the health care provider may decide to achieve full digitalization rapidly or slowly, depending on a patient's diagnosis, age, current condition, and other factors.

During digitalization, the patient's blood pressure, pulse, and respiratory rate are taken every 2 to 4 hours or as ordered by the health care provider. This time interval may be increased or decreased, depending on the patient's condition and the route of drug administration.

Serum levels (digoxin) may be ordered daily during the period of digitalization and periodically during maintenance therapy. Periodic electrocardiograms, serum electrolytes, hepatic and renal function tests, and other laboratory studies also may be ordered.

The patient is observed for signs of digitalis toxicity every 2 to 4 hours during digitalization and one or two times per day when a maintenance dose is being given. If digitalis toxicity develops, then the health care provider may discontinue digitalis use until all signs of toxicity are gone. If severe bradycardia occurs, then atropine (see Chapter 14) may be ordered. If digoxin has been given, then the health care provider may order blood tests to determine drug serum levels.

Diuretics (see Chapter 25) may be ordered for some patients receiving a cardiotonic drug. Diuretics and other conditions or factors, such as gastrointestinal suction, diarrhea, and old age, may produce low serum potassium levels (hypokalemia). The health care provider may order a potassium salt to be given orally or IV.

FACT CHECK
18-9   Why is it important for patients taking digoxin to have their renal function checked?
18-10   What is digitalization?
18-11   What form of digoxin is given for rapid digitalization and for maintenance therapy?

Educating the Patient and Family about Cardiotonic Drugs

In some instances, a cardiotonic may be prescribed for a prolonged period. Some patients may discontinue use of the drug, especially if they feel better and their original symptoms have been relieved. The patient and family members must understand that the prescribed drug must be taken exactly as directed by the health care provider.

The health care provider may want the patient to monitor his or her pulse rate daily during cardiotonic therapy. The

ALERT Rx

Hypokalemia and Digitalis Toxicity
Hypokalemia makes the heart muscle more sensitive to digitalis, thereby increasing the possibility of developing digitalis toxicity.

Patients with hypomagnesemia (low magnesium plasma levels) are at increased risk for digitalis toxicity. If low magnesium levels are detected, then the health care provider may prescribe magnesium replacement therapy.

KEY CONCEPTS

18-1 Monitoring Pulse Rate

When patients go home with digoxin, they need to monitor the pulse rate to prevent possible adverse reactions. They should be taught to perform the following steps:

- Use a watch with a second hand.
- Sit down and rest your nondominant arm on a table or chair armrest.
- Place the index and third fingers of your dominant hand just below the wrist bone on the thumb side of your nondominant arm.
- Feel for a beating or pulsing sensation. This is your pulse.
- Count the number of beats for 30 seconds (if the pulse is regular) and multiply by 2. If the pulse is irregular, then count the number of beats for 60 seconds.
- Record the number of beats of your pulse and keep a log of your reading.
- If you notice the pulse rate is more than 100 bpm or less than 60 bpm, then call your health care provider immediately.

patient or family member is shown the correct technique for taking the pulse (see Key Concepts 18-1). The health care provider may also want a patient to omit the next dose of the drug and call him or her if the pulse rate falls below a certain level. (These instructions should be emphasized as part of patient teaching.) Following are key points about taking a cardiotonic drug that the patient or family member should know.

- Do not discontinue use of this drug without first checking with your health care provider (unless instructed to do otherwise). Do not miss a dose and do not take an extra dose.
- Take this drug at the same time each day.
- Do not take antacids or nonprescription cough, cold, allergy, antidiarrheal, and diet (weight-reducing) drugs unless their use has been approved by your health care provider. Some of these drugs interfere with the action of the cardiotonic drug or cause other, potentially serious, problems.
- Carry an identification card describing the disease process and your medication regimen.
- Follow the dietary recommendations (if any) made by your health care provider.
- Your health care provider will closely monitor your drug therapy. Keep all appointments for visits or laboratory or diagnostic tests.

Chapter Review

KEY POINTS

- The cardiotonics are used to increase the efficiency and improve the contraction of the heart muscle, which leads to improved blood flow to all tissues of the body.
- Digitalis increases cardiac output through positive inotropic activity and decreases the conduction velocity through the AV and SA nodes in the heart.
- Digoxin is the most commonly used cardiotonic drug.
- There is a narrow margin of safety between the full therapeutic effects and the toxic effects of cardiotonic drugs. Even normal doses of a cardiotonic drug can cause toxic drug effects. Inamrinone and milrinone have inotropic actions and are used in the short-term management of severe heart failure that is not controlled by the digitalis preparations.

CRITICAL THINKING CASE STUDY

Digoxin—Maintenance Therapy

Mr. Brannen has been taking digoxin for 4 weeks and is in for a follow-up visit.

1. Which of the following questions should Mr. Brannen be asked to determine whether potentially serious side effects are occurring?
   a. Whether his appetite has changed
   b. Whether he is experiencing visual disturbances (blurred vision, disturbance in yellow/green vision, halo effect around dark objects)
   c. Whether he is experiencing muscle weakness
   d. All of the above

2. Mr. Brannen says that he thinks the digoxin is causing heartburn. When questioned, he admits that he is frequently consuming antacids to combat the heartburn. The correct response is
   a. antacids are fine; there is no cause for concern
   b. antacids should be avoided while on digoxin because they may interfere with the action of the digoxin
   c. excess stomach acid is a common side effect of digoxin use and may have to be tolerated; he should check with his health care provider
   d. ignore the symptom

3. What drug would be prescribed if digoxin toxicity develops?

4. Mr. Brannen's daughter asks why the dose of digoxin has changed from the time he started on the medication in the hospital until now. What should you tell her?

Review Questions

MULTIPLE CHOICE

1. Other terms for cardiotonics are
   a. cardiac glycosides and ACE inhibitors
   b. cardiac glycosides and digitalis glycosides
   c. digitalis glycosides and ACE inhibitors
   d. cardiac glycosides and β-blockers

2. Dosages for cardiotonics are individualized based on all of the following factors EXCEPT
   a. patient's renal function
   b. patient's age and ideal body weight
   c. patient's gender
   d. patient's other medications or medical problems
3. Inamrinone and milrinone are given by which route?
   a. Oral
   b. Buccal
   c. IM
   d. IV
4. The antidote for digoxin toxicity is
   a. Inocor
   b. Primacor
   c. Digibind
   d. Digitek

MATCHING

Match each drug listed with its use.

_____ 5. Digoxin
_____ 6. Inamrinone
_____ 7. Milrinone
_____ 8. Digoxin immune fab

a. used for short-term management of congestive heart failure in patients who have not responded to digitalis, diuretics, or vasodilators
b. used as an antidote for digoxin toxicity
c. used for atrial fibrillation and heart failure
d. used for acute decompensated heart failure

TRUE OR FALSE

_____ 9. Only certain conditions that impair the ability of the ventricles to pump blood can lead to heart failure.
_____ 10. Right ventricular dysfunction is the most common form of heart failure.
_____ 11. Toxic effects of digoxin will disappear rapidly if the drug is withheld.
_____ 12. Inamrinone and milrinone are drugs that cure heart failure.

FILL IN THE BLANKS

13. There is a _____ margin of safety between the full therapeutic effects and _____ effects of cardiotonic drugs.
14. Digoxin has a _____ onset and a _____ duration of action.
15. Thyroid hormones may _____ the effectiveness of digoxin, requiring a _____ dose of the drug.
16. _____ is an adverse reaction of digoxin immune fab.

SHORT ANSWERS

17. What are the symptoms of LVD?
18. What happens when a cardiotonic drug is taken with food?
19. How does rapid digitalization differ from gradual digitalization?
20. Why is it important to take a careful drug history for a patient receiving digoxin?

Web Activities

1. Go to the American Heart Association (AHA) Web site (www.heart.org) and conduct a search on heart failure.
   a. What are some lifestyle changes that you could recommend for a patient with heart failure to help them alleviate symptoms and improve their quality of life?
   b. Flu and pneumonia pose additional risks to patients with heart failure. What are some tips you could advise them to do to stay well?
2. Return to the AHA home page and click on the general topic of "What's New." Write a brief statement summarizing any new information on the topic of "Heart News."

SUMMARY DRUG TABLE Cardiotonics and Miscellaneous Inotropic Drugs (left, generic; right, trade)

Comprehensive Summary Drug Tables, including uses, adverses effects, dosages, and pregnancy classifications, are provided on the companion website, http://thePoint.lww.com/PharmacologyHP2e

Cardiotonics	
digoxin *di-jox'-in*	Lanoxin, *generic*
Miscellaneous Inotropic Drugs	
inamrinone lactate *in-am'-ri-none*	*generic*
milrinone lactate *mill'-ri-none*	*generic*
Antidote Digoxin Specific	
digoxin immune fab (ovine)	Digibind; DigiFab

19

Antiarrhythmic Drugs

CHAPTER OBJECTIVES

On completion of this chapter, students will be able to:

1. Define the chapter's key terms.
2. Identify common arrhythmias.
3. Describe the classes of antiarrhythmics.
4. Explain how the antiarrhythmics work.
5. Describe the uses and general drug actions for each class of antiarrhythmics.
6. Describe common adverse reactions of antiarrhythmics.
7. Describe common contraindications, precautions, and interactions of each class of antiarrhythmics.
8. Discuss important points to keep in mind when educating the patient or family members about the use of an antiarrhythmic drug.

KEY TERMS

action potential—an electrical impulse that passes from cell to cell in the myocardium, stimulating fibers to shorten and causing muscular contraction (systole)

arrhythmia—a disturbance or irregularity in the heart rate or rhythm, or both

blockade effect—the action of antiarrhythmic drugs blocking stimulation of β-receptors of the heart by adrenergic neurohormones

cinchonism—a term for quinidine toxicity characterized by ringing in the ears (tinnitus), hearing loss, headache, nausea, dizziness, vertigo, and light-headedness

depolarization—the movement of a stimulus passing along the nerve; the positive ions move from outside the cell into the cell, and the negative ions move from inside the cell to outside the cell

polarization—the point at which positive ions on the outside and negative ions on the inside of the cell membrane are in equilibrium

proarrhythmic effect—the development of a new arrhythmia or the worsening of an existing arrhythmia caused by an antiarrhythmic drug

refractory period—the period between transmissions of nerve impulses along a nerve fiber

repolarization—the movement back to the original state of positive and negative ions after a stimulus passes along the nerve fiber; the positive ions are on the outside and the negative ions on the inside of the nerve cell

CHAPTER OVERVIEW

Drug classes covered in this chapter are:

- Class I antiarrhythmic drugs
- Class II antiarrhythmic drugs
- Class III antiarrhythmic drugs
- Class IV antiarrhythmic drugs
- Miscellaneous drugs

Drugs by classification are listed on page 196.

thePOINT RESOURCES

- Comprehensive Summary Drug Tables
- Lippincott's Interactive Tutorials: Drugs Affecting the Cardiovascular System
- Interactive Practice and Review
- Monographs of Most Commonly Prescribed Drugs

Antiarrhythmic drugs are primarily used to treat cardiac arrhythmias. A cardiac **arrhythmia** is a disturbance or irregularity in the heart rate or rhythm, or both, which may require use of one of the antiarrhythmic drugs. Examples of cardiac arrhythmias are listed in Table 19-1.

An arrhythmia may occur as a result of heart disease or from a disorder that affects cardiovascular function. Conditions such as emotional stress, hypoxia, and electrolyte imbalance also may trigger an arrhythmia. An electrocardiogram (ECG) provides a record of the electrical activity of the heart. Careful interpretation of the ECG along with a thorough physical assessment is necessary to determine the cause and type of arrhythmia. The goal of antiarrhythmic drug therapy is to restore normal cardiac function and to prevent life-threatening arrhythmias.

Antiarrhythmic Drugs

Actions of Antiarrhythmic Drugs

Cardiac muscle (myocardium) has properties of both nerve and muscle. Some cardiac arrhythmias are caused by the generation of an abnormal number of electrical impulses (stimuli). Table 19-1 describes common types of arrhythmias. These abnormal impulses may come from the sinoatrial (SA) node or may be generated in other areas of the myocardium.

Antiarrhythmic drugs are classified according to their effects on the action potential of cardiac cells and their presumed mechanism of action. There are four basic classifications of antiarrhythmic drugs with several subclasses and a few miscellaneous antiarrhythmics. Drugs in each class have certain similarities, yet each drug has subtle differences that make it unique.

FACT CHECK

19-1   What is a cardiac arrhythmia?
19-2   What are the most common types of arrhythmias?
19-3   Which arrhythmia will result in death if not treated immediately? Why?

Class I Antiarrhythmic Drugs

Class I antiarrhythmic drugs, such as disopyramide, have a membrane-stabilizing or anesthetic effect on the cells of the myocardium. Class I antiarrhythmic drugs contain the largest number of drugs of the four classifications. Because the actions differ slightly, they are subdivided into classes I-A, I-B, and I-C.

Class I-A Drugs

The drugs quinidine, procainamide, and disopyramide are examples of class I-A drugs. Quinidine depresses myocardial excitability, which is the ability of the myocardium to respond to an electrical stimulus. Because the ability of the myocardium to respond to some but not all electrical stimuli is depressed, the pulse rate decreases and the arrhythmia is corrected. Quinidine also prolongs the refractory (resting) period and decreases the height and rate of the action potential of the impulses traveling through the myocardium.

All cells are electrically polarized, with the inside of the cell more negatively charged than the outside. The difference in electrical charge is called the resting membrane potential. Nerve and muscle cells are excitable, and the resting membrane potential can change in response to electrochemical stimuli. The **action potential** is an electrical impulse that passes from cell to cell in the myocardium, stimulating the fibers to shorten, causing muscular contraction (systole). After the action potential passes, the fibers relax and return to their resting length (diastole). An action potential generated in one part of the myocardium passes almost simultaneously through all of the fibers, causing rapid contraction.

Only one impulse can pass along a nerve fiber at any given time. After the passage of an impulse, there is a brief pause, or interval, before the next impulse can pass along the nerve fiber. This pause is called the **refractory period**, which is the period between the transmission of nerve impulses along a nerve fiber. When the refractory period is lengthened, the number of impulses traveling along a nerve fiber within a given time is decreased. For example, a patient has a pulse rate of 120 bpm. If the refractory period between each impulse is lengthened and the height and rate of the rise of action potential are decreased, then fewer impulses would be generated each minute, and the pulse rate would decrease. Procainamide is

---

TABLE 19-1   Common Types of Arrhythmias

Arrhythmia	Description
Atrial flutter	Rapid contraction of the atria (up to 300 bpm) at a rate too rapid for the ventricles to pump efficiently
Atrial fibrillation	Irregular and rapid atrial contraction, resulting in a quivering of the atria and causing an irregular and inefficient ventricular contraction
Premature ventricular contractions	Beats originating in the ventricles instead of the SA node in the atria, causing the ventricles to contract before the atria and resulting in a decrease in the amount of blood pumped to the body
Ventricular tachycardia	A rapid heartbeat with a rate of more than 100 bpm, usually originating in the ventricles
Ventricular fibrillation	Rapid disorganized contractions of the ventricles resulting in the inability of the heart to pump any blood to the body, which will result in death unless treated immediately

thought to act by decreasing the rate of diastolic depolarization in the ventricles, decreasing the rate and height of the action potential and increasing the fibrillation threshold. Disopyramide (Norpace) decreases the rate of depolarization of myocardial fibers during the diastolic phase of the cardiac cycle, prolongs the refractory period, and decreases the rate of rise of the action potential.

Nerve cells have positive ions on the outside and negative ions on the inside of the cell membrane when they are at rest (Fig. 19-1). This is called **polarization**. When a stimulus passes along the nerve, the positive ions move from outside the cell into the cell, and the negative ions move from inside the cell to outside the cell. This movement of ions is called **depolarization**. Unless positive ions move into and negative ions move out of a nerve cell, a stimulus (or impulse) cannot pass along the nerve fiber. Once the stimulus has passed along the nerve fiber, the positive and negative ions move back to their original place. This movement is called **repolarization**. When the rate of depolarization is decreased, the stimulus must literally wait for this process before it can pass along the nerve fiber. Decreasing the rate of depolarization therefore decreases the number of impulses that can pass along a nerve fiber during a specific time period.

Class I-B Drugs

Lidocaine (Xylocaine), the representative class I-B drug, raises the threshold in the ventricular myocardium. The threshold is the lowest-intensity stimulus that will cause a response in a nerve fiber. A stimulus must be of a specific intensity (strength, amplitude) to pass along a given nerve fiber (Fig. 19-2).

For example, let us say a certain nerve fiber has a threshold of 10. If a stimulus rated as 9 reaches the fiber, then it will not pass along the fiber because its intensity is lower than the fiber's threshold of 10. If a stimulus of 14 reaches the fiber,

however, then it will pass along the fiber because its intensity is greater than the fiber's threshold of 10. If the threshold of a fiber is raised from 10 to 15, then only those stimuli greater than 15 can pass along the nerve fiber.

Some cardiac arrhythmias result from too many stimuli present in the myocardium. Some of these are weak or of low intensity but are still able to excite myocardial tissue. Lidocaine, by raising the threshold of myocardial fibers, reduces the number of stimuli that can pass along these fibers and therefore decreases the pulse rate and corrects the arrhythmia. Mexiletine is another antiarrhythmic drug with actions similar to those of lidocaine.

Class 1-C Drugs

Flecainide (Tambocor) and propafenone (Rythmol) are examples of class I-C drugs. These drugs have a direct stabilizing action on the myocardium, decreasing the height and rate of rise of cardiac action potentials, thus slowing conduction in all parts of the heart.

Class II Antiarrhythmic Drugs

Class II antiarrhythmic drugs include β-adrenergic blocking drugs, such as acebutolol (Sectral), esmolol (Brevibloc), and propranolol. These drugs also decrease myocardial response to epinephrine and norepinephrine (adrenergic neurohormones) because of their ability to block stimulation of β-receptors of the heart (see Chapter 21). Adrenergic neurohormones stimulate the β-receptors of the myocardium and therefore increase the heart rate. Blocking the effect of these neurohormones decreases the heart rate. This is called a **blockade effect**.

Class III Antiarrhythmic Drugs

Amiodarone (Cordarone) appears to act directly on the cardiac cell membrane, prolonging the refractory period and

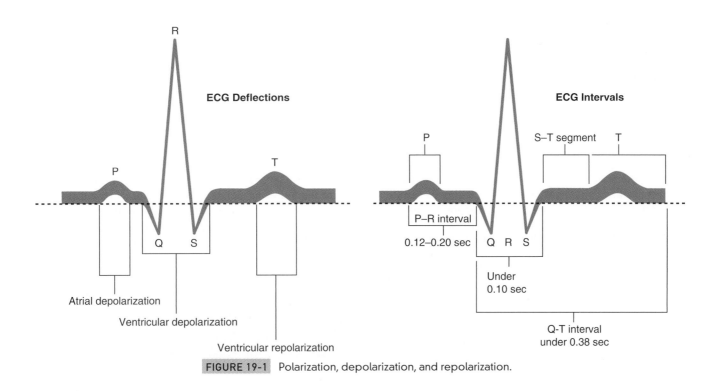

FIGURE 19-1 Polarization, depolarization, and repolarization.

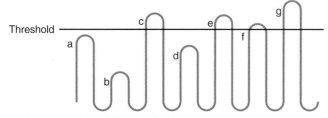

A stimulus must reach the threshold to cause a response in a nerve fiber. Note that stimuli **a**, **b**, and **d** do not reach the threshold; therefore, they do not cause a response in a nerve fiber. Stimuli **c**, **e**, **f**, and **g** do reach and surpass the threshold, resulting in stimulation of nerve fiber.

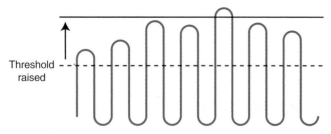

After receiving lidocaine hydrochloride (Xylocaine HCl), the threshold is raised to a higher level, allowing fewer stimuli to reach the threshold. This results in decreased stimulation of the nerve fiber and prevents conduction of the nerve impulses causing the arrthythmia.

FIGURE 19-2   The threshold phenomenon.

repolarization and increasing the ventricular fibrillation threshold. Other class III antiarrhythmic drugs include ibutilide (Corvert) and dofetilide (Tikosyn). These two drugs are used to convert atrial fibrillation or flutter to a normal sinus rhythm. Ibutilide acts by prolonging the action potential, producing a mild slowing of the sinus rate and atrioventricular (AV) conduction. Dofetilide selectively blocks potassium channels, widens the QRS complex, and prolongs the action potential. The drug has no effect on calcium channels or cardiac contraction. Another class III antiarrhythmic is sotalol, which blocks the β-receptors in the heart, causing a slowing of the heart rate and prolonging the action potential

Class IV Antiarrhythmic Drugs

Class IV antiarrhythmic drugs include verapamil (Calan) and the other calcium channel blockers. Calcium channel blockers produce their antiarrhythmic action by inhibiting the movement of calcium through channels across the myocardial cell membranes and vascular smooth muscle. Contraction of cardiac and vascular smooth muscle depends on the movement of calcium ions into these cells through specific ion channels. By reducing the calcium flow, conduction through the SA and AV nodes is slowed and the refractory period is prolonged, resulting in suppression of the arrhythmia. The calcium channel blockers are also called slow channel blockers or calcium antagonists. Two calcium channel blockers used as antiarrhythmics are verapamil and diltiazem.

Other Antiarrhythmic Drugs

In addition to the class I, II, III, and IV antiarrhythmics, several miscellaneous drugs are used for arrhythmias. These drugs include adenosine (Adenocard), dronedarone (Multaq), and digoxin (Lanoxin).

FACT CHECK

19-4   What are the classes and subclasses of antiarrhythmic drugs?
19-5   How do calcium channel blockers produce antiarrhythmic actions?

Uses of Antiarrhythmic Drugs

In general, antiarrhythmic drugs are used to prevent and treat cardiac arrhythmias such as premature ventricular contractions (PVCs), ventricular tachycardia (VT), premature atrial contractions, paroxysmal atrial tachycardia, atrial fibrillation, and atrial flutter. Some of the antiarrhythmic drugs are also used for other conditions. For example, propranolol may also be used for patients with myocardial infarction. This drug has reduced the risk of death and repeated myocardial infarctions in those surviving the acute phase of a myocardial infarction. Additional uses include control of tachycardia in those with pheochromocytoma (a tumor of the adrenal gland that secretes excessive amounts of norepinephrine), migraine headaches, angina pectoris caused by atherosclerosis, and hypertrophic subaortic stenosis.

Adverse Reactions of Antiarrhythmic Drugs

General adverse reactions common to most antiarrhythmic drugs include light-headedness, weakness, hypotension, bradycardia, and drowsiness. All antiarrhythmic drugs may cause new arrhythmias or worsen existing arrhythmias, even though they are administered to resolve an existing arrhythmia. This phenomenon is called the **proarrhythmic effect**. This effect ranges from an increase in frequency of PVCs, to the development of more severe VT, to ventricular fibrillation, and may lead to death. Proarrhythmic effects may occur at any time but occur more often if an excessive dosage is given, if the preexisting arrhythmia is life threatening, or if the drug is given IV.

The most common adverse reactions of quinidine include nausea, vomiting, abdominal pain, diarrhea, or anorexia. **Cinchonism** is the term used to describe quinidine toxicity, which occurs with high blood levels of quinidine. The occurrence of any of the following signs or symptoms of cinchonism must be reported: ringing in the ears (tinnitus), hearing loss, headache, nausea, dizziness, vertigo, and light-headedness. These symptoms may appear after a single dose of quinidine has been administered.

FACT CHECK

19-6   What are antiarrhythmic drugs generally used for?
19-7   What is the proarrhythmic effect?

Contraindications, Precautions, and Interactions of Antiarrhythmic Drugs

- Antiarrhythmic drugs are contraindicated in patients with a known hypersensitivity and during lactation.
- Antiarrhythmic drugs are contraindicated in patients with second- or third-degree AV block (if the patient has no artificial pacemaker), severe CHF, aortic stenosis, hypotension, or cardiogenic shock.
- Quinidine and procainamide are contraindicated in patients with myasthenia gravis (see Chapter 13).
- All antiarrhythmic drugs are used cautiously in patients with renal or hepatic disease. When renal or hepatic dysfunction is present, a dosage reduction may be necessary. All patients should be observed for renal and hepatic dysfunction.
- Quinidine and procainamide are used cautiously in patients with CHF.
- Disopyramide is used cautiously in patients with CHF, myasthenia gravis, or glaucoma and in men with prostate enlargement.
- Disopyramide, which has anticholinergic effects, may cause urinary retention. Urinary output is monitored closely, especially during the initial period of therapy. If a patient's fluid intake is sufficient but the output is low, then the lower abdomen is palpated for bladder distention. If urinary retention occurs, then catheterization may be necessary.
- During the first few weeks of disopyramide therapy, postural hypotension may occur. The patient is advised

to make position changes slowly. In some instances, a patient may require assistance in getting out of the bed or chair.
- Verapamil is used cautiously in patients with a history of serious ventricular arrhythmias or CHF. Electrolyte disturbances such as hypokalemia, hyperkalemia, or hypomagnesemia may alter the effects of antiarrhythmic drugs. The patient's electrolytes are monitored frequently and imbalances corrected as soon as possible.
- When two antiarrhythmic drugs are administered concurrently, the patient may experience additive effects and is at increased risk for drug toxicity.
- When quinidine and procainamide are administered with digitalis, the risk of digitalis toxicity is increased.
- The pharmacologic effects of procainamide may be increased when procainamide is administered with quinidine.
- When quinidine is administered with barbiturates or cimetidine, quinidine serum levels may be increased. When quinidine is administered with verapamil, the patient has an increased risk of hypotensive effects. When quinidine is administered with disopyramide, the patient has an increased risk of increased disopyramide blood levels and/or decreased serum quinidine levels.
- Propranolol may increase procainamide plasma levels.
- Additive cholinergic effects may occur when procainamide is administered with other drugs with anticholinergic effects. There is the potential for additive cardiodepressant effects when procainamide is administered with lidocaine.
- When a β-blocker, such as propranolol, is administered with lidocaine, the patient has an increased risk of lidocaine toxicity.
- Propranolol may alter the effectiveness of insulin or oral hypoglycemic drugs. Dosage adjustments may be necessary.
- Dofetilide is not administered with cimetidine because dofetilide plasma levels may be increased by as much as 50%. When treatment for gastric disorders is necessary, patients receiving dofetilide should take omeprazole, ranitidine, or antacids as an alternative to cimetidine.
- Verapamil may cause an additive hypotensive effect when administered with other antihypertensives, alcohol, or nitrates. Verapamil increases plasma digoxin levels and may cause bradycardia or CHF.

CONSIDERATIONS | Older adults

LIFESPAN

Adverse Reactions to Antiarrhythmic Drugs
When older adults take antiarrhythmic drugs, they are at greater risk for adverse reactions such as the development of additional arrhythmias or aggravation of existing arrhythmias, hypotension, and congestive heart failure (CHF). A dosage reduction may be indicated. Careful monitoring is necessary for early identification and management of adverse reactions. The health care provider monitors the intake and output and reports any signs of CHF, such as increase in weight, decrease in urinary output, or shortness of breath.

- Dronedarone should not be taken with grapefruit juice, but it should be taken with a meal.
- Dronedarone may have an additive effect when taken with β-blockers, calcium channel blockers, and class I and III antiarrhythmics.

Patient Management Issues with Antiarrhythmic Drugs

The health care provider performs initial preadministration assessments before starting therapy with any of the antiarrhythmic drugs. These assessments include taking blood pressure, pulse, and respiratory rates and assessing the patient's general condition.

It is important that each patient taking an antiarrhythmic drug be assessed with cardiac monitoring before therapy begins and thereafter to determine if the patient is experiencing a therapeutic response to the drug, developing another arrhythmia, or experiencing worsening of the original arrhythmia.

The health care provider may also order laboratory and diagnostic tests, renal and hepatic function tests, a complete blood count, serum enzymes, and serum electrolytes. An ECG may be performed to provide baseline data for comparison during therapy.

When interacting with a patient being treated for an arrhythmia, any significant changes should be reported immediately to the health care provider, including a change in blood pressure, pulse rate, or rhythm; respiratory difficulty; a change in respiratory rate or rhythm; or a change in the patient's general condition.

FACT CHECK

19-8   How does renal or hepatic dysfunction affect the dosage of an antiarrhythmic drug?

19-9   Which electrolyte disturbances may alter the effects of antiarrhythmic drugs?

19-10 What significant changes in a patient's condition should be reported to the health care provider?

Educating the Patient and Family about Antiarrhythmic Drugs

The adverse drug effects that may occur with use of the antiarrhythmic drug are explained to the patient and family. To ensure compliance with the prescribed drug regimen, the importance of taking these drugs exactly as prescribed is emphasized. It may be necessary to teach patients or their family members how to take their pulse rate. The patient is advised to report any changes in the pulse rate or rhythm to the health care provider. Key Concepts 19-1 reviews self-monitoring of the pulse rate with antiarrhythmic therapy.

Following are key points about antiarrhythmic drugs that the patient and family should know:

- Take the drug at the prescribed intervals. Do not omit a dose or increase or decrease the dose unless advised to do so by your health care provider. Do not stop taking the drug unless advised to do so by your health care provider.
- Do not take any nonprescription drug unless your health care provider has approved it.
- Do not drink alcoholic beverages or smoke unless these have been approved by your health care provider.
- Follow the directions on the drug label, such as taking the drug with food or swallowing whole.
- Do not attempt to drive or perform hazardous tasks if you feel light-headed or dizzy.
- If you experience dry mouth, then take frequent sips of water, allow ice chips to dissolve in your mouth, or chew (sugar-free) gum.
- Remember that the wax matrix of sustained-release tablets of procainamide is not absorbed by the body and may be seen in the stool. This is normal.
- Keep all appointments with your health care provider, clinic, or laboratory because your therapy needs to be closely monitored.

KEY CONCEPTS

19-1   Self-Monitoring Pulse Rate with Antiarrhythmic Therapy

The health care provider:

- Explains the purpose of self-monitoring of pulse rate when receiving antiarrhythmic therapy
- Instructs the patient about the importance of drug therapy and taking drug exactly as prescribed
- Provides written instruction for monitoring pulse rate (see Key Concepts Box 18-1: Monitoring Pulse Rate)
- Encourages self-monitoring before each dose
- Reviews acceptable pulse rate ranges for taking the drug, both verbally and in writing
- Encourages recording of pulse rates in a log
- Emphasizes need to notify the health care provider should the pulse rate fall outside acceptable range or the rhythm changes
- Reassures the patient that results of therapy will be monitored by periodic laboratory and diagnostic tests and follow-up visits with the health care provider
- Assists with arrangements for follow-up as necessary

Chapter Review

KEY POINTS

- Antiarrhythmic drugs are primarily used to treat cardiac arrhythmias. An arrhythmia may occur as a result of heart disease or from a disorder that affects cardiovascular function. Conditions such as emotional stress, hypoxia, and electrolyte imbalance also may trigger an arrhythmia.
- Class I antiarrhythmic drugs have a membrane-stabilizing or anesthetic effect on the cells of the myocardium, making them valuable in treating cardiac arrhythmias.
- Class II antiarrhythmic drugs include β-adrenergic blocking drugs, such as acebutolol (Sectral), esmolol (Brevibloc), and propranolol, which also decrease myocardial response to epinephrine and norepinephrine (adrenergic neurohormones) by their ability to block stimulation of β-receptors of the heart
- Class III antiarrhythmic drugs have different mechanisms of action. Amiodarone, dofetilide, ibutilide, and sotalol are all class III antiarrhythmics.
- Class IV antiarrhythmic drugs are calcium channel blockers and include verapamil and diltiazem.
- The miscellaneous antiarrhythmic drugs are adenosine, dronedarone, and digoxin.
- General adverse reactions common to most antiarrhythmic drugs include light-headedness, weakness, hypotension, bradycardia, and drowsiness.

CRITICAL THINKING CASE STUDY

Atrial Fibrillation

Mr. Russell is admitted to the hospital for an atrial fibrillation.

1. Upon discharge, he is prescribed quinidine gluconate. What class of antiarrhythmic is quinidine gluconate?
   a. Class I
   b. Class II
   c. Class III
   d. Class IV
2. You see Mr. Russell 2 weeks after discharge and he is complaining about his hearing. You ask him to describe his hearing problems and he describes a ringing in his ears. What is this called?
3. What should you tell Mr. Russell?
   a. The ringing is a normal adverse effect associated with quinidine, and it will go away over time.
   b. The ringing is a normal adverse effect associated with quinidine, but he should probably contact his physician.
   c. The ringing is a sign of quinidine toxicity and the health care provider should be notified immediately.
   d. The ringing is a sign of quinidine toxicity and he should stop taking the medication.
4. Are there other antiarrhythmics in the same class that do not have this as a side effect? If so, which ones?

Review Questions

MULTIPLE CHOICE

1. All of the following are true about premature ventricular contractions EXCEPT
   a. cause the ventricles to contract before the atria
   b. result in decreased amount of blood pumped to the body
   c. originate in the ventricles
   d. originate in the atria
2. Class II antiarrhythmic drugs include
   a. α-adrenergic blocking drugs
   b. β-adrenergic blocking drugs
   c. calcium channel blocking drugs
   d. none of the above
3. The blockade effect is produced by
   a. class I antiarrhythmic drugs
   b. class II antiarrhythmic drugs
   c. class III antiarrhythmic drugs
   d. class IV antiarrhythmic drugs
4. Patients taking antiarrhythmic drugs may need to be instructed on how to monitor
   a. blood pressure
   b. temperature
   c. pulse rate
   d. all of the above

MATCHING

_____ 5. acebutolol   a. Corvert
_____ 6. adenosine   b. Betapace
_____ 7. amiodarone   c. Sectral
_____ 8. dofetilide   d. Cordarone
_____ 9. esmolol   e. Rythmol
_____ 10. ibutilide   f. Tikosyn
_____ 11. propafenone   g. Adenocard
_____ 12. sotalol   h. Brevibloc

TRUE OR FALSE

_____ 13. An arrhythmia can be triggered by emotional stress, hypoxia, and electrolyte imbalance.
_____ 14. Ventricular fibrillation is a rapid heartbeat with a rate of more than 100 bpm, usually originating in the ventricles.
_____ 15. Antiarrhythmic drugs are not used for patients with myocardial infarction.
_____ 16. All antiarrhythmic drugs may cause new arrhythmias or worsen existing arrhythmias.

FILL IN THE BLANKS

17. _____ is an irregular and rapid atrial contraction, resulting in a quivering of the atria and causing irregular ventricular contraction.
18. Calcium channel blockers are also called _____ or _____.

19. All antiarrhythmic drugs are used with caution in patients with _____ or _____ disease.

20. When two antiarrhythmic drugs are administered concurrently, the patient may experience _____ _____ and is at increased risk for _____ _____.

21. _____ is a miscellaneous antiarrhythmic used intravenously to treat paroxysmal supraventricular tachycardia.

SHORT ANSWERS

22. What are the goals of antiarrhythmic drug therapy?
23. How are antiarrhythmic drugs classified?
24. Although proarrhythmic effects may occur at any time during therapy, under what circumstances are they most likely to occur?
25. What is the blockade effect?

Web Activities

1. Go to the Mayo Clinic Web site (www.mayoclinic.org) and conduct a search on heart arrhythmias.
   a. What are risk factors for developing an arrhythmia?
   b. What are some lifestyle changes that a patient can make to keep the heart healthy?
2. Go to the National Heart, Lung, and Blood Institute Web site (www.nhlbi.nih.gov) and conduct a search for arrhythmia.
   a. What are some tips for patients with arrhythmias as it relates to ongoing care?
   b. What are some key points about arrhythmias?

SUMMARY DRUG TABLE Antiarrhythmic Drugs
(left, generic; right, trade)

Comprehensive Summary Drug Tables, including uses, adverses effects, dosages, and pregnancy classifications, are provided on the companion website, http://thePoint.lww.com/PharmacologyHP2e

Class I	
disopyramide *dye-soe-peer'-a-mide*	Norpace, Norpace CR, *generic*
flecainide *fle-kay'-nide*	Tambocor, *generic*
lidocaine HCl *lye'-doe-kane*	Xylocaine, Xylocaine MPF, *generic*
mexiletine HCl *max-ill'-i-teen*	*generic*
procainamide HCl *proe-kane-a'-mide*	*generic*
propafenone HCl *proe-pa'9-a-non*	Rythmol, Rhythmol SR, *generic*
quinidine gluconate *kwin'-i-deen*	*generic*
quinidine sulfate *kwin'-i-deen*	*generic, generic CR*

Class II	
acebutolol *ah-see-byoo'-toe-lol*	Sectral, *generic*
esmolol HCl(*ez'-moe-lol*	Brevibloc, Brevibloc Double Strength, *generic*
propranolol *proe-pran'-oh-lole*	*generic*

Class III	
amiodarone *a-mee'-oh-da-rone*	Cordarone, Pacerone, *generic*
dofetilide *doe-fet'-il-ide*	Tikosyn
ibutilide *i-byoo'-ti-lide*	Corvert, *generic*
sotalol *soe'-ta-lole*	Betapace, Betapace AF, Sorine, *generic*

Class IV	
verapamil *ver-ap'-a-mil*	Calan, Calan SR, Covera-HS, Isoptin SR, Verelan, Verelan PM, *generic*
diltiazem *dil-tye'-a-zem*	

Miscellaneous Antiarrhythmics	
adenosine *a-den'-oh-seen*	Adenocard, Adenoscan, *generic*
dronedarone *droe-nab'-i-nol*	Multaq
digoxin *di-joks'-in*	Lanoxin, *generic*

20

Antianginal and Peripheral Vasodilating Drugs

CHAPTER OBJECTIVES

On completion of this chapter, students will be able to:

1. Define the chapter's key terms.
2. Describe the actions, uses, and common adverse reactions of nitrates.
3. Discuss patient management issues with nitrates.
4. Describe the actions, uses, and common adverse reactions of calcium channel blockers.
5. Discuss patient management issues with calcium channel blockers.
6. Discuss important points to keep in mind when educating patients and their families about the use of antianginal drugs.
7. Describe the actions, uses, and common adverse reactions of peripheral vasodilating drugs.
8. Discuss important points to keep in mind when educating patients and their families about the use of peripheral vasodilating drugs.

KEY TERMS

angina—a disorder often caused by atherosclerotic plaque formation in the coronary arteries, which causes decreased oxygen supply to the heart muscle and results in chest pain or pressure

atherosclerosis—a disease characterized by deposits of fatty plaques on the inner wall of arteries

intermittent claudication—a group of symptoms characterized by pain in the calf muscle of one or both legs, caused by walking and relieved by rest

lumen—the inside diameter of a vessel such as an artery

prophylaxis—prevention

transdermal system—a convenient form of drug administration in which the drug is impregnated in a pad and absorbed through the skin

vasodilation—an increase in the size of blood vessels, primarily small arteries and arterioles

CHAPTER OVERVIEW

Drug classes covered in this chapter are:

- Antianginal drugs
- Peripheral vasodilating drugs

Drugs by classification are listed on page 206.

thePOINT RESOURCES

- Comprehensive Summary Drug Tables
- Animations: Myocardial Blood Flow
- Lippincott's Interactive Tutorials: Drugs Affecting the Cardiovascular System
- Interactive Practice and Review
- Monographs of Most Commonly Prescribed Drugs

Diseases of the arteries can cause serious problems such as coronary artery disease, cerebral vascular disease, and peripheral vascular disease. Drug therapy for vascular diseases may include drugs that dilate blood vessels and thereby increase blood supply to an area.

Atherosclerosis is a disease characterized by deposits of fatty plaques on the inner wall of arteries. These deposits result in a narrowing of the **lumen** (inside diameter) of the artery and a decrease in blood supply to the area served by the artery (Fig. 20-1).

This chapter discusses two different types of drugs whose primary purpose is to increase blood supply to an area by dilating blood vessels: the antianginal and peripheral vasodilating drugs. Vasodilating drugs relax the smooth muscle layer of arterial blood vessels, which results in **vasodilation,** an increase in the size of blood vessels, primarily small arteries and arterioles. Because peripheral, cerebral, or coronary artery disease usually results in decreased blood flow to an area, drugs that dilate narrowed arterial blood vessels will increase the blood flow to the affected area. Increasing the blood flow to an area may result in complete or partial relief of symptoms. Vasodilating drugs sometimes relieve the symptoms of vascular disease, but in some cases, drug therapy provides only minimal and temporary relief. Many vasodilating drugs are also used to treat hypertension. Their use as antihypertensives is discussed in Chapter 21.

Antianginal Drugs

Angina is a disorder often caused by atherosclerotic plaque formation in the coronary arteries, which causes a decrease in the oxygen supply to the heart muscle and results in chest pain or pressure. Any activity that increases the workload of the heart, such as exercise or simply climbing stairs, can precipitate an angina attack. Antianginal drugs relieve chest pain or pressure by dilating the coronary arteries and increasing the blood supply to the myocardium. Figure 20-2 summarizes how various classes of antianginal drugs work.

Antianginal drugs include the nitrates and calcium channel blockers. Chapter 12 discusses adrenergic blocking drugs, which are also used to treat angina and other disorders.

FACT CHECK
20-1   How do antianginal drugs relieve chest pain?
20-2   Antianginal drugs include which two drugs classes?

NITRATES

Actions of Nitrates

The nitrates, such as isosorbide and nitroglycerin, have a direct relaxing effect on the smooth muscle layer of blood vessels. This increases the lumen of the artery or arteriole and increases the amount of blood flowing through these vessels. An increased blood flow results in an increased oxygen supply.

Uses of Nitrates

The nitrates are used to treat angina pectoris. Some of these drugs, such as isosorbide dinitrate (Isordil), are used for **prophylaxis** (prevention) and long-term treatment of angina, whereas others, such as sublingual nitroglycerin (Nitrostat), are used to relieve the pain of acute anginal attacks when they occur. Intravenous (IV) nitroglycerin is also used to control perioperative hypertension associated with surgical procedures.

Adverse Reactions of Nitrates

The nitrate antianginal drugs all have the same adverse reactions, although the intensity of some reactions may vary with the drug and the dose. A common adverse reaction is headache, especially early in therapy. Hypotension, dizziness, vertigo, and weakness may also occur. Flushing caused by dilation of small capillaries near the surface of the skin may also occur.

The nitrates are available in various forms, including sublingual and translingual forms. Some adverse reactions

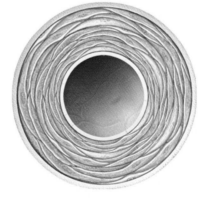
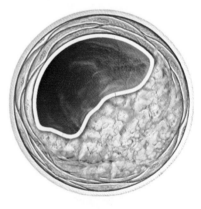

Normal vessel   Arteriosclerosis   Atherosclerosis

FIGURE 20-1   Schematic illustration of a plaque in atherosclerosis.

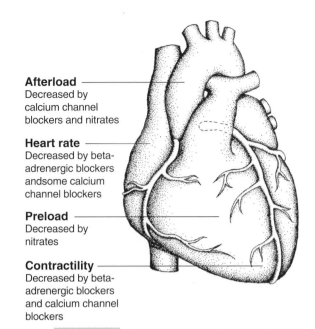

Afterload
Decreased by calcium channel blockers and nitrates

Heart rate
Decreased by beta-adrenergic blockers and some calcium channel blockers

Preload
Decreased by nitrates

Contractility
Decreased by beta-adrenergic blockers and calcium channel blockers

FIGURE 20-2   How antianginal drugs work.

result from the method of administration. For example, sublingual nitroglycerin may cause a local burning or tingling in the mouth. However, a patient must be aware that an absence of this effect does not indicate a decrease in the drug's potency. Contact dermatitis may occur from use of the transdermal delivery system.

In many instances, the adverse reactions associated with the nitrates lessen and often disappear with continued use of the drug. However, for some patients, these adverse reactions become severe, and the health care provider may lower the dose until symptoms subside. The dose may then be slowly increased if the lower dosage does not provide relief from the symptoms of angina.

FACT CHECK

20-3   What are nitrates used to treat?
20-4   What are the common adverse reactions of nitrates?

Contraindications, Precautions, and Interactions of Nitrates

- The nitrates are contraindicated in patients with a known hypersensitivity, severe anemia, closed-angle glaucoma, postural hypertension, cerebral hemorrhage, allergy to adhesive (transdermal system), or constrictive pericarditis.
- The nitrates are used cautiously in patients with severe hepatic or renal disease, severe head trauma, acute myocardial infarction, or hypothyroidism, and during lactation.
- If the nitrates are administered with the antihypertensives, alcohol, calcium channel blockers, or the phenothiazines, then there may be an increased hypotensive effect.

- When nitroglycerin is administered intravenously, the effects of heparin may be decreased. Increased nitrate serum concentrations may occur when the nitrates are administered with aspirin.

Patient Management Issues with Nitrates

Patients using nitrates are monitored for the frequency and severity of any episodes of angina pain. With treatment, episodes of angina should be eliminated or decrease in frequency and severity. Any chest pain that does not respond to three doses of nitroglycerin given every 5 minutes for 15 minutes should be reported to the health care provider.

The nitrates may be administered by the sublingual (under the tongue), buccal (between the cheek and gum), oral, IV, topical, or transdermal route. Absorption of sublingual and buccal forms depends on saliva. Dry mouth decreases absorption. For some individuals, the spray is more convenient than the small tablets placed under the tongue. The spray, however, should not be inhaled; the spray is directed from the canister onto or under the tongue.

Educating the Patient and Family about Nitrates

The patient and family must have a thorough understanding of the treatment of chest pain with an antianginal drug. These drugs are used either to prevent angina from occurring or to relieve the pain of angina. The therapeutic regimen (dose, time of day the drug is taken, how often to take the drug, how to take or apply the drug) is explained to the patient. Following are key points about nitrates that the patient or family should know.

- Do not drink alcohol unless it is permitted by your health care provider.
- Notify your health care provider if the drug does not relieve pain or if pain becomes more intense despite use of this drug.

ALERT ℞

Sublingual Nitroglycerin Doses

Nitroglycerin may also be administered by a metered spray canister that is used to abort an acute anginal attack. The canister meters each dose, delivering the same dose each time the canister top is depressed. The dose of sublingual nitroglycerin may be repeated every 5 minutes until pain is relieved or until the patient has received three doses in a 15-minute period.

The health care provider should be notified if a patient frequently has anginal pain, if the pain worsens, or if the pain is not relieved after three doses within a 15-minute period. A change in the dosage of the drug or other treatment may be necessary.

Nitroglycerin may also be administered in topical (ointment) form. The ointment is usually applied to the chest or back. Application sites are rotated to prevent inflammation of the skin. Areas that may be used for application include the chest (front and back), abdomen, and upper arms and legs.

ALERT Rx

Application of Nitroglycerin Ointment

Nitroglycerin ointment *must not* be rubbed into a patient's skin because this will immediately deliver a large amount of the drug through the skin. Care must be exercised in applying topical nitroglycerin. The ointment must not come in contact with the fingers or hands of the person applying the ointment, because the drug will be absorbed through his or her skin.

For many patients, nitroglycerin *transdermal systems* are convenient and easier to use because the drug is absorbed through the skin. In transdermal systems, the drug is impregnated in a pad. The pad is applied to the skin once per day for 10 to 14 hours.

Tolerance to the vascular and anginal effects of nitrates may develop, particularly in patients taking high dosages, those prescribed longer-acting products, and those on frequent dosing schedules. Patients using transdermal nitroglycerin patches are particularly prone to tolerance because the nitroglycerin is released at a constant rate, maintaining steady plasma concentrations.

Nitroglycerin is also available as oral tablets to be swallowed. The patient should take it on an empty stomach unless the health care provider orders otherwise. If the patient experiences nausea, then the health care provider should be notified. Taking the tablet or capsule with food may be ordered to relieve nausea. The sustained-release preparation must be swallowed, not crushed or chewed.

Because of the risk of developing tolerance to oral nitrates, the health care provider may prescribe a short-acting preparation two or three times daily or a sustained-release preparation once or twice daily.

Nitroglycerin is also available in IV form, administered by a health care provider.

- Keep an adequate supply of the drug on hand for situations such as vacations, bad weather conditions, and holidays.
- Keep a record of the frequency of acute anginal attacks (date, time of the attack, drug, and dose used to relieve the acute pain) and bring this record to each health care provider visit.

Nitrates

- Headache is a common adverse reaction but should decrease with continued therapy. If headache persists or becomes severe, then notify your health care provider because a change in dosage may be needed. Headache may be a marker of the drug's effectiveness. Do not try to avoid headaches by altering your treatment schedule because loss of headache may be associated with simultaneous loss of drug effectiveness. You may use aspirin or acetaminophen for headache relief.
- Do not change from one brand of nitrates to another without consulting your pharmacist or health care provider. Products manufactured by different companies may not be equally effective.

Oral nitrates

- When taking nitroglycerin for an acute attack of angina, sit or lie down. To relieve severe light-headedness or dizziness, lie down, elevate and move your extremities, and breathe deeply.
- Keep capsules and tablets in their original containers because nitroglycerin must be kept in a dark container and protected from exposure to light. Never mix this drug with any other drug in a container. Nitroglycerin will lose its potency in containers made of plastic or if mixed with other drugs.
- Always replace the cover or cap of the container as soon as the oral drug or ointment is removed from the container or tube. Replace caps or covers tightly because the drug deteriorates on contact with air.
- If your chest pain persists, changes character, increases in severity, or is not relieved by following the recommended dosing regimen, then seek prompt medical attention.

Sublingual or buccal administration

- Do not handle sublingual tablets any more than necessary.
- Check the expiration date on the container of sublingual tablets. If the expiration date has passed, then do not use the tablets. Instead, purchase a new supply. Unused tablets should be discarded 6 months after the original bottle is opened.
- Keep capsules and tablets in their original containers because nitroglycerin must be kept in a dark container and protected from exposure to light.
- Do not swallow or chew sublingual or transmucosal tablets; allow them to dissolve slowly. The tablet may cause a burning or tingling in your mouth, but the absence of this effect does not indicate a decrease in potency. Older adults are less likely to have this burning or tingling sensation.

Translingual/transmucosal

- The directions for use of translingual nitroglycerin are supplied with the product. Follow the instructions regarding using and cleaning the canister.
- This drug may be used prophylactically 5 to 10 minutes before engaging in activities that precipitate an attack.
- When using the transmucosal form, insert the tablet between the lip and gum above the incisors or between the cheek and gum.

Topical ointment or transdermal system

- Instructions for application of the topical ointment or transdermal system are provided with the product. Read these instructions carefully.
- Apply the topical ointment or transdermal system at approximately the same time each day.
- Be sure the area is clean and thoroughly dry before applying the topical ointment or transdermal system and rotate the application sites. Firmly press the patch to ensure contact with the skin. If the transdermal system comes off or becomes loose, then apply a new system.
- When using the topical ointment form or transdermal system, cleanse old application sites with soap and warm water as soon as the ointment or transdermal system is removed.

- To use the topical ointment, apply a thin layer on the skin using the paper applicator (you may need instructions regarding this technique). Do not touch the ointment with your fingers.
- Wash your hands before and after applying the ointment.

FACT CHECK

20-5 There may be increased hypotensive effects when nitrates are administered with which other drugs?

20-6 Why is it important for the person applying nitroglycerin ointment to avoid contact with the fingers or hands?

CALCIUM CHANNEL BLOCKERS

Actions of Calcium Channel Blockers

Systemic and coronary arteries are influenced by the movement of calcium across cell membranes of vascular smooth muscle. The contractions of cardiac and vascular smooth muscle depend on the movement of extracellular calcium ions through specific ion channels. Calcium channel blockers, such as amlodipine (Norvasc), diltiazem (Cardizem), nicardipine (Cardene), nifedipine (Procardia), and verapamil (Calan), inhibit the movement of calcium ions across cell membranes (Fig. 20-3). This results in less calcium

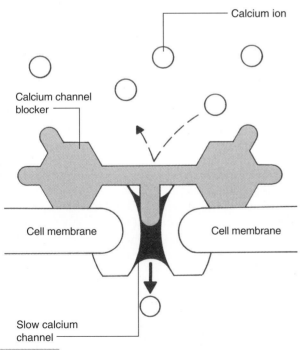

FIGURE 20-3 Calcium channel blockers work by inhibiting the movement of calcium ions across the cell membrane.

available for the transmission of nerve impulses. This drug action of the calcium channel blockers (also known as slow channel blockers) has several effects on the heart, including an effect on the smooth muscle of arteries and arterioles. These drugs dilate coronary arteries and arterioles, which in turn deliver more oxygen to cardiac muscle. Dilation of peripheral arteries reduces the workload of the heart. The end effect of these drug actions is the same as that of the nitrates.

Uses of Calcium Channel Blockers

Calcium channel blockers are primarily used to prevent anginal pain associated with certain forms of angina, such as vasospastic (Prinzmetal variant) angina and chronic stable angina. They are not used to stop anginal pain once it has occurred. When angina is caused by coronary artery spasm, these drugs are recommended when the patient cannot tolerate therapy with beta-adrenergic blocking drugs (see Chapter XX) or the nitrates. Calcium channel blockers used as antianginals are listed in the Summary Drug Table: Antianginal Drugs. Some calcium channel blocking drugs have additional uses. Verapamil affects the conduction system of the heart and may be used to treat cardiac arrhythmias. Diltiazem, nicardipine, nifedipine, and verapamil also are used in the treatment of essential hypertension (see Chapter 21).

Adverse Reactions of Calcium Channel Blockers

Adverse reactions to the calcium channel blocking drugs usually are not serious and rarely require discontinuation of the drug therapy. The more common adverse reactions include dizziness, light-headedness, nausea, diarrhea, constipation, peripheral edema, headache, bradycardia, flushing, dermatitis, skin rash, and nervousness.

When the drug regimen for angina pectoris is terminated, the drug dosage is gradually reduced to prevent withdrawal reactions. Abrupt withdrawal of a calcium channel blocker may cause an increase in chest pain. This phenomenon is called rebound angina and is most likely the result of the increased flow of calcium into cells, causing the coronary arteries to spasm. Therefore, calcium channel blockers are gradually withdrawn rather than discontinued abruptly.

ALERT ℞

Antianginal Drugs and Postural Hypotension

Patients having episodes of postural hypotension need help walking and with other activities. Patients experiencing episodes of postural hypotension are instructed to take the drug in a sitting or supine position and to remain in that position until symptoms disappear. Hypotension may be accompanied by paradoxical bradycardia and increased angina pectoris.

Contraindications, Precautions, and Interactions of Calcium Channel Blockers

- Calcium channel blockers are contraindicated in patients who are hypersensitive to them and in those with sick sinus syndrome, second-degree or third-degree AV block (except with a functioning pacemaker), hypotension (systolic pressure less than 90 mm Hg), ventricular dysfunction, or cardiogenic shock.
- Calcium channel blockers are used cautiously during lactation and in patients with congestive heart failure (CHF), hypotension, or renal or hepatic impairment.
- The effects of the calcium channel blockers are increased when administered with cimetidine or ranitidine.
- A decrease in effectiveness of the calcium channel blockers may occur when the agents are administered with phenobarbital or phenytoin.
- Calcium channel blockers have an antiplatelet effect (inhibition of platelet function) when administered with aspirin, causing easy bruising, petechiae (pinpoint purple–red spot caused by intradermal hemorrhage), and bleeding.
- An additive depressive effect on the myocardium occurs when a calcium channel blocker is administered with a beta-adrenergic blocking drug.
- When a calcium channel blocker is administered with digoxin, the patient has an increased risk for digitalis toxicity.

Patient Management Issues with Calcium Channel Blockers

Patients receiving calcium channel blockers should be monitored for signs of CHF, such as dyspnea, weight gain, peripheral edema, abnormal lung sounds (crackles or rales), and jugular vein distention. Any symptoms of CHF should be reported immediately to the health care provider.

With a few exceptions, calcium channel blockers may be taken without regard to meals. If gastrointestinal upset occurs, then the drug may be taken with meals. Verapamil frequently causes gastric upset and is routinely given with meals.

The calcium channel blockers are available in a variety of dosage forms. Some of the tablets may be crushed and mixed with food or liquids. However, the sustained-release tablets must be swallowed whole and should not be chewed or crushed. Some come in sustained-release forms in which

the tablet matrix is expelled in the stool. When nifedipine is ordered sublingually, the capsule is punctured with a sterile needle and the liquid squeezed under the tongue or in the buccal pouch.

Educating the Patient and Family about Calcium Channel Blockers

The patient and family members need a thorough understanding of how chest pain is treated with an antianginal drug. These drugs are used either to prevent angina from occurring or to relieve the pain of angina. The therapeutic regimen (dose, time of day the drug is taken, how often to take the drug, how to take or apply the drug) is explained to the patient. Following are key points about calcium channel blockers that the patient or family members should know.

- Do not chew or divide sustained-release tablets. Swallow them whole.
- Notify your health care provider if you experience any of the following: increased severity of chest pain or discomfort, irregular heartbeat, palpitations, nausea, shortness of breath, swelling of your hands or feet, or severe and prolonged episodes of light-headedness and dizziness.
- Make position changes slowly to minimize hypotensive effects.
- These drugs can cause dizziness or drowsiness. Do not drive or engage in hazardous activities until you know how you will respond to the drug.

FACT CHECK

20-7 How do calcium channel blockers act?
20-8 What are the primary uses of calcium channel blockers?

Peripheral Vasodilating Drugs

In contrast to antianginal drugs, which are used primarily for angina, the peripheral vasodilating drugs are given for disorders that affect blood vessels of the extremities. Unfortunately, although these drugs increase blood flow to nonischemic areas (areas with adequate blood flow), there is no conclusive evidence that blood flow is increased in ischemic areas (areas that lack adequate blood flow) that are in critical need of improved perfusion. Because of the lack of evidence of the effectiveness of the peripheral vasodilating drugs, most are labeled as "possibly effective" in the treatment of peripheral vascular disorders. These drugs are not as widely used now as they were in the past. Many peripheral dilating drugs are used for hypertension and are discussed in Chapter 21.

Actions of Peripheral Vasodilating Drugs

Peripheral vasodilating drugs, such as isoxsuprine, act on the smooth muscle layers of peripheral blood vessels, primarily by blocking alpha-adrenergic nerves and stimulating beta-adrenergic nerves. For a review of the effect of stimulation and blocking effects on adrenergic nerve fibers, see Chapters 11 and 12. Cilostazol (Pletal) inhibits platelet aggregation and dilates vascular beds, particularly in the femoral area. The exact mechanism of action is unknown.

Uses of Peripheral Vasodilating Drugs

Peripheral vasodilating drugs are chiefly used in the treatment of peripheral vascular diseases, such as Raynaud phenomenon. Short-term use is rarely beneficial or permanent. Improvement, if it occurs, takes place gradually during weeks of therapy.

The peripheral vasodilating drugs also have other uses, such as the relief of symptoms associated with cerebral vascular insufficiency. Some of these drugs are used for hypertension and will be discussed in Chapter 21.

Intermittent claudication is a group of symptoms characterized by pain in the calf muscle of one or both legs, caused by walking and relieved by rest. It is a manifestation of peripheral vascular disease, in which atherosclerotic lesions develop in the femoral artery, diminishing blood supply to the lower leg. Cilostazol (Pletal) is a phosphodiesterase II inhibitor (a drug that inhibits platelet aggregation and dilates vascular beds, particularly in the femoral area) used for the symptoms of intermittent claudication. This drug increases the walking distance possible in those with intermittent claudication. This drug is listed under Miscellaneous Drugs in the Summary Drug Table: Peripheral Vasodilators and Miscellaneous Vasodilating Drugs.

Adverse Reactions of Peripheral Vasodilating Drugs

Adverse reactions associated with these drugs are variable. Because these drugs dilate peripheral arteries, they may cause some degree of hypotension. They also cause a physiologic increase in the pulse rate (tachycardia). Some of these drugs also cause flushing of the skin, which can range from mild to moderately severe. Nausea, vomiting, flushing, headache, and dizziness may also occur with the use of these drugs.

Contraindications, Precautions, and Interactions of Peripheral Vasodilating Drugs

- The peripheral vasodilating drugs are contraindicated in patients with a known hypersensitivity, in women in the immediate postpartum period (isoxsuprine causes uterine relaxation), and in patients with arterial bleeding.
- These drugs are used cautiously in patients with bleeding tendencies, severe cerebrovascular or cardiovascular disease, or recent myocardial infarction.
- There are no significant drug–drug interactions.

Patient Management Issues with Peripheral Vasodilating Drugs

Therapeutic results may not occur immediately from the peripheral vasodilating drug. In some instances, results are minimal. The patient's involved extremities are assessed daily for changes in color and temperature, and the patient's comments regarding relief from pain or discomfort are recorded. Blood pressure and pulse should be monitored once or twice per day because these drugs may cause a decrease in blood pressure. The anticipated result of therapy for cerebral vascular disease is an improvement in the patient's mental status. When the drug is taken for intermittent claudication, a patient is assessed for increased walking distance without pain.

These drugs are often prescribed for outpatients. Positive results of therapy for a peripheral vascular disorder may include a decrease in pain, discomfort, and cramping; increased warmth in the extremities; and stronger peripheral pulses. Patients taking these drugs for relief of symptoms of peripheral vascular disorders often become discouraged about the lack of effectiveness of drug therapy. A patient may need to be encouraged to continue with the prescribed drug regimen and to follow the health care provider's recommendations regarding additional methods of treating the disorder. The patient is reminded that although signs of improvement may be rapid, improvement usually occurs slowly over many weeks. A patient's affected areas are examined at each visit to the health care provider's office, and the findings are recorded in a patient's record.

Educating the Patient and Family about Peripheral Vasodilating Drugs

To ensure compliance to the drug regimen, the patient and family members must understand that improvement will likely be gradual, although some improvement may be noted in a few days. The patient is encouraged to continue with drug therapy and to follow the health care provider's recommendations regarding care of the affected extremities even if improvement is slow. Following are key points about peripheral vasodilating drugs that patients and family members should know.

- If you experience nausea, vomiting, or diarrhea, then contact your health care provider. These drugs may also cause flushing, sweating, headache, tiredness, jaundice, skin rash, anorexia, and abdominal distress. Notify your health care provider if these effects become pronounced.
- Dizziness may occur. Avoid driving and other potentially dangerous tasks, as well as making sudden position changes. Dangle your legs over the side of the bed for a few minutes when getting up in the morning or after lying down. If dizziness persists, then contact your health care provider.
- Be careful when walking up or down stairs or when walking on ice, snow, a slick pavement, or slippery floors.

- Stop smoking.
- For peripheral vascular disease, follow your health care provider's recommendations regarding exercise, avoiding exposure to cold, keeping the extremities warm, and avoiding injury to the extremities.
- The therapeutic effects of drugs for peripheral vascular disease may not occur for 2 weeks and may take up to 12 weeks.
- Take cilostazol (Pletal) 30 minutes before or 2 hours after meals. Do not take the drug with grapefruit juice.

FACT CHECK

20-9 How do peripheral vasodilating drugs work?
20-10 What is the chief use of peripheral vasodilating drugs?

COMPLEMENTARY & ALTERNATIVE MEDICINE

L-Arginine

L-Arginine is an amino acid found in various foods that are commonly sold in health food specialty shops as a supplement capable of improving vascular health and sexual function in men. It is currently promoted in "medical food" form as a soy-based candy bar. As a supplement, L-arginine is marketed as a way to prevent heart disease, boost muscle growth, improve wound healing, and combat fatigue.

Oral doses of 9 to 30 g per day are well tolerated. No adverse reactions were reported in those taking 9 g per day. Higher doses may cause nausea and mild diarrhea. L-Arginine may exacerbate sickle cell crisis and should be used with caution in those with sickle cell anemia.

Chapter Review

KEY POINTS

- Antianginal drugs relieve chest pain or pressure by dilating coronary arteries, increasing the blood supply to the myocardium.
- The nitrates are used to treat angina pectoris. Some of these drugs are used for prophylaxis (prevention) and long-term treatment of angina, whereas others are used to relieve the pain of acute anginal attacks when they occur. A common adverse reaction of these drugs is headache, especially early in therapy. Hypotension, dizziness, vertigo, and weakness may also occur.
- Calcium channel blockers are primarily used to prevent anginal pain associated with certain forms of angina. They are not used to stop anginal pain once it has occurred. The more common adverse reactions include dizziness, light-headedness, nausea, diarrhea, constipation, peripheral edema, headache, bradycardia, flushing, dermatitis, skin rash, and nervousness.
- Peripheral vasodilating drugs are given for disorders that affect blood vessels of the extremities and are chiefly used in the treatment of peripheral vascular disease, Raynaud phenomenon, claudication, and cerebrovascular insufficiency. Short-term use is rarely beneficial or permanent. Adverse reactions associated with these drugs are variable.

CRITICAL THINKING CASE STUDY

Nitroglycerin

Mr. Bruce is sitting in the waiting room waiting for his appointment. He reaches into his pocket and gets his nitroglycerin, which has the name Nitrostat on the bottle. You observe this and offer to help.

1. How should Mr. Bruce take the sublingual nitroglycerin?
   a. Dissolve one tablet under the tongue at the first sign of the attack.
   b. Dissolve one tablet under the tongue at the first sign of the attack and repeat every 5 minutes until the attack resolves or he has taken three tablets in a 15-minute period.
   c. Use one or two sprays on or under the tongue every 5 minutes until the attack resolves or he has used the spray three times in a 15-minute period.
   d. Crush the tablet and put it under his tongue.
2. After Mr. Bruce takes the nitroglycerin, his symptoms resolve. What side effect should he expect to experience from the nitroglycerin?
   a. Headache
   b. Diarrhea
   c. Nausea/vomiting
   d. Weakness
   e. Constipation
3. The bottle of nitroglycerin that Mr. Bruce used had been previously opened. How long should he keep the unused tablets before he should discard the bottle and get a new supply?
4. What else is important for Mr. Bruce to know about handling his tablets?

Review Questions

MULTIPLE CHOICE

1. Calcium channel blockers
   a. constrict coronary arteries and arterioles
   b. dilate coronary arteries and arterioles
   c. are used to stop angina pain once it has occurred
   d. none of the above

2. Because peripheral vasodilating drugs dilate peripheral arteries, they may cause
   a. bradycardia
   b. hypokalemia
   c. hypotension
   d. hypertension

3. Which of the following drugs is used to treat intermittent claudication?
   a. Isoxsuprine
   b. Verapamil
   c. Amyl nitrite
   d. Cilostazol

4. What condition(s) may exist in older adults and require a reduction in dosage of antianginal drugs?
   a. Impaired renal function or heart disease
   b. Glaucoma
   c. Diabetes or hypoglycemia
   d. Rheumatoid arthritis

MATCHING

_____ 5. isosorbide mononitrate
_____ 6. isosorbide dinitrate
_____ 7. nitroglycerin
_____ 8. diltiazem
_____ 9. amlodipine
_____ 10. nicardipine
_____ 11. nifedipine
_____ 12. verapamil

a. Cardene SR
b. Calan SR
c. Minitran
d. Imdur
e. Procardia XL
f. Isordil
g. Cardizem
h. Norvasc

TRUE OR FALSE

_____ 13. Intravenous nitroglycerin is used to control perioperative hypertension associated with surgical procedures.

_____ 14. Patients have a decreased risk of digitalis toxicity when a calcium channel blocker is administered with digoxin.

_____ 15. Peripheral vasodilating drugs are given for disorders that affect blood vessels of the extremities.

_____ 16. Intermittent claudication is a manifestation of peripheral vascular disease in which blood supply to the lower leg is diminished.

FILL IN THE BLANKS

17. With some nitrates, the method of administration results in adverse effects. For example, _____ nitroglycerin may cause a local burning or tingling in the mouth, while _____ nitroglycerin may cause contact dermatitis.

18. One or two sprays of _____ _____ may be used to relieve angina, but no more than _____ metered doses are recommended within a 15-minute period.

19. Calcium channel blockers have a(n) _____ _____ when administered with aspirin.

20. Peripheral vasodilating drugs may cause _____, a physiologic increase in the pulse rate.

SHORT ANSWERS

21. Topical nitroglycerin is usually applied to which sites? Why is it important to rotate application sites?

22. Patients using what form of nitroglycerin are especially prone to tolerance? Why?

23. Patients receiving calcium channel blockers should be monitored for what signs of CHF?

24. What drug is used to treat intermittent claudication? How does it help this condition?

Web Activities

1. Go to the National Heart, Lung, and Blood Institute Web site (http://www.nhlbi.nih.gov/). Conduct a search on angina. What are the different types of angina? Who is at risk for angina?

2. Go to the Web site of the American Heart Association (www.americanheart.org). From the opening page, go to the Conditions page, then to the "More" section to find the article on Peripheral Artery Disease. What are the risk factors for Peripheral Artery Disease that a patient can control?

SUMMARY DRUG TABLE Antianginal Drugs
(left, generic; right, trade)

Comprehensive Summary Drug Tables, including uses, adverses effects, dosages, and pregnancy classifications, are provided on the companion website, http://thePoint.lww.com/PharmacologyHP2e

Nitrates	
amyl nitrite *am-il-nye-trite*	*generic*
isosorbide mononitrate *eye-soe-sor'-bide*	Imdur, Ismo, Monoket, *generic*
isosorbide dinitrate *eye-soe-sor'-bide*	Dilatrate-SR, Isochron, Isordil, Isordil Titradose, *generic*
nitroglycerin, IV *nye-troe-gli'-ser-in*	*generic*
nitroglycerin, sublingual *nye-troe-gli'-ser-in*	Nitrostat, *generic*
nitroglycerin, translingual *nye-troe-gli'-ser-in*	Nitrolingual, NitroMist
nitroglycerin, oral sustained-release *nye-troe-gli'-ser-in*	Nitro-Time, *generic*
nitroglycerin transdermal systems *nye-troe-gli'-ser-in*	Minitran, Nitro-Dur, *generic*
nitroglycerin, topical *nye-troe-gli'-ser in*	Nitro-Bid
Calcium Channel Blocking Drugs	
amlodipine *am-low'-dih-peen*	Norvasc, *generic*
diltiazem HCl *dil-tye'-a-zem*	Cardizem, Cardizem CD, Cardizem LA, Cartia XT, Matzim LA, Tatzia XT, Tiazac, *generic*
nicardipine HCl *nye-kar'-de-peen*	Cardene IV, Cardene SR, *generic*
nifedipine *nye-fed'-i-peen*	Adalat CC, Afeditab CR, Nifediac CC, Nifedical XL, Procardia, Procardia XL, *generic*
verapamil HCl *ver-ap'-a-mil*	Calan, Calan SR, Covera-HS, Isoptin SR, Verelan, Verelan PM, *generic*

SUMMARY DRUG TABLE Peripheral Vasodilators and Miscellaneous Vasodilating Drugs
(left, generic; right, trade)

Comprehensive Summary Drug Tables, including uses, adverses effects, dosages, and pregnancy classifications, are provided on the companion website, http://thePoint.lww.com/PharmacologyHP2e

cilostazol *sil-oh'-sta-zol*	Pletal, *generic*
isoxsuprine *eye-soks'-syoo-preen*	*generic*
papaverine *pa-pav'-er-een*	*generic*

21

Antihypertensive Drugs

CHAPTER OBJECTIVES

On completion of this chapter, students will be able to:

1. Define the chapter's key terms.
2. Identify normal blood pressure for adults and the different levels of hypertension.
3. Identify the different classes of drugs used to treat hypertension.
4. Identify the risk factors associated with hypertension.
5. Discuss the importance of systolic pressure.
6. Explain why blood pressure determinations are important during therapy with an antihypertensive drug.
7. Discuss common adverse reactions of antihypertensive drugs.
8. Discuss important points to keep in mind when educating the patient and family members about the use of antihypertensive drugs.

KEY TERMS

aldosterone—a hormone that promotes the retention of sodium and water, which may contribute to a rise in blood pressure

angiotensin-converting enzyme—a naturally occurring enzyme that converts angiotensin I to angiotensin II, which is a powerful vasoconstrictor

blood pressure—the force of the blood against the walls of the arteries

endogenous—substances normally manufactured by the body

essential hypertension—hypertension without a known cause

hypertension—usually defined as a systolic pressure more than 140 mm Hg or a diastolic pressure more than 90 mm Hg

hypokalemia—low blood potassium

hyponatremia—low blood sodium

isolated systolic hypertension—a condition of only an elevated systolic pressure

malignant hypertension—hypertension in which the diastolic pressure usually exceeds 130 mm Hg

secondary hypertension—hypertension in which a direct cause can be identified

CHAPTER OVERVIEW

Drug classes covered in this chapter are:

- Peripheral vasodilators
- β–Adrenergic blockers
- Antiadrenergics
- Calcium channel blockers
- Angiotensin-converting enzymes
- Angiotensin II receptor antagonists

Drugs by classification are listed on page 216.

thePOINT RESOURCES

- Comprehensive Summary Drug Tables
- Animations: Hypertension
- Lippincott's Interactive Tutorials: Drugs Affecting the Cardiovascular System
- Interactive Practice and Review
- Monographs of Most Commonly Prescribed Drugs

Blood pressure is the force of the blood against the walls of the arteries. Blood pressure rises and falls throughout the day. When the blood pressure stays elevated over time, the person is said to have hypertension. A systolic pressure less than 120 mm Hg and a diastolic blood pressure less than 80 mm Hg (120/80) are considered normal. **Hypertension**, often called high blood pressure, is usually defined as a systolic pressure more than 140 mm Hg and a diastolic pressure more than 90 mm Hg. Table 21-1 identifies normal blood pressure levels for adults and the different levels of hypertension. Patients in the prehypertension range require frequent blood pressure monitoring; patients with stage 1 or 2 hypertension should be under the care of a physician. Hypertension is serious because it causes the heart to work harder and contributes to atherosclerosis. It increases the risk of heart disease, congestive heart failure, kidney disease, blindness, and stroke.

Most cases of hypertension have no known cause. When there is no known cause, the term **essential hypertension** is used. Essential hypertension has been linked to certain risk factors such as diet and lifestyle. Key Concepts 21-1 identifies the risk factors associated with hypertension.

Essential hypertension cannot be cured but can be controlled. Many individuals experience hypertension as they grow older. For many older individuals, the systolic pressure gives the most accurate diagnosis of hypertension. Key Concepts 21-2 discusses the importance of systolic pressure.

Once essential hypertension develops, management of this disorder becomes a lifetime task. When a direct cause of the hypertension can be identified, the condition is described as **secondary hypertension**. Among the known causes of secondary hypertension, kidney disease ranks first, with tumors or other abnormalities of the adrenal glands following.

TABLE 21-1 Blood Pressure Levels for Adults

Category	Systolic* (in mm Hg)		Diastolic* (in mm Hg)
Normal	<120	and	<80
Prehypertension	120–139	or	80–89
Stage 1 hypertension	140–159	or	90–99
Stage 2 hypertension	≥160	or	≥100

*If systolic and diastolic pressures fall into different categories, then the patient's treatment status is the higher category.

From the Seventh Report of the Joint National Committee on Prevention, Detection, Evaluation and Treatment of High Blood Pressure, U.S. Department of Health and Human Services, May 2003. http://www.nhlbi.nih.gov/guidelines/hypertension/index.htm

In **malignant hypertension**, the diastolic pressure usually exceeds 130 mm Hg. Managing the medical condition causing secondary hypertension results in the patient regaining a normal blood pressure.

Malignant hypertension is a dangerous condition that develops rapidly and requires immediate medical attention. Patients with malignant hypertension experience organ damage as the result of hypertension. Target organs of hypertension include the heart, kidney, and eyes (retinopathy).

Most health care providers prescribe lifestyle changes for patients to reduce risk factors before prescribing drugs. The health care provider may recommend measures such as weight loss (if the patient is overweight), reduction of stress, regular aerobic exercise, quitting smoking (if applicable), and dietary changes such as a decrease in sodium (salt) intake. Most people with hypertension are "salt sensitive," which means that any salt or sodium more than the minimal bodily need is too much for them and leads to an increase in blood pressure. Stress-reducing techniques, such as relaxation techniques, meditation, and yoga, may also be a part of the treatment regimen.

When drug therapy is begun, the health care provider may first prescribe a diuretic (Chapter 25) or β-blocker (Chapter 12) because these drugs have been shown to be highly effective. However, as in many other diseases and conditions,

FACTS ABOUT . . .

Hypertension

- High blood pressure puts patients at risk for heart disease (first leading cause of death in the United States) and stroke (third leading cause of death in the United States).
- High blood pressure usually has no warning signs or symptoms, so many people are unaware that they even have it. It is often called the "silent killer."
- Approximately one out of every three adults has high blood pressure (31.3%).
- African Americans have a higher incidence of high blood pressure than whites and Mexican Americans. African Americans also develop it at an earlier age, and it is more prominent in men than women.
- More men under the age of 45 have hypertension than women, but more women over the age of 65 have hypertension. During their lifetime, the incidence is equal.

Source: Centers for Disease Control and Prevention

KEY CONCEPTS

21-1 Risk Factors for Hypertension

- Smoking
- Age (women older than 65 years and men older than 55 years of age)
- Obesity
- Diabetes
- Lack of physical activity
- Chronic alcohol consumption
- Family history of cardiovascular disease
- Sex (men and postmenopausal women)

there is no "best" single drug, drug combination, or medical regimen for treatment of hypertension. After examination and evaluation of the patient, the health care provider selects the antihypertensive drug and therapeutic regimen that will probably be most effective. Figure 21-1 shows an algorithm for the treatment of hypertension. In some instances, it may be necessary to change to another antihypertensive drug or add a second antihypertensive drug if the patient does not experience a response to therapy. The health care provider also recommends that a patient continue with stress reduction, dietary modification, and other lifestyle modifications important in the control of hypertension.

FACT CHECK

21-1 What is considered normal blood pressure for adults? Normal ≤ 120 mm Hg systolic and <80 mm Hg diastolic.

21-2 What are the different levels of hypertension?

21-3 What is the difference between essential hypertension and secondary hypertension?

Antihypertensive Drugs

The types of drugs used for the treatment of hypertension include

- Vasodilating drugs: for example, hydralazine (Apresoline) and minoxidil (Loniten)
- β-adrenergic blocking drugs: for example, atenolol (Tenormin), metoprolol (Lopressor), and propranolol (Inderal). Note that the generic names usually end in -lol.
- Antiadrenergic drugs (centrally acting): for example, guanabenz (Wytensin) and guanfacine (Tenex)
- Antiadrenergic drugs (peripherally acting): for example, guanadrel (Hylorel) and guanethidine (Ismelin)
- α-adrenergic blocking drugs: for example, doxazosin (Cardura) and prazosin (Minipress). Note that the generic names usually end in -zosin.
- Calcium channel blocking drugs: for example, amlodipine (Norvasc) and diltiazem (Cardizem)

- Angiotensin-converting enzyme (ACE) inhibitors: for example, captopril (Capoten), enalapril (Vasotec), and lisinopril (Prinivil). Note that the generic names usually end in -pril.
- Angiotensin II receptor antagonists: for example, irbesartan (Avapro), losartan (Cozaar), and valsartan (Diovan). Note that the generic names usually end in -sartan.
- Diuretics: for example, furosemide (Lasix) and hydrochlorothiazide (HydroDIURIL)

For additional information concerning antiadrenergic drugs (both centrally and peripherally acting) and α-adrenergic and β-adrenergic blocking drugs, see Chapter 12. For more information on calcium channel blockers, see Chapter 19. Information on vasodilating drugs and diuretics can be found in Chapters 20 and 25, respectively. Angiotensin-converting enzyme inhibitors and angiotensin II receptor antagonists are discussed in this chapter.

In addition to these antihypertensive drugs, many antihypertensive combinations are available. Some combination antihypertensive drugs combine an antihypertensive and a diuretic (Table 21-2). Other combination antihypertensive drugs combine two different antihypertensives (Table 21-3).

Actions of Antihypertensive Drugs

Many antihypertensive drugs lower the blood pressure by dilating or increasing the size of the arterial blood vessels (vasodilation). Vasodilation creates an increase in the lumen (the space or opening within an artery) of the arterial blood vessels, which in turn increases the amount of space available for the blood to circulate. Because blood volume (the amount of blood) remains relatively constant, an increase in the space in which the blood circulates (the blood vessels) lowers the pressure of the fluid (measured as blood pressure) in the blood vessels. Although the method by which antihypertensive drugs dilate blood vessels varies, the result remains basically the same. Antihypertensive drugs with vasodilating activity include:

- Adrenergic blocking drugs
- Antiadrenergic blocking drugs
- Calcium channel blocking drugs
- Vasodilating drugs

Another type of antihypertensive drug is the diuretic. The mechanism by which the diuretics reduce elevated blood pressure is unknown, but it is thought to be based, in part, on their ability to increase the excretion of sodium from the body through increased urine output. The actions and uses of diuretics are discussed in Chapter 25.

The mechanism of action of **angiotensin-converting enzyme** inhibitors is not fully understood. It is believed that these drugs may prevent (or inhibit) the activity of ACE, which converts angiotensin I to angiotensin II, a powerful vasoconstrictor. Both angiotensin I and ACE are normally manufactured by the body and are therefore called **endogenous** substances. The vasoconstricting activity of angiotensin II stimulates the secretion of the endogenous hormone aldosterone by the adrenal cortex. **Aldosterone** promotes the retention of sodium and water, which may contribute to a rise in blood pressure. By preventing the conversion of angiotensin I to angiotensin II, this chain of events is interrupted, sodium

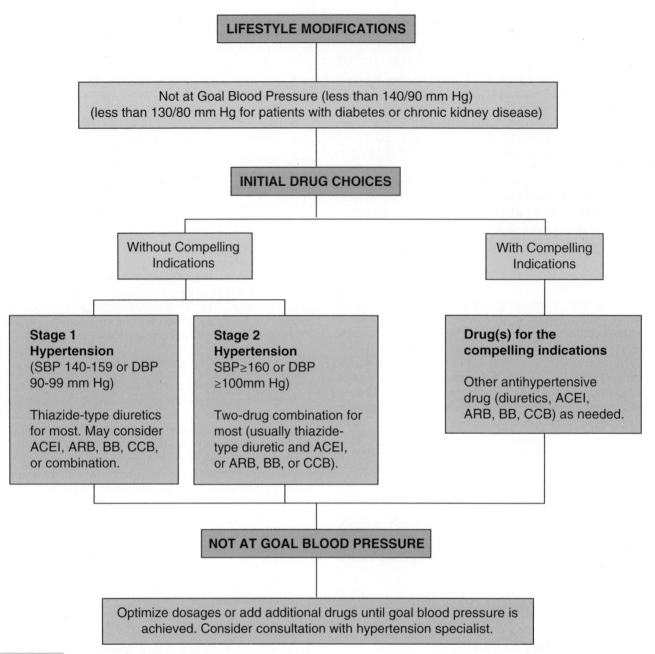

FIGURE 21-1 Algorithm for the treatment of hypertension. Compelling indications include HF, high risk for cardiovascular disease, post–myocardial infarction (MI), diabetes, stroke prevention, and chronic kidney disease. Key: DBP, diastolic blood pressure; SBP, systolic blood pressure; ACEI, ACE inhibitor; ARB, angiotensin receptor blocker; BB, β blocker; CCB, calcium channel blocker.

and water are not retained, and the blood pressure decreases. Angiotensin II receptor antagonists act to block the vasoconstrictor and aldosterone effects of angiotensin II at various receptor sites, resulting in a lowering of the blood pressure.

Uses of Antihypertensive Drugs

Antihypertensives are used in the treatment of hypertension. Although many antihypertensive drugs are available, not all drugs may work equally well in a given patient. In some instances, the health care provider may find it necessary to

prescribe a different antihypertensive drug when a patient experiences no response to therapy. Some antihypertensive drugs are used only in severe cases of hypertension and when other less potent drugs have failed to lower the blood pressure. At times, two antihypertensive drugs may be given together to achieve a better response (see Fig. 21-1).

Nitroprusside (Nitropress) is an example of an intravenous (IV) drug that may be used to treat hypertensive emergencies. A hypertensive emergency is a case of extremely high blood pressure that does not respond to conventional antihypertensive drug therapy.

TABLE 21-2　Examples of Selected Antihypertensive Combinations: Antihypertensive and Diuretic

Trade Name	Diuretic Constituent (mg)	Antihypertensive (mg)
(None)	Hydrochlorothiazide (25)	Propranolol (40 or 80)
Accuretic	Hydrochlorothiazide (12.5 or 25)	Quinapril (10 or 20)
Avalide	Hydrochlorothiazide (12.5 or 25)	Irbesartan (150 or 300)
Atacand	Hydrochlorothiazide (12.5 or 25)	Candesartan (16 or 32)
Benicar HCT	Hydrochlorothiazide (12.5 or 25)	Olmesartan (20 or 40)
Capozide 25/15	Hydrochlorothiazide (15)	Captopril (25)
Capozide 50/15	Hydrochlorothiazide (15)	Captopril (50)
Capozide 25/25	Hydrochlorothiazide (15)	Captopril (25)
Capozide 50/25	Hydrochlorothiazide (15)	Captopril (50)
Clorpress	Chlorthalidone (15)	Clonidine (0.1, 0.2, or 0.3)
Diovan	Hydrochlorothiazide (12.5 or 25)	Valsartan (80, 160, or 320)
Hyzaar	Hydrochlorothiazide (12.5 or 25)	Losartan (50 or 100)
Lopressor HCT 50/25	Hydrochlorothiazide (25)	Metoprolol (50)
Lopressor HCT 100/25	Hydrochlorothiazide (25)	Metoprolol (100)
Lopressor HCT 100/50	Hydrochlorothiazide (50)	Metoprolol (100)
Lotensin HCT	Hydrochlorothiazide (6.25, 12.5, or 25)	Benazeprin (5, 10, or 20)
Micardis HCT	Hydrochlorothiazide (12.5 or 25)	Telmisartan (40 or 80)
Minizide 5	Polythiazide (0.5)	Prazosin (5)
Prinzide	Hydrochlorothiazide (12.5 or 25)	Lisinopril (10 or 20)
Tenoretic 50	Chlorthalidone (25)	Atenolol (50)
Tenoretic 100	Chlorthalidone (25)	Atenolol (100)
Vaseretic	Hydrochlorothiazide (12.5 or 25)	Enalapril (5 or 10)
Zestoretic	Hydrochlorothiazide (12.5 or 25)	Lisinopril (10 or 20)
Ziac	Hydrochlorothiazide (6.25)	Bisoprolol (2.5, 5, or 10)

TABLE 21-3　Examples of Selected Antihypertensive Combinations: Two Antihypertensives

Trade Name	Antihypertensive Drug 1	Antihypertensive Drug 2
Tekamlo	Aliskiren 150 or 300 mg (direct renin inhibitor)	Amlodipine 5 or 10 mg (calcium channel blocker)
Valturna	Aliskiren 150 or 300 mg (direct renin inhibitor)	Valsartan 160 or 320 mg (angiotensin II receptor antagonist)
Lotrel	Amlodipine 2.5, 5, or 10 mg (calcium channel blocker)	Benazepril 10, 20, or 40 mg (ACE inhibitor)
Azor	Amlodipine 5 or 10 mg (calcium channel blocker)	Olmesartan 20 or 40 mg (angiotensin II receptor antagonist)
Exforge	Amlodipine 5 or 10 mg (calcium channel blocker)	Valsartan 160 or 30 mg (angiotensin II receptor antagonist)
Lexxel	ER tabs enalapril 5 mg (ACE inhibitor)	Felodipine 5 mg (calcium channel blocker)
Twynsta	Telmisartan 40 or 80 mg (angiotensin II receptor antagonist)	Amlodipine or 10 mg (calcium channel blocker)
Tarka	Trandolapril 1, 2, or 4 mg (ACE inhibitor)	Verapamil 180 or 240 mg (calcium channel blocker)

Adverse Reactions of Antihypertensive Drugs

When any antihypertensive drug is given, postural or orthostatic hypotension may occur in some patients, especially early in therapy. Postural hypotension is the occurrence of dizziness and light-headedness when the individual rises suddenly from a lying or sitting position. Orthostatic hypotension occurs when the individual has been standing in one place for a long time. These reactions can be prevented or minimized by having a patient rise slowly from a lying or sitting position and by avoiding standing in one place for a prolonged period.

Angiotensin-converting enzyme inhibitors often cause a nonproductive cough. The cough can be so bothersome that the drug must be discontinued.

FACT CHECK

21-4   What types of antihypertensive drugs have vasodilating activity?

21-5   What are two common adverse reactions that can occur with any type of antihypertensive drug?

A patient is observed for adverse drug reactions because their occurrence may require a change in the dose or the drug. The health care provider should be notified if any adverse reactions occur. In some instances, a patient may have to tolerate mild adverse reactions such as dry mouth or mild anorexia.

Electrolyte imbalances that may occur during therapy with a diuretic include **hyponatremia** (low blood sodium) and **hypokalemia** (low blood potassium), although other imbalances may also occur. See Chapter 45 for the signs and symptoms of electrolyte imbalances. The health care provider should be notified if any signs or symptoms of an electrolyte imbalance occur.

Contraindications, Precautions, and Interactions of Antihypertensives

- Antihypertensive drugs are contraindicated in patients with a known hypersensitivity to the individual drugs.
- When an antihypertensive is administered by a transdermal system (e.g., clonidine), the system is contraindicated if a patient is allergic to any component of the adhesive layer of the transdermal system.
- Antihypertensive drugs are used cautiously in patients with renal or hepatic impairment or electrolyte imbalances, during lactation and pregnancy, and in older patients.

ALERT Rx

Discontinuing Use of an Antihypertensive
Should it be necessary to discontinue antihypertensive therapy, withdrawal should never happen abruptly. The dosage is gradually reduced over 2 to 4 days to avoid rebound hypertension (a rapid rise in blood pressure).

- Angiotensin-converting enzyme inhibitors are used cautiously in patients with sodium depletion, hypovolemia, or coronary or cerebrovascular insufficiency and those receiving diuretic therapy or dialysis.
- Angiotensin II receptor agonists are used cautiously in patients with renal or hepatic dysfunction, hypovolemia, or volume or salt depletion and in patients receiving high doses of diuretics.
- The hypotensive effects of most antihypertensive drugs are increased when administered with diuretics and other antihypertensives.
- Many drugs can interact with antihypertensive drugs and decrease their effectiveness (e.g., antidepressants, monoamine oxidase inhibitors, antihistamines, and sympathomimetic bronchodilators). When ACE inhibitors are administered with nonsteroidal anti-inflammatory drugs (NSAIDs), their antihypertensive effect may be decreased. Absorption of ACE inhibitors may be decreased when administered with antacids.
- Administration of potassium-sparing diuretics or potassium supplements concurrently with ACE inhibitors may cause hyperkalemia.
- When angiotensin II receptor agonists are administered with NSAIDs or phenobarbital, their antihypertensive effects may be decreased.

FACT CHECK

21-6   Why is it important to avoid abruptly discontinuing antihypertensive therapy?

21-7   Which two electrolyte imbalances may commonly occur during diuretic therapy?

21-8   What happens when antihypertensive drugs are given with diuretics or other antihypertensives?

COMPLEMENTARY & ALTERNATIVE MEDICINE

Herbal Remedies

Various herbs and supplements, such as hawthorn extracts, garlic, onion, ginkgo biloba, vitamin E, and aspirin, may be used by herbalists for hypertension. Although these substances may lower blood pressure in some individuals, their use is not recommended because the effect is slight and usually too gentle to affect moderate to severe hypertension.

Potassium has been shown to be effective in preventing and controlling blood pressure. Diets that are rich in fruits and vegetables are good sources of potassium. It has been suggested that blood pressure can be significantly lowered by a diet high in magnesium, calcium, and potassium and low in sodium and fat. Patients should consult their health care provider before taking any herbal remedy.

CONSIDERATIONS | Older adults

Nitroprusside Sensitivity

Older adults are particularly sensitive to the hypotensive effects of nitroprusside. To minimize the hypotensive effects, the drug is initially given in lower dosages. Older adults require more frequent monitoring during the administration of nitroprusside.

Patient Management Issues with Antihypertensive Drugs

Before therapy with an antihypertensive drug is started, the health care provider obtains the blood pressure and pulse rate on both arms with a patient in standing, sitting, and lying positions. The health care provider also obtains a patient's weight, especially if a diuretic is part of therapy or if the health care provider prescribes a weight-loss regimen.

Monitoring and recording the blood pressure is an important part of patient management, especially early in therapy. The health care provider may need to adjust the dose of the drug upward or downward, try a different drug, or add another drug to the therapeutic regimen if a patient does not have an adequate response to drug therapy.

Each time the blood pressure is measured, the same arm and patient position (e.g., standing, sitting, or lying down) should be used. In some instances, the health care provider may order the blood pressure taken in one or more positions, such as standing and lying down.

The patient's weight is measured daily during the initial period of drug therapy. Patients taking an antihypertensive drug occasionally retain sodium and water, resulting in edema and weight gain. The patient's extremities are also examined for edema.

Educating the Patient and Family about Antihypertensive Drugs

Health care workers can do much to educate others about the importance of having their blood pressure checked periodically. This includes people of all ages because hypertension does not occur only in older individuals. Once hypertension is detected, patient teaching becomes an important factor in successfully returning the blood pressure to normal or near-normal levels.

To ensure lifetime compliance with the prescribed therapeutic regimen, the importance of drug therapy is emphasized, as well as other treatments recommended by the health care provider.

The health care provider may want the patient or family to monitor blood pressure during therapy. The health care provider teaches the technique of taking a blood pressure and pulse rate to the patient or family member, allowing sufficient time for supervised practice. The patient is instructed to keep a record of the blood pressure and to bring this record to each visit to the health care provider's office.

Many patients receiving antihypertensive therapy commonly receive more than one drug, placing them at risk for orthostatic hypotension. Patients are instructed to follow these measures:

- Change your position slowly.
- Sit at the edge of the bed or chair for a few minutes before standing up.
- Ask for help standing or walking when necessary.
- If you feel dizzy or light-headed, then sit or lie down immediately.
- Make sure to drink adequate amounts of fluid during the day.

Following are key points about antihypertensives that the patient or family members should know:

- Never discontinue use of this drug except on the advice of your health care provider. These drugs control but do not cure hypertension. Skipping doses of the drug or voluntarily discontinuing the drug may cause severe, rebound hypertension.
- Do not use any nonprescription drugs (some may contain drugs that are capable of increasing the blood pressure) unless approved by your health care provider.
- Do not drink alcohol unless its use has been approved by your health care provider.
- Take the drug as requested by your health care provider. Some drugs, such as captopril and moexipril, are usually taken 1 hour before or 2 hours after meals to enhance absorption.
- This drug may produce dizziness or light-headedness when rising suddenly from a sitting or lying position. To avoid these effects, rise slowly from a sitting or lying position.
- If the drug makes you drowsy, avoid hazardous tasks such as driving or performing tasks that require alertness. Drowsiness may disappear with time.
- If you feel weak or fatigued, contact your health care provider.
- Follow the diet restrictions recommended by your health care provider. Do not use salt substitutes unless a particular brand of salt substitute is approved by your health care provider.
- Notify your health care provider if your diastolic pressure suddenly increases to 130 mm Hg or higher; you may have malignant hypertension.

Chapter Review

KEY POINTS

- Hypertension is serious because it causes the heart to work harder and contributes to atherosclerosis. It increases the risk of heart disease, congestive heart failure, kidney disease, blindness, and stroke.
- Although many antihypertensive drugs are available, not all drugs may work equally well in a given patient.
- Antihypertensive drugs with vasodilating activity include adrenergic blocking drugs, antiadrenergic blocking drugs, calcium channel blocking drugs, and vasodilating drugs. Another type of antihypertensive drug is the diuretic.
- When any antihypertensive drug is given, postural or orthostatic hypotension may occur in some patients, especially early in therapy.
- Monitoring and recording the blood pressure is an important part of the ongoing assessment, especially early in therapy.

CRITICAL THINKING CASE STUDY

Treating Hypertension

Mrs. Ohlin has been diagnosed with hypertension. She has tried lifestyle modification, including diet modifications, but her hypertension is still not controlled.

1. Which classification of medication would you expect her physician to prescribe first?
   a. Diuretic
   b. β-blocker
   c. ACE inhibitor
   d. Calcium channel blocker
2. Mrs. Ohlin's physician prescribed medication, but it does not work. So her physician next prescribes lisinopril. What adverse effect should she watch for that could lead to a need for the medication to be discontinued?
3. Ms. Ohlin is visiting her dental hygienist to have her teeth cleaned, and she gets her blood pressure checked. The blood pressure reading is lower than normal. What question should the hygienist ask Mrs. Ohlin?
   a. How does she normally take her blood pressure?
   b. How is she taking her blood pressure medication?
   c. Has she done anything different today than she normally does before taking her blood pressure?
   d. All of the above

Review Questions

MULTIPLE CHOICE

1. All of the following antihypertensive drugs have vasodilating activity EXCEPT
   a. adrenergic blocking drugs
   b. antiadrenergic blocking drugs
   c. diuretics
   d. calcium channel blocking drugs

2. A patient receiving a diuretic drug is observed for the following adverse effect(s):
   a. Dehydration
   b. Dehydration and electrolyte imbalances
   c. Electrolyte imbalances
   d. Electrolyte imbalances and fluid volume excess
3. When discontinuing use of an antihypertensive drug, which of the following should occur?
   a. The blood pressure is monitored every hour for 8 hours after the drug therapy is discontinued.
   b. The drug dosage is gradually decreased during a period of 2 to 4 days to avoid rebound hypertension.
   c. The blood pressure and pulse are checked every 30 minutes after discontinuing the drug therapy.
   d. The dosage is tapered during a period of 2 weeks to prevent a return of hypertension.
4. Common adverse effects of nadolol (Corgard) include
   a. dizziness and impotence
   b. drowsiness, fatigue, and weakness
   c. dry mouth and a dry cough
   d. all of the above

MATCHING

Match each of the following drugs with their class.

_____ 5. losartan
_____ 6. fosinopril
_____ 7. hydralazine
_____ 8. clonidine
_____ 9. nitroprusside
_____ 10. propranolol
_____ 11. doxazosin
_____ 12. guanadrel
_____ 13. amlodipine

a. peripheral vasodilator
b. calcium channel blocking drug
c. centrally acting antiadrenergic
d. peripherally acting antiadrenergic
e. α-adrenergic blocking drug
f. ACE inhibitor
g. angiotensin II receptor antagonist
h. drugs for hypertensive crisis
i. β-adrenergic blocking drug

TRUE OR FALSE

_____ 14. Aldosterone promotes the excretion of sodium and water, which may contribute to a rise in blood pressure.
_____ 15. Peripherally acting antiadrenergics include guanadrel, guanethidine, and reserpine.
_____ 16. Clonidine is available in both oral and transdermal forms.
_____ 17. Because older adults are sensitive to the hypotensive effects of nitroprusside, the drug is initially given in a single large dose.

FILL IN THE BLANKS

18. In patients with _____, blood vessels become less flexible and stiffen, leading to cardiovascular disease and kidney damage.
19. Two drugs used for hypertensive crisis are _____ and _____.
20. Patients who do not drink enough while receiving diuretic therapy may experience _____.
21. Administering potassium-sparing diuretics or potassium supplements concurrently with ACE inhibitors may cause _____.

SHORT ANSWERS

22. What is malignant hypertension?
23. What are common drug types used to treat hypertension?
24. Why is it important to monitor the patient's blood pressure early during antihypertensive therapy?
25. How would you advise patients receiving antihypertensive therapy to avoid the effects of orthostatic hypotension?

Web Activities

1. Go to the National Heart, Lung, and Blood Institute Web site (http://www.nhlbi.nih.gov/). Conduct a search for "high blood pressure prevention." How can high blood pressure be prevented?
2. Go to the National Heart, Lung, and Blood Institute Web site (http://www.nhlbi.nih.gov/). Conduct a search for the "DASH Eating Plan." What are the key points about the DASH Eating Plan?

SUMMARY DRUG TABLE Antihypertensive Drugs (left, generic; right, trade)

Comprehensive Summary Drug Tables, including uses, adverses effects, dosages, and pregnancy classifications, are provided on the companion website, http://thePoint.lww.com/PharmacologyHP2e

Peripheral Vasodilators

Generic	Trade
epoprostenol *e-poe-prost'-en-ole*	Flolan, Veletri, *generic*
hydralazine HCl *hy-dral'-a-zeen*	*generic*
minoxidil *mi-nox'-i-dill*	*Rogaine, generic*
treprostinil *tre-prost'-in-il*	Remodulin (injection), Tyvaso (inhalation)

ß-Adrenergic Blocking Drugs

Generic	Trade
acebutolol HCl *a-se-byoo'-toe- lole*	Sectral, *generic*
atenolol *a-ten'-oh-lole*	Tenormin, *generic*
betaxolol HCl *be-tax'-oh-lol*	Betoptic-S (ophthalmic), Kerlone, *generic*
bisoprolol fumarate *bis-oh'-pro-lole*	Zebeta, *generic*
carteolol HCl *kar'-tee-oh-lole*	*generic*
esmolol HCl *es'-moe-lol*	Brevibloc, Brevibloc Double Strength, *generic*
metoprolol *me-toe'-proe-lole*	Lopressor, Toprol XL, *generic*
nadolol *nay'-doe-lole*	Corgard, *generic*
nebivolol *ne-biv'-oh-lole*	Bystolic
penbutolol sulfate *pen-byoo'-toe-lole*	Levatol
pindolol *pin'-doe-lole*	*generic*
propranolol HCl *proe-pran'-oh-lole*	Inderal LA, InnoPran XL, *generic*
timolol maleate *tim'-oh-lole*	Betimol, Istalol, Timoptic, Timoptic Ocudose, Timoptic-XE, *generic*

Antiadrenergics—Centrally Acting

Generic	Trade
clonidine HCl (oral) *kloe'-ni-deen*	Catapres, Duracion, Kapvay, Nexiclon XR, *generic*
clonidine HCl (transdermal) *kloe'-ni-deen*	Catapres-TTS-1, Catapres-TTS-2, Catapres-TTS-3, *generic*
guanabenz acetate *gwhan'-a-benz*	*generic*
guanfacine HCl *gwhan'-fa-seen*	Tenex, Intuniv, *generic*
methyldopa and methyldopate HCl *meth-ill-doe'-pa*	*generic*

Antiadrenergics—Peripherally Acting

Generic	Trade
doxazosin mesylate *doks-ay'-zoe-sin*	Cardura, Cardura XL, *generic*
prazosin HCl *praz'-oh-sin*	Minipress, *generic*
terazosin HCl *ter-ay'-zoe-sin*	*generic*
reserpine *re-ser'-peen*	*generic*

Angiotensin-Converting Enzyme Inhibitors

Generic	Trade
benazepril HCl *ben-a'-za-pril*	Lotensin, *generic*
captopril *kap'-toe-pril*	*generic*
enalapril *e-nal'-a-pril*	Vasotec
fosinopril sodium *foh-sin'-oh-pril*	*generic*
lisinopril *lyse-in'-oh-pril*	Prinivil, Zestril, *generic*
moexipril HCl *mo-ex'-ah-pril*	Univasc, *generic*
perindopril erbumine *pur-in'-doh-pril*	Aceon
quinapril HCl *kwin'-ah-pril*	Accupril, *generic*
ramipril *ra-mi'-prill*	Altace, *generic*
trandolapril *tran-doe'-la-pril*	Mavik, *generic*

Angiotensin II Receptor Antagonists

Generic	Trade
azilsartan	Edarbi
candesartan cilexetil *can-dah-sar'-tan*	Atacand
eprosartan mesylate *ep-row-sar'-tan*	Teveten
irbesartan *er-bah-sar'-tan*	Avapro
losartan potassium *low-sar'-tan*	Cozaar, *generic*
telmisartan *tell-mah-sar'-tan*	Micardis
valsartan *val-sar'-tan*	*Diovan*

Calcium Channel Blockers

Generic	Trade
amlodipine *am-loe'-di-peen*	Norvasc
clevidipine *klev-id'-i-peen*	Cleviprex
diltiazem *dil-tye'-a-zem*	Cardizem, Cardizem CD, Cardizem LA, Cartia XT, Dilacor XR, Matzim LA, Taztia XT, Tiazac, *generic*
felodipine *fe-loe-di-peen*	*generic*
isradipine *iz-ra'-di-peen*	DynaCirc CR, *generic*
nicardipine *nye-kar'-de-peen*	Cardene IV, Cardene SR, *generic*
nifedipine *nye-fed'-i-peen*	Adalat CC, Afeditab CR, Nifediac CC, Nifedical XL, Procardia, Procardia XL
nisoldipine *nye-sol'-di-peen*	Sular
verapamil *ver-ap'-a-mil*	Calan, Calan SR, Covera-HS, Isoptin SR, Verelan, Verelan PM, *generic*

Drugs Used for Hypertensive Crisis

Generic	Trade
fenoldopam mesylate *fe-nol'-doe-pam*	Corlopam, *generic*
nitroprusside sodium *nye-troe-pruss'-ide*	Nitropress

22

Antihyperlipidemic Drugs

CHAPTER OBJECTIVES

On completion of this chapter, students will be able to:

1. Define the chapter's key terms.
2. Discuss cholesterol, HDL, LDL, and triglyceride levels and how they contribute to the development of heart disease.
3. Discuss the general drug actions, uses, adverse reactions, contraindications, precautions, and interactions of antihyperlipidemic drugs.
4. Discuss important points to keep in mind when educating the patient or family member about the use of an antihyperlipidemic drug.

KEY TERMS

atherosclerosis—a disorder in which lipid deposits accumulate on the lining of the blood vessels, eventually producing degenerative changes and obstruction of blood flow

bile acid sequestrants—these drugs bind to bile acids to form an insoluble substance that cannot be absorbed by the intestine, so it is excreted in the feces

catalyst—a substance that accelerates a chemical reaction without itself undergoing a change

cholesterol—one of the lipids in the blood

high-density lipoproteins (HDL)—carry cholesterol from peripheral cells to the liver, where it is metabolized and excreted

HMG-CoA reductase inhibitor—an enzyme that is a catalyst in the manufacture of cholesterol

hyperlipidemia—an increase (hyper) in lipids (lipid), which are fats or fat-like substances, in the blood (-emia)

lipids—fats or fat-like substances in the blood

lipoprotein—a lipid-containing protein

low-density lipoproteins (LDL)—transport cholesterol to peripheral cells

rhabdomyolysis—a rare condition in which muscle damage results in the release of muscle cell contents into the bloodstream

triglycerides—a type of lipids in the blood

thePOINT RESOURCES

- Comprehensive Summary Drug Tables
- Lippincott's Interactive Tutorials: Drugs Affecting the Cardiovascular System
- Interactive Practice and Review
- Monographs of Most Commonly Prescribed Drugs

Hyperlipidemia is an increase (hyper) in the **lipids** (lipid), which are a group of fats or fat-like substances in the blood (-emia). **Cholesterol** and **triglycerides** are the two lipids in the blood. Elevation of one or both of these lipids results in hyperlipidemia. Serum cholesterol levels above 240 mg/dL and triglyceride levels above 150 mg/dL are associated with atherosclerosis. **Atherosclerosis** is a disorder in which lipid deposits accumulate on the lining of the blood vessels, eventually producing degenerative changes and obstruction of blood flow (Fig. 22-1). Atherosclerosis is considered to be a major contributor in the development of heart disease.

Triglycerides and cholesterides are insoluble in water and must be bound to a lipid-containing protein **(lipoprotein)** for transportation throughout the body. Although several lipoproteins are found in the blood, this chapter focuses on low-density lipoproteins (LDL), HDL, and cholesterol. **Low-density lipoproteins (LDL)** transport cholesterol to peripheral cells. When the cells have all the cholesterol they need, the excess cholesterol is discarded into the blood. This can result in a high blood level of cholesterol, which can penetrate the walls of the arteries, leading to atherosclerotic plaque formation. Elevated levels of LDL increase the risk for heart disease. The major protein constituent of LDL is apolipoprotein B. The function of apolipoprotein B is not well understood. However, the levels of apolipoprotein B correlate with familial combined hyperlipidemia, which is a genetic condition, and an increased risk of cardiovascular disease. **High-density lipoproteins (HDL)** take cholesterol from peripheral cells and bring it to the liver, where it is metabolized and excreted. The higher the level of HDL (the "good" lipoprotein), the lower the risk for development of atherosclerosis (Key Concepts 22-1).

Table 22-1 provides an analysis of LDL levels. HDL cholesterol protects against heart disease, so the higher the number, the better. An HDL level less than 40 mg/dL is low and considered a major risk factor for heart disease. Triglyceride levels that are borderline (150–199 mg/dL) or high (above 200 mg/dL) may require treatment in some individuals.

An increase in serum lipids is believed to contribute to or cause atherosclerosis, a disease characterized by deposits of fatty plaques on the inner walls of arteries. These deposits result in a narrowing of the lumen (inside diameter) of the artery and a decrease in blood supply to the area served by the artery. When these fatty deposits occur in the coronary arteries, the patient experiences coronary artery disease. Lowering blood cholesterol levels can arrest or reverse atherosclerosis in the vessels and can significantly decrease the person's risk for heart disease.

Hyperlipidemia, particularly elevated serum cholesterol and LDL levels, is a risk factor in the development of atherosclerotic heart disease. Other risk factors, besides cholesterol levels, play a role in the development of atherosclerotic heart disease, including

- Family history of early heart disease (father or brother before the age of 55 years and mother or sister before the age of 65 years)
- Cigarette smoking
- Hypertension (high blood pressure)
- Age (men older than 45 years and women older than 55 years)
- Low HDL levels
- Obesity
- Diabetes

In general, the higher one's LDL level and the more risk factors involved, the greater the risk for heart disease. The main goal of treatment in patients with hyperlipidemia is to lower the LDL to a level that will reduce their risk of heart disease (Box 22-1).

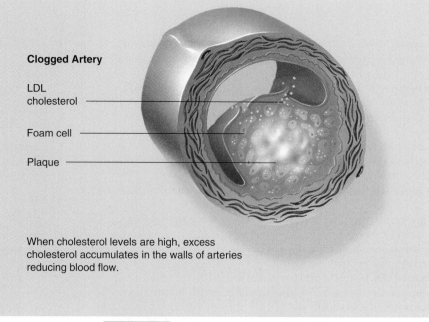

Clogged Artery

LDL cholesterol

Foam cell

Plaque

When cholesterol levels are high, excess cholesterol accumulates in the walls of arteries reducing blood flow.

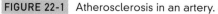

FIGURE 22-1   Atherosclerosis in an artery.

FACTS ABOUT . . .

Cholesterol

- 102.2 million Americans have a total cholesterol level of 200 mg/dL or higher, the point at which it becomes a cardiovascular risk factor.
- Coronary heart disease causes over 400,000 deaths in the United States each year, and approximately 17.6 million adults have coronary heart disease.
- Most people can raise their good cholesterol levels by eating a healthy diet, exercising, not smoking, and maintaining a healthy weight.
- The process leading to atherosclerosis can begin in children.
- Cholesterol levels are affected by genetics and eating habits.
- High cholesterol and atherosclerosis are not just a man's problem. While estrogen will aid in raising high-density lipoprotein (HDL) levels, women tend to have higher levels of triglycerides. As women age, and especially if they are overweight, their triglyceride and cholesterol levels will rise.

Source: American Heart Association

TABLE 22-1   Cholesterol Level Analysis

Total Cholesterol Level*	Category
<200 mg/dL	Desirable
200–239 mg/dL	Borderline
≥240 mg/dL	High
LDL Cholesterol Level*	LDL Cholesterol Category
≤100 mg/dL	Optimal
100–129 mg/dL	Near optimal/above optimal
130–159 mg/dL	Borderline high
160–189 mg/dL	High
≥190 mg/dL	Very high

*Cholesterol levels are measured in milligrams (mg) of cholesterol per deciliter (dL) of blood.

The health care provider may initially seek to control the cholesterol level by encouraging therapeutic life changes. This includes a cholesterol-lowering diet, physical activity, quitting smoking (if applicable), and weight management. The diet is a plan that is low in saturated fat and low in cholesterol. It includes less than 200 mg of dietary cholesterol per day. In addition, physical activity lasting at least 30 minutes each day is recommended. Walking at a brisk pace for 30 minutes per day 5 to 7 days per week can help raise the HDL and lower LDL. Added benefits of a healthy diet and exercise program include a reduction of body weight. If these lifestyle changes do not bring blood lipids to therapeutic levels, then the health care provider may add one of the antihyperlipidemic drugs to the treatment plan. The lifestyle changes are continued along with the drug regimen.

Antihyperlipidemic Drugs

In addition to controlling dietary intake of fat, particularly saturated fatty acids, antihyperlipidemic drug therapy is used to lower serum levels of cholesterol and triglycerides. The health care provider may use one drug or, in some instances, more than one antihyperlipidemic drug for those with poor response to therapy with a single drug. Three types of antihyperlipidemic drugs are currently in use, as well as two miscellaneous antihyperlipidemic drugs (see Summary Drug Table: Antihyperlipidemic Drugs for a complete listing of the drugs):

- Bile acid sequestrants
- HMG-CoA reductase inhibitors
- Fibric acid derivatives
- Ezetimibe
- Niacin

KEY CONCEPTS

22-1   Lipoprotein Profile/Lipid Panel

Because of HDL's protective properties against the development of atherosclerosis, it is desirable to see an increase in HDL and a decrease in LDL. A laboratory examination of blood lipids, called a lipoprotein profile or lipid panel, provides valuable information about a person's cholesterol levels, including

- Total cholesterol
- LDL (the harmful lipoprotein)
- HDL (the protective lipoprotein)
- Triglycerides

BOX 22.1

Assessing Risk for Cardiovascular Disease

A risk assessment tool using the data from the Framingham Heart Study can be used to estimate a 10-year risk for coronary heart disease. The tool is to be used in persons 20 years of age and older who do not currently have heart disease or diabetes. The tool uses age, gender, total cholesterol, HDL cholesterol, smoking habits, treatment for hypertension, and systolic blood pressure to calculate a person's risk of experiencing a myocardial infarction (heart attack) and coronary death within the next 10 years. For more details on the Framingham Heart Study, which is under the direction of the National Heart, Lung, and Blood Institute (NHLBI), visit http://www.framinghamheartstudy.org/.

The target levels for treatment are LDL less than 130 mg/dL, HDL greater than 40 mg/dL, and total cholesterol less than 200 mg/dL. If the patient's response to drug treatment is adequate, then lipid levels are monitored every 4 months. If the response is inadequate, then another drug or a combination of two drugs is used. Antihyperlipidemic drugs decrease cholesterol and triglyceride levels in several ways. Although the end result is a lower lipid blood level, each has a slightly different action.

FACT CHECK

22-1   What is atherosclerosis?
22-2   What is the desirable level of total cholesterol and the optimal level of LDL cholesterol?

BILE ACID SEQUESTRANTS

Actions of Bile Acid Sequestrants

Cholestyramine (Questran) and colestipol (Colestid) are examples of bile acid sequestrants. Bile, which is manufactured and secreted by the liver and stored in the gallbladder, emulsifies fat and lipids as they pass through the intestine. Once emulsified, fats and lipids are readily absorbed in the intestine. **Bile acid sequestrants** bind to bile acids to form an insoluble substance that cannot be absorbed by the intestine, so it is excreted in the feces. With increased loss of bile acids, the liver uses cholesterol to manufacture more bile. This is followed by a decrease in cholesterol levels.

Uses of Bile Acid Sequestrants

Bile acid sequestrants are used as adjunctive therapy for the reduction of elevated serum cholesterol in patients with hypercholesterolemia who do not have an adequate response to a diet and exercise program. Cholestyramine may also be used to relieve pruritus associated with partial biliary obstruction.

Adverse Reactions of Bile Acid Sequestrants

A common problem associated with bile acid sequestrants is constipation. Constipation may be severe and may occasionally result in fecal impaction. Hemorrhoids may be aggravated. Additional adverse reactions include vitamin A and D deficiencies, bleeding tendencies (including gastrointestinal bleeding) caused by a depletion of vitamin K, nausea, abdominal pain, and abdominal distention.

Contraindications, Precautions, and Interactions of Bile Acid Sequestrants

- Bile acid sequestrants are contraindicated in patients with known hypersensitivity to the drugs. Bile acid sequestrants are also contraindicated in those with complete biliary obstruction.
- These drugs are used cautiously in patients with a history of liver or kidney disease. Bile acid sequestrants are

ALERT ℞

Bile Acid Sequestrants and Constipation

Patients taking antihyperlipidemic drugs, particularly bile acid sequestrants, may experience constipation. The drugs can produce or severely worsen preexisting constipation. Patients are instructed to drink more fluids, eat foods high in dietary fiber, and exercise daily to help prevent constipation. If the problem persists or becomes severe, then a stool softener or laxative may be required. Some patients require a decreased dosage or discontinuation of the drug therapy. Because older adults are particularly prone to constipation when taking bile acid sequestrants, they should be monitored for hard dry stools, difficulty passing stools, and any reports of constipation. An accurate record of bowel movements should be kept.

used cautiously during lactation (decreased absorption of vitamins may affect the infant).
- Bile acids sequestrants, particularly cholestyramine, can decrease the absorption of numerous drugs. For this reason, bile acid sequestrants should be administered alone and other drugs given at least 1 hour before or 4 hours later.
- The patient has an increased risk of bleeding when bile acid sequestrants are administered with oral anticoagulants; the dosage of the anticoagulant is usually decreased.
- Bile acid sequestrants may bind with digoxin, thiazide diuretics, penicillin, propranolol, tetracyclines, folic acid, and thyroid hormones, resulting in decreased effects of these drugs.

FACT CHECK

22-3   How do bile acid sequestrants act?

HMG-COA REDUCTASE INHIBITORS

Actions of HMG-CoA Reductase Inhibitors

Another group of antihyperlipidemic drugs is called **HMG-CoA reductase inhibitors,** also known as "statins" because their generic names usually end in -statin. HMG-CoA (3-hydroxy-3-methylglutaryl coenzyme A) reductase is an enzyme that is a **catalyst** in the manufacture of cholesterol. (A catalyst is a substance that accelerates a chemical reaction without itself undergoing a change.) These drugs appear to inhibit the manufacture of cholesterol or promote the breakdown of cholesterol. This drug activity lowers the blood levels of cholesterol and serum triglycerides and increases blood levels of HDL. Examples of these drugs are fluvastatin (Lescol), lovastatin (Mevacor), and simvastatin (Zocor).

Uses of HMG-CoA Reductase Inhibitors

These drugs, along with a diet restricted in saturated fat and cholesterol, are used to treat hyperlipidemia when diet and other nonpharmacologic treatments alone have not resulted in lowered cholesterol levels.

Adverse Reactions of HMG-CoA Reductase Inhibitors

HMG-CoA reductase inhibitors are usually well tolerated. Adverse reactions, when they do occur, are often mild and transient and do not require discontinuing therapy. Common adverse reactions include nausea, vomiting, constipation, abdominal pain or cramps, and headache. A rare but more serious adverse reaction is rhabdomyolysis.

Contraindications, Precautions, and Interactions of HMG-CoA Reductase Inhibitors

- HMG-CoA reductase inhibitors are contraindicated in individuals with hypersensitivity to the drugs, patients with serious liver disorders, and during pregnancy and lactation.
- HMG-CoA reductase inhibitors are used cautiously in patients with a history of alcoholism, acute infection, hypotension, trauma, endocrine disorders, visual disturbances, or myopathy.
- HMG-CoA reductase inhibitors have an additive effect when used with bile acid sequestrants, which may provide an added benefit in treating hypercholesterolemia that does not respond to a single-drug regimen.
- The patient has an increased risk of myopathy (disorders of the striated muscle) if taking an HMG-CoA reductase inhibitor along with erythromycin, niacin, or cyclosporine.
- When the HMG-CoA reductase inhibitors are given with oral anticoagulants, the anticoagulant effect is increased.

FACT CHECK

22-4   How do HMG-CoA reductase inhibitors act?

FIBRIC ACID DERIVATIVES

Actions of Fibric Acid Derivatives

Fibric acid derivatives, the third group of antihyperlipidemic drugs, work in a variety of ways. Clofibrate (Atromid-S) acts to stimulate the liver to increase the breakdown of very-low-density lipoproteins (VLDL) to LDL, decreasing the liver synthesis of VLDL and inhibiting cholesterol formation. Fenofibrate (Tricor) acts by reducing VLDL and stimulating the catabolism of triglyceride-rich lipoproteins, resulting in a decrease in plasma triglyceride and cholesterol. Gemfibrozil (Lopid) increases the excretion of cholesterol in the feces and reduces the production of triglycerides by the liver, thus lowering serum lipid levels.

Uses of Fibric Acid Derivatives

Although fibric acid derivatives have antihyperlipidemic effects, their use varies depending on the drug. For example, clofibrate (Atromid-S) and gemfibrozil (Lopid) are used to treat individuals with very-high-serum triglyceride levels who have a risk of abdominal pain and pancreatitis and who do not experience a response to diet modifications. Clofibrate is not used to treat other types of hyperlipidemia and is not thought to be effective for prevention of coronary heart disease. Fenofibrate (Tricor) is used as adjunctive treatment for the reduction of LDL, total cholesterol, and triglycerides in patients with hyperlipidemia.

Adverse Reactions of Fibric Acid Derivatives

The adverse reactions of fibric acid derivatives include nausea, vomiting, gastrointestinal upset, and diarrhea. Clofibrate, fenofibrate, and gemfibrozil may increase cholesterol excretion into the bile, leading to cholelithiasis (stones in the gallbladder) or cholecystitis (inflammation of the gallbladder). If cholelithiasis occurs, then use of the drug is discontinued. Fenofibrate may also result in abnormal liver function tests, respiratory problems, back pain, and headache. Gemfibrozil may cause dyspepsia, skin rash, vertigo, and headache.

Contraindications, Precautions, and Interactions of Fibric Acid Derivatives

- Fibric acid derivatives are contraindicated in patients with hypersensitivity to the drugs and those with significant hepatic or renal dysfunction or primary biliary cirrhosis because these drugs may increase the already elevated cholesterol.
- The drugs are used cautiously during lactation and in patients with peptic ulcer disease or diabetes.
- Although rare, when a fibric acid derivative, particularly gemfibrozil, is given along with an HMG-CoA reductase inhibitor, the patient has an increased risk for rhabdomyolysis.
- When clofibrate, fenofibrate, or gemfibrozil is administered with anticoagulants, the patient is at an increased risk for bleeding.

ALERT Rx

Rhabdomyolysis

Antihyperlipidemic drugs, particularly HMG-CoA reductase inhibitors and fibric acid derivatives, have been associated with skeletal muscle effects leading to rhabdomyolysis. Rhabdomyolysis is a very rare condition in which muscle damage results in the release of muscle cell contents into the bloodstream. Rhabdomyolysis may precipitate renal dysfunction or acute renal failure. It is important to be alert for unexplained muscle pain, muscle tenderness, or weakness, especially if accompanied by malaise or fever. These symptoms should be reported to the health care provider because it may be necessary to discontinue the drug.

MISCELLANEOUS ANTIHYPERLIPIDEMIC DRUGS

Actions of Miscellaneous Antihyperlipidemics

Ezetimibe

Ezetimibe reduces blood cholesterol by inhibiting the absorption of cholesterol by the small intestine.

Niacin

The mechanism by which niacin (nicotinic acid) lowers blood lipids is not fully understood.

Uses of Miscellaneous Antihyperlipidemics

Ezetimibe

Ezetimibe reduces total cholesterol, LDL cholesterol, apolipoprotein B, and triglycerides and increases HDL cholesterol in patients with hypercholesterolemia. Administration of ezetimibe together with certain other antihyperlipidemic drugs provides better results than administration of the individual drugs by themselves. For example, administration of ezetimibe with an HMG-CoA reductase inhibitor is more effective in improving serum total cholesterol, LDL cholesterol, apolipoprotein B, triglycerides, and HDL cholesterol than either treatment alone. Also, administration of ezetimibe with the fibric acid derivative fenofibrate is more effective in improving serum total cholesterol, LDL cholesterol, apolipoprotein B, and non-HDL cholesterol in patients with mixed hyperlipemia as compared with either treatment alone.

Ezetimibe is also available in a combination product with simvastatin under the trade name Vytorin.

Niacin

Niacin is used as adjunctive therapy for the treatment of very-high-serum triglyceride levels in patients who present a risk of pancreatitis (inflammation of the pancreas) and who do not adequately respond to dietary control.

Adverse Reactions of Miscellaneous Antihyperlipidemics

Ezetimibe

Ezetimibe is generally well tolerated, whether administered alone or with an HMG-CoA reductase inhibitor. In general, adverse reactions were similar between ezetimibe administered with HMG-CoA reductase inhibitors and HMG-CoA reductase inhibitors alone. The same applies for ezetimibe administered in combination with other antihyperlipidemics.

However, elevated transaminase levels occurred slightly more often in patients receiving ezetimibe administered with HMG-CoA reductase inhibitors than in patients treated with HMG-CoA reductase inhibitors alone. Common adverse reactions of ezetimibe alone include back pain, diarrhea, abdominal pain, arthralgia, and sinusitis.

Common adverse reactions of ezetimibe with a statin include headache, upper respiratory infection, myalgia, and extremity pain.

Niacin

Niacin may cause nausea, vomiting, abdominal pain, diarrhea, severe generalized flushing of the skin, a sensation of warmth, and severe itching or tingling. Although these reactions are most often seen at higher dose levels, some patients may experience them even when small doses of nicotinic acid are administered. The sudden appearance of these reactions may frighten the patient. Taking an aspirin will help with the flushing. If the patient is in severe discomfort, then the health care provider should be notified immediately.

Contraindications, Precautions, and Interactions of Miscellaneous Antihyperlipidemics

Ezetimibe

- Ezetimibe is contraindicated in individuals with hypersensitivity to the drug.
- The combination of ezetimibe with an HMG-CoA reductase inhibitor is contraindicated in patients with active liver disease or unexplained persistent elevations in serum transaminases.

Niacin

- Niacin is contraindicated in patients with a known hypersensitivity to it and in those with active peptic ulcer, hepatic dysfunction, or arterial bleeding.
- The drug is used cautiously in patients with renal dysfunction, high alcohol consumption, unstable angina, and gout.

COMPLEMENTARY & ALTERNATIVE MEDICINE

Garlic

Garlic, an herb, is commonly used as a food product and an herbal supplement. Although garlic has many medicinal purposes, its positive effect on cardiovascular health is the most well known and has been extensively researched. Other benefits of garlic are that it helps to lower serum cholesterol and triglyceride levels, improves the ratio of HDL to LDL cholesterol, lowers blood pressure, and helps to prevent atherosclerosis.

Adverse reactions include mild stomach upset or irritation. Although no serious reactions have occurred in pregnant women taking garlic, its use is not recommended. Garlic is excreted in breast milk and may cause colic in some infants.

COMPLEMENTARY & ALTERNATIVE

MEDICINE

Fish Oil

Many individuals use fish oils to promote heart health. Oils from cold-water fish contain large amounts of omega-3 polyunsaturated fatty acids, eicosapentaenoic acid (EPA), and docosahexaenoic acid (DHA). These fatty acids may help reduce VLDL, triglycerides, and total cholesterol while increasing HDL or the "good" cholesterol.

The American Heart Association recommends eating fish at least twice each week as part of a normal diet. Fish that have the most omega-3 fatty acids include anchovy, bluefish, herring, mackerel, menhaden, mullet, salmon, sardines, sturgeon, trout, and tuna. A number of over-the-counter products containing fish oils are also available. These supplements are produced using salmon, halibut, herring, mackerel, and tuna, as well as cod liver and seal or whale blubber. A prescription-only product called Lovaza contains the omega-3 fatty acids, EPA, DHA, and Vitamin E in capsule form. Lovaza is taken with meals as either a single 4 g dose or as two 2 g doses. Any of the fish oil products should be combined with a lipid-lowering diet.

FACT CHECK

22-6   The combination of ezetimibe with an HMG-CoA reductase inhibitor is contraindicated in which patients?

22-7   How is niacin used?

COMPLEMENTARY & ALTERNATIVE

MEDICINE

Phytosterols

Phytosterols, also called plant sterols/stanols, are naturally occurring cholesterol-like molecules found in plants. In the intestine, they block the absorption of cholesterol. They have been shown to lower LDL without lowering HDL. As a result, they reduce the risk of heart disease. Dosages of 2 to 3 g of plant stanols per day have been shown to be effective. Many vegetables and fruits are naturally high in sterols. These include beets, brussel sprouts, cauliflower, onions, carrots, cabbage, yams, oranges, bananas, apples, cherries, peaches, and pears. Other high-sterol foods include cashews and other nuts, kidney beans, and vegetable oils. In addition, some foods come fortified with plant sterols, including regular and light margarines, yogurts, cheese, orange juice, granola bars, and whole grain bread.

ALERT ℞

Elevation of Blood Lipid Levels

Sometimes a paradoxical elevation of blood lipid levels occurs with drug therapy. Should this happen, the health care provider is notified, and a different antihyperlipidemic drug may be prescribed.

Patient Management Issues with Antihyperlipidemic Drugs

In many individuals, hyperlipidemia has no symptoms and the disorder is not discovered until laboratory tests reveal elevated cholesterol and triglyceride levels, elevated LDL levels, and decreased HDL levels. Serum cholesterol levels (i.e., a lipid profile) and liver function tests are obtained before the drugs are administered.

Patient assessment includes a dietary history, focusing on the types of foods in the patient's usual diet. Vital signs and weight are recorded. The patient's skin and eyelids are inspected for evidence of xanthomas (flat or elevated yellow deposits), which may occur in the more severe forms of hyperlipidemia.

Patients usually take these drugs as outpatients and then are seen by the health care provider for periodic monitoring. Blood cholesterol and triglyceride levels are monitored as a part of the ongoing therapy.

During therapy, vital signs and bowel functioning are assessed to watch for the adverse reaction constipation. Constipation may become serious if not treated.

Bile acid sequestrants may interfere with the digestion of fats and prevent the absorption of the fat-soluble vitamins (vitamins A, D, E, and K) and folic acid. When a bile acid sequestrant is used for long-term therapy, vitamins A and D may be given in a water-soluble form or administered parenterally. If the patient has bleeding tendencies as the result of vitamin K deficiency, then parenteral vitamin K is administered for immediate treatment, and oral vitamin K is given for prevention of a deficiency in the future.

Advise all patients starting therapy with ezetimibe of the risk of myopathy and tell them to promptly report any unexplained muscle pain, tenderness, or weakness.

Educating the Patient and Family about Antihyperlipidemic Drugs

It is essential to stress the importance of following the recommended diet because drug therapy alone cannot significantly lower cholesterol and triglyceride levels. If necessary, the patient or family member is referred to a teaching dietitian, a dietary teaching session, or a lecture provided by a hospital or community agency.

- When using diet and drugs to control high blood cholesterol levels, the health care provider does the following:
- Emphasizes that drug therapy alone will not significantly lower blood cholesterol levels
- Stresses importance of taking drug exactly as prescribed

- Reinforces the importance of adhering to the prescribed diet
- Provides a written copy of dietary plan and reviews its contents
- Answers the patient's questions and offers suggestions for ways to reduce dietary fat intake
- Reassures the patient that the results of therapy will be monitored by periodic laboratory and diagnostic tests and follow-up with the health care provider

Following are key points about antihyperlipidemic drugs the patient or family should know:

Bile Acid Sequestrants:

- Take the drug before meals unless your health care provider directs otherwise.
- Cholestyramine powder: The prescribed dose must be mixed in 4 to 6 fluid ounces of water or noncarbonated beverage and shaken vigorously. The powder can also be mixed with highly fluid soups or pulpy fruits (applesauce, crushed pineapple). The powder should not be ingested in its dry form. Other drugs are taken 1 hour before or 4 to 6 hours after cholestyramine. Cholestyramine is available combined with the artificial sweetener aspartame (Questran Light) for patients with diabetes or those concerned with weight gain.
- Colestipol granules: The prescribed dose must be mixed in liquids, soup, cereals, carbonated beverages, or pulpy fruits. Because the granules do not dissolve, the preparation should be slowly stirred until it is ready to drink. Take the entire drug, then rinse the glass with a small amount of water and drink it.
- Colesevelam: Mix the granules in liquids, soups, cereals, or pulpy fruits. Do not take it dry. Mix the prescribed amount in a glassful of liquid. Carbonated beverages should be stirred slowly in a large glass. The tablets are taken twice daily without regard to meals.
- Constipation, flatulence, nausea, and heartburn may occur and may disappear with continued therapy. Notify your health care provider if these effects become bothersome or if you experience unusual bleeding.

HMG-CoA Inhibitors:

- Take lovastatin once daily, preferably with the evening meal. Fluvastatin, pravastatin, and simvastatin are taken, without regard to meals, once daily in the evening or at bedtime.
- If fluvastatin or pravastatin is prescribed with a bile acid sequestrant, then take fluvastatin 2 hours after the bile acid sequestrant and pravastatin at least 4 hours afterward.
- Contact your health care provider as soon as possible if you experience nausea; vomiting; muscle pain, tenderness, or weakness; fever; upper respiratory infection; rash; itching; or extreme fatigue.

Fibric Acid Derivatives:

- Clofibrate: If you experience gastrointestinal upset, then take the drug with food. Notify your health care provider if you experience chest pain, shortness of breath, palpitations, nausea, vomiting, fever, chills, or sore throat.
- Gemfibrozil: Dizziness or blurred vision may occur. Observe caution when driving or performing hazardous tasks. Notify your health care provider if you experience epigastric pain, diarrhea, nausea, or vomiting.

Miscellaneous Antihyperlipidemics

- Ezetimibe: Take with or without food. If taken with an HMG-CoA reductase inhibitor or fenobibrate, the two drugs may be taken at the same time. If taken with a bile acid sequestrant, ezetimibe should be taken 2 hours before or 4 hours after the bile acid sequestrant.
- Niacin (nicotinic acid): Take this drug with meals. This drug may cause mild to severe facial flushing, a feeling of warmth, severe itching, or headache. These symptoms usually subside with continued therapy, but contact your health care provider as soon as possible if your symptoms are severe. Your health care provider may prescribe aspirin (325 mg) to be taken approximately 30 minutes before nicotinic acid to decrease the flushing reaction. If you become dizzy, avoid sudden changes in posture.

FACT CHECK

22-8 When teaching patients about antihyperlipidemic drugs, why should you emphasize the importance of following the recommended dietary guidelines?

Chapter Review

KEY POINTS

- Bile acid sequestrants are used as adjunctive therapy to reduce elevated serum cholesterol in patients with hypercholesterolemia who do not adequately respond to a diet and exercise program. Constipation is a common adverse effect. Bile acid sequestrants are contraindicated in those with complete biliary obstruction and are used cautiously in patients with a history of liver or kidney disease.
- HMG-CoA reductase inhibitors, along with a diet restricted in saturated fat and cholesterol, are used to treat hyperlipidemia when diet and other nonpharmacologic treatments alone have not resulted in lowered cholesterol levels. HMG-CoA reductase inhibitors are usually well tolerated. A rare but serious adverse reaction is rhabdomyolysis. HMG-CoA reductase inhibitors are contraindicated in individuals with a serious liver disorder.
- Although the fibric acid derivatives have antihyperlipidemic effects, their use varies depending on the drug. Clofibrate (Atromid-S) and gemfibrozil (Lopid) are used to treat individuals with very-high-serum triglyceride levels who have a risk of abdominal pain and pancreatitis and

who do not experience a response to diet modifications. Fibric acid derivatives are contraindicated in patients with significant hepatic or renal dysfunction or primary biliary cirrhosis because these drugs may increase the already elevated cholesterol.

- Ezetimibe is used as adjunctive therapy for the treatment of hypercholesterolemia and hyperlipidemia. Ezetimibe may be combined with an HMG-CoA reductase inhibitor (typically atorvastatin or simvastatin) or a fibric acid derivative (fenofibrate).

- Niacin is used as adjunctive therapy for the treatment of very-high-serum triglyceride levels in patients at risk for pancreatitis. Nicotinic acid may cause nausea, vomiting, abdominal pain, diarrhea, severe generalized flushing of the skin, a sensation of warmth, and severe itching or tingling.

CRITICAL THINKING CASE STUDY

Antihyperlipidemic Therapy

Mr. Caden, age 62, is taking Lipitor. He has questions about his exercise plan and the adverse effects he is experiencing.

1. Which of the following elements will most help his overall health?
   a. Lowering the amount of saturated fat he consumes
   b. Eating more fruits and vegetables
   c. Exercising at least 5 days per week
   d. All of the above; no single element alone is sufficient
2. Mr. Caden says he hates going to the gym to exercise and asks what other options you would suggest. You tell him the following:
   a. He must continue with heavy cardiovascular workouts.
   b. Walking at a brisk pace for at least 30 minutes per day 5 to 7 days per week has proven effective.
   c. Walking three times per week for 10 minutes at a brisk pace has proven effective.
   d. None of the above; exercise for someone on Lipitor is ineffective.
3. Mr. Caden is scheduled for a follow-up visit with his physician next week. He has been on Lipitor for approximately 6 weeks now. He does not understand why the physician has scheduled him for "lab work" at his next visit. What should you tell him?
4. At his next visit, Mr. Caden's physician decides to add Zetia to the Lipitor. Both of the medications are to be taken once daily. When should he take them?

Review Questions

MULTIPLE CHOICE

1. Lovastatin (Mevacor) is best taken
   a. once daily, preferably with the evening meal
   b. three times daily with meals
   c. at least 1 hour before or 2 hours after meals
   d. twice daily without regard to meals

2. HMG-CoA reductase inhibitors have an additive effect when used with
   a. bile acid sequestrants
   b. fibric acid derivatives
   c. niacin
   d. all of the above
3. A patient taking niacin reports flushing after each dose of the drug. Which of the following drugs might be prescribed to help alleviate the flushing?
   a. Demerol
   b. Aspirin
   c. Vitamin K
   d. Benadryl
4. A patient is at increased risk for bleeding if which of the following are administered with anticoagulants?
   a. Clofibrate
   b. Fenofibrate
   c. Gemfibrozil
   d. All of the above
5. A patient taking cholestyramine (Questran) who has vitamin K deficiency should
   a. be checked for bruising
   b. keep a record of fluid intake and output
   c. be monitored for myalgia
   d. keep a dietary record of foods eaten

MATCHING

_____ 6. cholestyramine   a. Zetia
_____ 7. simvastatin   b. Zocor
_____ 8. gemfibrozil   c. Mevacor
_____ 9. atorvastatin   d. Colestid
_____ 10. ezetemibe   e. Questran
_____ 11. rosuvastatin   f. Lipitor
_____ 12. colestipol   g. Lopid
_____ 13. lovastatin   h. Crestor

TRUE OR FALSE

_____ 14. Antihyperlipidemic drugs have been associated with skeletal muscle effects leading to rhabdomyolysis.
_____ 15. The lower the level of HDL, the lower the risk for development of atherosclerosis.
_____ 16. If a patient's initial response to treatment with an antihyperlipidemic drug is inadequate, then another drug or a combination of two drugs is used.
_____ 17. Patient teaching about drug and diet therapy for hyperlipidemia should emphasize that the medication alone will lower cholesterol levels.
_____ 18. A risk assessment tool for estimating a patient's 10-year risk for coronary heart disease can be used in patients who are 20 years of age or older and who have heart disease or diabetes.

FILL IN THE BLANKS

19. Elevated levels of _____ _____. lipoproteins increase the risk for heart disease.
20. _____ is the most common adverse reaction associated with bile acid sequestrants.

21. HMG-CoA reductase is an enzyme that is a(n) _____ in the manufacture of cholesterol.
22. Gemfibrozil is a fibric acid derivative that increases excretion of _____ in the feces and reduces the production of _____ by the liver.
23. _____ reduces blood cholesterol by inhibiting the absorption of cholesterol by the small intestine.

SHORT ANSWERS

24. What are the benefits of lowering blood cholesterol levels?
25. Because bile acid sequestrants can decrease the absorption of many drugs, how should they be administered?
26. What is a lipoprotein profile?
27. What are the common adverse reactions of niacin?

28. Why should HMG-CoA reductase inhibitors not be taken by a woman who is pregnant or nursing?

Web Activities

1. Go to the MedlinePlus Web site (http://medlineplus.gov). Click on "Health Topics" and search for cholesterol. Write a brief statement about one of the "Latest News" articles on the MedlinePlus site involving cholesterol.
2. Go to the National Heart, Lung, and Blood Institute Web site (www.nhlbi.nih.gov). Conduct a search for the Framingham Heart Study. Discuss the factors used to estimate risk of coronary heart disease in men and women. How are they similar and how are they different?

SUMMARY DRUG TABLE Antihyperlipidemic Drugs (left, generic; right, trade)

Comprehensive Summary Drug Tables, including uses, adverses effects, dosages, and pregnancy classifications, are provided on the companion website, http://thePoint.lww.com/PharmacologyHP2e

Bile Acid Sequestrants	
cholestyramine *koe-less'-tir-a-meen*	Prevalite, Questran, Questran Light, *generic*
colestipol HCl *koe-les'-ti-pole*	Colestid, *generic*
colesevelam HCl *ko-leh-sev'-eh-lam*	Welchol
HMG-CoA Reductase Inhibitors	
atorvastatin *ah-tor'-va-stah-tin*	Lipitor, *generic*
fluvastatin *flue-va-sta'-tin*	Lescol, Lescol XL
lovastatin *loe-va-sta'-tin*	Altoprev, Mevacor, *generic*
pitavastatin *pi-ta'-va-sta-tin*	Livalo
pravastatin *prah-va-sta'-tin*	Pravachol, *generic*

rosuvastatin *roe-soo-va-stat'-in*	Crestor
simvastatin *sim-va-stah'-tin*	Zocor, *generic*
Fibric Acid Derivatives	
fenofibrate *fen-oh-figh'-brate*	Tricor, Fenoglide, Lipofen, Lofibra, Triglide, Trilipix, Antara, *generic*
gemfibrozil *jem-fi'-broe-zil*	Lopid, *generic*
Miscellaneous Preparations	
ezetimibe *ez-et'-i-mibe*	Zetia
ezetimibe/simvastatin *ez-et'-i-mibe sim-va-stat'-in*	Vytorin
niacin *nye'-a-sin* (nicotinic acid)	Endur-Acin, Niacinol, Niacor, Niaspan, No Flush Niacin, Slo-Niacin, *generic*

23

Anticoagulant and Thrombolytic Drugs

CHAPTER OBJECTIVES

On completion of this chapter, students will be able to:

1. Define the chapter's key terms.

2. Discuss hemostasis and the blood-clotting pathway.

3. Discuss the similarities and differences among the adverse reactions of warfarin, heparin, and thrombolytics.

4. Explain how warfarin and heparin overdosages are managed.

5. Describe the general drug actions, uses, adverse reactions, contraindications, precautions, and interactions of anticoagulant and thrombolytic drugs.

6. Discuss important points to keep in mind when educating the patient or family members about the use of an anticoagulant and thrombolytic drug.

KEY TERMS

fibrinolytic drugs—another name for thrombolytic drugs
hemostasis—a process that stops bleeding in a blood vessel
prothrombin—a substance that is essential for the clotting of blood
thrombolytic drugs—drugs designed to dissolve blood clots that have already formed within a blood vessel
thrombosis—the formation of a clot
thrombus—blood clot

CHAPTER OVERVIEW

Drug classes covered in this chapter are:

- Anticoagulant drugs

- Thrombolytic drugs

Drugs by classification are listed on page 236.

thePOINT RESOURCES

- Comprehensive Summary Drug Tables

- Lippincott's Interactive Tutorials: Drugs Affecting the Cardiovascular System

- Interactive Practice and Review

- Monographs of Most Commonly Prescribed Drugs

Anticoagulants are used to prevent the formation and extension of a **thrombus** (blood clot). Anticoagulants have no direct effect on an existing thrombus and do not reverse any damage from the thrombus. However, once a thrombus has been established, anticoagulant therapy can prevent additional clots from forming. Although anticoagulants do not thin the blood, they are sometimes called blood thinners by patients. Anticoagulants are a group of drugs that include warfarin (a coumarin derivative) and heparin.

Whereas the anticoagulants prevent thrombus formation, **thrombolytic drugs** dissolve blood clots that have already formed within a blood vessel. These drugs can reopen blood vessels after they become occluded. Another term for thrombolytic drugs is **fibrinolytic drugs**. A basic understanding of hemostasis and thrombus formation is a foundation for understanding these drugs.

Hemostasis

Hemostasis is the body's process of stopping bleeding in a blood vessel. Normal hemostasis involves a complex process of extrinsic and intrinsic factors. Figure 23-1 shows the coagulation pathway and factors involved. The coagulation cascade is so named because as each factor is activated, it acts as a catalyst that enhances the next reaction, and the net result is a large collection of fibrin that forms a plug in the vessel. Fibrin is the insoluble protein that is essential to clot formation.

Thrombosis

Thrombosis is the formation of a clot. A thrombus may form in any vessel, artery, or vein when blood flow is impeded. For example, a venous thrombus can develop as the result of venous stasis (decreased blood flow), injury to the vessel wall, or altered blood coagulation. Venous thrombosis most often occurs in the lower extremities and is associated with venous stasis. Deep vein thrombosis occurs in the lower extremities and is the most common type of venous thrombosis. Arterial thrombosis can occur because of atherosclerosis or arrhythmias, such as atrial fibrillation. The thrombus may begin small, but fibrin, platelets, and red blood cells attach to the thrombus, increasing its size and shape. When a thrombus detaches from the wall of the vessel and is carried along through the bloodstream, it becomes an embolus. The embolus travels until it reaches a vessel that is too small to permit its passage. If the embolus goes to the lung and obstructs a pulmonary vessel, then it is called a pulmonary embolism. If the embolus occludes a vessel supplying blood to the heart, then it can cause a myocardial infarction. Anticoagulant drugs therefore are used prophylactically in patients who are at high risk for clot formation.

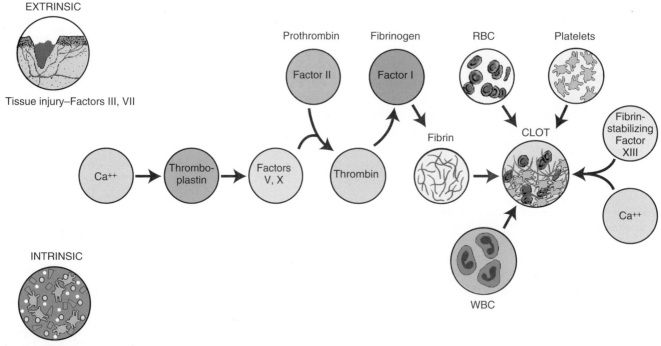

FIGURE 23-1 The blood-clotting pathway. Blood coagulation results in the formation of a stable fibrin clot. Formation of this clot involves a cascade of interactions of clotting factors, platelets, and other substances. Clotting factors exist in the blood in inactive form and must be converted to an active form before the next step in the clotting pathway can occur. Each factor is stimulated in turn until the process is complete and a fibrin clot is formed. In the intrinsic pathway, all of the components necessary for clot formation are in the circulating blood. Clot formation in the intrinsic pathway is initiated by factor XII. In the extrinsic pathway, coagulation is initiated by release of tissue thromboplastin, a factor not found in circulating blood.

Anticoagulants

WARFARIN

Warfarin (Coumadin), a coumarin derivative, is the only oral anticoagulant available at this time. Warfarin can also be administered parenterally. Because it can be given orally, it is the drug of choice for patients requiring long-term therapy with an anticoagulant. Peak activity is reached 1.5 to 3 days after therapy is initiated.

All anticoagulants interfere with the clotting mechanism of the blood. Warfarin interferes with the manufacturing of vitamin K–dependent clotting factors by the liver. This results in the depletion of clotting factors II (prothrombin), VII, IX, and X.

Actions of Warfarin

It is the depletion of **prothrombin** (see Fig. 23-1), a substance that is essential for the clotting of blood, that accounts for most of the action of warfarin.

Uses of Warfarin

Warfarin is used for

- Prevention (prophylaxis) and treatment of deep vein thrombosis
- Prevention and treatment of atrial fibrillation with embolization
- Prevention and treatment of pulmonary embolism
- As part of the treatment of myocardial infarction
- Prevention of thrombus formation after valve replacement

Adverse Reactions of Warfarin

The principal adverse reaction of warfarin is bleeding, which may range from very mild to severe. Bleeding may be seen in many areas of the body, such as the bladder, bowel, stomach, uterus, and mucous membranes (Key Concepts 23-1). Other

KEY CONCEPTS

23-1   Bleeding in Patients Receiving Warfarin

Bleeding can occur any time during therapy with warfarin, even when the patient's PT appears to be within a safe limit. (Prothrombin time is a test of the blood's clotting time. International normalized ratio is another measure of clotting time.) All health care team members should be made aware of any patient receiving warfarin and help observe for bleeding.

adverse reactions are rare but may include alopecia (loss of hair) and abdominal cramping.

Warfarin Overdosage

Symptoms of warfarin overdosage include

- Blood in the stool (melena)
- Petechiae (pinpoint-size red hemorrhagic spots on the skin)
- Oozing from superficial injuries, such as cuts from shaving or bleeding from the gums after brushing the teeth
- Excessive menstrual bleeding

Any adverse reactions or evidence of bleeding must be immediately reported to the health care provider. Because warfarin interferes with the synthesis of vitamin K_1–dependent clotting factors, the administration of vitamin K_1 reverses the effects of warfarin by providing the necessary ingredient to enhance clot formation and stop bleeding. However, withholding one or two doses of warfarin may quickly bring the PT to an acceptable level. The PT generally returns to a safe level within 6 hours of administration of vitamin K_1. Administration of whole blood or plasma may be necessary if severe bleeding occurs because the vitamin K_1 is delayed.

Contraindications, Precautions, and Interactions of Warfarin

- Warfarin is contraindicated in patients with a known hypersensitivity, hemorrhagic disease, tuberculosis, leukemia, uncontrolled hypertension, gastrointestinal ulcers, recent surgery of the eye or central nervous system, aneurysms, or severe renal or hepatic disease, and during pregnancy and lactation.
- Use during pregnancy (pregnancy category X) can cause fetal death.
- Warfarin is used cautiously in patients with fever, heart failure, diarrhea, malignancy, hypertension, renal or hepatic disease, psychoses, or depression. Women of childbearing age must use a reliable contraceptive to prevent pregnancy.
- The effects of warfarin may increase when administered with acetaminophen, NSAIDs, beta blockers, disulfiram, isoniazid, chloral hydrate, loop diuretics, aminoglycosides, cimetidine, tetracyclines, and cephalosporins.

- Oral contraceptives, ascorbic acid, barbiturates, diuretics, and vitamin K decrease the effects of warfarin.
- Because the effects of warfarin are influenced by many drugs, the patient should notify the health care provider when taking a new drug or discontinuing use of any drug, both prescription and over-the-counter preparations.

Patient Management Issues with Warfarin

Before the first dose of warfarin is administered, the patient is questioned about all drugs taken during the previous 2 to 3 weeks.

Because deep vein thrombosis usually occurs in the leg, the health care provider examines the patient's legs for color and skin temperature. The rate and strength of the pedal pulse are checked, noting any difference between the affected leg and the unaffected leg. Areas of redness or tenderness are noted. The affected leg may appear edematous and exhibit a positive Homans sign (pain in the calf when the foot is dorsiflexed). A positive Homans sign is suggestive of deep vein thrombosis.

During the course of therapy, a patient is continually assessed for any signs of bleeding and hemorrhage. Areas of assessment include the gums, nose, stools, urine, or nasogastric drainage.

Patients receiving warfarin for the first time often require daily adjustment of the dose.

Educating the Patient and Family about Warfarin

The health care provider gives a full explanation of the drug regimen to patients taking warfarin, including an explanation of the problems that can occur during therapy. A thorough review of the dose regimen, possible adverse drug reactions, and early signs of bleeding tendencies helps a patient cooperate with the prescribed therapy. Following are key points about warfarin that the patient and family members should know:

- Follow the dosage schedule prescribed by your health care provider.
- You will have periodic blood tests to monitor your condition. Keep all health care provider and laboratory appointments because dosage changes may be necessary during therapy.
- Do not take or stop taking other drugs except on the advice of your health care provider. This includes nonprescription drugs as well as those prescribed by your health care provider or dentist.
- Inform your dentist and other health care providers of your therapy with this drug before any treatment or procedure is started or drugs are prescribed.
- Take the drug at the same time each day.
- Do not drink alcohol unless it is approved by your health care provider. You should limit intake of foods high in vitamin K, such as green leafy vegetables, beans, broccoli, cabbage, cauliflower, cheese, fish, and yogurt.
- If you see evidence of bleeding, such as unusual bleeding or bruising, bleeding gums, blood in the urine or stool, black stool, or diarrhea, then omit the next dose of the drug and contact your health care provider immediately.
- Use a soft toothbrush and consult a dentist regarding routine oral hygiene, including the use of dental floss. Use an electric razor when possible to avoid small skin cuts.
- Wear or carry identification, such as a medical alert tag, to inform medical personnel and others of your therapy with this drug.

ALERT Rx

Vitamin K

Studies indicate that diet can influence patients' PT. In patients receiving warfarin, a diet high in vitamin K may increase the risk of clot formation. A diet low in vitamin K may increase the risk of hemorrhage. Significant changes in vitamin K intake may necessitate warfarin dosage adjustment. The key to vitamin K management for patients receiving warfarin is maintaining a consistent daily intake of vitamin K. To avoid large fluctuations in vitamin K intake, patients receiving warfarin should be aware of the vitamin K content of food. For example, green leafy vegetables and some vegetable oils (soybean and canola oil) are high in vitamin K. Root vegetables, fruits, cereals, dairy products, and meats are generally low in vitamin K.

Although the drug is most often administered orally, warfarin injection may be used as an alternative route for patients who are unable to receive oral drugs. The IV dosage is the same as that for the oral drug.

ALERT Rx

Warfarin Interaction

Warfarin has a narrow therapeutic index (the difference between the minimum therapeutic and minimum toxic drug concentrations is small), making any interactions very important. Warfarin interacts with many herbal remedies. For example, warfarin should not be combined with any of the following herbs because they may have additive or synergistic activity and increase the risk for bleeding: celery, chamomile, clove, dong quai, feverfew, garlic, ginger, ginkgo biloba, ginseng, green tea, onion, passion flower, red clover, St. John's wort, and turmeric.

FACT CHECK

23-3 Why is warfarin the drug of choice for patients requiring long-term anticoagulant therapy?

23-4 Which drugs decrease the effects of warfarin?

23-5 What are the symptoms of warfarin overdosage?

HEPARIN AND LOW-MOLECULAR-WEIGHT HEPARINS

Heparin preparations to prevent clot formation are available as heparin sodium and the low-molecular-weight heparins (LMWHs) (fractionated heparins). Heparin is not a single drug, but rather a mixture of high- and low-molecular-weight drugs. Drugs with low molecular weights are available as LMWH. Examples of LMWHs are dalteparin (Fragmin), enoxaparin (Lovenox), and tinzaparin (Innohep). Low-molecular-weight heparins produce very stable responses when administered at the recommended doses. Because of this stability, frequent laboratory monitoring is not necessary. In addition, bleeding is less likely to occur with LMWHs than with heparin sodium.

Actions of Heparin

Heparin inhibits the formation of fibrin clots, inhibits the conversion of fibrinogen to fibrin, and inactivates several of the factors necessary for the clotting of blood. Heparin cannot be taken orally because it is inactivated by gastric acid in the stomach; therefore, it must be given by injection. Heparin has no effect on clots that have already formed and aids only in preventing the formation of new blood clots (thrombi). The LMWHs act to inhibit clotting reactions by binding to antithrombin III, which inhibits the synthesis of factor Xa and the formation of thrombin.

Uses of Heparin

Heparin is used for

- Prevention and treatment of venous thrombosis, pulmonary embolism, and peripheral arterial embolism
- Atrial fibrillation with embolus formation
- Prevention of postoperative venous thrombosis and pulmonary embolism in certain patients undergoing surgical procedures, such as major abdominal surgery
- Prevention of clotting in arterial and heart surgery, in blood transfusions and dialysis procedures, and in blood samples for laboratory purposes
- Prevention of a repeat cerebral thrombosis in some patients who have experienced a stroke
- Treatment of coronary occlusion, acute myocardial infarction, and peripheral arterial embolism

ALERT Rx

Signs and Symptoms of Patient Bleeding
Bleeding at virtually any site can occur during therapy with any heparin preparation, even the LMWHs. A patient's vital signs are monitored every 2 to 4 hours or as ordered by the health care provider. Evidence of bleeding should be immediately reported: bleeding gums, epistaxis (nosebleed), easy bruising, black tarry stools, hematuria (blood in the urine), oozing from wounds or IV sites, or a decrease in blood pressure.

- Prevention of clotting in equipment used for extracorporeal (outside the body) blood circulation
- Treatment of disseminated intravascular coagulation, a severe hemorrhagic disorder
- Maintenance of patency of IV catheters (very low doses of 10 to 100 units)

The LMWHs are used to prevent deep vein thrombosis after certain surgical procedures, such as hip or knee replacement surgery or abdominal surgery. These drugs are also used for ischemic complications of unstable angina and myocardial infarction.

Adverse Reactions of Heparin

Hemorrhage is the chief complication of heparin administration. Hemorrhage can range from minor local bruising to major hemorrhaging from any organ. Thrombocytopenia (low levels of platelets in the blood) may occur, causing bleeding from the small capillaries and resulting in easy bruising, petechiae, and hemorrhage into the tissues.

Other adverse reactions include local irritation when heparin is given by SC injection. Hypersensitivity reactions may also occur with any route of administration and include fever, chills, and urticaria. More serious hypersensitivity reactions include an asthma-like reaction and an anaphylactoid reaction.

The LMWHs cause fewer adverse reactions than heparin. Bleeding related to the LMWHs is possible but has generally been low.

Heparin Overdosage

If a patient has a significant decrease in blood pressure or increase in pulse rate, then the health care provider should be

CONSIDERATIONS | Older adults

LIFESPAN

Heparin-Related Bleeding
Bleeding is more common in individuals older than 60 years (particularly older women) when heparin is administered. Older patients should be carefully monitored for evidence of bleeding.

notified because this may indicate internal bleeding. Because hemorrhage may begin as a slight bleeding or bruising tendency, the patient is frequently observed for these. At times, hemorrhage can occur without warning. If bleeding should occur, then the health care provider may decrease the dose, discontinue the heparin therapy for a time, or order the administration of protamine sulfate.

In most instances, discontinuation of the drug is sufficient and corrects the overdosage because the duration of action of heparin is short. However, if hemorrhaging is severe, then the health care provider may order protamine sulfate, the specific heparin antagonist or antidote. Protamine sulfate is also used to treat overdosage of the LMWHs. Protamine sulfate has an immediate onset of action and a duration of 2 hours. It counteracts the effects of heparin. The drug is given slowly via the IV route during a period of 10 minutes.

Contraindications, Precautions, and Interactions of Heparin

- Heparin preparations are contraindicated in patients with a known hypersensitivity, active bleeding (except when caused by disseminated intravascular coagulation), hemorrhagic disorders, severe thrombocytopenia, or recent surgery (except for the LMWHs used after certain surgical procedures to prevent thromboembolic complications).
- The LMWHs are contraindicated in patients with a hypersensitivity to the drug, to heparin, or to pork products, and in inpatients with active bleeding or thrombocytopenia.
- Treatment with heparin preparations is approached cautiously in the elderly; in patients with severe renal or kidney disease, diabetes, diabetic retinopathy, ulcer disease, or uncontrolled hypertension; and in all patients with a potential site for bleeding or hemorrhage.
- The LMWHs are used with caution in patients who are at increased risk for hemorrhage, such as those with severe uncontrolled hypertension, diabetic

retinopathy, bacterial endocarditis, congenital or acquired bleeding disorders, gastrointestinal disease, or hemorrhagic stroke, and in patients soon after brain, spinal, or ophthalmologic surgery.
- When heparin is administered with a nonsteroidal anti-inflammatory drug (NSAID), aspirin, penicillin, or cephalosporin, there may be an increase in clotting times, thereby increasing the risk for bleeding.
- During heparin administration, serum transaminase (aspartate, alanine) levels may be falsely elevated; careful interpretation is required because these laboratory tests may be used to help diagnose certain disorders, such as liver disease or myocardial infarction.
- Protamine sulfate, a heparin antagonist, is incompatible with certain antibiotics such as penicillin and the cephalosporins.
- Use of the LMWHs with any of these drugs may increase the risk of bleeding: aspirin, salicylates, NSAIDs, and thrombolytics.

Patient Management Issues with Heparin

The most commonly used test to monitor heparin's effects is activated partial thromboplastin time (APTT). Blood is drawn for laboratory studies before giving the first dose of heparin to obtain baseline data. The dosage of heparin is adjusted according to daily APTT monitoring. Periodic platelet counts, hematocrit, and tests for occult blood in the stool should also be performed throughout the course of heparin therapy.

Patients receiving heparin require close observation and careful monitoring. It is also important that a patient be monitored for any indication of hypersensitivity reaction. Reactions, such as chills, fever, or hives, are reported to the health care provider. When heparin is given to prevent the formation of a thrombus, a patient is observed for signs of thrombus formation every 2 to 4 hours. Because the signs and symptoms of thrombus formation vary and depend on the area or organ involved, the health care provider should evaluate and report any symptom the patient may have or any change in a patient's condition.

Heparin preparations, unlike warfarin, must be given by the parenteral route, preferably subcutaneously or IV. The onset of anticoagulation is almost immediate after a single dose. Maximum effects occur within 10 minutes of administration. Clotting time returns to normal within 4 hours unless subsequent doses are given. Heparin may be given by intermittent IV administration, continuous IV infusion, and the SC route. Intramuscular administration is avoided because of the possibility of the development of local irritation, pain, or hematoma (a collection of blood in the tissue).

Educating the Patient and Family about Heparin

Although heparin is given in the hospital, the LMWHs can be administered at home by a home health care provider, the patient, or a family member. The patient or a family member is taught how to administer the drug by the SC route. Prefilled syringes are available, making administration more convenient. The health care provider instructs the patient to apply firm pressure after the injection to prevent hematoma formation. Each time the drug is given, all recent injection sites are inspected for signs of inflammation (redness, swelling, tenderness) and hematoma formation. Following are key points about heparin that the patient and family members should know:

- Report any signs of active bleeding to your health care provider immediately.
- Regular blood tests are critical for safe monitoring of the drug's effects (except the LMWHs).
- Avoid any IM injections while receiving anticoagulant therapy.
- Use a soft toothbrush when cleaning your teeth and use an electric razor for shaving (to avoid nicks and cuts).
- Do not take any prescription or nonprescription drugs without consulting your health care provider. Drugs containing alcohol, aspirin, or ibuprofen may alter the effects of heparin.
- Advise your dentist or other health care providers that you are on anticoagulant therapy before any procedure or surgery.
- Carry appropriate identification with information concerning your drug therapy, or wear a medical alert tag at all times.

FACT CHECK

23-6   How does heparin act?
23-7   What are the adverse reactions of heparin?
23-8   What are the contraindications for use of LMWHs?

Thrombolytic Drugs

Thrombolytics are drugs that dissolve certain types of blood clots and reopen blood vessels after they have been occluded. Examples of thrombolytics include alteplase recombinant (Activase), reteplase recombinant (Retavase), tenecteplase (TNKase), and urokinase (Abbokinase). Before these drugs are used, their potential benefits must be carefully weighed against the potential dangers of bleeding.

Actions of Thrombolytic Drugs

Although the exact action of different thrombolytic drugs vary slightly, all these drugs break down fibrin clots by converting plasminogen to plasmin (fibrinolysin). Plasmin is an enzyme that breaks down the fibrin of a blood clot. This reopens blood vessels after their occlusion and thereby prevents tissue necrosis.

Uses of Thrombolytic Drugs

Thrombolytic drugs are used to treat an acute myocardial infarction by lysing (dissolving) a blood clot in a coronary artery. These drugs are also effective in lysing clots causing pulmonary embolism and deep vein thrombosis. Urokinase is also used to treat pulmonary embolism and to clear IV catheter cannulas obstructed by a blood clot.

ALERT R_x

Combining Heparin and a Thrombolytic Drug

Heparin may be given along with or after administration of a thrombolytic drug to prevent another thrombus from forming. However, administration of an anticoagulant increases the risk for bleeding. The patient must be monitored closely for internal and external bleeding.

If uncontrolled bleeding is noted or if the bleeding appears to be internal, then the drug is stopped and the health care provider is notified immediately. Vital signs are monitored every hour or more frequently for at least 48 hours after the drug is discontinued. The health care provider should be notified if there is a marked change in any of the patient's vital signs. Any signs of an allergic (hypersensitivity) reaction, such as difficulty breathing, wheezing, hives, skin rash, or hypotension, are reported immediately to the health care provider.

Adverse Reactions of Thrombolytic Drugs

Bleeding is the most common adverse reaction seen with the use of thrombolytic drugs. Bleeding may be internal and involve areas such as the gastrointestinal tract, genitourinary tract, or the brain. Bleeding may also be external (superficial) and may occur in areas of broken skin, such as venipuncture sites and recent surgical wounds. Allergic reactions may also occur.

Bleeding is the most common adverse reaction. Throughout therapy with a thrombolytic drug, the patient is monitored for signs of bleeding and hemorrhage (see earlier discussion of warfarin). Internal bleeding may occur in the gastrointestinal tract, genitourinary tract, intracranial sites, or respiratory tract. Symptoms of internal bleeding may include abdominal pain, coffee-ground emesis, black tarry stools, hematuria, joint pain, and spitting or coughing up of blood. Superficial bleeding may occur at venous or arterial puncture sites or recent surgical incision sites. As fibrin is lysed during therapy, bleeding from recent injection sites may occur. All potential bleeding sites (including catheter insertions sites, arterial and venous puncture sites, cutdown sites, and needle puncture sites) are carefully monitored.

Contraindications, Precautions, and Interactions of Thrombolytic Drugs

- Thrombolytic drugs are contraindicated in patients with known hypersensitivity, active bleeding, history of stroke, aneurysm, or recent intracranial surgery.
- These drugs are used cautiously in patients who have recently undergone major surgery (within 10 days or less), such as coronary artery bypass graft, or experienced stroke, trauma, vaginal or cesarean section delivery, gastrointestinal bleeding, or trauma within the past 10 days; those who have hypertension, diabetic retinopathy, or any condition in which bleeding is a significant possibility; and patients currently receiving oral anticoagulants.

- Administration of a thrombolytic drug along with aspirin, dipyridamole, or an anticoagulant may increase the risk of bleeding.

Patient Management Issues with Thrombolytic Drugs

The patient's history is checked for any conditions that might contraindicate the use of a thrombolytic drug, including any history of bleeding tendencies, heart disease, or allergic reactions to any drugs. In addition, a history of any drugs currently being taken is obtained. Most of these patients are admitted or transferred to an intensive care unit because close monitoring is necessary for 48 hours or more after therapy begins.

During drug therapy, the patient must also be continually assessed for an anaphylactic reaction (difficulty breathing, wheezing, fever, swelling around the eyes, hives, or itching).

For optimal therapeutic effect, the thrombolytic drugs are used as soon as possible after the formation of a thrombus, preferably within 4 to 6 hours or as soon as possible after the symptoms are identified. The greatest benefit occurs when the drugs are administered within 4 hours, but studies indicate that significant benefit can still occur when the drug is used within the first 24 hours.

Educating the Patient and Family about Thrombolytic Drugs

Following are key points about thrombolytic drugs that the patient and family members should know:

- It is normal for the health care team to continuously monitor you before and after administering the drug to watch for any potential adverse effects.
- Report any evidence of hypersensitivity reaction (rash, difficulty breathing) or evidence of bleeding or bruising to your health care provider.
- Bed rest is important during therapy.

FACT CHECK

23-9   How are thrombolytic drugs used for patients with acute myocardial infarction?

23-10   What is the most common adverse reaction of thrombolytic drugs?

Chapter Review

KEY POINTS

- Anticoagulants include warfarin (a coumarin derivative) and fractionated and unfractionated heparin.
- Warfarin (Coumadin) is the only oral anticoagulant available at this time. The principal adverse reaction of warfarin is bleeding, which may range from very mild to severe. Warfarin is contraindicated in patients with known hypersensitivity to the drug, hemorrhagic disease, tuberculosis, leukemia, uncontrolled hypertension, gastrointestinal ulcers, recent surgery of the eye or central nervous system, aneurysms, or severe renal or hepatic disease, and during pregnancy and lactation. Use during pregnancy can cause fetal death.
- Heparin inhibits the formation of fibrin clots, inhibits the conversion of fibrinogen to fibrin, and inactivates several of the factors necessary for the clotting of blood. Hemorrhage is the chief complication of heparin administration. Heparin preparations are contraindicated in patients with known hypersensitivity to the drug, active bleeding (except when caused by disseminated intravascular coagulation), hemorrhagic disorders, severe thrombocytopenia, or recent surgery (except for the LMWHs used after certain surgical procedures to prevent thromboembolic complications) and during pregnancy.
- Thrombolytics are a group of drugs used to dissolve certain types of blood clots and reopen blood vessels after they have been occluded. Bleeding is the most common adverse reaction seen with the use of these drugs. Bleeding may be internal and involve areas such as the gastrointestinal tract, genitourinary tract, and the brain. Thrombolytic drugs are contraindicated in patients with

known hypersensitivity, active bleeding, history of stroke, aneurysm, or recent intracranial surgery.

CRITICAL THINKING CASE STUDY
Warfarin Therapy

Mr. Harris, age 72 years, is a widower who has lived alone since his wife died 5 years ago. He has been prescribed warfarin to take at home after his dismissal from the hospital. Mr. Harris has questions about caring for himself to prevent any complications with his treatment.

1.   Mr. Harris wonders about potential adverse effects. You tell him the following:
   a.   Side effects are minimal but may include diarrhea.
   b.   Bleeding is the only adverse reaction.
   c.   Bleeding is the principal adverse reaction, and although other adverse reactions are rare, abdominal cramping and alopecia may occur.
   d.   None of the above.
2.   Mr. Harris asks if he needs to modify his diet in any way because of warfarin use. He should be told
   a.   not to drink alcohol unless his health care provider approves it
   b.   not to drink alcohol or eat lots of foods high in vitamin K
   c.   not to take vitamin supplements containing vitamin B_{12}, which can impact the absorption of warfarin
   d.   that there are no known dietary restrictions
3.   Mr. Harris wonders aloud whether he will remember how the doctor told him to take his warfarin

because the dose on Monday, Wednesday, and Friday is different from the dose on Tuesday, Thursday, and Saturday. He is not supposed to take a dose on Sunday at all. How can you help him?

Review Questions

MULTIPLE CHOICE

1. Urokinase is used for which of the following?
   a. Acute myocardial infarction
   b. Clear IV catheter cannulas obstructed by a blood clot
   c. Acute management of heparin overdosage
   d. Deep vein thrombosis
2. The patient receiving heparin has an increased risk for bleeding when also taking
   a. allopurinol
   b. an NSAID
   c. digoxin
   d. furosemide
3. In which of the following situations would a LMWH be prescribed?
   a. To prevent deep vein thrombosis
   b. To treat disseminated intravascular coagulation
   c. To prevent hemorrhage
   d. To treat atrial fibrillation
4. Bleeding associated with thrombolytic drugs may involve which of the following areas?
   a. Brain
   b. Gastrointestinal tract
   c. Genitourinary tract
   d. All of the above
5. If severe hemorrhage occurs in a patient taking heparin, the health care provider is likely to order
   a. administration of protamine sulfate
   b. administration of vitamin K
   c. administration of a decreased dosage of heparin
   d. none of the above
6. What should you instruct a patient taking warfarin to do if they notice bleeding gums or blood in the urine or stool?
   a. Do not take any action as this is a normal adverse reaction of warfarin.
   b. Take the next dose of warfarin but contact the health care provider.
   c. Skip the next dose of warfarin and contact the health care provider immediately.
   d. Increase intake of foods high in vitamin K.

MATCHING

_____ 7. warfarin
_____ 8. dalteparin
_____ 9. enoxaparin
_____ 10. tinzaparin
_____ 11. phytonadione
_____ 12. alteplase
_____ 13. reteplase
_____ 14. tenecteplase
_____ 15. urokinase

a. Retavase
b. Mephyton
c. Kinlytic
d. Lovenox
e. TNKase
f. Coumadin
g. Fragmin
h. Activase
i. Innohep

TRUE OR FALSE

_____ 16. If uncontrolled bleeding occurs while a patient is receiving a thrombolytic drug, then the patient may receive whole blood, packed red cells, or fresh frozen plasma.
_____ 17. Because LMWHs produce unstable responses, frequent laboratory monitoring is required.
_____ 18. For patients taking thrombolytic drugs, bed rest is important during therapy.
_____ 19. Hemostasis is the body's process of stopping clotting in a blood vessel.
_____ 20. Heparin preparations may be given by either the oral or parenteral routes.
_____ 21. For the best therapeutic effect, thrombolytic drugs should be given within 4 hours after the formation of a thrombus.

FILL IN THE BLANKS

22. Patients taking heparin should avoid _____ injections.
23. _____ _____ thrombosis is the most common type of venous thrombosis and occurs in the _____ _____.
24. Administration of a thrombolytic drug with aspirin, dipyridamole, or an anticoagulant may increase the risk of _____.
25. _____ interferes with the manufacturing of vitamin K–dependent clotting factors by the liver.
26. Administration of heparin with an NSAID, aspirin, penicillin, or cephalosporin may _____ clotting times.
27. An embolus occurs when a(n) _____ detaches from the vessel wall and is carried along through the bloodstream.

SHORT ANSWERS

28. What is warfarin used for?
29. What kind of equipment should be readily available when protamine sulfate is administered and why?
30. What are some of the uses of heparin?
31. How do thrombolytic drugs act?

Web Activities

1. Go to the National Library of Medicine Web site (http://www.nlm.nih.gov) and conduct a search for sources of vitamin K. What are common food sources of vitamin K? Where is vitamin K made in the body?
2. Go to the Agency for Healthcare Research and Quality Web site (http://www.ahrq.gov) and conduct a search for warfarin. How do anticoagulants (often referred to as blood thinners by patients) work? Why is it important to take them correctly?

SUMMARY DRUG TABLE Anticoagulants
(left, generic; right, trade)

Comprehensive Summary Drug Tables, including uses, adverses effects, dosages, and pregnancy classifications, are provided on the companion website, http://thePoint.lww.com/PharmacologyHP2e

Coumadin	
warfarin sodium *war'-far-in*	Coumadin, Jantoven, *generic*
Unfractionated Heparin	
heparin *hep'-ah-rin*	*generic*
Low-Molecular-Weight Heparins	
dalteparin sodium *dal-tep'-a-rin*	Fragmin
enoxaparin sodium *en-ocks'-a-par-in*	Lovenox
tinzaparin sodium *ten-zah'-pear-in*	Innohep

Anticoagulant Antagonists	
phytonadione (vitamin K) *fye-toe-na-dye'-on*	Mephyton, generic
protamine sulfate *proe'-ta-meen*	*generic*
alteplase, recombinant *al'-te-plaz*	Activase, Cathflo Activase
reteplase, recombinant *ret'-ah-plaze*	Retavase, Retavase Half-Kit
tenecteplase *teh-nek'-ti-plaze*	TNKase
urokinase *yoor-oh'-kye-nase*	Kinlytic

24

Antianemia Drugs

CHAPTER OBJECTIVES

On completion of this chapter, students will be able to:

1. Define the chapter's key terms.
2. Explain th e differences between the types of anemias.
3. Describe the general drug actions, uses, adverse reactions, contraindications, precautions, and interactions of antianemia drugs.
4. Compare and contrast the most common adverse reactions of drugs used for the various types of anemias.
5. Match the antianemic drug with the appropriate type of anemia that it is used to treat.
6. Explain folinic acid rescue or leucovorin rescue.
7. Discuss important points to keep in mind when educating the patient or family members about the use of an antianemia drug.

KEY TERMS

anemia—a decrease in the number of red blood cells (RBCs), a decrease in the amount of hemoglobin in RBCs, or both a decrease in the number of RBCs and hemoglobin

folinic acid or leucovorin rescue—the technique of administering leucovorin after a large dose of methotrexate to rescue normal cells and allow them to survive

intrinsic factor—a substance produced by cells in the stomach that is necessary for the absorption of vitamin B_{12} in the intestine

iron deficiency anemia—condition that results when the body does not have enough iron to supply the body's needs

megaloblastic anemia—a type of anemia that results from a deficiency of folic acid and certain other causes

pernicious anemia—a type of megaloblastic anemia that results from a deficiency of intrinsic factor

CHAPTER OVERVIEW

Drug classes covered in this chapter are:

- Antianemia drugs

Drugs by classification are listed on page 244.

thePOINT RESOURCES

- Comprehensive Summary Drug Tables
- Lippincott's Interactive Tutorials: Drugs Affecting the Cardiovascular System
- Interactive Practice and Review
- Monographs of Most Commonly Prescribed Drugs

Anemia is a decrease in the number of red blood cells (RBCs), a decrease in the amount of hemoglobin in RBCs, or both. Anemia occurs when there is an insufficient amount of hemoglobin to deliver oxygen to the tissues. There are various types and causes of anemia. For example, anemia can result from blood loss, excessive destruction of RBCs, inadequate production of RBCs, or deficits in various nutrients, such as in iron deficiency anemia. Once the type and cause have been identified in a patient, the health care provider selects the appropriate treatment.

The anemias discussed in this chapter include iron deficiency anemia, anemia in patients with chronic renal disease, pernicious anemia, and anemia resulting from a folic acid deficiency. Table 24-1 defines these anemias.

Antianemia Drugs

DRUGS FOR IRON DEFICIENCY ANEMIA

Iron deficiency anemia is by far the most common type of anemia. Iron is a component of hemoglobin, which is present in RBCs. It is the iron in the hemoglobin of RBCs that takes oxygen from the lungs and carries it to all body tissues. Iron is stored in the body and is found mainly in the reticuloendothelial cells of the liver, spleen, and bone marrow. When the body does not have enough iron to supply the body's needs, the resulting condition is **iron deficiency anemia.**

Actions of Drugs for Iron Deficiency Anemia

Iron preparations act by elevating the serum iron concentration, which replenishes hemoglobin and depleted iron stores.

Uses of Drugs for Iron Deficiency Anemia

Iron salts, such as ferrous sulfate or ferrous gluconate, are used in the treatment of iron deficiency anemia, which occurs when there is a loss of iron that is greater than the available iron stored in the body.

Iron dextran is a parenteral iron that is also used for the treatment of iron deficiency anemia. It is primarily used when the patient cannot take oral drugs or when the patient experiences

ALERT Rx

Parenteral Iron
Parenteral iron has resulted in fatal anaphylactic-type reactions. Any of the following adverse reactions are reported to the health care provider: dyspnea, urticaria, rashes, itching, or fever.

gastrointestinal intolerance to oral iron administration. Other iron preparations, both oral and parenteral, for iron deficiency anemia can be found in the Summary Drug Table: Drugs Used in the Treatment of Anemia.

Adverse Reactions of Drugs for Iron Deficiency Anemia

Iron salts occasionally cause gastrointestinal irritation, nausea, vomiting, constipation, diarrhea, headache, backache, and allergic reactions. The stools may appear darker or black. Iron dextran is given by the parenteral route. Hypersensitivity reactions, including fatal anaphylactic reactions, have been reported with the use of this form of iron. Additional adverse reactions include soreness, inflammation, and sterile abscesses at the intramuscular (IM) injection site. Intravenous (IV) administration may result in phlebitis at the injection site. When iron is administered by IM injection, a brown discoloration of the skin may occur. Patients with rheumatoid arthritis may experience an acute exacerbation of joint pain, and swelling may occur when iron dextran is administered.

Contraindications, Precautions, and Interactions of Drugs for Iron Deficiency Anemia

- Drugs used to treat anemia are contraindicated in patients with known hypersensitivity to the drug or any component of the drug.
- Iron compounds are contraindicated in patients with any anemia except iron deficiency anemia.
- Iron compounds are used cautiously in patients with tartrazine or sulfite sensitivity because some iron compounds contain these substances.

TABLE 24-1   Anemias

Type of Anemia	Description
Iron deficiency	Anemia characterized by an inadequate amount of iron in the body to produce hemoglobin
Anemia in chronic renal failure (CRF)	Anemia resulting from a reduced production of erythropoietin, a hormone secreted by the kidney that stimulates the production of RBCs
Pernicious anemia	Anemia resulting from lack of secretions by the gastric mucosa of the intrinsic factor essential to the formation of RBCs and the absorption of vitamin B_{12}
Folic acid deficiency	A slowly progressive type of anemia occurring because of the lack of folic acid, a component necessary in the formation of RBCs

- Iron dextran is used cautiously in patients with cardiovascular disease, a history of asthma or allergies, or rheumatoid arthritis (may exacerbate joint pain).
- The absorption of oral iron is decreased when the agent is administered with an antacid, tetracycline, penicillamine, or fluoroquinolone.
- When iron is administered with levothyroxine, the effectiveness of levothyroxine may be decreased.
- When administered orally, iron decreases the absorption of levodopa.
- Ascorbic acid increases the absorption of oral iron.
- Iron dextran administered concurrently with chloramphenicol increases serum iron levels.

FACT CHECK

24-1 What is iron deficiency anemia?
24-2 What are the common adverse reactions of oral, IV, and IM administration of iron salts?

DRUGS FOR ANEMIA ASSOCIATED WITH CHRONIC RENAL FAILURE

Anemia may occur in patients with chronic renal failure because the kidneys do not produce enough erythropoietin. Erythropoietin is a glycoprotein hormone synthesized mainly in the kidneys and used to stimulate and regulate the production of erythrocytes or RBCs. Failure to produce the needed erythrocytes results in anemia. Two examples of drugs used to treat anemia associated with chronic renal failure are epoetin alfa (Epogen) and darbepoetin alfa (Aranesp).

Actions of Drugs for Anemia Associated with Chronic Renal Failure

Epoetin alfa is a drug that is produced using recombinant DNA technology. Epoetin alfa acts in a manner similar to that of natural erythropoietin. Darbepoetin alfa (Aranesp) is an erythropoiesis-stimulating protein produced in Chinese hamster ovary cells using recombinant DNA technology. Darbepoetin stimulates erythropoiesis by the same manner as natural erythropoietin. These drugs elevate or maintain RBC levels and decrease the need for transfusions.

Uses of Drugs for Anemia Associated with Chronic Renal Failure

Epoetin alfa is used to treat anemia associated with chronic renal failure, anemia in patients with cancer who are receiving chemotherapy, and anemia in patients who are undergoing elective nonvascular surgery.

Darbepoetin is used to treat anemia associated with chronic renal failure in patients receiving dialysis, as well as other patients.

Adverse Reactions of Drugs for Anemia Associated with Chronic Renal Failure

Epoetin alfa (erythropoietin [EPO]) and darbepoetin alfa are usually well tolerated. The most common adverse reactions include hypertension, headache, tachycardia, nausea, vomiting, diarrhea, skin rashes, fever, myalgia, and skin reaction at the injection site.

Contraindications, Precautions, and Interactions of Drugs for Anemia Associated with Chronic Renal Failure

- Epoetin alfa is contraindicated in patients with uncontrolled hypertension, those needing an emergency transfusion, or those with a hypersensitivity to human albumin.
- Darbepoetin alfa (Aranesp) is contraindicated in patients with uncontrolled hypertension or in those allergic to the drug.
- Epoetin alfa and darbepoetin alfa are used with caution in patients with hypertension, heart disease, congestive heart failure, or a history of seizures.
- Both of these drugs are used cautiously during lactation.

FACT CHECK

24-3 How are epoetin alfa and darbepoetin alfa produced, and what are their uses?

DRUGS FOR FOLIC ACID DEFICIENCY ANEMIA

Folic acid is required for the manufacture of RBCs in the bone marrow. Folic acid is found in green leafy vegetables, fish, meat, poultry, and whole grains. A deficiency of folic acid results in **megaloblastic anemia.** Megaloblastic anemia is characterized by the presence of large, abnormal, immature erythrocytes circulating in the blood.

Actions of Drugs for Folic Acid Deficiency Anemia

Although not related to anemia, studies indicate there is a decreased risk for neural tube defects if folic acid is taken before conception and during early pregnancy. Neural tube defects occur during early pregnancy, when the embryonic folds forming the spinal cord and brain join together. Defects of this type include anencephaly (congenital absence of brain and spinal cord), spina bifida (defect of the spinal cord), and meningocele (a sac-like protrusion of the meninges in the spinal cord or skull).

Leucovorin "rescues" normal cells from the destruction caused by methotrexate and allows them to survive. This technique of administering leucovorin after a large dose of methotrexate is called **folinic acid rescue** or **leucovorin rescue.**

Uses of Drugs for Folic Acid Deficiency Anemia

Folic acid is used in the treatment of megaloblastic anemias that are caused by a deficiency of folic acid. The U.S. Public Health Service recommends the use of folic acid for all women of childbearing age to decrease the incidence of neural tube defects. Dosages during pregnancy and lactation are as great as 1 mg per day.

Leucovorin is a derivative (and active reduced form) of folic acid. The oral and parenteral forms of this drug are used in the treatment of megaloblastic anemia. Leucovorin may also be used to diminish the hematologic effects of (intentional) massive doses of methotrexate, a drug used in the treatment of certain types of cancer (see Chapter 41). Occasionally, high doses of methotrexate are administered to select patients. Leucovorin is then used either at the same time or after the methotrexate has been given to decrease the toxic effects of the methotrexate.

Adverse Reactions of Drugs for Folic Acid Deficiency Anemia

Few adverse reactions are associated with the administration of folic acid and leucovorin. Rarely, parenteral administration may result in allergic hypersensitivity.

Contraindications, Precautions, and Interactions of Drugs for Folic Acid Deficiency Anemia

- Folic acid and leucovorin are contraindicated for the treatment of pernicious anemia or for other anemias for which vitamin B_{12} is deficient.
- Pregnant women are more likely to experience folate deficiency because folic acid requirements are increased during pregnancy. Pregnant women with a folate deficiency are at increased risk for complications of pregnancy and fetal abnormalities.
- Use of aminosalicylic with folic acid may decrease serum folate levels.
- Folic acid utilization is decreased when folate is administered with methotrexate.
- Signs of folic acid deficiency may occur when sulfasalazine is administered concurrently.
- An increase in seizure activity may occur when folic acid is administered with a hydantoin. Leucovorin decreases the effectiveness of anticonvulsants. The patient has an increased risk of 5-fluorouracil toxicity when that drug is administered with leucovorin.

FACT CHECK

24-4   What is megaloblastic anemia?
24-5   What are the contraindications for folic acid and leucovorin?

DRUGS FOR PERNICIOUS ANEMIA

Vitamin B_{12} is essential for growth, cell reproduction, the manufacture of myelin (which surrounds some nerve fibers), and blood cell manufacture. The substance called **intrinsic factor,** which is produced by cells in the stomach, is necessary for the absorption of vitamin B_{12} in the intestine. A deficiency of intrinsic factor results in abnormal formation of erythrocytes because of the body's failure to absorb vitamin B_{12}, a necessary component for blood cell formation. The resulting anemia is a type of megaloblastic anemia called **pernicious anemia**.

Actions of Drugs for Pernicious Anemia

Vitamin B_{12} (cyanocobalamin) acts by replenishing the diminished level of vitamin B_{12} in the body.

Uses of Drugs for Pernicious Anemia

Vitamin B_{12} (cyanocobalamin) is used to treat a vitamin B_{12} deficiency. A vitamin B_{12} deficiency may be seen in

- Strict vegetarians
- People who have had a total gastrectomy or subtotal gastric resection (when the cells producing intrinsic factor are totally or partially removed)
- People who have intestinal diseases, such as ulcerative colitis or sprue
- People who have gastric carcinoma
- People who have a congenital decrease in the number of gastric cells secreting intrinsic factor

Vitamin B_{12} is also used to perform the Schilling test, which is used to diagnose pernicious anemia.

Adverse Reactions of Drugs for Pernicious Anemia

Mild diarrhea and itching have been reported with the administration of vitamin B_{12}. Other adverse reactions include a marked increase in RBC production, edema, headache, dizziness, anxiety, ataxia, nervousness.

ALERT ℞

Pernicious Anemia
Pernicious anemia must be diagnosed and treated as soon as possible because a vitamin B_{12} deficiency that is allowed to progress for more than 3 months may result in degenerative lesions of the spinal cord.

Vitamin B_{12} deficiency caused by a low dietary intake of vitamin B_{12} is rare because the vitamin is found in meats, milk, eggs, and cheese. Because the body can store this vitamin, a deficiency from any cause will not occur for 5 to 6 years.

Contraindications, Precautions, and Interactions of Drugs for Pernicious Anemia

- Vitamin B$_{12}$ is contraindicated in patients allergic to cobalt.
- Vitamin B$_{12}$ is administered cautiously in patients with pulmonary disease and anemia.
- Alcohol, aminosalicylic acid, neomycin, and colchicine may decrease the absorption of oral vitamin B$_{12}$.

FACT CHECK

24-6 What nutritional advice would you recommend for a patient with pernicious anemia?

Patient Management Issues with Antianemia Drugs

Laboratory tests are often used to determine the type, severity, and possible cause of anemia. Sometimes, it is easy to identify the cause of the anemia, but in some instances, the cause of the anemia is obscure.

Vital signs are taken to provide a baseline during therapy. Patients may be evaluated for their ability to perform the activities of daily living. General symptoms of anemia include fatigue, shortness of breath, sore tongue, headache, and pallor (Key Concepts 24-1).

If iron dextran is to be given, then an allergy history is necessary because this drug is given only with caution to those with significant allergies or asthma. The patient's weight and hemoglobin level are required for calculating the dosage.

A patient on iron salt therapy should be told that the color of the stool will become darker or black. If diarrhea or constipation occurs, then the health care provider must be notified.

Patients being given iron dextran should be told that they might feel soreness at the injection site. Injection sites are checked daily for signs of inflammation, swelling, or abscess formation.

For patients receiving therapy for iron deficiency anemia, a balanced diet with an emphasis on foods that are high in iron (e.g., organ meats, lean red meats, cereals, dried beans, and green leafy vegetables), folic acid (e.g., green leafy vegetables, liver, and yeast), or vitamin B$_{12}$ (e.g., beef, pork, organ meats, eggs, milk, and milk products) is recommended. The amount of food eaten at meals is monitored. If the patient's appetite is poor or if the patient's eating habits are inadequate to maintain

normal nutrition, then consultation with the dietitian may be necessary. Small portions of food may be more appealing than large or moderate portions. A pleasant atmosphere and ample time for eating help encourage good eating habits.

Educating the Patient and Family about Antianemia Drugs

Following are key points about antianemia drugs that the patient and family members should know.

Iron Salt

- Take this drug with water on an empty stomach. If you experience gastrointestinal upset, then take the drug with food or meals.
- Do not take antacids, tetracyclines, penicillamine, or fluoroquinolones at the same time or 2 hours before or after taking iron without first checking with your health care provider.
- This drug may cause a darkening of your stools, constipation, or diarrhea. To help decrease the constipating effects of iron, increase fluid intake (if permitted), eat a high-fiber diet, and increase physical activity. If constipation or diarrhea becomes severe, then contact your health care provider.
- Mix the liquid iron preparation with water or juice and drink it through a straw to prevent staining of your teeth.
- Do not indiscriminately use advertised iron products. If you have a true iron deficiency, then its cause must be determined and your therapy should be guided by a health care provider.
- Have periodic blood tests during therapy to determine how you are responding to treatment.
- Patients with rheumatoid arthritis may experience an acute exacerbation of joint pain, and swelling may occur with iron dextran therapy.

Epoetin Alfa

- Strict compliance with antihypertensive drug regimen is important if you are being treated for known hypertension during epoetin therapy.
- Report to your health care provider any numbness, tingling of extremities, severe headache, dyspnea, chest pain, dizziness, fatigue, joint pain, nausea, vomiting, or diarrhea. Joint pain may occur but can be controlled with analgesics.
- Keep all your appointments for blood testing, which is necessary to determine the effects of the drug on the blood count and to determine the correct dosage.

Folic Acid

- Avoid the use of multivitamin preparations unless they are approved by your health care provider.
- Follow the diet recommended by your health care provider because both the diet and the drug are necessary to correct a folic acid deficiency.

Leucovorin

- Megaloblastic anemia: Adhere to the diet prescribed by your health care provider. If the purchase of foods high

KEY CONCEPTS

24-1 Monitoring Antianemia Drug Therapy

All patients receiving antianemia drugs are monitored for relief of the symptoms of anemia (fatigue, shortness of breath, sore tongue, headache, pallor). Some patients may note a relief of symptoms after a few days of therapy. Periodic laboratory tests are necessary to monitor the results of therapy.

in protein (which can be expensive) becomes a problem, then discuss this with your health care provider.

- Folinic acid rescue: Take this drug at the exact prescribed intervals. If nausea and vomiting occur, then contact your health care provider immediately.

Vitamin B$_{12}$

- Nutritional deficiency of vitamin B$_{12}$: Eat a balanced diet that includes seafood, eggs, meats, and dairy products.
- Pernicious anemia: Lifetime therapy is necessary. Eat a balanced diet that includes seafood, eggs, meats, and

dairy products. Try to avoid contact with people who have infections, and report any signs of infection to your health care provider immediately because an increase in dosage may be necessary.

- Adhere to the treatment regimen and keep all appointments with your health care provider. The drug is given at periodic intervals (usually monthly for life). In some instances, parenteral self-administration or parenteral administration by a family member is allowed (instruction in administration is necessary).

Chapter Review

KEY POINTS

- Iron deficiency anemia is by far the most common type of anemia.
- Iron salts, such as ferrous sulfate or ferrous gluconate, are used in the treatment of iron deficiency anemia, which occurs when there is a loss of iron that is greater than the available iron stored in the body. Iron salts occasionally cause gastrointestinal irritation, nausea, vomiting, constipation, diarrhea, headache, backache, and allergic reactions.
- Iron compounds are contraindicated in patients with any anemia except iron deficiency anemia.
- Anemia may occur in patients with chronic renal failure as the result of the inability of the kidney to produce erythropoietin. Epoetin alfa is used to treat anemia associated with chronic renal failure, anemia in patients with cancer who are receiving chemotherapy, and anemia in patients who are undergoing elective nonvascular surgery. Darbepoetin is used to treat anemia associated with chronic renal failure in patients receiving dialysis and other patients.
- The most common adverse reactions include hypertension, headache, tachycardia, nausea, vomiting, diarrhea, skin rashes, fever, myalgia, and skin reaction at the injection site.
- Folic acid is required for the manufacture of RBCs in the bone marrow. Folic acid is used in the treatment of megaloblastic anemias that are caused by a deficiency of folic acid. Folic acid and leucovorin are contraindicated for the treatment of pernicious anemia or for other anemias for which vitamin B$_{12}$ is deficient.
- A deficiency of the intrinsic factor results in abnormal formation of erythrocytes because of the body's failure to absorb vitamin B$_{12}$, a necessary component for blood cell formation. The resulting anemia is pernicious anemia. There is a decreased risk for neural tube defects if folic acid is taken before conception and during early pregnancy. Folic acid and leucovorin are contraindicated for the treatment of pernicious anemia or for other anemias for which vitamin B$_{12}$ is deficient.

CRITICAL THINKING CASE STUDY

Newly Diagnosed Anemia

Mrs. Bruce, who is a regular patient at the medical clinic where you work, complains that she has been feeling fatigued, short of breath, and having headaches.

1. What should you tell Mrs. Bruce?
   a. Her symptoms are consistent with anemia and she should see her physician.
   b. Her symptoms are consistent with anemia and she should start taking an iron preparation.
   c. Her symptoms are consistent with anemia and she should start taking folic acid.
   d. Her symptoms are consistent with anemia and she should start taking vitamin B$_{12}$.
2. Mrs. Bruce sees her physician and is diagnosed with megaloblastic anemia. Which of the following would you expect her physician to prescribe?
   a. Ferrous sulfate
   b. Folic acid
   c. Cyanocobalamin
   d. Erythropoietin alfa
3. What types of food contain folic acid?

Review Questions

MULTIPLE CHOICE

1. Which is the most common type of anemia?
   a. Iron deficiency anemia
   b. Folic acid anemia
   c. Pernicious anemia
   d. Megaloblastic anemia
2. Which of the following substances would decrease the absorption of oral iron?
   a. Antacids
   b. Levothyroxine
   c. Ascorbic acid
   d. Vitamin B$_{12}$

3. A patient with iron deficiency anemia who experiences GI intolerance to oral iron administration would likely be prescribed
   a. epoetin alfa
   b. iron dextran
   c. ferrous gluconate
   d. ferrous sulfate

4. A patient with anemia associated with chronic renal failure is undergoing dialysis. Which of the following antianemia drugs would most likely be prescribed?
   a. epoetin alfa
   b. darbepoetin alfa
   c. epogen
   d. all of the above

MATCHING

Match the drug on the left with the correct use on the right.

_____ 5. darbepoetin alfa a. Iron deficiency anemia
_____ 6. ferrous sulfate b. Anemia associated with
_____ 7. cyanocobalamin   chronic renal failure
_____ 8. leucovorin c. Megaloblastic anemia
_____ 9. folic acid d. Pernicious anemia
                        e. Folinic acid rescue

TRUE OR FALSE

_____ 10. Epoetin alfa and darbepoetin alfa lower RBC levels and increase the need for transfusions.
_____ 11. Folic acid deficiency results in megaloblastic anemia.
_____ 12. Iron salt should be taken with water on an empty stomach.

_____ 13. Patients receiving vitamin B_{12} should be told that stools may become darker or black.

FILL IN THE BLANKS

14. _____ is a substance produced by cells in the stomach that is necessary for the absorption of vitamin B_{12} in the intestine.
15. Oral administration of iron decreases the absorption of _____ .
16. Fatal _____ reactions have been reported with the use of iron _____ .
17. Increased seizure activity may occur when folic acid is administered with a _____ .

SHORT ANSWERS

18. Describe the four types of anemias discussed in the chapter.
19. What is leucovorin rescue?
20. A vitamin B_{12} deficiency may be seen in which types of patients?
21. What are the contraindications for epoetin alfa?

Web Activities

1. Go to the Web site of the Spina Bifida Association (www.spinabifidaassociation.org). Who is at risk for spina bifida? What can be done to reduce the risk?
2. Go to the Office of Dietary Supplements Web site (http://ods.od.nih.gov). Conduct a search for vitamin B_{12}. How much vitamin B_{12} do you need per day? What foods provide vitamin B_{12}?

SUMMARY DRUG TABLE Antianemia Drugs
(left, generic; right, trade)

Comprehensive Summary Drug Tables, including uses, adverses effects, dosages, and pregnancy classifications, are provided on the companion website, http:// thePoint.lww.com/PharmacologyHP2e

darbepoetin alfa *dar-bah-poe-e'-tin*	Aranesp
epoetin alfa (erythropoietin [EPO]) *e-po-e'-tin*	Epogen, Procrit
ferrous fumarate (33% elemental iron) *fair'-us*	Femiron, Ferrimin 150, Ferrocite, Ferro-Sequels, Hemocyte, Nephro-Fer, *generic*
ferrous gluconate (11.6% elemental iron) *fair'-us*	Fergon, *generic*
ferrous sulfate (20% elemental iron) *fair'-us*	Enfamil Fer-In-Sol, Feosol, Feratab, Fer-Iron, FeroSul, Slow FE, *generic*
folic acid *foe'-lik*	Folvite (Rx), Deplin (Rx), DuLeek-Dp (Rx), ViloFane-Dp (Rx), *generic* (Rx and OTC)
iron dextran	DexFerrum (Rx), Elite Iron (OTC), Feosol (OTC), Icar (OTC), Infed (Rx), Ircon (OTC), *generic*
iron sucrose	Venofer
leucovorin calcium *loo-koe-vor'-in*	*generic*
sodium ferric gluconate complex	Ferrlecit
vitamin B$_{12}$ (cyanocobalamin) *sye-an-oh-koe- bal'-a-min*	Calomist (Rx), Nascobal (Rx), Rapid B-12 Energy (OTC), *generic* (Rx, OTC)

VI

DRUGS THAT AFFECT THE URINARY SYSTEM

25

Diuretics

CHAPTER OBJECTIVES

On completion of this chapter, students will be able to:

1. Define the chapter's key terms.
2. Explain how and where diuretics work.
3. Compare and contrast the actions and uses of the various diuretics.
4. Identify common fluid and electrolyte imbalances associated with the various diuretic categories and explain the signs and symptoms of each.
5. Identify common adverse reactions associated with the various diuretic categories.
6. Identify common contraindications, precautions, and interactions of diuretics.
7. Discuss important points to keep in mind when educating the patient or family members about the use of diuretics.
8. Identify which diuretic categories should be cautious of potassium intake and the signs and symptoms of hypokalemia and hyperkalemia that the patient and family members should watch for.

KEY TERMS

dehydration—loss of too much water from the body
diuretic—a drug that increases the secretion of urine (water, electrolytes, and waste products) by the kidneys
edema—retention of excess fluid
filtrate—fluid removed from the blood through kidney function
hyperkalemia—high blood level of potassium
nephron—long tubular structure that is the functional part of the kidney

CHAPTER OVERVIEW

Drug classes covered in this chapter are:

- Carbonic anhydrase inhibitors
- Loop diuretics
- Osmotic diuretics
- Potassium-sparing diuretics
- Thiazides and related diuretics

Drugs by classification are listed on page 255.

thePOINT RESOURCES

- Comprehensive Summary Drug Tables
- Animations: Edema; Renal Function
- Lippincott's Interactive Tutorials: Drugs Affecting the Cardiovascular System
- Interactive Practice and Review
- Monographs of Most Commonly Prescribed Drugs

A **diuretic** is a drug that increases the secretion of urine (i.e., water, electrolytes, and waste products) by the kidneys. The different types of diuretic drugs are

- Carbonic anhydrase inhibitors
- Loop diuretics
- Osmotic diuretics
- Potassium-sparing diuretics
- Thiazides and related diuretics

The Summary Drug Table: Diuretics lists examples of the different types of diuretic drugs. Most diuretics act on the tubules of the kidney **nephron** (Fig. 25-1), the functional unit of the kidney. Each kidney contains approximately one million nephrons, which filter the bloodstream to remove waste products. During this process, water and electrolytes are also selectively removed. The **filtrate** (the fluid removed from the blood) normally contains ions (potassium, sodium, chloride), waste products (ammonia, urea), water, and, at times, other substances that are being excreted, such as drugs. The filtrate then passes through the proximal tubule, the loop of Henle, and the distal tubules. At these points, selective reabsorption of amino acids, glucose, some electrolytes, and water occurs. Ions and water that are required by the body to maintain fluid

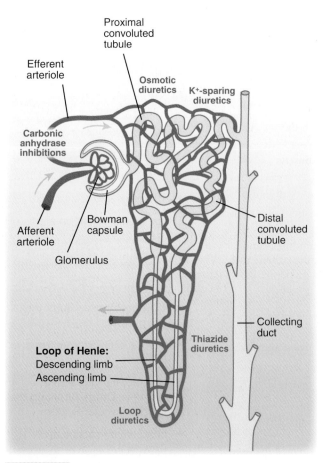

FIGURE 25-1 The nephron is the functional unit of the kidney. Note the various tubules, the site of most diuretic activity. The loop of Henle is the site of action for the loop diuretics. Thiazide diuretics act at the ascending portion of the loop of Henle and the distal tube of the nephron.

and electrolyte balance are returned to the bloodstream by means of the minute capillaries that surround the distal and proximal tubules and the loop of Henle. Ions and water that are not needed are excreted in the urine.

Diuretics are used for a variety of medical disorders (Key Concepts 25-1). In some instances, hypertension may be treated with the administration of an antihypertensive drug and a diuretic. The diuretics used for this combination therapy include loop diuretics and thiazides and related diuretics.

FACT CHECK

25-1   What is edema and what conditions cause it?
25-2   How do diuretics reduce edema?

Carbonic Anhydrase Inhibitors

Actions of Carbonic Anhydrase Inhibitors

Carbonic anhydrase is an enzyme that produces free hydrogen ions, which are then exchanged for sodium ions in the kidney tubules. Carbonic anhydrase inhibitors inhibit the action of the enzyme carbonic anhydrase. This effect results in the excretion of sodium, potassium, bicarbonate, and water. Carbonic anhydrase inhibitors also decrease the production of aqueous humor in the eye, which in turn decreases intraocular pressure (the pressure within the eye).

Uses of Carbonic Anhydrase Inhibitors

Glaucoma causes an increase in intraocular pressure that, if left untreated, can result in blindness. Normally the eye is filled with aqueous humor in an amount that is carefully regulated to maintain the shape of the eyeball. In glaucoma, aqueous humor is increased, which causes the intraocular pressure to rise and can, without treatment, damage the retina.

Acetazolamide (Diamox) is used in the treatment of simple (open-angle) glaucoma, secondary glaucoma, and preoperatively in acute angle-closure glaucoma when the intraocular pressure is to be lowered before surgery. These drugs are also used in the treatment of edema caused by congestive heart failure, drug-induced edema, and some forms of epilepsy. Methazolamide (Neptazane) is used in the treatment of glaucoma.

Adverse Reactions of Carbonic Anhydrase Inhibitors

Adverse reactions associated with short-term therapy with carbonic anhydrase inhibitors are rare. Long-term use of these drugs may result in drowsiness, fatigue, headache, malaise, seizures, irritability, decreased libido, vertigo, confusion, hyperuricemia, hyperchloremia, paresthesia (numbness, tingling), photosensitivity reactions (exaggerated sunburn reaction when the skin is exposed to sunlight or ultraviolet light), and crystalluria (crystals in the urine). On occasion, acidosis may occur, and oral sodium bicarbonate may be used to correct this imbalance.

Contraindications, Precautions, and Interactions of Carbonic Anhydrase Inhibitors

- Carbonic anhydrase inhibitors are contraindicated in patients with known hypersensitivity, electrolyte imbalances, severe kidney or liver dysfunction, or anuria and for long-term use in patients with chronic noncongestive angle-closure glaucoma (may mask worsening glaucoma).
- Diuretics are used cautiously in patients with renal dysfunction.
- The patient has an increased risk of cyclosporine toxicity when the drug is administered with acetazolamide.
- Decreased serum and urine concentrations of primidone occur when the drug is administered with acetazolamide.

> **FACT CHECK**
> **25-3** What are the uses of carbonic anhydrase inhibitors?

Loop Diuretics

Actions of Loop Diuretics

Loop diuretics, furosemide (Lasix) and ethacrynic acid (Edecrin), increase the excretion of sodium and chloride by inhibiting reabsorption of these ions in the distal and proximal tubules and in the loop of Henle. This mechanism of action at these three sites appears to increase their effectiveness as diuretics. Torsemide (Demadex) also increases urinary excretion of sodium, chloride, and water but acts primarily in the ascending portion of the loop of Henle. Bumetanide (Bumex) primarily increases the excretion of chloride but also has some sodium-excreting ability. This drug acts primarily on the proximal tubule of the nephron.

Uses of Loop Diuretics

Loop diuretics are used in the treatment of edema associated with chronic heart failure, cirrhosis of the liver, and renal disease. These drugs are particularly useful when a greater diuretic effect is desired. Furosemide is the drug of choice when a rapid diuresis is needed or if a patient has renal insufficiency. Furosemide and torsemide are also used to treat hypertension. Ethacrynic acid is also used for the short-term management of ascites (accumulation of serous fluid in the peritoneal cavity) caused by a malignancy, idiopathic edema, or lymphedema.

Adverse Reactions of Loop Diuretics

Adverse reactions seen with loop diuretics may include anorexia, nausea, vomiting, dizziness, rash, postural or orthostatic hypotension, photosensitivity reactions, and glycosuria (glucose in the urine). Patients with diabetes who take these drugs may experience an elevated blood glucose level.

Contraindications, Precautions, and Interactions of Loop Diuretics

- Loop diuretics are contraindicated in patients with known hypersensitivity to loop diuretics or to sulfonamides, severe electrolyte imbalances, hepatic coma, or anuria and in infants (ethacrynic acid).
- Loop diuretics are used cautiously in patients with renal dysfunction.
- Furosemide should be used cautiously in children and in patients with liver disease, diabetes, lupus erythematosus (may exacerbate or activate the disease), or diarrhea.
- Patients with sensitivity to sulfonamides may have allergic reactions to furosemide, torsemide, or bumetanide.
- Loop diuretics may increase the effectiveness of anticoagulants or thrombolytics.
- There is an increased risk of glycoside toxicity and digitalis-induced arrhythmias if a patient experiences hypokalemia (low blood potassium) while taking a loop diuretic.
- Ototoxicity (damage to the hearing organs from a toxic substance) is more likely to occur if a loop diuretic is given with an aminoglycoside.
- Plasma levels of propranolol may increase when the drug is administered with furosemide.
- The patient has an increased risk of lithium toxicity when it is administered with a loop diuretic.
- Hydantoins (phenytoin) may reduce the diuretic effects of furosemide.
- The effects of loop diuretics may be decreased when they are administered with a nonsteroidal anti-inflammatory drug (NSAID).

> **FACT CHECK**
> **25-4** How do loop diuretics act?

Osmotic Diuretics

Actions of Osmotic Diuretics

Osmotic diuretics increase the density of the filtrate in the glomerulus (see Fig. 25-1). This prevents selective reabsorption of water, which allows the water to be excreted. Sodium and chloride excretion is also increased.

Uses of Osmotic Diuretics

Mannitol (Osmitrol) is used for the promotion of diuresis in the prevention and treatment of the oliguric phase (low urine production) of acute renal failure, as well as for the reduction of intraocular pressure and the treatment of cerebral edema. Urea (Ureaphil) is used to reduce cerebral edema and to reduce intraocular pressure.

Adverse Reactions of Osmotic Diuretics

The osmotic diuretics urea and mannitol are administered IV. Administration by the IV route may result in a rapid fluid and electrolyte imbalance, especially when these drugs are administered before surgery to a patient in a fasting state.

Contraindications, Precautions, and Interactions of Osmotic Diuretics

- Osmotic diuretics are contraindicated in patients with known hypersensitivity to the drugs, electrolyte imbalances, severe dehydration, or anuria and those who experience progressive renal damage after using mannitol.
- Mannitol is contraindicated in patients with active intracranial bleeding (except during craniotomy).
- Osmotic diuretics are used cautiously in patients with renal or kidney impairment or electrolyte imbalances.

FACT CHECK

25-5 What adverse reaction may occur with IV administration of osmotic diuretics?

Potassium-Sparing Diuretics

Actions of Potassium-Sparing Diuretics

Potassium-sparing diuretics work in either of two ways. Triamterene (Dyrenium) and amiloride (Midamor) depress the reabsorption of sodium in the kidney tubules, therefore increasing sodium and water excretion. Both drugs additionally depress the excretion of potassium and therefore are called potassium-sparing (or potassium-saving) diuretics. Spironolactone (Aldactone), also a potassium-sparing diuretic, antagonizes the action of aldosterone. Aldosterone, a hormone produced by the adrenal cortex, enhances the reabsorption of sodium in the distal convoluted tubules of the kidney. When this activity of aldosterone is blocked, sodium (but not potassium) and water are excreted.

Uses of Potassium-Sparing Diuretics

Amiloride (Midamor) is used in the treatment of chronic heart failure and hypertension and is often used with a thiazide diuretic. Spironolactone and triamterene are also used in the treatment of hypertension and edema caused by chronic heart failure, cirrhosis, and the nephrotic syndrome. Amiloride, spironolactone, and triamterene are also available with hydrochlorothiazide, a thiazide diuretic that enhances the antihypertensive and diuretic effects of the drug combination while still conserving potassium.

Adverse Reactions of Potassium-Sparing Diuretics

Hyperkalemia (increased potassium in the blood), a serious event, may occur with the administration of potassium-sparing diuretics (Key Concepts 25-2). Hyperkalemia is most likely to occur in patients with an inadequate fluid intake and urine output, those with diabetes or renal disease, the

KEY CONCEPTS

25-2 Potassium Intake and Diuretics

All diuretics can cause hypokalemia except the potassium-sparing ones, which can cause hyperkalemia. Patients taking any diuretics except the potassium-sparing ones will usually also take potassium supplements. However, patients on potassium-sparing diuretics must be careful about the amount of potassium they take in, especially in their diet.

elderly, and severely ill patients. In patients taking spironolactone, gynecomastia (breast enlargement in the male) may occur. This reaction appears to be related to both dosage and duration of therapy. The gynecomastia usually reverses when therapy is discontinued, but in rare instances some breast enlargement may remain.

When a potassium-sparing diuretic and a thiazide diuretic are given together, the adverse reactions associated with both drugs may occur.

Contraindications, Precautions, and Interactions of Potassium-Sparing Diuretics

- Potassium-sparing diuretics are contraindicated in patients with known hypersensitivity to the drugs, serious electrolyte imbalances, significant renal impairment, or anuria and those receiving another potassium-sparing diuretic.
- Potassium-sparing diuretics are contraindicated in patients with hyperkalemia and are not recommended for children.
- Potassium-sparing diuretics are used cautiously in patients with renal or kidney impairment.
- Potassium-sparing diuretics are used cautiously in patients with liver disease, diabetes, or gout.
- When a potassium-sparing diuretic is administered to a patient taking an angiotensin-converting enzyme (ACE) inhibitor (see Chapter 21), the patient has an increased risk for hyperkalemia.
- When a potassium-sparing diuretic is administered with a potassium preparation, severe hyperkalemia may occur, possibly causing a cardiac arrhythmia or cardiac arrest.
- When spironolactone is administered with an anticoagulant drug or NSAID, the anticoagulant or NSAID has decreased effectiveness.
- When spironolactone or triamterene is administered with an ACE inhibitor, significant hyperkalemia may occur.

FACT CHECK

25-6 What are the two ways that potassium-sparing diuretics work?

25-7 Patients taking potassium-sparing diuretics are at risk for which electrolyte imbalance? What are the symptoms of this disorder?

Thiazides and Related Diuretics

Actions of Thiazides and Related Diuretics

Thiazides and related diuretics inhibit the reabsorption of sodium and chloride ions in the ascending portion of the loop of Henle and the early distal tubule of the nephron. This action results in the excretion of sodium, chloride, and water.

Uses of Thiazides and Related Diuretics

Thiazides and related diuretics are used in the treatment of hypertension, edema caused by chronic heart failure, hepatic cirrhosis, corticosteroid and estrogen therapy, and renal dysfunction.

Adverse Reactions of Thiazides and Related Diuretics

Thiazides and related diuretics may be associated with numerous adverse reactions. However, many patients take these drugs without experiencing adverse reactions other than excessive fluid and electrolyte loss, which often can be corrected with an adequate fluid intake, a balanced diet, supplemental oral electrolytes, or ingesting foods or fluids high in the electrolytes that are being lost. Some of the adverse reactions that may occur, include gastric irritation, abdominal bloating, reduced libido, dizziness, vertigo, headache, photosensitivity, and weakness.

Contraindications, Precautions, and Interactions of Thiazides and Related Diuretics

- Thiazide diuretics are contraindicated in patients with known hypersensitivity to thiazides or related diuretics, electrolyte imbalances, renal decompensation, hepatic coma, or anuria.
- A cross-sensitivity reaction may occur with thiazides and sulfonamides. Some of the thiazide diuretics contain tartrazine, which may cause allergic reactions or bronchial asthma in individuals sensitive to tartrazine.
- These drugs should be used cautiously in children and in patients with liver or kidney disease, lupus erythematosus (may exacerbate or activate the disease), or diabetes.
- Concurrent use of thiazides with allopurinol may increase the incidence of hypersensitivity to allopurinol.
- The effects of anesthetics may be increased by thiazide administration.
- The effects of anticoagulants may be diminished when administered with a thiazide diuretic.
- Because thiazide diuretics may raise blood uric acid levels, dosage adjustments of antigout drugs may be necessary.
- Thiazide diuretics may prolong antineoplastic-induced leukopenia.
- Hyperglycemia may occur when a thiazide is administered with an antidiabetic drug.
- Synergistic effects may occur when a thiazide diuretic is administered concurrently with a loop diuretic, causing profound diuresis (excretion of urine) and serious electrolyte abnormalities.

ALERT Rx

Common Drug Interactions: Additive Hypotensive Effects

Additive hypotensive effects occur when alcohol, other antihypertensive drugs, or nitrates are given with the following diuretics:
Loop diuretics
Osmotic diuretics
Potassium-sparing diuretics
Thiazides

- There is an increased risk of glycoside toxicity if a patient experiences hypokalemia while taking a thiazide diuretic.
- The administration of a thiazide diuretic and a digitalis glycoside may result in cardiac arrhythmias.

FACT CHECK

25-8   How are thiazides and related diuretics used?

Patient Management Issues with Diuretics

Before the first dose of a diuretic is given, the purpose of the drug, when diuresis may be expected to occur, and how long diuresis will last are explained to the patient (Table 25-1). These

TABLE 25-1   Examples of Onset and Duration of Activity of Diuretics

Drug	Onset	Duration of Activity
Acetazolamide tablets	1–1.5 h	8–12 h
Sustained-release capsules	2 h	18–24 h
IV	2 min	4–5 h
Amiloride	2 h	24 h
Bumetanide	30–60 min	4–6 h
Ethacrynic acid		
PO	Within 30 min	6–8 h
IV	Within 5 min	2 h
Furosemide		
PO	Within 1 h	6–8 h
IV	Within 5 min	2 h
Mannitol (IV)	30–60 min	6–8 h
Spironolactone	24–48 h	48–72 h
Thiazides and related diuretics	1–2 h	Varies*
Triamterene	2–4 h	12–16 h
Urea (V)	30–45 min	5–6 h

*Duration varies with drug used. Average duration is 12–24 h with polythiazide and chlorthalidone. Indapamide has a duration of more than 24 h.

KEY CONCEPTS

25-3   Electrolyte Imbalance

The most common adverse reaction of diuretics is the loss of fluid and electrolytes (see Signs and Symptoms Box), especially during initial therapy. In some patients, the diuretic effect is moderate, whereas in others a large volume of fluid is lost. Regardless of the amount of fluid lost, there is always the possibility of excessive electrolyte loss, which is potentially serious.

The most common imbalances are a loss of potassium and water. Other electrolytes, such as magnesium, sodium, and chlorides, are also lost. When too much potassium is lost, hypokalemia (low blood level of potassium) occurs. In certain patients, such as those also receiving a digitalis glycoside or those with a cardiac arrhythmia, hypokalemia may cause a more serious arrhythmia. Hypokalemia is treated with potassium supplements or foods with high potassium content or by changing the diuretic to a potassium-sparing diuretic. In addition to hypokalemia, patients taking loop diuretics are prone to magnesium deficiency (see Signs and Symptoms Box). If too much water is lost, then **dehydration** occurs, which also can be serious, especially in elderly patients.

drugs are administered early in the day to prevent nighttime sleep disturbances caused by frequent urination.

Patients with Edema. Patients with edema caused by heart failure or other causes are weighed daily or as ordered by the health care provider to monitor fluid loss. A weight loss of approximately 2 lb per day is desirable to prevent dehydration and electrolyte imbalances (Key Concepts 25-3). Fluid intake and output are measured and recorded every 8 hours. A critically ill patient or a patient with renal disease may require more frequent measurements of urinary output. Blood pressure, pulse, and respiratory rate are taken every 4 hours or as ordered by the health care provider. Areas of edema are examined daily to evaluate the effectiveness of drug therapy.

Patients with Hypertension. The blood pressure, pulse, and respiratory rate of patients with hypertension receiving a diuretic, or a diuretic along with an antihypertensive drug, are taken before the administration of the drug. More frequent monitoring may be necessary if the patient is critically ill or the blood pressure excessively high.

Carbonic Anhydrase Inhibitors

If a carbonic anhydrase inhibitor is given for glaucoma, then the patient's response to drug therapy (relief of eye pain) is monitored every 2 hours. The health care provider should be notified immediately if eye pain increases or if it has not begun to decrease 3 to 4 hours after the first dose. If the patient has acute closed-angle glaucoma, then the pupils of the affected eye are checked every 2 hours for dilation and response to light. A patient who can walk but has reduced

vision because of glaucoma may need help walking and with self-care activities.

If a carbonic anhydrase inhibitor is being given to control epileptic seizures, then the patient is checked frequently for the occurrence of seizures, especially early in therapy and in patients known to experience seizures frequently. If a seizure does occur, then it should be documented in the patient's chart, including time of onset and duration. Accurate descriptions of seizures help the health care provider plan future therapy and adjust drug dosages as needed.

Loop Diuretics

Because loop diuretics may cause GI upset, they should generally be taken with food or milk. However, torsemide may be given without regard to meals, and ethacrynic acid should be given after a meal. The health care provider should be notified if muscle weakness, cramps, nausea, or dizziness occurs. Patients should be advised to rise slowly in order to avoid orthostatic hypotension.

In patients with diabetes mellitus, urine glucose tests may be affected because these drugs may increase blood glucose levels. Some patients may experience photosensitivity, so provide teaching about the use of sunscreens or protective clothing during exposure to ultraviolet light or sunlight. Patients with hypertension should be instructed to avoid medications that may increase blood pressure, including over-the-counter (OTC) appetite suppressants and cold remedies.

Osmotic Diuretics

When an osmotic is prescribed, the disease or disorder and the symptoms being treated are closely monitored. For example, if the patient has a low urinary output and the osmotic diuretic is given to increase urinary output, then the intake and output ratio and symptoms the patient is experiencing are recorded. In addition, the patient is weighed and vital signs are taken before starting drug therapy.

Mannitol is administered only IV. The patient's urine output is monitored hourly.

When a patient is receiving the osmotic diuretic mannitol or urea for treatment of increased intracranial pressure caused by cerebral edema, the blood pressure, pulse, and respiratory rate are monitored every 30 to 60 minutes or as ordered by the health care provider. Any increase in blood pressure, decrease in the pulse or respiratory rate, or any change in the patient's neurologic status should be reported.

ALERT ℞

Potassium-Sparing Diuretics and Hyperkalemia

Patients taking potassium-sparing diuretics are at risk for hyperkalemia. Symptoms of hyperkalemia include paresthesia (numbness, tingling, or prickling sensation), muscular weakness, fatigue, flaccid paralysis of the extremities, bradycardia, shock, and electrocardiographic (ECG) abnormalities (see Signs and Symptoms Box for additional symptoms). The drug is discontinued and the health care provider notified immediately if the patient experiences these symptoms.

Potassium-Sparing Diuretics

Patients taking potassium-sparing diuretics are at risk for hyperkalemia. Serum potassium levels are monitored frequently, particularly during initial treatment.

SIGNS & SYMPTOMS

Common Fluid and Electrolyte Imbalances Associated with Diuretic Therapy

Dehydration (Excessive Water Loss)

- Thirst
- Poor skin turgor
- Dry mucous membranes
- Weakness
- Dizziness
- Fever
- Low urine output

Hyponatremia (Excessive Loss of Sodium)

- Cold, clammy skin
- Decreased skin turgor
- Confusion
- Hypotension
- Irritability
- Tachycardia

Hypomagnesemia (Low Levels of Magnesium)

- Leg and foot cramps
- Hypertension
- Tachycardia
- Neuromuscular irritability
- Tremor
- Hyperactive deep tendon reflexes
- Confusion
- Visual or auditory hallucinations
- Paresthesias

Hypokalemia (Low Blood Potassium)

- Anorexia
- Nausea
- Vomiting
- Depression
- Confusion
- Cardiac arrhythmias
- Impaired thought processes
- Drowsiness

Hyperkalemia (High Blood Potassium)

- Irritability
- Anxiety
- Confusion
- Nausea
- Diarrhea
- Cardiac arrhythmias
- Abdominal distress

CONSIDERATIONS | Older adults

LIFESPAN

Older Patients and Electrolyte Imbalances

Older adults are particularly prone to fluid volume deficits and electrolyte imbalances (see Signs and Symptoms Box) while taking a diuretic. An older adult is carefully monitored for hypokalemia (when taking a loop or thiazide diuretic) and hyperkalemia (with a potassium-sparing diuretic).

Thiazide and Related Diuretics

When thiazide diuretics are administered, the patient's renal function is monitored periodically. These drugs may precipitate azotemia (accumulation of nitrogenous wastes in the blood). If the patient's level of nonprotein nitrogen or blood urea nitrogen rises, then the health care provider may consider withholding or discontinuing the drug. In addition, serum uric acid concentrations are monitored periodically during treatment with thiazide diuretics because these drugs may precipitate an acute attack of gout. The patient also is monitored for joint pain or discomfort. Because hyperglycemia may occur, insulin or oral antidiabetic drug dosages may require alterations. Serum glucose concentrations are monitored periodically.

Educating the Patient and Family about Diuretics

The patient or a family member should be given a full explanation of the prescribed drug therapy, including when to take the drug (diuretics taken once per day are best taken early in the morning), if the drug is to be taken with food, and the importance of following the dosage schedule. The onset and duration of the drug's diuretic effect are also explained. The patient and family must also be made aware of the signs and symptoms of fluid and electrolyte imbalances and adverse reactions that may occur when using a diuretic. To ensure compliance with the prescribed drug regimen, the importance of diuretic therapy in the treatment of the patient's disorder should be emphasized. Following are key points about diuretics that the patient and family members should know.

- Do not stop taking the drug and do not skip doses except on the advice of your health care provider.
- If you experience gastrointestinal upset, take the drug with food or milk.

ALERT ℞

Warning Signs of Fluid and Electrolyte Imbalance

Warning signs of a fluid and electrolyte imbalance include dry mouth, thirst, weakness, lethargy, drowsiness, restlessness, muscle pains or cramps, confusion, gastrointestinal disturbances, hypotension, oliguria (decreased urinary output), tachycardia, and seizures

COMPLEMENTARY & ALTERNATIVE MEDICINE

Diuretics

Numerous herbal diuretics are available as OTC products. Most plants and herbal extracts available as OTC diuretics are nontoxic. However, most are either ineffective or no more effective than caffeine. The following are some of the herbals reported to have diuretic activity: celery, chicory, sassafras, juniper berries, St. John's wort, foxglove, horsetail, licorice, dandelion, digitalis purpurea, ephedra, hibiscus, parsley, and elderberry.

There is very little and in many instances no scientific evidence to justify the use of these plants as diuretics. For example, dandelion root is a popular preparation once thought to be a strong diuretic, but scientific research has found dandelion root, although safe, to be ineffective as a diuretic. No herbal diuretic should be taken unless approved by the health care provider.

Diuretic teas such as juniper berries and shave grass or horsetail should be avoided. Juniper berries have been associated with renal damage, and horsetail contains severely toxic compounds. Teas with ephedrine should also be avoided, especially by individuals with hypertension.

- Take the drug early in the morning (with a once-a-day dosage) unless directed otherwise to minimize the effects on nighttime sleep. Twice-a-day dosing should be administered early in the morning (e.g., 7.00 AM) and early afternoon (e.g., 2.00 PM) or as directed by your health care provider. These drugs initially cause more frequent urination, which should subside after a few weeks.
- Avoid alcohol and nonprescription drugs unless your health care provider approves. Hypertensive patients should be careful to avoid medications that increase blood pressure, such as OTC drugs for appetite suppression or cold symptoms.
- Notify your health care provider if you experience any of the following: muscle cramps or weakness, dizziness, nausea, vomiting, diarrhea, restlessness, excessive thirst, general weakness, rapid pulse, increased heart rate or pulse, or gastrointestinal distress.
- If you feel dizzy or weak, be careful while driving or performing hazardous tasks, rise slowly from a sitting or lying position, and avoid standing in one place for an extended time.
- Weigh yourself weekly or as recommended by your health care provider. Keep a record of these weekly weights and contact your health care provider if your weight loss exceeds 3 to 5 lb per week.
- If your health care provider recommends foods or fluids high in potassium, then eat the amount recommended. Do not exceed this amount or eliminate these foods

BOX 25.1

High-Potassium Foods

- *Meats:* beef, chicken, pork, turkey, veal
- *Seafood:* flounder, haddock, halibut, salmon, flounder, canned sardines, scallops, tuna
- *Fruits:* apricots, bananas, dates, raisins, fresh orange juice, tomato juice, oranges, dried fruit, cantaloupe, peaches, prunes, avocado
- *Vegetables:* carrots, lima beans, potatoes, radishes, spinach, sweet potatoes, tomatoes
- *Other:* gingersnaps, graham crackers, molasses, peanuts, peanut butter, coffee, tea, nuts

from your diet for more than 1 day, except when told to do so by your health care provider (Box 25-1).
- After a time, the diuretic effect of the drug may be minimal because most of the body's excess fluid has been removed. Continue taking the drug as directed to prevent further accumulation of fluid.
- If you are taking a thiazide or related diuretic, loop diuretic, potassium-sparing diuretic, carbonic anhydrase inhibitor, or triamterene, then avoid exposure to sunlight or ultraviolet light (sunlamps, tanning beds) because exposure may cause exaggerated sunburn (photosensitivity reaction). Wear sunscreen and protective clothing until your tolerance is determined.
- If you are taking a loop or thiazide diuretic and have diabetes mellitus, your blood glucometer test results for glucose may be elevated or your urine positive for glucose. Contact your health care provider if the results of your home testing of blood glucose levels increase or if your urine tests positive for glucose.
- If you are taking a thiazide diuretic, it may cause gout attacks. Contact your health care provider if you experience significant, sudden joint pain.
- If you are taking a carbonic anhydrase inhibitor for glaucoma, contact your health care provider immediately if your eye pain is not relieved or if it increases. If you are being treated for seizures, a family member should keep a record of all seizures that occur. Bring this record to your health care provider at your next visit. Contact your health care provider immediately if your seizures increase.

TABLE 25-2 Combination Diuretics

Generic Name	Trade Name
amiloride/HCTZ	Moduretic
spironolactone/HCTZ	Aldactazide
triamterene/HCTZ	Maxzide, Dyazide

Chapter Review

KEY POINTS

- Diuretics are used for a variety of medical disorders. Diuretics are administered early in the day to prevent any nighttime sleep disturbance caused by increased urination.

- Carbonic anhydrase inhibitors cause the excretion of sodium, potassium, bicarbonate, and water. These drugs are commonly used in the treatment of glaucoma. Carbonic anhydrase inhibitors are contraindicated in patients with known hypersensitivity, electrolyte imbalances, severe kidney or liver dysfunction, or anuria and for long-term use in chronic noncongestive angle-closure glaucoma.

- Loop diuretics, furosemide (Lasix) and ethacrynic acid (Edecrin), increase the excretion of sodium and chloride by inhibiting reabsorption of these ions in the distal and proximal tubules and in the loop of Henle. Loop diuretics are used to treat edema associated with chronic heart failure, cirrhosis of the liver, and renal disease. These drugs are contraindicated in patients with known hypersensitivity to loop diuretics or to sulfonamides, severe electrolyte imbalances, hepatic coma, or anuria and in infants (ethacrynic acid).

- Osmotic diuretics increase the density of the filtrate in the glomerulus (Fig. 25-1), thereby preventing selective reabsorption of water. Sodium and chloride excretion is increased. Administration by the IV route may result in a rapid fluid and electrolyte imbalance, especially when these drugs are administered before surgery to a patient in a fasting state.

- Potassium-sparing diuretics work in two ways. Triamterene (Dyrenium) and amiloride (Midamor) depress the reabsorption of sodium, therefore increasing sodium and water excretion. Both drugs depress the excretion of potassium and therefore are called potassium-sparing (or potassium-saving) diuretics. Spironolactone (Aldactone), also a potassium-sparing diuretic, antagonizes the action of aldosterone, causing sodium (but not potassium) and water to be excreted. Hyperkalemia, a serious event, may occur with the administration of potassium-sparing diuretics.

- Thiazides and related diuretics inhibit the reabsorption of sodium and chloride. Thiazides and related diuretics are used to treat hypertension, edema caused by chronic heart failure, hepatic cirrhosis, corticosteroid and estrogen therapy, and renal dysfunction. Thiazide diuretics are contraindicated in patients with known hypersensitivity to thiazides or related diuretics, electrolyte imbalances, renal decompensation, hepatic coma, or anuria.

CRITICAL THINKING CASE STUDIES

CASE 1

A Diuretic for Hypertension

Mr. Rodriguez, age 68 years, is taking amiloride for hypertension. He and his wife have stopped by the clinic for a routine blood pressure check. Mrs. Rodriguez states that her husband has been confused and very irritable for the past 2 days. He reports nausea and has had several "loose" stools.

1. Mrs. Rodriguez asks about the adverse effects of amiloride. She should be told that
   a. irritability and confusion are not caused by amiloride unless it is combined with certain other drugs
   b. nausea and loose stools may be adverse reactions to amiloride
   c. there are no known adverse effects of amiloride use
   d. both a and b are correct
2. You ask Mrs. Rodriguez if her husband is taking any other prescription drug. She nods and says ACE inhibitor. You know the health care provider has already considered that
   a. amiloride and ACE inhibitors have no known interactive effects
   b. there is an increased risk of hyperkalemia when the two drugs are combined
   c. there is an increased risk of hypokalemia when the two drugs are combined
   d. none of the above
3. Mr. Rodriguez asks if he should change his diet in any way because of his prescription drug use. He should be told
   a. do not drink alcohol unless his health care provider approves it
   b. when taking both an ACE inhibitor and amiloride, avoid foods high in potassium
   c. drinking adequate fluids is an important component of diuretic use
   d. all of the above
4. Mrs. Rodriguez asks which foods are high in potassium. What should you tell her?

CASE 2

A Diuretic for Intraocular Pressure

Mrs. Salzman was recently diagnosed with glaucoma and was given a prescription for acetazolamide. However, at her follow-up appointment, she stated that she does not understand why she is taking a diuretic for her eye.

1. How does acetazolamide help treat glaucoma?
   a. It reduces the production of aqueous humor in the eye, which decreases intraocular pressure.
   b. It reduces the amount of sodium in the aqueous humor in the eye, thus drawing water out and decreasing intraocular pressure.
   c. It increases the production of aqueous humor in the eye, which decreases intraocular pressure.
   d. It reduces the amount of potassium in the aqueous humor in the eye, thus drawing water out and decreasing intraocular pressure.
2. Which other diuretic(s) is/are also used for glaucoma or reduction of intraocular pressure?
   a. Methazolamide
   b. Mannitol
   c. Urea
   d. All of the above

3. Mrs. Salzman asks if she has to watch her diet because her friend who takes a diuretic has to eat a special diet. Although she cannot remember the specifics, she knows it has something to do with potassium. What do you tell her?

Review Questions

MULTIPLE CHOICE

1. Which of the following drugs would be used for edema due to CHF?
   a. mannitol
   b. methazolamide
   c. bumetanide
   d. all of the above
2. Which of the following drugs has the longest onset and duration of activity?
   a. spironolactone
   b. triamterene
   c. mannitol
   d. furosemide
3. Which of the following adverse reactions would most likely be seen in patients on long-term therapy with acetazolamide?
   a. Constipation
   b. Nausea and vomiting
   c. Crystalluria
   d. None of the above
4. When a diuretic is being given for heart failure, which of the following would be most indicative of an effective response to diuretic therapy?
   a. Low urine flow
   b. Daily weight loss of 2 lb
   c. Increased blood pressure
   d. Increasing edema in the legs and feet
5. Which electrolyte imbalance would most likely develop in a patient receiving a loop or thiazide diuretic?
   a. Hypernatremia
   b. Hyponatremia
   c. Hyperkalemia
   d. Hypokalemia
6. Which of the following foods should patients include in their daily diet to prevent hypokalemia?
   a. Green beans
   b. Apples
   c. Bananas
   d. Corn

MATCHING

Match each drug's brand name with its generic name.
_____ 7. acetazolamide   a. Ureaphil
_____ 8. furosemide   b. Demadex
_____ 9. mannitol   c. Aldactone
_____ 10. amiloride   d. Diamox
_____ 11. chlorothiazide   e. Zaroxolyn
_____ 12. spironolactone   f. Neptazane
_____ 13. metolazone   g. Midamor
_____ 14. methazolamide   h. Diuril
_____ 15. urea   i. Osmitrol
_____ 16. torsemide   j. Lasix

Match each drug with its classification.
_____ 17. Carbonic anhydrase inhibitor   a. mannitol
_____ 18. Loop   b. amiloride
_____ 19. Osmotic   c. acetazolamide
_____ 20. Potassium-sparing   d. indapamide
_____ 21. Thiazide   e. furosemide

TRUE OR FALSE

_____ 22. A patient taking an ACE inhibitor who receives amiloride is at increased risk for hyperkalemia.
_____ 23. Diuretics effectively increase the amount of fluid in body tissues.
_____ 24. A patient with diabetes who is taking a loop or thiazide diuretic may have increased blood glucose levels.
_____ 25. Potassium-sparing diuretics are typically given to control epileptic seizures.

FILL IN THE BLANKS

26. Mannitol is a(n) _____ diuretic that is used to reduce _____ pressure.
27. _____, a loop diuretic, should be used with caution in patients with lupus erythematosus.
28. A patient taking a diuretic who has leg and foot cramps, hypertension, neuromuscular irritability, and hallucinations is likely experiencing _____, an electrolyte disturbance.
29. Gout attacks may occur in patients taking _____ diuretics.

SHORT ANSWERS

30. What are the different types of diuretic drugs?
31. What are the most common fluid and electrolyte imbalances that patients taking diuretics may experience? Briefly explain each.
32. Why should patients taking certain diuretics avoid exposure to sunlight or ultraviolet light? What would you recommend to avoid this problem?
33. Initial diuretic therapy may cause more frequent urination, disturbing a patient's nighttime sleep. How would you instruct a patient to take the drug to minimize these effects?

Web Activities

1. Go to the National Library of Medicine Web site (www.nlm.nih.gov) and conduct a search on "heart failure." How does fluid intake and diuretic therapy help with the treatment of heart failure?
2. On the same Web site, conduct a search on "edema." Where does edema usually occur in the body? What are some causes of edema?

SUMMARY DRUG TABLE Diuretics
(left, generic; right, trade)

Comprehensive Summary Drug Tables, including uses, adverses effects, dosages, and pregnancy classifications, are provided on the companion website, http://thePoint.lww. com/PharmacologyHP2e

Carbonic Anhydrase Inhibitors	
acetazolamide *a-set-a-zole'-a-mide*	Diamox Sequels, *generic*
methazolamide *meth-a-zoe'-la-mide*	Neptazane, *generic*

Loop Diuretics	
bumetanide *byoo-met'-a-nide*	*generic*
ethacrynic acid *eth-a-krin-ik*	Edecrin, Edecrin Sodium
furosemide *fur-oh'-se-mide*	Lasix, *generic*
torsemide *tor'-se-myde*	Demadex, *generic*

Osmotic Diuretics	
mannitol *man'-i-tole*	Osmitrol, Resectisol, *generic*
urea *your-ee'-a*	Ureaphil

Potassium-Sparing Diuretics	
amiloride hydrochloride *a-mill'-oh-ride*	Midamor, *generic*
spironolactone *speer-on-oh-lak'-tone*	Aldactone, *generic*

Potassium-Sparing Diuretics	
triamterene *trye-am'-ter-een*	Dyrenium

Thiazides and Related Diuretics	
chlorothiazide *klor-oh-thye'-a-zide*	Diuril, Diuril IV, *generic*
chlorthalidone *klor-thal'-l-done*	Thalitone, *generic*
hydrochlorothiazide *hye-droe-klor-oh- thye'-a-zide*	Microzide, *generic*
indapamide *in-dap'-a-mide*	*generic*

Thiazides and Related Diuretics	
methyclothiazide *meth-i-kloe-thye'-a-zide*	*generic*
metolazone *me-tole'-a-zone*	Zaroxolyn, *generic*

26

Urinary Anti-Infectives

CHAPTER OBJECTIVES

On completion of this chapter, students will be able to:

1. Define the chapter's key terms.
2. Describe the general drug actions, uses, adverse reactions, contraindications, precautions, and interactions of urinary anti-infectives.
3. Discuss important points to keep in mind when educating the patient or family members about the use of urinary anti-infectives.

KEY TERMS

anti-infective—a drug used to treat infection
bactericidal—a drug that kills bacteria
bacteriostatic—a drug or agent that slows or retards bacteria
dysuria—burning and pain upon urination
urinary tract infection—an infection caused by pathogenic microorganisms of one or more structures of the urinary tract; commonly abbreviated as UTI
urinary frequency—frequent urination day and night
urinary urgency—sudden strong need to urinate

CHAPTER OVERVIEW

Drug classes covered in this chapter are:

- Urinary anti-infectives

Drugs by classification are listed on page 262.

thePOINT RESOURCES

- Comprehensive Summary Drug Tables
- Lippincott's Interactive Tutorials: Drugs Used to Treat Infections
- Interactive Practice and Review
- Monographs of Most Commonly Prescribed Drugs

This chapter discusses anti-infective drugs used to treat urinary tract infections. Urinary system infections may involve the bladder (cystitis), prostate gland (prostatitis), kidney and renal pelvis (pyelonephritis), or the urethra (urethritis) (Fig. 26-1).

Urinary tract infection (UTI) is an infection caused by pathogenic microorganisms of one or more structures of the urinary tract. The most common structure affected is the bladder (Key Concepts 26-1).

Urinary Anti-Infectives

Some drugs used in the treatment of UTIs do not belong to the antibiotic or sulfonamide groups of drugs. The drugs discussed in this chapter are **anti-infectives** (against infection) used in the treatment of UTIs. These drugs have an effect on bacteria in the urinary tract. Taken orally or by parenteral route, the drugs do not achieve significant levels in the bloodstream and are of no value in the treatment of systemic infections. They are primarily excreted by the kidneys and exert their major antibacterial effects in the urine (see Summary Drug Table: Urinary Anti-Infectives).

Examples of urinary anti-infectives include doripenem (Doribax), fosfomycin (Monurol), nitrofurantoin (Furadantin), and trimethoprim (Primsol). The anti-infectives work on various strains of bacteria. In addition to the anti-infectives, methenamine is an antiseptic used for UTIs.

Additional drugs can be used in the treatment of UTIs. Examples of these drugs include penicillins, cephalosporins, fluoroquinolones, tetracyclines, aminoglycosides, and sulfonamides (see Chapter 35). Combination drugs are also available.

FACT CHECK

26-1 What are the symptoms of a UTI affecting the bladder?

KEY CONCEPTS

26-1 UTI Symptoms

Symptoms of a UTI of the bladder (cystitis) include urinary urgency, urinary frequency, dysuria, a feeling of incomplete voiding after urination, and pain caused by spasm in the region of the bladder and lower abdominal area. Urinary tract infections are most common in females. However, males with indwelling catheters or other urinary disorders may also suffer from UTIs.

Actions, Uses, and Adverse Reactions of Urinary Anti-Infectives

All of the anti-infectives are used to treat UTIs caused by strains of susceptible bacteria.

Doripenem

Doripenem is a carbapenem antibiotic. It has bactericidal activity. It is indicated for complicated UTIs. It is given by IV infusion over 1 hour.

The most common adverse reactions associated with doripenem are nausea, diarrhea, and anemia. Since it is given intravenously, phlebitis may also occur.

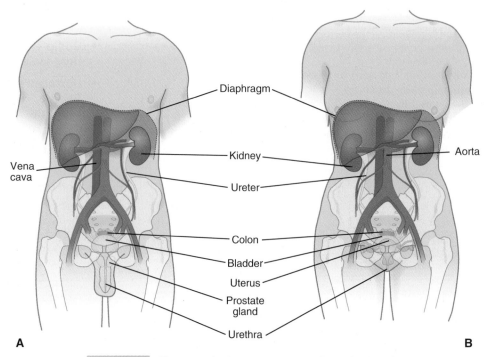

A **B**

FIGURE 26-1 The normal urinary system. A, male and B, female.

Fosfomycin

Fosfomycin is a bactericidal that interferes with bacterial cell wall synthesis. Fosfomycin is used for UTIs caused by microorganisms susceptible to its effects.

Adverse reactions of fosfomycin include headache, nausea, diarrhea, and vaginitis.

Methenamine and Methenamine Salts

Methenamine and methenamine salts are not antibiotics but are antiseptics that inhibit the growth of bacteria by sterilizing the urine. These drugs break down and form ammonia and formaldehyde, which are bactericidal. Acid salts (mandelate and hippurate) have some nonspecific bacteriostatic activity and help to maintain low urine pH, which inhibits bacterial growth.

Use of methenamine and methenamine salts may result in gastrointestinal disturbances, such as anorexia, nausea, vomiting, stomatitis, and cramps. Large doses may result in burning on urination and bladder irritation.

Nitrofurantoin

Nitrofurantoin may be **bacteriostatic** (slows or retards the multiplication of bacteria) or **bactericidal** (destroys bacteria), depending on the concentration of the drug in the urine. Nitrofurantoin is used to treat UTIs caused by strains of bacteria susceptible to it.

Nitrofurantoin use may result in nausea, headache, and flatulence. However, it may also result in other adverse reactions that range in severity from mild to severe and include vomiting, anorexia, rash, peripheral neuropathy, brown discoloration of the urine, and hypersensitivity reactions, which may range from mild to severe. Acute and chronic pulmonary reactions may occur.

Trimethoprim

Trimethoprim interferes with the ability of bacteria to metabolize folinic acid. Trimethoprim is also included in combination with sulfamethoxazole (Bactrim, Septra), which may also be used for UTIs.

The most common adverse reaction associated with trimethoprim is diarrhea. However, trimethoprim use may also result in rash, pruritus, exfoliative dermatitis, abdominal pain, and vomiting. When trimethoprim is combined with sulfamethoxazole (Bactrim), the adverse effects of the sulfonamide may also occur.

ALERT ℞

Pulmonary Reactions with Nitrofurantoin
Pulmonary reactions have been reported with the use of nitrofurantoin and may occur within hours and up to 3 weeks after therapy with this drug begins. Signs and symptoms of an acute pulmonary reaction include dyspnea (difficulty breathing), chest pain, cough, fever, and chills. If these reactions occur, then the health care provider is contacted immediately and the next dose of the drug is not taken until the patient is seen by the health care provider. Signs and symptoms of chronic pulmonary reactions, which may occur with prolonged therapy, include dyspnea, nonproductive cough, and malaise.

The adverse reactions of other anti-infectives, such as sulfonamides, penicillins, fluoroquinolones, tetracyclines, aminoglycosides, and cephalosporins are covered in other chapters.

FACT CHECK

26-2 What is the difference between a drug that is bacteriostatic and one that is bactericidal? Which urinary anti-infective drug may be both?

Contraindications, Precautions, and Interactions of Urinary Anti-Infectives

Doripenem

- Doripenem is contraindicated in patients with hypersensitivity to β-lactams.
- Dosage adjustment is required in patients with moderate or severe renal function impairment.
- Probenecid increases the plasma concentrations of doripenem. They should not be administered together.
- Doripenem may reduce the blood level of valproic acid.

Fosfomycin

- Fosfomycin is contraindicated in patients with a hypersensitivity to the drug.
- Fosfomycin is used cautiously during lactation.
- Lowered plasma concentration and urinary tract excretion occur when fosfomycin is administered with metoclopramide.

Methenamine and Methenamine Salts

- Methenamine is contraindicated in patients with hypersensitivity to the drug or a liver condition and during lactation.
- Patients who are allergic to tartrazine should not take methenamine hippurate (Hiprex).
- The drug is used cautiously in patients with liver or kidney disease or gout (may cause crystals to form in the urine).
- No serious interactions have been reported.
- An increased urinary pH decreases the effectiveness of methenamine. Therefore, to avoid raising the urine pH when taking methenamine, the patient should not use antacids containing sodium bicarbonate or sodium carbonate.

Nitrofurantoin

- Nitrofurantoin is contraindicated in patients with kidney disease or hypersensitivity to the drug and in lactating women.
- The drug is also used with caution in patients with a glucose-6-phosphate dehydrogenase deficiency, anemia, or diabetes.
- There is a decreased absorption of nitrofurantoin when the drug is administered with magnesium trisilicate or magaldrate.
- When nitrofurantoin is administered with anticholinergics, there is a delay in the rate at which nitrofurantoin leaves the stomach, increasing the amount absorbed.

Trimethoprim

- Trimethoprim is contraindicated in patients with a hypersensitivity to the drug or a lowered creatinine clearance (rate at which creatinine is excreted from the urine over time).
- The drug is used cautiously in patients with liver or kidney disease and in patients with megaloblastic anemia caused by folate deficiency.
- Trimethoprim is not recommended during lactation.
- No significant interactions have been reported.

FACT CHECK

26-3 Chronic pulmonary reactions may occur with prolonged therapy with nitrofurantoin. What are the signs and symptoms?

Patient Management Issues with Urinary Anti-Infectives

When a UTI is diagnosed, sensitivity tests are performed to determine bacterial sensitivity to drugs (antibiotics and urinary anti-infectives) that may control the infection. The color and appearance of the patient's urine and vital signs are recorded, and a urine sample is obtained for culture and sensitivity before the first dose of the drug is given.

Most UTIs are treated on an outpatient basis, and hospitalization usually is not required. Urinary tract infections may occur in hospitalized or nursing home patients with an indwelling urethral catheter or a disorder such as a stone in the urinary tract.

The patient's response to therapy is monitored daily. If after several days the symptoms have not improved or have become worse, then the health care provider is notified as soon as possible. Periodic urinalysis and urine culture and sensitivity tests may be ordered to monitor the effects of drug therapy.

Educating the Patient and Family about Urinary Anti-Infectives

Following are key points about urinary anti-infectives and miscellaneous urinary drugs that the patient and family members should know.

- Take the drug with food or meals (nitrofurantoin must be taken with food or milk). If you experience stomach upset despite taking the drug with food, contact your health care provider.
- Take the drug at the prescribed intervals and complete the full course of therapy. Do not stop taking the drug when your symptoms disappear unless directed to do so by your health care provider.
- Continue therapy until all of the drug is finished or until your health care provider discontinues the therapy.
- Try to drink fluids every hour. Drinking extra fluids aids in the physical removal of bacteria from your urinary tract and is an important part of treatment. When your fluid intake is increased, your urine should appear clear or barely yellow.

- Continue your increased fluid intake even when your symptoms subside.
- Notify your health care provider if your urine output is low, your urine appears dark or concentrated during the daytime, or your symptoms do not improve after 3 to 4 days.
- If you are elderly, you may have a decreased thirst sensation, but it is important nonetheless to increase fluid intake.
- If you experience drowsiness or dizziness, avoid driving and performing tasks that require alertness.
- During therapy with this drug, do not drink alcoholic beverages and do not take any nonprescription drug unless your health care provider approves it.
- Fosfomycin comes in dry form as a one-dose packet to be dissolved in 90 to 120 mL water (not hot water). Drink it immediately after mixing with food to prevent gastric upset.
- Methenamine and methenamine salts: Avoid excessive intake of citrus products, milk, and milk products. Increase intake of vitamin C and drink prune juice to acidify the urine.
- Nitrofurantoin: Take this drug with food or milk to improve absorption. Continue therapy for at least 1 week or for 3 days after the urine shows no signs of infection. Notify your health care provider immediately if you experience any of the following: fever, chills, cough, shortness of breath, chest pain, or difficulty breathing. Do not take the next dose of the drug until you talk with your health care provider. The urine may appear brown during therapy with this drug; this is not abnormal.

FACT CHECK

26-4 What instructions would you give a patient taking urinary anti-infectives regarding fluid intake? Why?

FACT CHECK

26-5 How do cranberries help prevent UTIs?

COMPLEMENTARY & ALTERNATIVE MEDICINE

Cranberry

Cranberry juice has long been recommended for preventing and treating UTIs. Clinical studies have confirmed that cranberry juice is beneficial to individuals with frequent UTIs. Cranberries inhibit bacteria from attaching to the walls of the urinary tract. Cranberry juice and capsules have no contraindications, no known adverse reactions, and no drug interactions.

Although cranberry may help to prevent the occurrence and relieve the symptoms of a UTI, no evidence suggests it works as a cure. If a UTI is thought to be present, then it is necessary to seek medical treatment.

Chapter Review

KEY POINTS

- A UTI is an infection caused by pathogenic microorganisms of one or more structures of the urinary tract. The most common structure affected is the bladder, with the urethra, prostate, and kidney also affected.
- Anti-infectives are used in the treatment of UTIs and have an effect on bacteria in the urinary tract. Taken orally or by parenteral route, they do not achieve significant levels in the bloodstream and are of no value in the treatment of systemic infections.
- Examples of urinary anti-infectives include doripenem (Doribax), fosfomycin (Monurol), nitrofurantoin (Furadantin), and trimethoprim (Primsol).
- Each drug works best on certain strains of bacteria. When a UTI is diagnosed, sensitivity tests are performed to determine bacterial sensitivity to drugs (antibiotics and urinary anti-infectives) that may control the infection.
- When any of these drugs is administered, the patient is monitored for a reduction in symptoms such as dysuria, urinary frequency, urgency, nocturia, and relief of any pain associated with irritation of the lower urinary tract.

CRITICAL THINKING CASE STUDY

Treating Urinary Tract Infections

Ms. Elliott, 42 years old, had a UTI 8 weeks ago. She failed to see her health care provider for a follow-up urine sample 2 weeks after completing her course of drug therapy. Ms. Elliot is now seeing her health care provider because her symptoms of a UTI have recurred. The health care provider suspects that Ms. Elliott may not have followed treatment instructions.

1. What course of action is taken to determine whether Ms. Elliott's UTI has recurred?
   a. A review of symptoms
   b. Laboratory testing of a urine sample
   c. Ask Ms. Elliott whether she completed the full course of drug therapy
   d. All of the above
2. Ms. Elliott is confirmed to have a UTI. What information should be reviewed with Ms. Elliott to ensure successful treatment?
   a. Drink plenty of fluids until the pain subsides
   b. Drink plenty of fluids throughout the course of treatment
   c. Emphasize the importance of follow-up visits and laboratory tests
   d. b and c
3. Ms. Elliott asks about the effectiveness of cranberry juice for treating UTIs. She is told
   a. clinical studies confirm its effectiveness in treating and preventing UTIs
   b. cranberry juice is a reliable substitute for drug therapy
   c. cranberry juice is effective in the treatment of dental plaque in the mouth but has little therapeutic value for UTIs
   d. none of the above

4. What signs and symptoms should Ms. Elliott look for in the future that would indicate she has a UTI?

Review Questions

MULTIPLE CHOICE

1. Nitrofurantoin (Macrodantin) is best taken
   a. with food
   b. no longer than 7 days
   c. without regard to food
   d. no longer than 2 days
2. When taking methenamine (Mandelamine), the patient is advised to
   a. use an antacid before taking the drug
   b. take an antacid immediately after taking the drug
   c. avoid antacids containing sodium bicarbonate or sodium carbonate
   d. avoid the use of antacids 1 hour before or 2 hours after taking the drug
3. What instruction would be most important to give a patient prescribed fosfomycin (Monurol)?
   a. Drink one to two glasses of cranberry juice daily to promote healing of the urinary tract.
   b. You may take the drug without regard to meals.
   c. This drug comes in a one-dose packet that must be dissolved in 90 mL or more of fluids.
   d. This drug may cause mental confusion.
4. Which of the following drugs may be given parenterally?
   a. fosfomycin
   b. doripenem
   c. nitrofurantoin
   d. none of the above

MATCHING

_____ 5. doripenem	a.	Macrobid
_____ 6. fosfomycin	b.	Septra
_____ 7. methenamine	c.	Hiprex
_____ 8. nitrofurantoin	d.	Monurol
_____ 9. trimethoprim	e.	Doribax
_____ 10. trimethoprim/Sulfamethoxazole	f.	Primsol

TRUE OR FALSE

_____ 11. Acute or chronic pulmonary reactions may occur in patients taking cinoxacin.

_____ 12. When a UTI is diagnosed, sensitivity tests are performed to determine bacterial sensitivity to drugs that may control the infection.

_____ 13. Increased urinary pH decreases the effectiveness of methenamine.

_____ 14. Cranberries may help to cure UTIs.

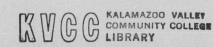

FILL IN THE BLANKS

15. _____ is contraindicated in patients with known hypersensitivity to the drug or a lowered creatinine clearance.
16. Because _____ is given intravenously, phlebitis is a potential adverse reaction.
17. A patient experiencing brown discoloration of the urine is likely taking the drug _____.
18. An anti-infective that is _____ kills the bacteria, whereas an anti-infective that is _____ slows or retards the bacteria.

SHORT ANSWERS

19. Once a UTI is diagnosed, how does the health care provider determine which drug to use?
20. Patients taking nitrofurantoin may experience acute pulmonary reactions. What are the signs and symptoms? What should be done if this occurs?

Web Activities

1. Go to the National Kidney and Urologic Disease Information Clearinghouse Web site (http://kidney.niddk.nih.gov) and conduct a search for "What I need to know about my child's urinary tract infection." What are some points that a parent should remember?
2. Go to the Mayo Clinic Web site (www.mayoclinic.com) and conduct a search for UTI. What are the risk factors for developing a UTI?

SUMMARY DRUG TABLE Urinary Anti-Infectives
(left, generic; right, trade)

Comprehensive Summary Drug Tables, including uses, adverses effects, dosages, and pregnancy classifications, are provided on the companion website, http://thePoint.lww.com/PharmacologyHP2e

doripenem *dore-i-pen'-em*	Doribax
fosfomycin tromethamine *foss-fo-my'-sin* *tro-meth-a-meen*	Monurol
methenamine *meth-en'-a-meen*	Hiprex, Urex, Methenamine Mandelate, *Methenamine Hippurate*
nitrofurantoin *nye-troe-fyoor- an'-toyn*	Furadantin, Macrobid, Macrodantin, *generic*
trimethoprim *trye-meth'-oh-prim*	Primsol, *generic*
trimethoprim and sulfamethoxazole (TMP–SMZ) *trye-meth'-oh-prim* *sul-fa-meth-ox'-a-zole*	Bactrim, Bactrim DS, Septra DS, Sulfatrim, *generic*

*The term *generic* indicates the drug is available in generic form.

27

Miscellaneous Urinary Drugs

CHAPTER OBJECTIVES

On completion of this chapter, students will be able to:

1. Define the chapter's key terms.
2. Describe the general drug actions, uses, adverse reactions, contraindications, precautions, and interactions of miscellaneous urinary drugs.
3. Discuss important points to keep in mind when educating the patient or family members about the use of miscellaneous urinary drugs.

KEY TERMS

overactive bladder—involuntary contractions of the detrusor, or bladder, muscle
urge incontinence—accidental loss of urine caused by a sudden and unstoppable need to urinate

CHAPTER OVERVIEW

Drug classes covered in this chapter are:

- Miscellaneous urinary drugs

Drugs by classification are listed on page 266.

The drugs reviewed in this chapter are used to relieve the symptoms associated with **overactive bladder** (involuntary contractions of the detrusor, or bladder, muscle) and to help control the discomfort associated with irritation of the lower urinary tract mucosa caused by infection, trauma, surgery, and endoscopic procedures. Symptoms of an overactive bladder include urinary urgency, urinary frequency, and urge incontinence, which is an accidental loss of urine caused by a sudden and unstoppable need to urinate.

Miscellaneous Urinary Drugs

The miscellaneous urinary drugs include several anticholinergic drugs and a urinary analgesic.

Actions, Uses, and Adverse Reactions of Miscellaneous Urinary Drugs

Anticholinergics

A number of anticholinergics are used to treat overactive bladder. These drugs counteract smooth muscle spasms of the urinary tract by relaxing the detrusor and other muscles through action at the parasympathetic receptors. The anticholinergics are used to relieve symptoms of dysuria (painful or difficult urination), urinary urgency (a strong and sudden desire to urinate), nocturia (excessive urination during the night), lower abdominal pain, frequency, and **urge incontinence** (accidental loss of urine caused by a sudden and unstoppable urge to void). The anticholinergics can cause a variety of adverse reactions; however, dry mouth and constipation are the two most common, particularly in the elderly. Some of the newer anticholinergics, such as tolterodine, act more specifically on the bladder, so their adverse reactions are less pronounced than other anticholinergic drugs.

The anticholinergics include darifenacin, fesoterodine, flavoxate, oxybutynin, solifenacin, tolterodine, and trospium.

Phenazopyridine

Phenazopyridine (Pyridium) is a dye that exerts a topical analgesic effect on the lining of the urinary tract. It has no anti-infective activity. Phenazopyridine is available as a separate urinary analgesic drug but is also included in some urinary anti-infective combination drugs. It is used to relieve the pain, burning, urgency, frequency, and irritation caused by infection, trauma, catheters, or surgical procedures of the urinary tract. Adverse reactions may include headache, rash, and gastrointestinal upset. Phenazopyridine may cause a red–orange discoloration of the urine and may stain fabrics or contact lenses, but this is normal and subsides when the drug is discontinued. Phenazopyridine is available both by prescription and over the counter.

FACT CHECK

27-1 Which drugs have parasympathetic action?
27-2 What are the most common adverse effects associated with anticholinergics?
27-3 Which drug has a topical analgesic effect on the urinary tract lining?

ALERT Rx

Phenazopyridine
When used in combination with an antibacterial drug to treat a urinary tract infection, phenazopyridine should not be administered for more than 2 days, because it may mask the symptoms of a more serious disorder.

Contraindications, Precautions, and Interactions of Miscellaneous Urinary Drugs

Anticholinergics

* The anticholinergics are contraindicated in patients with intestinal or gastric blockage, abdominal bleeding, or urinary tract blockage.
* They are used cautiously in patients with glaucoma and during lactation.
* No significant interactions with other drugs have been reported.
* Oxybutynin is contraindicated in patients with a hypersensitivity to the drug, glaucoma, partial or complete blockage of the gastrointestinal tract, myasthenia gravis, or urinary tract obstruction.
* Oxybutynin is used cautiously in patients with kidney or liver disease, heart failure, irregular or rapid heart rate, hypertension, or enlarged prostate.
* Phenothiazines are less effective when administered with oxybutynin.
* Haloperidol may have a decreased response and cause an increased risk of tardive dyskinesia (involuntary movements of face and/or extremities) when administered with oxybutynin.

Phenazopyridine

* Phenazopyridine is contraindicated in patients with renal impairment or undiagnosed urinary tract pain.
* Phenazopyridine is used cautiously during lactation.
* Phenazopyridine treats the symptom of pain but does not treat the cause of the disorder. No significant interactions have been reported.

Patient Management Issues with Miscellaneous Urinary Drugs

When the miscellaneous drugs are administered, patient symptoms such as pain, urinary frequency, and bladder distension are recorded to provide a baseline for future assessment. The patient is monitored for a reduction in symptoms such as dysuria (painful or difficult urination), urinary frequency, urgency, nocturia (excessive urination at night), and relief of pain associated with irritation of the lower urinary tract.

Educating the Patient and Family about Miscellaneous Urinary Drugs

Following are key points about miscellaneous urinary drugs that the patient and family members should know.

- For dry mouth, suck on hard candy, sugarless lozenges, or small pieces of ice, and brush your teeth regularly.
- These drugs may cause drowsiness or blurred vision. Do not drive or operate dangerous machinery or participate in any activity that requires full mental alertness until you know how the medication affects you.
- If you experience constipation, drink plenty of fluids, eat a high-fiber diet, and exercise (if your condition allows). If constipation persists, your health care provider may prescribe a mild laxative or stool softener.
- Anticholinergics: These drugs are used only to treat symptoms; other drugs are given to treat the cause.
- Oxybutynin: Take this drug with or without food. Oxybutynin (Ditropan XL) contains an outer coating that may not disintegrate and which may be seen in the stool. This is not a cause for concern. This drug can cause heat prostration (fever and heat stroke caused by decreased sweating) in high temperatures. If you live in a hot climate or will be exposed to high temperatures, take appropriate precautions.
- Phenazopyridine: This drug may cause a red–orange discoloration of the urine and may stain fabrics or contact lenses. This is normal. Take the drug after meals. Do not take this drug for more than 2 days if you are also taking an antibiotic for the treatment of a urinary tract infection.
- Tolterodine: If you experience difficulty voiding, take the drug immediately after voiding. If urinating is difficult or your pain persists, notify your health care provider.

FACT CHECK

27-4 What should the patient know about Ditropan XL?
27-5 Why should phenazopyridine not be administered for more than 2 days in a patient taking an antibiotic for a urinary tract infection?

Chapter Review

KEY POINTS

- Symptoms of an overactive bladder include urinary urgency, urinary frequency, and urge incontinence.
- Many of the drugs used to treat overactive bladder are anticholinergics, which relax the smooth muscle of the bladder. The newer anticholinergics act more specifically on the bladder and have less pronounced adverse reactions than those of the older anticholinergics.
- The most common adverse effects of the anticholinergics are dry mouth and constipation.
- Phenazopyridine is a urinary analgesic. It will relieve the symptoms of pain, burning, urgency, frequency, and irritation caused by infection, trauma, catheters, or surgical procedures of the urinary tract.
- The most common adverse effect of phenazopyridine is urine discoloration, which stains.

CRITICAL THINKING CASE STUDY

Overactive Bladder

Ms. Windham was recently diagnosed with overactive bladder. She has been prescribed tolterodine.

1. What type of drug is tolterodine?
   a. Anticholinergic
   b. Urinary analgesic
   c. Anti-infective
   d. None of the above
2. Given the drug's classification, what would you expect to be the most common adverse effects?
3. Ms. Windham comments to you that she has trouble remembering her evening dose since most of her medications are taken once a day in the morning. What could you suggest?

Review Questions

MULTIPLE CHOICE

1. Which of the following would be included in the information provided to a patient taking phenazopyridine (Pyridium)?
   a. There is a danger of heat prostration or heat stroke when taking phenazopyridine in a hot climate.
   b. This drug may turn the urine dark brown, which is an indication of a serious condition and should be reported immediately.
   c. This drug may cause photosensitivity; take precautions when out in the sun by wearing sunscreen, a hat, and long-sleeved shirts for protection.
   d. This drug may turn the urine red–orange; this is a normal occurrence that will disappear when the drug is discontinued.
2. Which of the following are potential adverse effects of Ditropan?
   a. Arrhythmia
   b. Yellow discoloration of the skin
   c. Blurred vision
   d. Photosensitivity
3. Patients who live in a hot climate should take precautions to avoid heat prostration when taking
   a. flavoxate
   b. oxybutynin
   c. tolterodine
   d. phenazopyridine

4. Tolterodine is an anticholinergic drug that acts more specifically on the bladder, so its adverse reactions are
   a. more pronounced than other anticholinergic drugs
   b. less pronounced than other anticholinergic drugs
   c. the same as other anticholinergic drugs
   d. none of the above

MATCHING

_____ 5. darifenacin
_____ 6. fesoterodine
_____ 7. phenazopyridine (OTC)
_____ 8. oxybutynin
_____ 9. phenazopyridine (Rx)
_____ 10. solifenacin
_____ 11. tolterodine
_____ 12. trospium

a. AZO Standard
b. Ditropan
c. Detrol
d. Enablex
e. Pyridium
f. Sanctura
g. Toviaz
h. VESIcare

TRUE OR FALSE

_____ 13. Phenazopyridine may cause anticholinergic reactions such as dry mouth, drowsiness, and decreased sweating.
_____ 14. Neurogenic bladder is caused by a nervous system abnormality.
_____ 15. Both oxybutynin and tolterodine are available in extended release form.
_____ 16. Symptoms of urge incontinence include painful urination.

FILL IN THE BLANKS

17. _____ is contraindicated in patients with uncontrolled narrow-angle glaucoma.
18. Patients should not take _____ for more than 2 days if they are also taking an antibiotic for a urinary tract infection.
19. _____ is used to treat bladder instability caused by a neurogenic bladder.
20. A patient who urinates frequently during the night is experiencing _____ and will likely be prescribed _____ to relieve the symptoms.

SHORT ANSWERS

21. How do the anticholinergics work?
22. Which of the miscellaneous urinary drugs has no anti-infective activity?
23. What would you recommend for patients who are experiencing dry mouth and constipation from their anticholinergic medication?

Web Activities

1. Go to Mayo Clinic Web site (www.mayoclinic.com) and conduct a search for "Overactive Bladder." What are the risk factors for developing overactive bladder?
2. Go to ClinicalTrials.gov. Are there any current clinical trials being conducted for overactive bladder? Write a brief description of your findings.

SUMMARY DRUG TABLE   Miscellaneous Urinary Drugs (left, generic; right, trade)

Comprehensive Summary Drug Tables, including uses, adverses effects, dosages, and pregnancy classifications, are provided on the companion website, http://thePoint.lww.com/PharmacologyHP2e

darifenacin *dar-i-fen'-a-sin*	Enablex
fesoterodine *fes-oh-ter'-oh-deen*	Toviaz
flavoxate HCl *la-voks'-ate*	*generic*
oxybutynin chloride *ox-i-byoo'-ti-nin*	Gelnique, Ditropan XL, Oxytrol, *Generic*
phenazopyridine HCl *fen-az-oh-peer'-i-dee*	AZO Standard, Azo-Dine, Baridium, Pyridium (Rx), Re-Azo, *generic*
solifenacin *sol-i-fen'-a-sin*	VESIcare
tolterodine tartrate *toll-tear'-oh-dyne*	Detrol, Detrol LA
trospium *trose'-pee-um*	Sanctura, Sanctura XR, *generic*

28

Drugs That Affect the Stomach and Pancreas

CHAPTER OVERVIEW

Drug classes covered in this chapter are

- Antacids
- Antiflatulents
- Histamine H$_2$ antagonists
- Proton pump inhibitors
- Anticholinergics
- Gastrointestinal stimulants
- Digestive enzymes
- Emetics
- Miscellaneous drugs that affect the stomach

Drugs by classification are listed on page 281.

CHAPTER OBJECTIVES

On completion of this chapter, students will be able to:

1. Define the chapter's key terms.
2. List the different classifications of drugs that affect the stomach.
3. Describe the actions and uses of antacids.
4. Describe the different ways that antacids interfere with the actions of other medications.
5. Describe the action of antiflatulents.
6. Compare and contrast the different drugs used to treat gastric and duodenal ulcers.
7. Describe the different treatment regimens for *H. pylori*.
8. Describe the actions and uses of anticholinergics, GI stimulants, and digestive enzymes in treating stomach disorders.
9. Identify when to use an emetic.
10. Describe the actions and uses of bismuth subsalicylate, misoprostol, and Carafate.
11. Discuss important points to keep in mind when educating the patient or family members about the use of drugs that affect the stomach and pancreas.

KEY TERMS

antacids—drugs that neutralize or reduce the acidity of stomach and duodenal contents

antiflatulents—drugs that remove flatus or gas in the stomach and small intestine

colic—spasmodic pains in the abdomen; in infants, this often presents with crying and irritability due to a variety of causes, such as swallowing of air, emotional upset, or overfeeding

thePOINT RESOURCES

- Comprehensive Summary Drug Tables
- Animation: General Digestion
- Lippincott's Interactive Tutorials: Drugs Affecting the Gastrointestinal System
- Interactive Practice and Review
- Monographs of Most Commonly Prescribed Drugs

emetic—a drug that induces vomiting
gastric stasis—failure to move food normally out of the stomach, also called gastroparesis
gastroesophageal reflux disease—a reflux or backup of gastric contents into the esophagus
Helicobacter pylori—bacteria that cause a type of chronic gastritis and peptic and duodenal ulcers
hydrochloric acid—a substance the stomach secretes that aids in the digestive process

hypersecretory—excessive gastric secretion of hydrochloric acid
paralytic ileus—lack of peristalsis or movement of the intestines
proton pump inhibitors—drugs with antisecretory properties

The gastrointestinal (GI) tract begins in the mouth, extends through the stomach and intestines, and terminates at the anus. This chapter will focus specifically on drugs that affect the stomach, as well as those that affect the pancreas. The drugs presented in this chapter include antacids, antiflatulents, histamine H_2 antagonists, proton pump inhibitors (PPIs), anticholinergics, GI tract stimulants, digestive enzymes, emetics, and miscellaneous drugs. Some of the more common preparations are listed in the Summary Drug Table: Drugs That Affect the Stomach and Pancreas.

Antacids

Actions of Antacids

Some of the cells of the stomach secrete **hydrochloric acid**, a substance that aids in the initial digestive process. **Antacids** (against acids) neutralize or reduce the acidity of stomach and duodenal contents by combining with hydrochloric acid and producing salt and water. Examples of antacids include aluminum hydroxide, calcium carbonate, magaldrate, and magnesia or magnesium hydroxide. Some antacid products contain a single active ingredient, while others contain two or more antacids. Table 28-1 lists the combination antacid products.

Uses of Antacids

Antacids are used in the treatment of hyperacidity problems such as heartburn, gastroesophageal reflux, sour stomach, and acid indigestion and in the medical treatment of peptic ulcer (Fig. 28-1). Many antacid preparations contain more than one ingredient. Additional uses for calcium carbonate include treating calcium deficiency states such as menopausal osteoporosis. Magnesium salts may be used in the treatment of magnesium deficiencies or magnesium depletion from malnutrition, restricted diet, or alcoholism.

Adverse Reactions of Antacids

The magnesium- and sodium-containing antacids may have a laxative effect and produce diarrhea. Aluminum- and calcium-containing products tend to produce constipation. Combination products are available. The advantage of a combination product, such as one that combines magnesium and aluminum, is that the adverse reactions are minimized. Since aluminum causes constipation and magnesium causes diarrhea, a combination product that contains both aluminum and magnesium should result in an overall adverse reaction of little change on the patient's bowel movements.

Some of the less common but more serious adverse reactions include:

- **Aluminum-containing antacids:** constipation, intestinal impaction, anorexia, weakness, tremors, and bone pain
- **Magnesium-containing antacids:** severe diarrhea, dehydration, and hypermagnesemia (nausea, vomiting, hypotension, decreased respirations)
- **Calcium-containing antacids:** rebound hyperacidity, metabolic alkalosis, hypercalcemia, vomiting, confusion, headache, renal calculi, and neurologic impairment
- **Sodium bicarbonate:** systemic alkalosis and rebound hypersecretion

Although antacids have the potential for serious adverse reactions, they have a wide margin of safety, especially when used as prescribed.

Contraindications, Precautions, and Interactions of Antacids

- Antacids are contraindicated in patients with severe abdominal pain of unknown cause and during lactation.
- Sodium-containing antacids are contraindicated in patients with cardiovascular problems, such as hypertension or congestive heart failure, and in patients on sodium-restricted diets.
- Calcium-containing antacids are contraindicated in patients with renal calculi or hypercalcemia.
- Aluminum-containing antacids are used cautiously in patients with gastric outlet obstruction.
- Magnesium- and aluminum-containing antacids are used cautiously in patients with decreased kidney function.
- Calcium-containing antacids are used cautiously in patients with respiratory insufficiency, renal impairment, or cardiac disease.
- The following drugs have a decreased pharmacologic effect when administered with an antacid: corticosteroids, digoxin, chlorpromazine, oral iron products, isoniazid, phenothiazines, ranitidine, phenytoin, valproic acid, and tetracyclines. Key Concepts 28-1 describes how antacids may interfere with other drugs.

Patient Management Issues with Antacids

Antacids should not be given within 2 hours before or after administration of other oral drugs. Liquid antacid preparations must be shaken thoroughly immediately before

TABLE 28-1   Antacid Combinations

	Drugs	Brand Name(s)
Tablets and Capsules	Magnesium hydroxide/calcium carbonate	Rolaids, Rolaids Extra Strength, Rolaids Multi-Symptom, Calcium Rich Rolaids Mylanta Antacid, Mylanta Ultra
	Aluminum hydroxide/magnesium hydroxide	Mintox
	Calcium carbonate/simethicone	Maalox Advanced Maximum Strength, Maalox Max Maximum Strength, Maalox Plus Antigas Junior Gas-Ban Gas-X with Maalox Extra Strength Titralac Plus
	Calcium carbonate/magnesium carbonate	Mylagen
	Calcium/magnesium/simethicone	Rolaids Plus Gas Relief
	Alginic acid	Gaviscon
	Magnesium hydroxide/calcium carbonate/ simethicone	Advanced Formula Di-Gel
	Magaldrate/simethicone	Riopan Plus, Riopan Plus Double Strength
Liquids	Aluminum hydroxide/magnesium hydroxide/ simethicone	Maalox Advanced Regular Strength, Maalox Regular Strength, Maalox Maximum Strength Multi-Symptom, Maalox Advanced Maximum Strength Mylanta, Mylanta Extra Strength
	Aluminum hydroxide/magnesium carbonate	Gaviscon Liquid, Gaviscon Extra Strength Relief Formula
	Calcium carbonate/simethicone	Titralac Plus
	Magnesium hydroxide/calcium carbonate	Mylanta Supreme
Powders/Effervescent Tablets	Sodium bicarbonate/citric acid/potassium bicarbonate	Alka-Seltzer Gold
	Sodium bicarbonate/aspirin/citric acid	Alka-Seltzer, Original Alka-Seltzer, Extra Strength Alka-Seltzer
	Sodium bicarbonate/citric acid	Alka-Seltzer Heartburn
	H_2 antagonist combinations	Pepcid Complete, Tums Dual Action
	Famotidine/calcium carbonate/magnesium hydroxide	

KEY CONCEPTS

28-1   How Antacids Interfere with Other Drugs

Antacids may interfere with other drugs in three ways:
1. By increasing the gastric pH, which causes a decrease in absorption of weakly acidic drugs and results in a decreased drug effect (e.g., digoxin, phenytoin, chlorpromazine, and isoniazid)
2. By absorbing or binding drugs to their surface, resulting in a decrease in the amount of drug being absorbed into the bloodstream (e.g., tetracycline)
3. By affecting the rate of drug elimination by increasing urinary pH (e.g., the excretion of salicylates is increased, whereas excretion of quinidine and amphetamines is decreased)

administration. If tablets are given, the patient is told to chew the tablets thoroughly before swallowing and to then drink a full glass of water or milk. Liquid antacids are followed by a small amount of water. The health care provider should be notified if the patient dislikes the taste of the antacid or has difficulty chewing the tablet form. A flavored antacid may be ordered if the taste is a problem, and a liquid form may be ordered if the patient has difficulty chewing a tablet.

ALERT Rx

Antacid Interaction with Other Drugs
Because of the possibility of an antacid interfering with the activity of other oral drugs, no oral drug should be administered within 2 hours of an antacid.

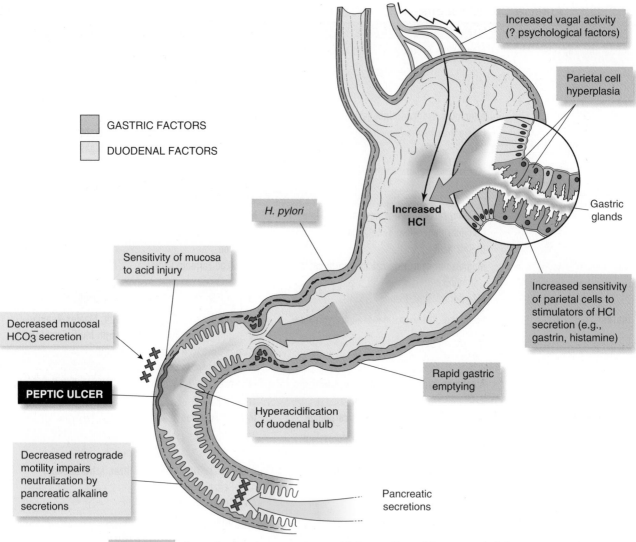

GASTRIC FACTORS

DUODENAL FACTORS

Increased vagal activity (? psychological factors)

Parietal cell hyperplasia

H. pylori

Increased HCl

Gastric glands

Sensitivity of mucosa to acid injury

Decreased mucosal HCO₃⁻ secretion

Increased sensitivity of parietal cells to stimulators of HCl secretion (e.g., gastrin, histamine)

PEPTIC ULCER

Rapid gastric emptying

Hyperacidification of duodenal bulb

Decreased retrograde motility impairs neutralization by pancreatic alkaline secretions

Pancreatic secretions

FIGURE 28-1 A peptic ulcer is an erosion and inflammation of the stomach lining.

Educating the Patient and Family about Antacids

Following are key points about antacids that the patient and family members should know:

- Do not use the drug indiscriminately. Check with your health care provider before using an antacid if you have other medical problems, such as a cardiac condition, because some laxatives contain sodium.
- Chew tablets thoroughly before swallowing and then drink a full glass of water.
- Allow effervescent tablets to completely dissolve in water. Allow most of the bubbling to stop before drinking.
- Follow the dosage schedule recommended by your health care provider. Do not increase the frequency of use or the dose if your symptoms become worse; instead, see your health care provider as soon as possible.

- Antacids impair the absorption of some drugs. Do not take other drugs within 2 hours before or after taking the antacid unless your health care provider recommends use of an antacid with the drug.
- If your pain or discomfort remains the same or becomes worse, if your stools turn black, or if you vomit a substance that resembles coffee grounds, then contact your health care provider as soon as possible.
- Antacids may change the color of your stool (white, white streaks); this is normal.
- Magnesium-containing products may produce a laxative effect and may cause diarrhea; aluminum- or calcium-containing antacids may cause constipation.
- If you take too much antacid, then it may cause your stomach to secrete excess stomach acid. Consult your health care provider or pharmacist about an appropriate dose. Do not use the maximum dose for more than 2 weeks, except under the supervision of your health care provider.

Antiflatulents

Actions of Antiflatulents

Simethicone (Mylicon) and charcoal are used as **antiflatulents** (reducing flatus or gas in the stomach and small intestine). Simethicone has a defoaming action that disperses and prevents the formation of mucus-surrounded gas pockets in the intestine. Charcoal is an absorbent that reduces the amount of intestinal gas.

Uses of Antiflatulents

Antiflatulents are used for the relief of painful symptoms of excess gas in the digestive tract. These drugs are useful as adjunctive treatment for any condition in which gas retention is a problem (e.g., postoperative gaseous distention, **colic**, air swallowing, dyspepsia, peptic ulcer, irritable colon, or diverticulosis). Charcoal may also be used to prevent nonspecific pruritus (itching) associated with kidney dialysis treatment and as an antidote in poisoning. Simethicone is included in some antacid products (see Table 28-1).

Adverse Reactions of Antiflatulents

Adverse reactions with simethicone are uncommon but may include diarrhea, vomiting, and abdominal pain. Activated charcoal will cause fecal discoloration.

Contraindications, Precautions, and Interactions of Antiflatulents

- Antiflatulents are contraindicated in patients with known hypersensitivity to any components of the drug.
- A decreased effectiveness of other drugs may occur because of adsorption by charcoal, which can also adsorb other drugs in the GI tract.
- There are no known interactions with simethicone.

Patient Management Issues with Antiflatulents

Activated charcoal can adsorb drugs while they are in the GI tract. Charcoal is administered 2 hours before or 1 hour after other medications. If diarrhea persists or lasts longer than 2 days or is accompanied by fever, then the health care provider should be notified. Simethicone is administered after each meal and at bedtime.

Educating the Patient and Family about Antiflatulents

Following are key points about antiflatulents that the patient and family members should know.

- Take simethicone after each meal and at bedtime.
- Take charcoal 2 hours before or 1 hour after meals.
- Notify your health care provider if your symptoms are not relieved within several days.

Histamine H$_2$ Antagonists

Actions of Histamine H2 Antagonists

These drugs inhibit the action of histamine at histamine H$_2$ receptor cells of the stomach, which then reduces the secretion of gastric acid and reduces total pepsin output. The decrease in acid allows ulcerated areas to heal. Examples of histamine H$_2$ antagonists include cimetidine (Tagamet HB), famotidine (Pepcid), nizatidine (Axid), and ranitidine (Zantac).

Uses of Histamine H$_2$ Antagonists

Histamine H$_2$ antagonists are used for the medical treatment of gastric and duodenal ulcers, gastric **hypersecretory** (excessive gastric secretion of hydrochloric acid) conditions, and gastroesophageal reflux disease (GERD). They are also all available over-the-counter to treat heartburn. These drugs may also be used to prevent stress-related ulcers and acute upper GI tract bleeding in critically ill patients.

Adverse Reactions of Histamine H$_2$ Antagonists

Adverse reactions of histamine H$_2$ antagonists include dizziness, somnolence (a tendency to sleep), headache, diarrhea, and impotence (reversible when the drug is discontinued). Adverse reactions are usually mild and transient.

CONSIDERATIONS | Older adults

LIFESPAN

H₂ Antagonists

Because older adults are particularly sensitive to the effects of histamine H₂ antagonists, they must be carefully monitored for confusion and dizziness, which increase the risk for falls. These patients often need help walking and with self-care activities. Throw rugs or small pieces of furniture should be removed. Any change in the patient's orientation should be reported to the health care provider.

Contraindications, Precautions, and Interactions of Histamine H₂ Antagonists

- Histamine H₂ antagonists are contraindicated in patients with a known hypersensitivity.
- These drugs are used cautiously in patients with renal or hepatic impairment and in severely ill or debilitated patients.
- Cimetidine is used cautiously in patients with diabetes.
- Histamine H₂ antagonists are used cautiously in older adults because they may cause confusion, and a dosage reduction may be required.
- Histamine antagonists should be used with caution during lactation.
- Many drugs may interact with H₂ antagonists, but only some of the more common interactions can be described here. Cimetidine has more drug interactions than the other H₂ antagonists.
- Antacids and metoclopramide may decrease absorption of H₂ antagonists if administered concurrently.
- Concurrent use of cimetidine and digoxin may decrease serum digoxin levels.
- The patient may have a decreased white blood cell count when an H₂ antagonist is administered along with an alkylating drug or antimetabolite.
- The patient has an increased risk for toxicity of oral anticoagulants, phenytoin, quinidine, lidocaine, or theophylline when administered with H₂ antagonists.
- Concurrent use of cimetidine and morphine increases the risk of respiratory depression.

Patient Management Issues with Histamine H₂ Antagonists

Ranitidine and oral cimetidine are administered before or with meals and at bedtime. Nizatidine and famotidine are given in single doses at bedtime or with twice-per-day doses in the morning and at bedtime. These drugs may be given concurrently with an antacid for more rapid onset of action by the antacid until the H₂ antagonist can be absorbed and begin working. Pepcid is available over the counter in a combination product called Pepcid Complete, which contains famotidine, calcium carbonate, and magnesium hydroxide.

Educating the Patient and Family about Histamine H₂ Antagonists

Following are key points about histamine H₂ antagonists that the patient and family members should know.

- Keep your health care provider informed of relief of pain or discomfort.
- Take as directed on the prescription container, for example, with meals or at bedtime.
- Follow your health care provider's recommendations regarding additional treatment such as eliminating certain foods or avoiding the use of alcohol and additional drugs such as antacids.
- If you become drowsy, then avoid driving or performing other hazardous tasks.
- Notify your health care provider of the following adverse reactions: sore throat, rash, fever, unusual bleeding, black or tarry stools, easy bruising, or confusion.
- Regular follow-up appointments are required while taking these drugs. These drugs may need to be taken for 4 to 6 weeks or longer.
- With cimetidine, inform your health care provider if you smoke. Cigarette smoking may decrease the effectiveness of the drug.

FACT CHECK

28-4 What are the four common histamine H₂ antagonists?

28-5 Which H₂ antagonist has the most drug interactions?

Proton Pump Inhibitors

Actions of Proton Pump Inhibitors

Proton pump inhibitors, such as lansoprazole, omeprazole, pantoprazole, and rabeprazole, belong to a group of drugs with antisecretory properties. These drugs suppress gastric acid secretion by blocking the last step of acid production, the production of gastric acid by the gastric mucosa. Omeprazole is also available in a combination product with sodium bicarbonate, both prescription (Zegerid) and over-the-counter (Zegerid OTC).

Uses of Proton Pump Inhibitors

Proton pump inhibitors are used for treatment or symptomatic relief of various gastric disorders including gastric and duodenal ulcers, GERD, or pathological hypersecretory conditions. Painful, persistent heartburn 2 or more days per week may indicate acid reflux disease, which can erode the delicate lining of the esophagus, causing erosive esophagitis. Proton pump inhibitors may provide 24-hour relief from the heartburn associated with GERD or erosive esophagitis while healing occurs.

Proton pump inhibitors are particularly important in the treatment of *Helicobacter pylori (H.pylori)* in patients with active duodenal ulcers. *Helicobacter pylori* have been implicated as bacteria that cause a type of chronic vgastritis and in a large number of cases of peptic and duodenal ulcers. Infection with *H. pylori* is often treated with a triple-drug treatment regimen, such as one of the PPIs and two anti-infectives. The standard treatment for *H. pylori* in the United States is a 10- to 14-day treatment regimen with clarithromycin, a PPI, and either amoxicillin or metronidazole. Another treatment regimen includes bismuth subsalicylate plus two anti-infective drugs. Helidac, a treatment regimen of three drugs (bismuth subsalicylate, metronidazole, and tetracycline), may be given along with a histamine H_2 antagonist or a PPI to treat disorders of the GI tract infected with *H. pylori*. Such quadruple therapies tend to have lower compliance than triple therapies. Table 28-2 lists various combinations used in the treatment of *H. pylori*. Additional information concerning the anti-infectives listed is in Chapter 35.

TABLE 28-2 *H. pylori* Therapy: Current First-Line Regimens Supported by the American College of Gastroenterology

Drug	Dose
H. pylori Triple Therapy for 10 to 14 days	
PPI	Once daily or BID (depends on drug chosen)
Clarithromycin	500 mg BID
Amoxicillin	1000 mg BID
------- or --------	
PPI	Once or BID (depends on drug chosen)
Clarithromycin	500 mg BID
Metronidazole	500 mg BID
H. pylori Quadruple Therapy for 10 to 14 days	
Bismuth subsalicylate	525 mg 4 times/d
Metronidazole	250 mg 4 times/d
Tetracycline	500 mg 4 times/d
Ranitidine or	150 mg BID or
PPI	Once or twice daily (depends on drug chosen)
Alternative Regimen	
PPI	BID for 5 d
Amoxicillin	1000 mg BID for 5 d
Followed by:	Followed by:
PPI	BID for 5 d
Clarithromycin	500 mg BID for 5 d
Tinidazole	500 mg BID for 5 d

Source: American College of Gastroenterology Guideline on the Management of *Helicobacter pylori* Infection. http://www.acg.gi.org/physicians/guidelines/ManagementofHpylori.pdf

Adverse Reactions of Proton Pump Inhibitors

The most common adverse reactions of PPIs include headache, diarrhea, and abdominal pain. Other less common adverse reactions include nausea, flatulence, constipation, and dry mouth.

Contraindications, Precautions, and Interactions of Proton Pump Inhibitors

- Proton pump inhibitors are contraindicated in patients who have a known hypersensitivity.
- Proton pump inhibitors are used cautiously in older adults and in patients with liver disease.
- There is a decreased absorption of lansoprazole when it is administered with sucralfate.
- Lansoprazole may decrease the effects of ketoconazole, iron salts, and digoxin.
- When lansoprazole is administered with theophylline, there is an increase in theophylline clearance, requiring dosage changes of theophylline.
- When omeprazole is administered with clarithromycin, there is a risk for an increase in plasma levels of both drugs.
- Omeprazole may prolong the elimination of warfarin when the two drugs are administered together.
- Increased serum levels and the risk for toxicity of benzodiazepines, phenytoin, and warfarin may occur if any of these drugs is used with omeprazole.

Patient Management Issues with Proton Pump Inhibitors

Omeprazole is taken before meals. The drug should be swallowed whole and not chewed or crushed. Esomeprazole must be swallowed whole and taken at least 1 hour before meals. For patients who have difficulty swallowing, the capsule may be broken open and the granules mixed lightly with applesauce and eaten immediately without chewing. Likewise, lansoprazole may be sprinkled on approximately one tablespoon of applesauce, cottage cheese, pudding, yogurt, or strained pears. The drug may also be administered through a nasogastric tube. The granules are mixed with a small amount of apple juice and injected through a tube. The tube is flushed with fluid afterward.

Educating the Patient and Family about Proton Pump Inhibitors and *H. pylori* Combination Drugs

Following are key points about PPIs and *H. pylori* combination drugs that the patient and family members should know.

Proton Pump Inhibitors

- Esomeprazole: Swallow whole at least 1 hour before eating. If you have difficulty swallowing, then the capsule may be opened and the granules sprinkled on a small amount of applesauce.
- Omeprazole: Swallow tablets whole; do not chew them. You will take this drug for up to 8 weeks or a prolonged period. Regular medical checkups are required.
- Lansoprazole: Take before meals. Swallow the capsules whole. You should not chew, open, or crush them. If you

have difficulty swallowing the capsule, then open and sprinkle granules on gelatin or applesauce. You will need regular medical checkups while taking this drug.

H. pylori Combination Drugs

- Helidac: Each dose includes four tablets: two round, chewable, pink tablets (bismuth); one white tablet (metronidazole); and one pale orange and white capsule (tetracycline). Take each dose four times per day with meals and at bedtime for 14 days. Chew and swallow the bismuth subsalicylate tablets; swallow the metronidazole tablet and tetracycline capsule with a full glass of water. Take prescribed H₂ antagonist therapy as directed. Drink an adequate amount of fluid to reduce the risk of esophageal irritation and ulceration. Missed doses may be made up by continuing the formal dosing schedule until the medication is gone. Do not take double doses. If you miss more than four doses, contact your health care provider.
- Bismuth subsalicylate: Immediately report any symptoms of salicylate toxicity (ringing in the ears, rapid respirations) to your health care provider. Chew tablets thoroughly or dissolve them in the mouth. Do not swallow tablets whole. Stools may become dark; this is normal and will disappear when the drug therapy is discontinued. Do not take this drug with aspirin or aspirin products.

FACT CHECK
28-6 What is a key use of PPIs?

Anticholinergics

Actions of Anticholinergics

Anticholinergics (cholinergic blocking drugs) reduce gastric motility and decrease the amount of acid secreted by the stomach (see Chapter 14). Examples of anticholinergics used for GI tract disorders include propantheline and glycopyrrolate (Robinul).

Uses of Anticholinergics

Specific anticholinergic drugs are occasionally used in the medical treatment of peptic ulcer. These drugs have been largely replaced by histamine H₂ antagonists, which appear to be more effective and have fewer adverse drug reactions.

Adverse Reactions of Anticholinergics

Dry mouth, blurred vision, urinary hesitancy, urinary retention, nausea, vomiting, palpitations, and headache are some of the adverse reactions that may occur with anticholinergic drugs (see Chapter 14).

Contraindications, Precautions, and Interactions of Anticholinergic Drugs

Contraindications, precautions, and interactions of anticholinergic drugs are discussed in Chapter 14.

Patient Management Issues with Anticholinergics

Patient management issues with anticholinergic drugs are discussed in Chapter 14.

Educating the Patient and Family about Anticholinergics

Following are key points about anticholinergics that the patient and family members should know:

- If your eyes become sensitive to light (photophobia), wear sunglasses when outside, keep rooms dimly lit, and schedule outdoor activities (when necessary) before taking the first dose, such as early in the morning.
- If you experience dry mouth, then take frequent sips of cool water during the day, several sips of water before taking oral drugs, and frequent sips of water during meals.
- Constipation may be avoided by drinking plenty of fluids during the day.
- Drowsiness may occur with these drugs. Schedule tasks requiring alertness during times when drowsiness does not occur, such as early in the morning before taking the first dose of the drug.

FACT CHECK
28-7 How do anticholinergics work?

Gastrointestinal Stimulants

Actions of Gastrointestinal Stimulants

Metoclopramide (Reglan) and dexpanthenol increase the strength of the spontaneous movement of the upper GI tract. The exact mode of action of these drugs is unclear.

Uses of Gastrointestinal Stimulants

Oral preparations of metoclopramide are used in the treatment of symptomatic **gastroesophageal reflux disease** (a reflux or backup of gastric contents into the esophagus) and **gastric stasis** (failure to move food normally out of the stomach) in patients with diabetes. This drug is given intravenously to prevent nausea and vomiting associated with cancer chemotherapy and intramuscularly to prevent nausea and vomiting during the immediate postoperative period. Dexpanthenol may be given intramuscularly immediately after major abdominal surgery to reduce the risk of **paralytic ileus** (lack of peristalsis or movement of the intestines).

Adverse Reactions of Gastrointestinal Stimulants

The adverse reactions of metoclopramide are usually mild. Higher doses or prolonged administration may produce central nervous system (CNS) symptoms, such as drowsiness, dizziness, Parkinson-like symptoms (tremor, mask-like facial expression, muscle rigidity), depression, facial grimacing, motor restlessness,

- Take metoclopramide 30 minutes before meals. If you experience drowsiness or dizziness, then be cautious while driving or performing hazardous tasks.
- Immediately report any of the following signs: difficulty speaking or swallowing; a mask-like facial expression; shuffling gait; muscle rigidity or tremors; uncontrolled movements of the mouth, face, or extremities; and uncontrolled chewing or unusual movements of the tongue.

Digestive Enzymes

Actions of Digestive Enzymes

The enzymes pancreatin and pancrelipase, which are manufactured and secreted by the pancreas, are responsible for the breakdown and digestion of fats, starches, and proteins in food. Pancrelipase is available as an oral supplement.

Uses of Digestive Enzymes

Pancrelipase is prescribed as a replacement therapy for those with pancreatic enzyme insufficiency. Conditions or diseases that may cause a decrease in or absence of pancreatic digestive enzymes include cystic fibrosis, chronic pancreatitis, cancer of the pancreas, malabsorption syndrome, surgical removal of all or part of the stomach, and surgical removal of all or part of the pancreas.

Adverse Reactions of Digestive Enzymes

Few adverse reactions have been reported with the use of digestive enzymes; however, high doses may cause nausea and diarrhea.

Contraindications, Precautions, and Interactions of Digestive Enzymes

- Digestive enzymes are contraindicated in patients with a hypersensitivity to hog or cow proteins and in patients with acute pancreatitis.
- The digestive enzymes are used cautiously in patients with asthma (an acute asthmatic attack can occur) and hyperuricemia (increased concentrations of uric acid in the blood) and during lactation.
- Calcium carbonate or magnesium hydroxide antacids may decrease the effectiveness of the digestive enzymes.
- When administered concurrently with an iron preparation, the digestive enzymes decrease the absorption of oral iron preparations.

Patient Management Issues with Digestive Enzymes

Pancrelipase is taken before or with meals and with plenty of fluids. When digestive enzymes are given in capsule or

and involuntary movements of the eyes, face, or limbs. Dexpanthenol administration may cause nausea, vomiting, diarrhea, hypotension, or colic (spasms of the colon). If drowsiness or dizziness occurs when taking metoclopramide, then the patient will need help walking and with self-care activities.

Contraindications, Precautions, and Interactions of Gastrointestinal Stimulants

- Gastrointestinal tract stimulants are contraindicated in patients with a known hypersensitivity, GI tract obstruction, gastric perforation or hemorrhage, or epilepsy.
- These drugs are secreted in breast milk and should not be used during lactation and are used cautiously in patients with diabetes and cardiovascular disease.
- The effects of metoclopramide are compromised by concurrent administration of anticholinergics or narcotic analgesics.
- Metoclopramide may decrease the absorption of digoxin and cimetidine and increase absorption of acetaminophen, tetracyclines, and levodopa. Metoclopramide may alter the body's insulin requirements.

Patient Management Issues with Gastrointestinal Stimulants

The administration of oral metoclopramide should be carefully timed to occur 30 minutes before each meal. Dexpanthenol is administered intramuscularly, and the patient is told that an intestinal colic may occur within 30 minutes. This is not abnormal and will pass within a short time.

Educating the Patient and Family about Gastrointestinal Stimulants

Following are key points about GI stimulants that the patient and family members should know.

enteric-coated tablet form, the patient is instructed not to bite or chew the capsule or tablet. If the patient has difficulty swallowing, then the capsule can be opened and sprinkled on a small amount of soft food that does not need to be chewed served at room temperature, such as applesauce or flavored gelatin.

Educating the Patient and Family about Digestive Enzymes

Following are key points about digestive enzymes that the patient and family members should know:

- Take the drugs as directed by your health care provider. Do not exceed the recommended dose.
- Do not chew tablets or capsules. Swallow the whole form of the drug quickly while sitting upright to improve swallowing and to prevent mouth and throat irritation. Eat immediately after taking the drug.
- If the capsules are difficult to swallow, then you may open them and sprinkle the contents over small quantities of food but not with hot foods. You should eat all the food sprinkled with the powder without chewing.
- Do not change brands without consulting with your health care provider or pharmacist.
- Do not inhale the powder dosage form or powder from capsules because it may irritate the skin or mucous membranes.

FACT CHECK

28-10   What is pancrelipase and what does it do?

Emetics

Actions of Emetics

The **emetic** (a drug that induces vomiting) ipecac causes vomiting because of its local irritating effect on the stomach and by stimulating the vomiting center in the medulla.

Uses of Emetics

Emetics are used to cause vomiting to empty the stomach rapidly when an individual has accidentally or intentionally ingested a poison or drug overdose. Not all poison ingestions or drug overdoses are treated with emetics.

Adverse Reactions of Emetics

There are few adverse reactions to ipecac aside from the effects associated emesis. Although not an adverse reaction, a danger associated with any emetic is the aspiration (inhalation) of stomach contents.

Contraindications, Precautions, and Interactions of Emetics

- Emetics are contraindicated in patients who are unconscious, semiconscious, or convulsing and in poisonings

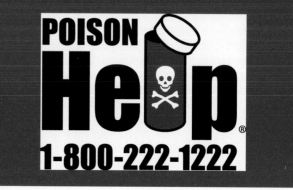

ALERT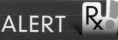

Emetic Administration and Poison Control
Untrained health care workers should never administer an emetic without first consulting poison control. The national poison control center number is 1-800-222-1222, and it will direct the call to one of the 57 poison control centers in the United States.

caused by corrosive substances, such as strong acids or petroleum products.
- Activated charcoal may absorb ipecac, negating its effects.

Patient Management Issues with Emetics

Before an emetic is given, it is extremely important to know the chemicals or substances the patient ingested, the time they were ingested, and what symptoms occurred before seeking medical treatment. This information is often obtained from a family member or friend. The health care provider may also contact the local poison control center for more information. (From American Association of Poison Control Centers, www.aapcc.org).

The patient's blood pressure, pulse, and respiratory rate are measured, and a brief physical examination is performed to determine what other damages or injuries, if any, may have occurred.

After the administration of an emetic, the patient is closely observed for signs of shock, respiratory depression, or other signs and symptoms associated with the specific poison or drug.

Educating the Patient and Family about Emetics

Following are key points about emetics that the patient and family members should know:

- Ipecac is available without a prescription for use at home. The instructions for use and the recommended dose are printed on the label.
- Read the directions on the label and be familiar with these instructions before an emergency occurs.
- In case of accidental or intentional poisoning, contact the nearest poison control center before using or giving this drug. Not all poisonings can be treated with this drug.

- Do not give this drug to anyone who is semiconscious, unconscious, or convulsing.
- Vomiting should occur in 20 to 30 minutes after taking this drug. Seek medical attention immediately after contacting the poison control center and giving this drug.

FACT CHECK

28-11 How does ipecac work?

Miscellaneous Drugs That Affect the Stomach

Actions of Miscellaneous Drugs That Affect the Stomach

Miscellaneous drugs include bismuth subsalicylate, misoprostol, and sucralfate.

Bismuth disrupts the integrity of the bacterial cell wall. Misoprostol (Cytotec) inhibits gastric acid secretion and increases the protective property of the mucosal lining of the GI tract by increasing the production of mucus by the lining of the tract. Sucralfate (Carafate) exerts a local action on the lining of the stomach. The drug forms a complex with the fluid from the inflamed tissue of the stomach lining. This complex forms a protective layer over a duodenal ulcer, thus aiding in healing of the ulcer. The exact mechanism of action of these drugs is unknown.

Uses of Miscellaneous Drugs That Affect the Stomach

Bismuth subsalicylate is used in combination with other drugs to treat gastric and duodenal ulcers caused by *H. pylori* bacteria. Misoprostol is used to prevent gastric ulcers in those taking aspirin or nonsteroidal anti-inflammatory drugs in high doses for a prolonged time. Sucralfate is used in the treatment of duodenal ulcers.

Adverse Reactions of Miscellaneous Drugs That Affect the Stomach

Adverse reactions of bismuth subsalicylate include a temporary and harmless darkening of the tongue and stool and constipation. Salicylate toxicity (e.g., tinnitus and rapid respirations; see Chapter 8) may also occur, particularly when the drug is used for an extended period of time.

The adverse reactions of sucralfate are usually mild, but constipation may occur in some patients. Misoprostol administration may result in diarrhea, abdominal pain, nausea, GI tract distress, and vomiting.

Contraindications, Precautions, and Interactions of Miscellaneous Drugs That Affect the Stomach

- Miscellaneous GI tract drugs are given with caution to patients with a known hypersensitivity.

- Misoprostol is contraindicated in those with an allergy to prostaglandins and during pregnancy and lactation.
- Misoprostol is used cautiously in women of childbearing age.
- Sucralfate is used with caution during lactation.
- A patient has an increased risk of diarrhea when taking misoprostol along with a magnesium-containing antacid.
- When bismuth subsalicylate is administered with an aspirin-containing drug, the patient is at risk for salicylate toxicity.
- The patient has an increased risk of toxicity of valproic acid and methotrexate and decreased effectiveness of corticosteroids when these agents are administered with bismuth subsalicylate.
- Patients taking medication for anticoagulation, diabetes, gout, or arthritis should consult their health care provider prior to taking bismuth subsalicylate.

Patient Management Issues with Miscellaneous Drugs That Affect the Stomach

Bismuth subsalicylate liquid should be shaken well before using. The chewable tablets must be chewed or allowed to dissolve in the mouth. If the tongue appears to have a black growth, it will go away when the drug is discontinued. Brushing the tongue will temporarily remove the black. The stool may appear black as well.

Misoprostol is intended to be taken along with aspirin or a nonsteroidal antiinflammatory drug (NSAID). It should be taken for the duration of the NSAID therapy.

Sucralfate should be taken four times daily on an empty stomach. Antacids should be taken within one-half hour before or after sucralfate.

Educating the Patient and Family about Miscellaneous Drugs That Affect the Stomach

Following are key points about miscellaneous drugs that the patient and family members should know:

- Misoprostol: Take this drug four times per day with meals and at bedtime. Continue to take the NSAID while taking misoprostol. Take it with meals to decrease the severity of diarrhea. Taking antacids before or after misoprostol may decrease the pain. Avoid magnesium-containing antacids because of the risk of increasing the diarrhea.
- Misoprostol may cause spontaneous abortion. Women of childbearing age must use a reliable contraceptive while taking this drug. If pregnancy is suspected, then discontinue use and notify your health care provider. Report severe menstrual pain, bleeding, or spotting.
- Sucralfate: Take on an empty stomach 1 hour before meals. Antacids may be taken for pain but not within 30 minutes before or after sucralfate. Your sucralfate dosage will continue for 4 to 8 weeks. Keep all follow-up appointments with your health care provider.

MEDICINE

FACT CHECK

28-12   What are the contraindications of misoprostol?

COMPLEMENTARY & ALTERNATIVE

MEDICINE

Ginger

Ginger is a medicinal herb derived from the root of the ginger plant. Ginger is usually taken to reduce nausea, vomiting, and indigestion. Clinical studies suggest that ginger is effective in preventing the nausea associated with motion sickness, seasickness, and anesthesia.

Ginger is not recommended for morning sickness associated with pregnancy or for patients with gallstones or hypertension. Small amounts present in food preparation are generally regarded as safe. Further, it is suggested that medicinal use of ginger should cease 2 to 3 weeks before surgery to reduce the risk of bleeding. The only known side effects of ginger are heartburn and heightened taste sensitivity.

COMPLEMENTARY & ALTERNATIVE

MEDICINE

Chamomile

Chamomile reduces flatulence and diarrhea caused by a nervous stomach and reduces stomach upset.

It is available in pill, liquid, and tea formulations. When used as a tea, chamomile appears to produce an antispasmodic effect on the smooth muscle of the GI tract and to protect against the development of stomach ulcers. Although the herb is generally safe and nontoxic, the tea is prepared from the pollen-filled flower heads and has resulted in mild symptoms of contact dermatitis to severe anaphylactic reactions in individuals hypersensitive to ragweed, asters, and chrysanthemums.

Chapter Review

KEY POINTS

- Antacids neutralize or reduce the acidity of stomach and duodenal contents by combining with hydrochloric acid and producing salt and water. They are used in the treatment of hyperacidity, such as heartburn, gastroesophageal reflux, sour stomach, acid indigestion, and in the medical treatment of peptic ulcer.
- Anticholinergics reduce gastric motility and decrease the amount of acid secreted by the stomach. Specific anticholinergic drugs are occasionally used in the medical treatment of peptic ulcer. Dry mouth, blurred vision, urinary hesitancy, urinary retention, nausea, vomiting, palpitations, and headache are some of the adverse reactions that may occur.
- Gastrointestinal stimulants increase the strength of the spontaneous movement of the upper GI tract. Metoclopramide is used in the treatment of symptomatic GERD and gastric stasis in patients with diabetes. Dexpanthenol may be given immediately after major abdominal surgery to reduce the risk of paralytic ileus.
- Histamine H_2 antagonists inhibit the action of histamine at histamine H_2 receptor cells of the stomach, which then reduces the secretion of gastric acid and reduces total pepsin output. The decrease in acid allows the ulcerated areas to heal. These drugs are used mainly to treat gastric and duodenal ulcers, gastric hypersecretory conditions, and GERD.
- Antiflatulents are used for the relief of painful symptoms of excess gas in the digestive tract. These drugs are useful as

adjunctive treatment of any condition in which gas retention may be a problem. Simethicone (Mylicon) and charcoal are both antiflatulents. Simethicone has a defoaming action that disperses and prevents the formation of mucus-surrounded gas pockets in the intestine. Charcoal is an absorbent that reduces the amount of intestinal gas.
- The digestive enzymes pancreatin and pancrelipase, which are manufactured and secreted by the pancreas, are responsible for the breakdown of fats and starches in food. Pancrelipase is available as an oral supplement and is prescribed as replacement therapy for those with pancreatic enzyme insufficiency.
- Emetics are used to cause vomiting to empty the stomach rapidly when an individual has accidentally or intentionally ingested a poison or drug overdose. Not all poison ingestions or drug overdoses are treated with emetics.
- Proton pump inhibitors suppress gastric acid secretion by blocking the last step of acid production and are used for treatment or symptomatic relief of various gastric disorders including gastric and duodenal ulcers, GERD, or pathological hypersecretory conditions.
- Proton pump inhibitors are particularly important in the treatment of *H. pylori*, which has been implicated as a cause of a type of chronic gastritis and most cases of peptic and duodenal ulcers. These drugs are often used in combination therapy for the treatment of *H. pylori* in patients with duodenal ulcers.
- Miscellaneous GI tract drugs include bismuth subsalicylate, misoprostol, and sucralfate. Bismuth disrupts the integrity of the bacterial cell wall. It is used in combination

with other drugs to treat gastric and duodenal ulcers caused by *H. pylori* bacteria.

- Misoprostol (Cytotec) inhibits gastric acid secretion and increases the protective property of the mucosal lining of the GI tract by increasing the production of mucus by the lining of the tract. It is used to prevent gastric ulcers in those taking aspirin or nonsteroidal anti-inflammatory drugs in high doses for a prolonged time.
- Sucralfate (Carafate) exerts a local action on the lining of the stomach, forming a protective layer over a duodenal ulcer, thus aiding in healing of the ulcer. It is used in the treatment of duodenal ulcer.

CRITICAL THINKING CASE STUDIES

CASE 1

Treating Heartburn

Mr. Gee has been experiencing frequent heartburn, especially after eating foods that are spicy or greasy. He asks you about over-the-counter products that are available to treat heartburn.

1. Which of the following is a product that is available over the counter for the treatment of heartburn?
   a. Antacids
   b. H2 antagonists
   c. Proton pump inhibitors
   d. All of the above
2. Mr. Gee decides to begin with an antacid. He notices that some contain only one active ingredient, while others contain two or more. He asks about the advantages of taking a product with two active ingredients. What should you tell him?
3. How should Mr. Gee take the antacid?
   a. Once daily at bedtime
   b. Immediately before eating the spicy or greasy food
   c. Between meals and at bedtime
   d. None of the above
4. Mr. Gee mentions that he has also been experiencing gas. What are some drugs that are commonly used to relieve gas?

CASE 2

Triple Therapy for *H. pylori*

Mr. Tim has been diagnosed with *H. pylori*. His physician has recommended that he begin a triple therapy treatment.

1. Which of the following would NOT be part of a triple therapy?
   a. Clarithromycin
   b. PPI
   c. Amoxicillin
   d. H2 antagonist
2. How long will Mr. Tim likely have to take the therapy?
   a. 5 days
   b. 7 days
   c. 10 to 14 days
   d. 4 to 6 weeks
3. Mr. Tim is particularly curious about the proton pump inhibitor and wants to know how it works. What would you tell him?

Review Questions

MULTIPLE CHOICE

1. Oral metoclopramide should be taken
   a. during early morning
   b. at bedtime
   c. 30 minutes before each meal
   d. 30 minutes after each meal
2. Histamine H_2 antagonists are used for all of the following EXCEPT
   a. gastric and duodenal ulcers
   b. paralytic ileus
   c. gastric hypersecretory conditions
   d. acute upper GI bleeding in critically ill patients
3. When an anticholinergic drug is prescribed for the treatment of a peptic ulcer, which of the following adverse reactions may occur?
   a. Dry mouth, urinary retention
   b. Edema, tachycardia
   c. Weight gain, increased respiratory rate
   d. Diarrhea, anorexia
4. The absorption of oral iron preparations is decreased when administered concurrently with
   a. emetics
   b. antacids
   c. digestive enzymes
   d. none of the above
5. Which drug is most likely prescribed for treatment of a patient experiencing erosive esophagitis?
   a. esomeprazole
   b. ipecac
   c. metoclopramide
   d. simethicone
6. Which of the following drugs is pregnancy category X and should not be taken by a pregnant woman?
   a. famotidine
   b. dexpanthenol
   c. sucralfate
   d. misoprostol

MATCHING

Match each drug to its correct category.

_____ 7. esomeprazole	a. Antiflatulent
_____ 8. calcium carbonate	b. Digestive enzyme
_____ 9. hyoscyamine	c. Emetic
_____ 10. dexpanthenol	d. Antacid
_____ 11. ranitidine	e. H_2 antagonist
_____ 12. simethicone	f. Proton pump inhibitor
_____ 13. pancrelipase	g. Anticholinergic
_____ 14. ipecac	h. GI stimulant

Match each drug's generic name to its brand name.

_____ 15. lansoprazole	a. Pepcid
_____ 16. dicyclomine	b. Creon
_____ 17. metoclopramide	c. Protonix
_____ 18. famotidine	d. Mylanta Gas
_____ 19. pancrelipase	e. Axid
_____ 20. simethicone	f. Prevacid
_____ 21. nizatidine	g. Bentyl
_____ 22. pantoprazole	h. Reglan

TRUE OR FALSE

_____ 23. Cimetidine is the H$_2$ antagonist that causes the most drug interactions.

_____ 24. The enzyme pancreatin is administered intravenously.

_____ 25. Propantheline is used to treat *H. pylori* in patients with duodenal ulcers.

_____ 26. Emetics are always administered to patients who overdose on drugs.

_____ 27. To treat calcium deficiency, a patient with menopausal osteoporosis may take the antacid calcium carbonate.

_____ 28. Common adverse reactions that occur with proton pump inhibitors include headache, diarrhea, and abdominal pain.

FILL IN THE BLANKS

29. When a(n) _____ is administered, there is a danger that the patient may aspirate the stomach contents because of vomiting.

30. _____ is a common adverse reaction of aluminum hydroxide gel.

31. Concurrent use of cimetidine and digoxin may _____ serum digoxin levels.

32. A patient experiencing paralytic ileus would likely be prescribed _____ for this condition.

33. Salicylate toxicity may occur if a patient is taking aspirin and _____ _____, a drug used to treat nausea, diarrhea, indigestion, and heartburn.

34. _____ _____ are contraindicated in patients with hypersensitivity to hog or cow proteins.

SHORT ANSWERS

35. Why are histamine H2 antagonists used cautiously in older adults?

36. Which drugs have a decreased pharmacological effect when administered with an antacid?

37. What conditions or diseases may cause pancreatic enzyme insufficiency?

38. What is misoprostol used to treat?

39. When is the antiflatulent simethicone administered?

40. When are emetics contraindicated?

Web Activities

1. Go to the Centers for Disease Control and Prevention Web site (www.cdc.gov) and follow the links through "Health Topics A–Z" to look for information about peptic ulcers. What is *H. pylori*, and what percentage of the people in the world are thought to be infected? How does *H. pylori* increase the risk of developing peptic ulcer disease?

2. Go to the Mayo Clinic Web site (www.mayoclinic. com) and conduct a search for GERD. What is GERD? What are some lifestyle changes and home remedies for treating GERD?

SUMMARY DRUG TABLE Drugs That Affect the Stomach and Pancreas (left, generic; right, trade)

Comprehensive Summary Drug Tables, including uses, adverses effects, dosages, and pregnancy classifications, are provided on the companion website, http://thePoint.lww.com/PharmacologyHP2e

Antacids

aluminum hydroxide *a-loo'-mi-num*	Alternagel, *generic*
calcium carbonate *kal'-see-um*	Alka-Mints, Cal-Gest, Maalox, Antacid Barrier Maximum Strength, Maalox Children's, Maalox Quick Dissolve, Pepto-Bismol Children's, Rolaids Extra strength, Tums, Tums E-X, Tums Ultra, *generic*
magnesia (magnesium hydroxide) *mag-nee'-zee-ah*	Phillips' Milk of Magnesia, Phillips' Chewable, Pedia-Lax, Dulcolax, *generic*
magnesium oxide *mag-nee'-zee-um*	Mag-200, Mag-Ox 400, Maox 420, Mag-G, Magonate, Magtrate, Maginex, Slow-Mag, Mag-Tab SR, Uro-Mag, Mag-Caps, Magonate Natal, MagonateMaginex, DS, *generic*
sodium bicarbonate *sow'-dee-um*	*generic*

Antiflatulents

alpha-D-galactosidase	Beano, Gas-X Prevention
charcoal *char'-kole*	Charcoal Plus DS, CharcoCaps, *generic*
simethicone *sigh-meth'-ih-kohn*	Alka-Seltzer Anti-Gas, Bicarsim, Bicarsim Forte, Gas-X, Gas-X Children's, Gas-X Extra-Strength, Gas-X Infant Drops, Gas-X Ultra Strength, Little Tummys Gas Relief, Mylanta Gas, Mylanta Gas Relief Maximum Strength, Mylicon, Mylicon Infants Gas Relief, Phazyme, *generic*

Histamine H² Antagonists

cimetidine *sye-met'-i-deen*	Tagamet HB (OTC), *generic*
famotidine *fa-moe'-ti-deen*	Pepcid, Pepcid AC (OTC), *generic*
nizatidine *ni-za'-ti-deen*	Axid, Axid AR (OTC), *generic*
ranitidine *ra-nye'-te-deen*	Zantac, Zantac 150 Maximum Strength (OTC), Zantac 75 (OTC), *generic*

Proton Pump Inhibitors

deslansoprazole	Dexilant
esomeprazole *ess-oh-me'-pra-zol*	Nexium, Nexium I.V.
lansoprazole *lan-soe'-pra-zole*	Prevacid, Prevacid 24 HR (OTC), Prevacid SoluTab, *generic*
omeprazole *oh-me'-pra-zol*	Prilosec, Prilosec OTC, *generic*

pantoprazole sodium *pan-to'-pray-zol*	Protonix, *generic*
rabeprazole sodium *rah-beh'-pray-zol*	Aciphex

Combination PPI

omeprazole/sodium bicarbonate *oh-me'-pra-zol*	Zegerid, Zegerid OTC

Anticholinergics

glycopyrrolate *gly-ko-pie'-roll-ate*	Cuvposa, Robinul, Robinul Forte, *generic*
hyoscyamine sulfate *hi'-o-si-ah-meen*	Anaspaz, HyoMax, HyoMax-DT, HyoMax-FT, HyoMax-SL, HyoMax-SR, Levbid, Levsin, Levinsin/SL, NuLev, Symax, Symax Duotab, Symax FasTabs, Symax-SI, Symax-SR, *generic*
mepenzolate bromide *me-pin-zo'-late*	Cantil
methscopolamine bromide *meth-sco-pol'-a-meen*	Pamine Pamine Forte, Pamine FQ
propantheline bromide *proe-pan'-the-leen*	*generic*
dexpanthenol *dex-pan'-the-nole*	*generic*

Gastrointestinal Stimulants

metoclopramide *met-oh-kloe-pra'-mide*	Metozolv ODT, Reglan, *generic*

Digestive Enzymes

pancrelipase *pan-kre-li'-pase*	Creon, Pancrelipase, Zenpep, Dygase, Lipram, Pancreaze, Pancrecarb, Ultrase, Viokase

Emetics

ipecac syrup *ip'-e-kak*	*generic*
bismuth subsalicylate *biz'-muth*	B.F.I, Devrom, Kaopectate, Kaopectate Extra-Strength, Kola-Pectin DS, Pepto-Bismol, Pepto-Bismol Maximum Strength, *generic*
misoprostol *mye-soe-prost'-ole*	Cytotec, *generic*
sucralfate *soo-kral'-fate*	Carafate, *generic*

29

Drugs That Affect the Gallbladder and Intestines

KEY TERMS

constipation—a condition where bowel movements are infrequent or incomplete

Crohn disease—chronic enteritis in the terminal ileum; symptoms include fever, diarrhea, cramping, abdominal pain, and weight loss

thePOINT RESOURCES

- Comprehensive Summary Drug Tables
- Animation: General Digestion
- Lippincott's Interactive Tutorials: Drugs Affecting the Gastrointestinal System
- Interactive Practice and Review
- Monographs of Most Commonly Prescribed Drugs

Chapter 28 discussed drugs that affect the stomach and pancreas. This chapter continues the discussion of drugs that affect the gastrointestinal (GI) tract, with coverage of drugs that affect the lower part of the GI system, specifically the gallbladder and intestines.

The drugs presented in this chapter include gallstone-solubilizing drugs, antidiarrheals, laxatives, and miscellaneous drugs. Some of the more common preparations are listed in the Summary Drug Table: Drugs That Affect the Gallbladder and Intestines.

Gallstone-Solubilizing Drugs

Actions of Gallstone-Solubilizing Drugs

Gallstone-solubilizing (gallstone-dissolving) drugs, such as ursodiol (Actigall) and chenodiol (Chenodal), suppress the manufacture of cholesterol and cholic acid by the liver. This may ultimately result in a decrease in the size of radiolucent gallstones. Figure 29-1 displays common sites of gallstones.

Uses of Gallstone-Solubilizing Drugs

These drugs are used in the nonsurgical treatment of radiolucent gallstones. They are not effective for all types of gallstones and require many months of use to produce results. Because of the potential toxic effects associated with long-term use, these drugs are recommended only for carefully selected and closely monitored patients.

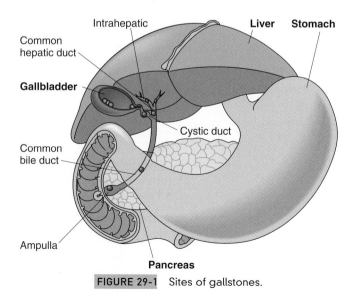

FIGURE 29-1 Sites of gallstones.

Adverse Reactions of Gallstone-Solubilizing Drugs

Diarrhea, cramps, nausea, and vomiting are common adverse drug reactions with these drugs. A reduction in the dose may reduce or eliminate these problems. Prolonged use of these drugs may result in hepatotoxicity (toxic to the liver).

Contraindications, Precautions, and Interactions of Gallstone-Solubilizing Drugs

- Ursodiol and chenodiol are used cautiously in patients with a known hypersensitivity to them or to bile salts and in patients with liver impairment, calcified stones, radiopaque stones or radiolucent bile pigment stones, severe acute cholecystitis, biliary obstruction, or gallstone pancreatitis.
- Ursodiol is used cautiously during lactation.
- Absorption of ursodiol is decreased if the agent is taken with bile acid–sequestering drugs or aluminum-containing antacids.
- Clofibrate, estrogens, and oral contraceptives increase hepatic cholesterol secretion, encourage cholesterol gallstone formation, and may counteract the effectiveness of ursodiol.
- Chenodiol is a pregnancy category X drug. It is not known if chenodiol is excreted in breast milk; therefore, it should be used cautiously.
- Chenodiol absorption is reduced if it is taken with aluminum-based antacids and bile acid sequestrants.
- Chenodiol effectiveness may be decreased when taken with clofibrate and oral contraceptives.
- Warfarin when taken with chenodiol may result in a prolonged prothrombin time and possible hemorrhage. The warfarin dose may need to be adjusted or the chenodiol discontinued.

Patient Management Issues with Gallstone-Solubilizing Drugs

Since these drugs are potentially hepatotoxic, it is very important that the patient have routine liver function test performed.

Educating the Patient and Family about Gallstone-Solubilizing Drugs

Following are key points about gallstone-solubilizing drugs the patient and family members should know:

- Periodic laboratory tests (liver function studies) and ultrasound or radiologic examinations of the gallbladder may be scheduled by your health care provider.
- If you experience diarrhea, then contact your health care provider. If symptoms of gallbladder disease (pain, nausea,

or vomiting) occur, then immediately contact your health care provider.

- Never take these drugs with aluminum-containing antacids. If you need an antacid, then take it 2 to 3 hours after ursodiol or chenodiol.

Antidiarrheals

Actions of Antidiarrheals

Antidiarrheals decrease intestinal peristalsis, which is usually increased in a patient with **diarrhea.** Examples of these drugs include difenoxin with atropine (Motofen), diphenoxylate with atropine (Lomotil), and loperamide (Imodium). Motofen is a schedule IV drug, Lomotil is a schedule V drug, and Imodium is not a controlled substance and is available as both a prescription and an over-the-counter drug.

Uses of Antidiarrheals

Antidiarrheals are used in the treatment of diarrhea.

Adverse Reactions of Antidiarrheals

Diphenoxylate use may result in anorexia, nausea, vomiting, constipation, rash, dizziness, drowsiness, sedation, euphoria, and headache. This is a narcotic-related drug that has no analgesic activity but has sedative and euphoric effects and a potential for drug dependence. To discourage abuse, it is combined with atropine (an anticholinergic or cholinergic blocking drug), which causes dry mouth and other mild adverse reactions. Loperamide is not a narcotic-related drug, and minimal adverse reactions are associated with its use. Occasionally, abdominal discomfort, pain, and distention occur, but these symptoms also occur with severe diarrhea and are difficult to distinguish from an adverse drug reaction.

Contraindications, Precautions, and Interactions of Antidiarrheals

- These drugs are contraindicated in patients whose diarrhea is associated with organisms that can harm the intestinal mucosa (*Escherichia coli*, *Salmonella*, *Shigella*) and in patients with pseudomembranous colitis, abdominal pain of unknown origin, or obstructive jaundice.
- Antidiarrheals are used cautiously in patients with severe liver disease or inflammatory bowel disease.
- Antidiarrheals should be used cautiously during lactation.
- Antidiarrheals cause an additive central nervous system depression when administered with alcohol, antihistamines, narcotics, and sedatives or hypnotics.
- The patient has additive cholinergic effects when they are administered with other drugs having anticholinergic activity, such as antidepressants or antihistamines.
- Concurrent use of an antidiarrheal with a monoamine oxidase inhibitor increases the risk of a hypertensive crisis.

Patient Management Issues with Antidiarrheals

The health care provider may request these drugs to be given after each loose bowel movement. Each bowel movement is inspected before a decision is made to administer the drug.

Drowsiness or dizziness may occur, and the patient may need help walking and with self-care activities. For chronic diarrhea, the patient is encouraged to drink extra fluids. Fluids such as weak tea, water, bouillon, or a commercial electrolyte preparation may be used. Fluid intake and output should be closely monitored. In some instances, the health care provider may prescribe an oral electrolyte supplement to replace electrolytes lost by frequent loose stools. For perianal irritation caused by loose stools, the area may be cleaned with mild soap and water after each bowel movement, dried with a soft cloth, and an emollient applied, such as petrolatum.

Educating the Patient and Family about Antidiarrheals

Following are key points about antidiarrheals that the patient and family members should know:

- Do not exceed the recommended dosage.
- The drug may cause drowsiness. Be cautious when you are driving or performing other hazardous tasks.

- Do not drink alcohol or use other central nervous system depressants (tranquilizers, sleeping pills) and other non-prescription drugs unless use has been approved by your health care provider.
- Notify your health care provider if diarrhea persists or becomes more severe.

Laxatives

Actions of Laxatives

There are various types of laxatives (see the Summary Drug Table: Drugs That Affect the Gallbladder and Intestines). The action of each laxative is somewhat different, but they produce the same result: the relief of **constipation** (Key Concepts 29-1).

- **Bulk-producing laxatives** are not digested by the body and therefore add bulk and water to the contents of the intestines. The added bulk in the intestines stimulates peristalsis, moves the products of digestion through the intestine, and encourages evacuation of the stool. Examples of bulk-forming laxatives are psyllium (Metamucil) and polycarbophil (FiberCon). These laxatives have an onset of action within 12 to 24 hours but may take up to 3 days.
- **Emollient laxatives** lubricate the intestinal walls and soften the stool, thereby enhancing passage of fecal material. Mineral oil is an emollient laxative. These laxatives have an onset of action within 6 to 8 hours.
- **Fecal softeners** promote water retention in the fecal mass and soften the stool. One difference between emollient laxatives and fecal softeners is that the emollient laxatives do not promote the retention of water in the stool. Examples of fecal softeners include docusate sodium (Colace) and docusate calcium (Kaopectate Stool Softener). The stool softeners have an onset of action between 24 and 72 hours.
- **Hyperosmolar drugs** dehydrate local tissues, which causes irritation and increased peristalsis, with consequent

KEY CONCEPTS

29-1 Understanding Constipation

Constipation is having fewer than three bowel movements per week. Stools are usually hard and dry. They are small in size and difficult to eliminate. Patients who are constipated may find it painful to have a bowel movement. Bowel habits vary from person to person. People often say they are constipated but do not match the definition described here.

evacuation of the fecal mass. Glycerin is a hyperosmolar drug. These laxatives have an onset of action within 24 to 48 hours when taken orally and within 15 minutes to an hour if used rectally.

- **Irritant or stimulant laxatives** increase peristalsis by direct action on the intestine. Senna (Senokot) is an irritant laxative. These laxatives have an onset of action within 6 to 12 hours if taken orally, within 15 to 60 minutes as a suppository, and within 3 to 5 minutes as an enema.
- **Saline laxatives** attract or pull water into the intestine, thereby increasing pressure in the intestine, followed by an increase in peristalsis. Magnesium hydroxide (Milk of Magnesia) is a saline laxative. These laxatives have an onset of action within 30 minutes to 3 hours.

Uses of Laxatives

A laxative is most often prescribed for short-term relief or prevention of constipation. Certain stimulant, emollient, and saline laxatives are used to empty the colon for rectal and bowel examinations. Fecal softeners or mineral oil are used to prevent constipation in patients who should not strain during defecation, such as after anorectal surgery or a myocardial infarction. Psyllium may be used in patients with irritable bowel syndrome and diverticular disease. Polycarbophil may be prescribed for constipation or diarrhea associated with irritable bowel syndrome and diverticulosis. Mineral oil is useful for the relief of fecal impaction. Docusate is used to prevent dry, hard stools.

Constipation may occur as an adverse drug reaction to some drugs, such as narcotic analgesics. When the patient has constipation as an adverse reaction to another drug, the health care provider may prescribe a stool softener or another laxative to prevent constipation during the drug therapy.

Adverse Reactions of Laxatives

Laxative use, especially high doses or prolonged use, can cause diarrhea and a loss of water and electrolytes. For some patients, this may be a serious adverse reaction. Laxatives may also cause abdominal pain or discomfort, nausea, vomiting, perianal irritation, flatulence, and cramps. Prolonged use of a laxative can result in serious electrolyte imbalances. Some laxatives, such as the irritant or stimulant laxatives, may result in a "laxative habit," that is, a dependency on a laxative to have a bowel movement. Some of these products contain tartrazine, which may cause allergic-type reactions (including bronchial asthma) in susceptible individuals.

Obstruction of the esophagus, stomach, small intestine, and colon may occur when bulk-forming laxatives are administered without adequate fluid intake or in patients with intestinal stenosis (narrowing).

Contraindications, Precautions, and Interactions of Laxatives

- Laxatives are contraindicated in patients with a known hypersensitivity and those with persistent abdominal pain, nausea, or vomiting of unknown cause or signs of acute appendicitis, fecal impaction, intestinal obstruction, or acute hepatitis.
- These drugs must be used only as directed because excessive or prolonged use may cause dependence.

- Magnesium hydroxide is used cautiously in patients with any degree of renal impairment.
- Laxatives are used cautiously in patients with rectal bleeding, and during lactation.
- Mineral oil may impair the GI tract absorption of fat-soluble vitamins (A, D, E, and K).
- Laxatives may reduce absorption of other drugs present in the GI tract by combining with them chemically or hastening their passage through the intestinal tract.
- When surfactants are administered with mineral oil, surfactants may increase mineral oil absorption.
- Milk, antacids, H$_2$ antagonists, and proton pump inhibitors should not be administered 1 to 2 hours before bisacodyl tablets, because the enteric coating may dissolve early (before reaching the intestinal tract), resulting in gastric lining irritation or dyspepsia and decreasing the laxative effect of the drug.

Patient Management Issues with Laxatives

Bulk-producing or fecal-softening laxatives are taken with a full glass of water or juice. A bulk-producing laxative is followed by an additional full glass of water. An increase in foods high in fiber is encouraged to prevent a repeat of the problem. Mineral oil is preferably given to the patient with an empty stomach in the evening. Laxatives in powder, flake, or granule form are mixed or stirred immediately before administration. The laxative may have an unpleasant or salty taste that may be disguised by chilling, adding to juice, or pouring over cracked ice.

If excessive bowel movements or severe prolonged diarrhea occur, or if the laxative is ineffective, then the health care provider should be notified.

Magnesium citrate can be chilled and mixed with lemon juice or other fruit juices to help mask the objectionable taste.

Educating the Patient and Family about Laxatives

Following are key points about laxatives that the patient and family members should know:

- Avoid long-term use of many of these products, except the bulk-forming laxatives and stool softeners, unless use of the product has been recommended by your health care provider. Long-term use may result in the "laxative habit," which is a dependence on a laxative to have a bowel movement. Constipation may also occur with overuse of these drugs. Read and follow the directions on the label.
- Avoid long-term use of mineral oil. Daily use of this product may interfere with the absorption of some vitamins (vitamins A, D, E, and K). Take it when your stomach is empty, preferably at bedtime.
- Do not use these products if you are having abdominal pain, nausea, or vomiting.
- Notify your health care provider if your constipation is not relieved or if rectal bleeding or other symptoms occur.
- To avoid constipation, drink plenty of fluids, get exercise, and eat foods high in bulk or roughage.
- Bulk-producing or fecal-softening laxatives: Drink a full

glass of water or juice, followed by more glasses of fluid in the next few hours.
- Bisacodyl (Dulcolax): Do not chew the tablets or take them within 1 hour of taking an antacid or milk.
- Senna: Your urine may turn pink-red, red-violet, red-brown, yellow-brown, or black when taking this drug.

FACT CHECK

29-5 What are the different types of laxatives?
29-6 How do laxatives affect other drugs present in the GI tract?

Bowel Evacuants

Actions of Bowel Evacuants

These oral solutions induce diarrhea and result in a rapid cleansing of the bowel.

Uses of Bowel Evacuants

Polyethylene glycol (PEG) solution is used to treat constipation. Polyethylene glycol with electrolytes is used as a bowel cleansing prior to a GI exam, such as a colonoscopy.

Adverse Reactions of Bowel Evacuants

The most common adverse reactions associated with the bowel evacuants are nausea, abdominal fullness, and bloating.

Contraindications, Precautions, and Interactions of Bowel Evacuants

- Polyethylene glycol is contraindicated in patients known to be allergic to PEG.
- Bowel evacuants should not be used if the patient has a known or suspected GI obstruction, gastric retention, bowel perforation, toxic colitis, megacolon, or ileus.
- These drugs should be used with caution in patients with ulcerative colitis.
- It is possible for patients who are unconscious or semiconscious to experience regurgitation or aspiration during use.
- Any medications taken within 1 hour of initiating bowel evacuant therapy may be flushed from the GI tract.

Patient Management Issues with Bowel Evacuants

If the adverse reactions become severe, patients should contact their health care provider. The bowel prep should be performed exactly as prescribed. Failure to do so could result in the procedure being rescheduled. Prolonged, frequent, or excessive use may result in an electrolyte balance and "laxative habit."

Educating the Patient and Family about Bowel Evacuants

Following are key points about bowel evacuants that the patient and family members should know.

- Patients should be educated about good defecatory habits.
- Patients should incorporate diet and lifestyle changes to prevent constipation, including eating a high fiber diet, drinking plenty of fluids, and exercising regularly.
- Polyethylene glycol should be dissolved in 8 ounces of water.
- It may take 2 to 4 days before PEG produces a bowel movement.

FACT CHECK

29-7 What are uses of the bowel evacuants?

Miscellaneous Drugs

Actions of Miscellaneous Drugs

Miscellaneous GI tract drugs include balsalazide, infliximab, mesalamine, olsalazine, sulfasalazine, lubiprostone, and orlistat.

Mesalamine (Asacol), balsalazide (Colazal), olsalazine (Dipentum), and sulfasalazine (Azulfidine) exert a topical anti-inflammatory effect in the bowel. The exact mechanism of action of these drugs is unknown. Infliximab neutralizes the biological activity of tumor necrosis factor-alpha (TNFalpha). In **Crohn disease,** it decreases the infiltration of inflammatory cell and TNFalpha production in the areas of the intestine that are inflamed. Lubiprostone (Amitiza) increases intestinal motility by acting on the chloride channel activator which increases chloride-rich intestinal fluid secretion. Orlistat inhibits lipase in the stomach and small intestine, which prevents the breakdown of dietary fat. The undigested triglycerides are not absorbed but instead pass through the intestines.

Dicyclomine is an anticholinergic that acts on the cholinergic receptors on the smooth muscle in the GI tract and slows GI motility.

Uses of Miscellaneous Drugs

Mesalamine is used in the treatment of chronic inflammatory bowel disease. Olsalazine is used in the treatment of **ulcerative colitis** (Fig. 29-2) in those allergic to sulfasalazine. Sulfasalazine is used in the treatment of Crohn disease and ulcerative colitis. Balsalazide is used in the treatment of mild to moderate ulcerative colitis. Lubiprostone is used to treat chronic idiopathic constipation and irritable bowel syndrome with constipation. Orlistat is used for obesity management. Infliximab is used for a variety of GI disorders including Crohn disease and ulcerative colitis. Dicyclomine is used for irritable bowel syndrome.

Adverse Reactions of Miscellaneous Drugs

Oral administration of balsalazide, olsalazine, and sulfasalazine may cause abdominal pain, nausea, headache, and diarrhea. Oral administration of mesalamine may cause headache, abdominal cramps, nausea, tiredness, weakness, malaise, and fatigue. Sulfasalazine is a sulfonamide with adverse reactions that are the same as for the sulfonamide drugs (see Chapter 35). The adverse reactions associated with rectal administration are less than those with oral administration, but headache, abdominal discomfort, flu-like syndrome, and weakness may still occur. Lubiprostone

causes similar adverse reactions to the other miscellaneous drugs; they include headache, diarrhea, abdominal pain, and nausea. Since orlistat prevents the absorption of intestinal fat, the adverse reactions are related to the passage of the fat through the intestine. Adverse reactions of orlistat include fatty or oily stools, fecal incontinence, fecal urgency, flatus (gas) with discharge, increased defecation, oily evacuation, and oily spotting. Infliximab may cause myalgia, fever, and increased susceptibility to infections. Since it is injected, it may also cause infusion-site reactions. Dicyclomine causes adverse reactions similar to the other anticholinergics discussed in Chapter 14. These adverse reactions include dry mouth, dizziness, and blurred vision.

Contraindications, Precautions, and Interactions of Miscellaneous Drugs

- The miscellaneous GI tract drugs are given with caution to patients with a known hypersensitivity.
- In addition, mesalamine, balsalazide, olsalazine, and sulfasalazine are contraindicated in patients who have hypersensitivity to the sulfonamides and salicylates or intestinal obstruction, and in children younger than 2 years.
- There is a possible cross-sensitivity of mesalamine, olsalazine, and sulfasalazine with furosemide, sulfonylurea antidiabetic drugs, and carbonic anhydrase inhibitors.
- Sulfasalazine may increase the risk of toxicity of oral hypoglycemic drugs, zidovudine, methotrexate, and phenytoin. There is also an increased risk of crystalluria (the excretion of crystalline materials in the urine) when sulfasalazine is administered with methenamine. A decrease in the absorption of iron and folic acid may occur when these agents are administered with sulfasalazine.
- Patients who are using infliximab should not receive live vaccines during infliximab therapy.
- Orlistat will interfere with the body's absorption of fat-soluble vitamins (A, D, E, and K). Patients should take a multivitamin daily, 2 hours before or after orlistat.
- Lubiprostone is contraindicated in patients with a known hypersensitivity to the drug, mechanical GI obstruction, and severe diarrhea.
- Lubiprostone should be used with caution in patients with moderate to severe hepatic disease.
- Dicyclomine should be used with caution in hot or humid environments. It can cause heat prostration because it decreases the sweating mechanism.
- Dicyclomine is contraindicated in patients with ulcerative colitis, myasthenia gravis, and glaucoma and in those with a GI or urinary obstruction.
- Dicyclomine should be used with caution in patients with an existing cardiovascular disease.

Patient Management Issues with Miscellaneous Drugs

The dosage forms should be swallowed whole, unless they are capsules that can be opened and sprinkled on food. If the patient's condition does not improve or adverse reactions worsen, the health care provider should be contacted.

Sulfasalazine may discolor the urine to an orange-yellow color. This is normal and will go away when the drug is discontinued. Lubiprostone may cause dyspnea within an hour of the first dose. The symptoms should resolve but may reappear

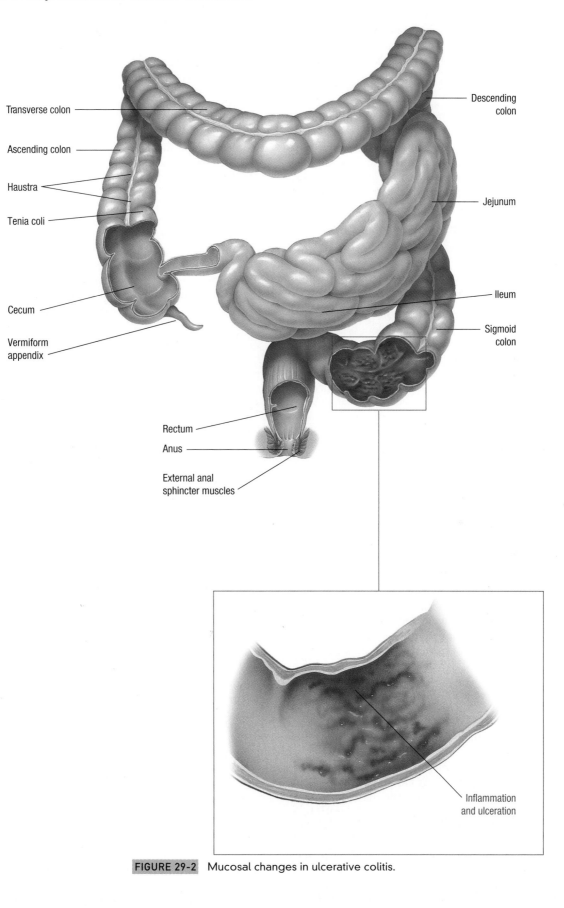

FIGURE 29-2 Mucosal changes in ulcerative colitis.

with repeat dosing. If the symptoms do not resolve, the health care provider should be contacted. Patients taking infliximab who develop signs and symptoms of infection should seek medical attention immediately. Orlistat should be combined with a reduced-calorie and low-fat diet. Orlistat is only indicated for obese patients with a BMI of 30 kg/m^2 or more or 27 kg/m^2 in patients with other risk factors (diabetes, dyslipidemia).

Patients taking mesalamine should have regular blood tests to evaluate a complete blood count and liver function.

Dicyclomine may cause dry mouth. This can be resolved by sucking on hard candy or ice chips or using an artificial saliva product. It may also cause dry eyes, which can be resolved with lubricating drops or artificial tears.

Educating the Patient and Family about Miscellaneous Drugs

Following are key points about miscellaneous drugs that the patient and family members should know.

- Olsalazine: If you experience diarrhea, then contact your health care provider as soon as possible.
- Mesalamine: Swallow the tablets whole; do not chew them. Partially intact tablets may be found in the stool; if this occurs, you should notify your health care provider. To use the suppository, remove the foil wrapper and immediately insert the pointed end of the suppository into the rectum without using force. For the suspension form, instructions are included with the product. Shake well, remove the protective sheath from the applicator tip, and gently insert the tip into the rectum.

- Balsalazide: Swallow the capsules whole. The capsule may be opened and the contents sprinkled on soft food, such as applesauce, and taken without chewing.
- Infliximab: Patients and family members should be instructed on aseptic technique and how to properly reconstitute vials and deliver infusions if it will be done at home. Infusions should be administered over at least 2 hours.
- Sulfasalazine: Take after meals. The enteric-coated tablets should be swallowed whole. Urine may be discolored orange-yellow.
- Lubiprostone: The capsules should be taken twice daily with food and water.
- Orlistat: Orlistat should be taken one capsule with each main meal that contains fat, up to three times a day. It may be taken during the meal or up to 1 hour after the meal. Meals should not include more than 30% of calories from fat. Orlistat will interfere with the body's absorption of fat-soluble vitamins (A, D, E, and K). Patients should take a multivitamin daily.

FACT CHECK

29-8 Which of the miscellaneous drugs are used to treat ulcerative colitis?

29-9 Which of the miscellaneous drugs are used to treat chronic inflammatory bowel disease?

29-10 Orlistat interferes with the absorption of which vitamins?

Chapter Review

KEY POINTS

- Gallstone-solubilizing drugs are used in the nonsurgical treatment of radiolucent gallstones. They are not effective for all types of gallstones and require many months of use to produce results. Because of the potential toxic effects with long-term use, these drugs are recommended for only carefully selected and closely monitored patients.
- Antidiarrheals are used to treat diarrhea by decreasing intestinal peristalsis. Diphenoxylate is a narcotic-related drug. Loperamide is not a narcotic-related drug, and minimal adverse reactions are associated with its use. Antidiarrheal drugs are contraindicated in children younger than 2 years.
- A laxative is used primarily for the short-term relief or prevention of constipation. Certain stimulant, emollient, and saline laxatives are used to evacuate the colon for rectal and bowel examinations. The action of each laxative is somewhat different, but they produce the same result: the relief of constipation. Laxative use, especially high doses or use over a long time, can cause diarrhea and a loss of water and electrolytes. For some patients, this may be a serious adverse reaction.
- Bowel evacuants are used for constipation and bowel cleansing before a GI examination. PEG-ES (CoLyte,

GoLYTELY) is used to cleanse the colon prior to a GI exam. These solutions must be mixed and consumed using a specific schedule usually the day preceding the GI exam. Polyethylene glycol (MiraLAX) is used to treat constipation. Polyethylene glycol must be mixed with water prior to consumption.
- Miscellaneous GI tract drugs include balsalazide, mesalamine, olsalazine, sulfasalazine, infliximab, lubiprostone, and orlistat. Mesalamine (Asacol), balsalazide (Colazal), olsalazine (Dipentum), and sulfasalazine (Azulfidine) exert a topical anti-inflammatory effect in the bowel. The exact mechanism of action of these drugs is unknown.
- Balsalazide is used to treat ulcerative colitis. Mesalamine is used in the treatment of chronic inflammatory bowel disease. Olsalazine is used in the treatment of ulcerative colitis in those allergic to sulfasalazine. Sulfasalazine is used in the treatment of Crohn disease and ulcerative colitis.
- Lubiprostone (Amitiza) is an infusion used to treat chronic idiopathic constipation and irritable bowel syndrome with constipation. It is administered via a 2-hour IV infusion.
- Orlistat is available by prescription (Xenical) and over the counter (Alli) for the management of obesity. Orlistat binds fat in the intestines and therefore has numerous

adverse reactions associated with the bound fat moving through the GI tract.

CRITICAL THINKING CASE STUDIES

CASE 1
Diarrhea

Mr. Eldridge developed diarrhea yesterday. He calls the clinic where you work and asks for a prescription. He is informed that Imodium A-D (loperamide) is available over the counter and he should purchase it.

1. He calls back and asks how to take the Imodium A-D. He cannot read the print on the box because it is too small. What should you tell him?
    a. Take two tablets (10 mg) now, then one tablet (5 mg) every 3 hours as needed.
    b. Take one tablet (5 mg) now, then one tablet four times daily as needed.
    c. Take two tablets (4 mg) now, then one tablet (2 mg) after each loose bowel movement.
    d. Take two tablets (4 mg) now, then two tablets every 3 hours as needed.
2. Which of the following is NOT an expected adverse reaction of loperamide?
    a. Abdominal pain
    b. Constipation
    c. Nausea
    d. Headache
3. Mr. Eldridge's 18-month-old granddaughter is visiting and has developed diarrhea as well. Can she take the liquid Imodium A-D?

CASE 2
Constipation

Ms. Tira, one of the regular patients at the clinic where you work, has come for her monthly visit. While there, she complains that she is constipated.

1. When you ask Ms. Tira to explain her symptoms, she states that she normally has a bowel movement every morning but didn't today. Is this constipation?
2. During your discussion, Ms. Tira states that she hasn't been as regular lately as in the past. Her diet and exercise regimens have changed because of her arthritis. Which of the following drugs, used routinely, would help to make her bowel movements more regular?
    a. Magnesium citrate
    b. Psyllium
    c. Mineral oil
    d. Glycerin
3. Ms. Tira is concerned that she needs to have a bowel movement today. How long will it take for a bulk-forming laxative to work?
    a. 8 hours (overnight)
    b. 12 hours
    c. 48 hours
    d. 72 hours

4. Ms. Tira states that her friend takes Carter's Little Pills every day and asks if that would be a better option because it will work faster. What should you tell her?

Review Questions

MULTIPLE CHOICE

1. Which of the following laxatives are used to prepare patients for rectal and bowel examinations?
    a. Stimulant laxatives
    b. Emollient laxatives
    c. Saline laxatives
    d. All of the above
2. Fecal softeners relieve constipation by
    a. stimulating the walls of the intestine
    b. promoting the retention of sodium in the fecal mass
    c. promoting water retention in the fecal mass
    d. lubricating the intestinal walls
3. When ursodiol is prescribed, the patient should be advised to
    a. avoid aluminum-containing antacids
    b. take the medication at bedtime
    c. wear sunglasses if light sensitivity occurs
    d. none of the above
4. Antidiarrheal drugs are administered
    a. hourly until diarrhea ceases
    b. after each loose bowel movement
    c. with food
    d. twice per day, in the morning and at bedtime

MATCHING

Match each medication with its correct classification.

_____ 5. loperamide	a. Bowel evacuant
_____ 6. ursodiol	b. Hyperosmotic laxative
_____ 7. magnesium citrate	c. Antidiarrheal
_____ 8. bisacodyl	d. Fecal softener/surfactant
_____ 9. psyllium	e. Bulk-forming laxative
_____ 10. mineral oil	f. Emollient
_____ 11. docusate	g. Saline laxative
_____ 12. glycerin	h. Irritant/stimulant laxative
_____ 13. polyethylene glycol	i. Gallstone-solubilizing agent

Match each drug's generic name with its correct brand name.

_____ 14. diphenoxylate/ atropine	a. Kondremul Plain
_____ 15. ursodiol	b. Azulfidine
_____ 16. magnesium hydroxide	c. Remicade
_____ 17. sennosides	d. Actigall
_____ 18. polycarbophil	e. Amitiza
_____ 19. mineral oil	f. Lomotil
_____ 20. docusate sodium	g. Phillips' Milk of Magnesia
_____ 21. infliximab	h. Colace
_____ 22. sulfasalazine	i. Senna Smooth
_____ 23. lubiprostone	j. FiberCon

TRUE OR FALSE

_____ 24. Gallstone-solubilizing drugs are used for non-surgical treatment of all types of gallstones.

_____ 25. You should instruct a patient taking mesalamine to swallow the tablet whole.

_____ 26. The antidiarrheal drug loperamide is not a narcotic-related drug.

_____ 27. A patient taking a laxative may experience constipation as an adverse drug reaction.

FILL IN THE BLANKS

28. _____ laxatives lubricate the intestinal walls and soften the stool.

29. A patient taking antidepressants or antihistamines may experience additive cholinergic effects when _____ are administered.

30. Stimulant laxatives increase _____ by acting directly on the intestine.

31. _____ is available as a suspension enema, rectal suppository, or tablet.

SHORT ANSWERS

32. Why is the antidiarrheal diphenoxylate combined with atropine?

33. What can occur with prolonged use of laxatives or use of high doses?

34. What are the most common adverse reactions associated with orlistat?

Web Activities

1. Go to the National Digestive Disease Information Clearinghouse Web site (digestive.niddk.nih.gov) and conduct a search on constipation. What are common causes of constipation?

2. On the same Web site, conduct a search on diarrhea. What is diarrhea and what are common causes of diarrhea?

SUMMARY DRUG TABLE DRUGS That Affect the Gallbladder and Intestines (left, generic; right, trade)

Comprehensive Summary Drug Tables, including uses, adverses effects, dosages, and pregnancy classifications, are provided on the companion website, http://thePoint.lww.com/PharmacologyHP2e

Gallstone-Solubilizing Agent	
chenodiol *kee-noe-dye'-ole*	Chenodal
ursodiol *ur-soe-dye'-ole*	Actigall, Urso 250, Urso Forte, *generic*

Antidiarrheals	
difenoxin HCl with atropine *dye-fen-ox'-in a'-troe-peen*	Motofen (CIV)
diphenoxylate HCl with atropine sulfate *di-fen-ox'-i'-late*	Logen, Lomanate, Lomotil, Lonox, *generic (CV)*
loperamide HCl *loe-per'-a-mide*	Imodium A-D (OTC), *generic (Rx and OTC)*

LAXATIVES	

Saline Laxatives	
magnesium citrate *mag-nee'-zhum sit'-rate*	*generic*
magnesium hydroxide *mag-nee'-zhum hye-droks'-ide*	Pedia-Lax, Phillips' Milk of Magnesia, Phillips' Milk of Magnesia Concentrated, *generic*
magnesium oxide *mag-nee'-zhum oks'-ide*	Phillips' Cramp-Free, Uro-Mag 140, Mag-Ox, *generic*
magnesium sulfate *mag-nee'-zhum sul'-fate*	*generic*

Irritant or Stimulant Laxatives	
sennosides *sen'-oh-sides*	Black Draught, Correctol Herbal Tea, Dr. Edwards' Olive Laxative, Evac-U-Gen, Ex-Lax, Ex-Lax Maximum Strength, Little Tummys Laxative, Medi-Lax, Perdiem Overnight Relief, Senna Smooth, SennaCon, Senna-Ex, Senno, Senexon Senna-Max, Senokot, Senokot XTRA
bisacodyl *bis-a-koe'-dill*	Bisac-Evac, Carter's Little Pills, Correctol, Dulcolax, Dulcolax Bowel-Prep Kit, Ex-Lax Ultra, Feen-A-mint, Fleet, *generic*

Bulk-Producing Laxatives	
psyllium *sill'-l-um*	Evac, Konsyl, Konsyl-D, Metamucil, Metamucil Fiber Singles, Metamucil MultiHealth Fiber, Metamucil Smooth Texture, Reguloid,
polycarbophil *pol-i-kar'-boe-fil*	Equalactin, FiberCon, FiberGen, Fiber-Lax, Konsyl Fiber

Emollients	
mineral oil	Kondremul Plain, *generic*

Fecal Softeners/Surfactants	
docusate sodium *dok'-yoo-sate*	Colace, Correctol Extra Gentle, Docusil, Docusoft-S, DocuSol Mini, DOK, Dulcolax Stool Softener, Enemeez Mini, Pedia-Lax, Phillips' Liqui-Gels, Phillips' Stool Softener, Sof-Lax, *generic*
docusate calcium *dok'-yoo-sate*	Kaopectate Stool Softener, *generic*

Hyperosmotic Agents	
glycerin *gli'-ser-in*	Fleet Liquid Glycerin Suppositories, Introl, Ora-Blend, Ora-Sweet, PCCA Sweet-SF, Pedia-Lax, Sani-Supp *generic*
lactulose *lak-tyoo-los*	Kristalose, *generic*

Bowel Evacuants	
polyethylene glycol-electrolyte solution (PEG-ES) *pol-e-eth-i-leen*	CoLyte, GoLYTELY, OCL, MoviPrep, NuLYTELY, TriLyte, GaviLyte, OCL, *generic*
polyethylene glycol (PEG) solution *pol-i-eth'-i-leen gly'-kol*	Dulcolax Balance, GaviLAX, GlycoLax, MiraLAX, *generic*

Miscellaneous	
balsalazide disodium *bal-sal'-a-zyde*	Colazal, *generic*
infliximab *in-flicks'-ih-mab*	Remicade
mesalamine *me-sal'-a-meen*	Apriso, Asacol, Asacol HD, Canasa, Lialda, Pentasa, Rowasa, SF Rowasa, *generic*
olsalazine sodium *ole-sal'-a-zeen*	Dipentum
sulfasalazine *sul-fa-sal'-a-zeen*	Azulfidine, Azulfidine EN-Tabs, *generic*
lubiprostone *loo-bi-pros'-tone*	Amitiza
orlistat *or'-li-stat*	Alli (OTC), Xenical (Rx)

Anticholinergics	
atropine sulfate *a'-troe-peen*	AtroPen, Isopto Atropine, Sal-Tropine, *generic*
dicyclomine HCl *dye-sye-klo'-meen*	Bentyl, *generic*

30

Antidiabetic Drugs

CHAPTER OBJECTIVES

On completion of this chapter, students will be able to:

1. Define the chapter's key terms.
2. Describe the differences between type 1 and type 2 diabetes and how they are treated.
3. Identify the signs and symptoms of type 1 diabetes.
4. Identify risk factors for type 2 diabetes.
5. List the various classifications of insulin preparations and explain the differences in onset, peak, and duration for each.
6. Identify drugs that are used to elevate glucose levels in patients experiencing hypoglycemia.
7. Compare and contrast the varied actions of the antidiabetic drugs.
8. Identify common adverse reactions for each drug category.
9. Discuss dosing parameters specific to each drug category with relation to timing and whether the drugs should be taken with or without food or meals.
10. Discuss important points to keep in mind when educating the patient or family members about the use of antidiabetic drugs.

KEY TERMS

diabetes mellitus—a chronic disorder characterized either by insufficient insulin production in the β-cells of the pancreas or by cellular resistance to insulin

diabetic ketoacidosis—a potentially life-threatening deficiency of insulin (hypoinsulinism), resulting in severe hyperglycemia and requiring prompt diagnosis and treatment

glucagon—a hormone produced by the α-cells of the pancreas that increases blood sugar by stimulating the conversion of glycogen to glucose in the liver

glucometer—a device used to monitor blood glucose levels

hyperglycemia—elevated blood glucose level

hypoglycemia—low blood glucose level

CHAPTER OVERVIEW

Drug classes covered in this chapter are:

- Insulin
- Antidiabetic drugs
- Glucose elevating agents

Drugs by classification are listed on page 310.

thePOINT RESOURCES

- Comprehensive Summary Drug Tables
- Animation: Diabetes
- Lippincott's Interactive Tutorials: Drugs Affecting the Endocrine System
- Interactive Practice and Review
- Monographs of Most Commonly Prescribed Drugs

insulin—a hormone produced by the pancreas that helps maintain blood glucose levels within normal limits
lipodystrophy—atrophy of subcutaneous fat
polydipsia—increased thirst
polyphagia—increased appetite

polyuria—increased urination
secondary failure—a gradual increase in blood sugar levels that can be caused by an increase in the severity of diabetes or a decreased response to a drug

nsulin, a hormone produced by the pancreas, acts to maintain blood glucose levels within normal limits. This is accomplished by the release of small amounts of insulin into the bloodstream throughout the day in response to changes in blood glucose levels. Insulin is essential for using glucose in cellular metabolism and for the metabolism of protein and fat (Fig. 30-1).

Diabetes mellitus is a complicated, chronic disorder characterized either by insufficient insulin production in the β-cells of the pancreas or by cellular resistance to insulin. Insulin insufficiency results in elevated blood glucose levels or hyperglycemia. Individuals with diabetes are at greater risk for a number of disorders, including myocardial infarction, cerebrovascular accident (stroke), blindness, kidney disease, and lower limb amputations.

Insulin and the oral antidiabetic drugs, along with diet and exercise, are the cornerstones of treatment for diabetes mellitus. They are used to prevent episodes of hyperglycemia and to normalize carbohydrate metabolism.
There are two major types of diabetes mellitus:

- Type 1 (Formerly known as insulin-dependent diabetes mellitus, juvenile diabetes, juvenile-onset diabetes, and brittle diabetes)
- Type 2 (Formerly known as non-insulin-dependent diabetes mellitus, maturity-onset diabetes, adult-onset diabetes, and stable diabetes)

Those with type 1 diabetes produce insulin in insufficient amounts and therefore must have insulin supplementation to survive. Type 1 diabetes usually has a rapid onset, occurs before the age of 20 years, produces more severe symptoms than type 2 diabetes, and is more difficult to control. Major symptoms of type 1 diabetes include hyperglycemia, **polydipsia** (increased thirst), **polyphagia** (increased appetite), **polyuria** (increased urination), and weight loss. Treatment of type 1 diabetes is particularly difficult because of the lack of insulin production by the pancreas. Treatment requires a strict regimen that typically includes a carefully calculated diet, planned physical activity, home glucose testing several times per day, and multiple daily insulin injections.

Approximately 90% to 95% of adults with diabetes have type 2. Those with type 2 either have a decreased production of insulin by the β-cells of the pancreas or have a decreased sensitivity of the cells to insulin, making the cells insulin resistant. Although type 2 diabetes may occur at any age, the disorder occurs most often after the age of 40 years. The onset of type 2 diabetes is usually insidious, and the symptoms are less severe than in type 1 diabetes mellitus. Because it tends to be more stable, it is easier to control than type 1 diabetes. Risk factors for type 2 diabetes include

- Obesity
- Older age
- Family history of diabetes
- History of gestational diabetes (diabetes that develops during pregnancy but disappears when pregnancy is over)
- Impaired glucose tolerance
- Minimal or no physical activity
- Race/ethnicity (more common in blacks, Hispanic/Latino Americans, American Indians, and some Asian Americans)

Obesity is thought to contribute to type 2 diabetes by placing additional stress on the pancreas, which makes it less able to respond and produce adequate insulin to meet the body's metabolic needs.

Many individuals with type 2 diabetes are able to control the disorder with diet, exercise, and antidiabetic drugs.

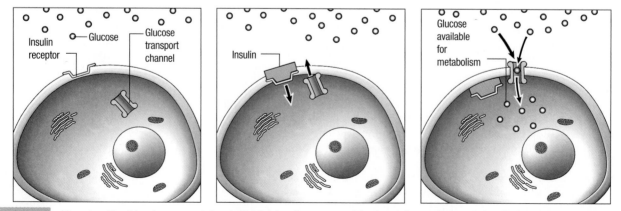

FIGURE 30-1　How insulin aids glucose uptake. A. Available glucose outside the cell membrane. B. Insulin binds with receptors on the cell membrane, activating glucose transport channels. C. Glucose enters the cell through the transport channels and is used for metabolism and energy production.

However, approximately 40% of those with type 2 diabetes do not have a good response to the antidiabetic drugs and require the addition of insulin to control the diabetes.

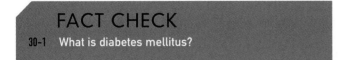

FACT CHECK

30-1 What is diabetes mellitus?

Insulin

Insulin is a hormone manufactured by the β-cells of the pancreas. It is the principal hormone required for the proper use of glucose (carbohydrate) by the body. Insulin also controls the storage and use of amino acids and fatty acids. Insulin lowers blood glucose levels by inhibiting liver glucose production.

Insulin was originally developed from purified extracts from beef and pork pancreas because it was biologically similar to human insulin. However, these animal-source insulins are no longer used today. Synthetic insulins, including human insulin or insulin analogs, have replaced them.

Human insulin is derived from a biosynthetic process using strains of *Escherichia coli* (a nonpathogenic colon bacteria). Insulin analogs, like insulin lispro and insulin aspart, are newer forms of human insulin made by using recombinant DNA technology and are structurally similar to human insulin.

Actions of Insulin

Insulin appears to activate a process that helps glucose molecules enter the cells of striated muscle and adipose tissue (see Fig. 30-1). Insulin also stimulates the synthesis of glycogen by the liver. In addition, insulin promotes protein synthesis and helps the body store fat by preventing its breakdown for energy.

Various insulin preparations have been developed with a more gradual onset and prolonged duration of effect. Insulin preparations are classified as rapid-acting, short-acting,

TABLE 30-1   Insulin Preparations

Types of Insulin	Trade Name	Activity		
		Onset (h)	Peak (h)	Duration (h)
Rapid-Acting Insulins insulin lispro (insulin analog) *in'-soo-lin lye'-spror*	Humalog (Rx), Humalog Mix 50/50, Humalog Mix 75/25	0.25	0.5–1.5	2–5
insulin aspart solution (insulin analog) *in'-soo-lin as'-part*	NovoLog (Rx)	0.25	1–3	3–5
insulin glulisine *in'-soo-lin gloo-lis'-een*	Apidra (Rx), Apidra OptiClik, Apidra SoloStar	0.3	1	1.5–2.5
Short-Acting Insulins insulin injection (regular) *in'-soo-lin*	Humulin R (OTC), Novolin R (OTC), Novolin R InnoLet, Novolin R PenFill	0.5–1	2–5	8–12
Intermediate-Acting Insulin isophane insulin suspension (NPH)	Humulin N Pen (OTC), Novolin N (OTC), Novolin N Innolet, Novolin N PenFill	1–1.5	4–12	Up to 24
Long-Acting Insulins insulin detemir	Levemir	1–2	6–8	Up to 24
insulin glargine solution *in'-soo-lin glar'-jeen*	Levemir FlexPen Lantus (Rx), Lantus OptiClik, Lantus SoloStar	1	None	Up to 24
Mixed Insulins 70% isophane insulin suspension (NPH) and 30% insulin injections (regular)	Humulin 70/30 (OTC), Novolin 70/30 (OTC)	0.5	1–3	8–12
50% isophane insulin suspension (NPH) and 30% insulin injection (regular)	Humulin 50/50	0.5	1–3	8–12
70% insulin aspart protamine suspension and 30% insulin aspart solution	Novolog 70/30 (Rx)	10–20 min	1–4	Up to 24
High-Potency Insulin insulin injection concentrated	Humulin R U-500 (Rx)	IV:15 min Subcutaneously: 0.5	IV:15–30 min Subcutaneously: 2.5–5	IV:30–60 min Subcutaneously: 8–12

TABLE 30-2   Hypoglycemia versus Hyperglycemia

Symptoms	Hypoglycemia (Insulin Reaction)	Hyperglycemia (Diabetic Coma, Ketoacidosis)
Onset	Sudden	Gradual (hours or days)
Blood glucose	<60 mg/dL	>200 mg/dL
Central nervous system	Fatigue, weakness, nervousness, agitation, confusion, headache, diplopia, convulsions, dizziness, unconsciousness	Drowsiness, dim vision
Respirations	Normal to rapid, shallow	Deep, rapid (air hunger)
Gastrointestinal	Hunger, nausea	Thirst, nausea, vomiting, abdominal pain, loss of appetite, excessive urination
Skin	Pale, moist, cool, diaphoretic	Dry, flushed, warm
Pulse	Normal or uncharacteristic	Rapid, weak
Miscellaneous	Numbness, tingling of the lips or tongue	Acetone breath

intermediate-acting, or long-acting. Table 30-1 gives information concerning the onset, peak, and duration of various insulins.

Uses of Insulin

Insulin is necessary for controlling type 1 diabetes that is caused by a marked decrease in the amount of insulin produced by the pancreas. Insulin is also used to control the more severe and complicated forms of type 2 diabetes. However, many patients can control type 2 diabetes with diet and exercise alone or with diet, exercise, and an antidiabetic drug (see later section). Insulin may also be used in the treatment of severe diabetic ketoacidosis (a type of metabolic acidosis caused by an accumulation of ketone bodies in the blood) or diabetic coma. Insulin is also used in combination with glucose to treat hypokalemia by shifting potassium from the blood into the cells.

FACT CHECK

30-2   What does insulin do in the body?
30-3   How are insulin preparations classified?

Adverse Reactions of Insulin

The two major adverse reactions seen with insulin administration are **hypoglycemia** (low blood glucose or sugar) and **hyperglycemia** (elevated blood glucose or sugar). The symptoms of hypoglycemia and hyperglycemia are listed in Table 30-2.

Hypoglycemia may occur when there is too much insulin in the bloodstream in relation to the available glucose (hyperinsulinism). Hypoglycemia may occur

- When the patient eats too little food
- When the insulin dose is incorrectly measured and is greater than that prescribed
- When the patient drastically increases physical activity

Hyperglycemia may occur if there is too little insulin in the bloodstream in relation to the available glucose (hypoinsulinism). Hyperglycemia may occur

- When the patient eats too much food
- When too little or no insulin is used
- When the patient experiences emotional stress, infection, surgery, pregnancy, or an acute illness

A patient can also become insulin resistant because of the development of antibodies against insulin.

Diabetic ketoacidosis, a severe form of hypoinsulinism, is described in Key Concepts 30-1.

Hypoglycemic Reactions

Close observation of a patient with diabetes is important, especially when diabetes is newly diagnosed, the insulin dosage is changed, or the patient is pregnant, has a medical illness or has had surgery, or fails to adhere to the prescribed diet.

KEY CONCEPTS

30-1   Understanding Diabetic Ketoacidosis

Diabetic ketoacidosis is a potentially life-threatening deficiency of insulin (hypoinsulinism), resulting in severe hyperglycemia. Dangerously high levels of glucose build up in the blood (hyperglycemia). The body, unable to use the glucose but needing energy, begins to break down fat for energy. As fats are broken down, the liver produces ketones. As more and more fat is used for energy, higher levels of ketones accumulate in the blood. This increase in ketones disrupts the acid–base balance within the body, leading to diabetic ketoacidosis. This condition is treated with fluids, correction of acidosis and hypotension, and low doses of regular insulin.

Episodes of hypoglycemia are corrected as soon as the symptoms are recognized.

Methods of ending a hypoglycemic reaction include taking one or more of the following:

- Orange juice or other fruit juice
- Hard candy or honey
- Commercial glucose products
- **Glucagon** by the subcutaneous, intramuscular, or intravenous route
- Glucose 10% or 50% via intravenous route

Use of any one or more of these methods for terminating a hypoglycemic reaction depends on the written order of the health care provider or hospital policy. Oral fluids or substances (such as candy) used to terminate a hypoglycemic reaction should never be given to a patient without intact swallowing and gag reflexes. Absence of these reflexes may result in aspiration of the oral fluid or substance into the lungs, which can result in extremely serious consequences and even death. If a patient's swallowing and gag reflexes are absent, or if the patient is unconscious, then glucose or glucagon is given by the parenteral route. Agents used to elevate glucose are included in the Summary Drug Table: Glucose Elevating Agents.

The health care provider should be notified of any hypoglycemic reaction, the substance and amount used to terminate the reaction, blood samples drawn (if any), the length of time required for the symptoms of hypoglycemia to disappear, and the current status of the patient. After a hypoglycemic reaction, the patient is closely observed for additional hypoglycemic reactions.

FACT CHECK

30-4   What are the two major adverse reactions of insulin administration?

30-5   If a patient is experiencing a hypoglycemic reaction, what should they do?

Contraindications, Precautions, and Interactions of Insulin

- Insulin is contraindicated in patients with hypersensitivity to any ingredient of the product and when a patient is hypoglycemic.
- Insulin is used cautiously in patients with liver or kidney disease.
- Insulin appears to inhibit milk production in lactating women and could interfere with breast-feeding.

Lactating women may require adjustment of their insulin dose and diet.

When certain drugs are administered with insulin, a decrease or increase in hypoglycemic effect can occur. Following are some drugs that decrease the hypoglycemic effect of insulin:

- AIDS antivirals
- Albuterol
- Contraceptives, oral
- Corticosteroids
- Diltiazem
- Diuretics
- Dobutamine
- Epinephrine
- Estrogens
- Lithium
- Morphine sulfate
- Niacin
- Phenothiazines
- Thyroid hormones

Following are some drugs that, when administered with insulin, may increase the hypoglycemic effect of insulin:

- Alcohol
- Angiotensin-converting enzyme inhibitors
- Antidiabetic drugs, oral
- β–Blocking drugs
- Calcium
- Clonidine
- Disopyramide
- Lithium
- Monoamine oxidase inhibitors (MAOIs)
- Salicylates
- Sulfonamides
- Tetracycline

Patient Management Issues with Insulin

The number of daily insulin injections, the dosage, times of administration, and diet and exercise require continual monitoring. Dosage adjustments may be necessary when changing types of insulin, particularly when changing from the single-peak to the more pure Humulin insulins.

The patient is assessed for signs and symptoms of hypoglycemia and hyperglycemia throughout insulin therapy. A patient on insulin is particularly prone to hypoglycemic reactions at the time of peak insulin action or when the patient has not eaten for some time or has skipped a meal. Patients in acute care settings have frequent blood glucose monitoring. Testing usually occurs before meals and at bedtime.

There is no standard dose of insulin as there is for most other drugs. Insulin dosage is highly individualized. Some patients achieve the best control with one injection of insulin per day; others may require two or more injections per day. In addition, two different types of insulin may be combined, such as a rapid-acting and a long-acting preparation. The number of insulin injections, dosage, times of administration, and type of insulin are determined by the health care provider after careful evaluation of a patient's metabolic needs and response to therapy.

Insulin must be given parenterally, usually subcutaneously. Insulin cannot be administered orally because it is a protein and is readily destroyed in the gastrointestinal tract. Regular insulin is the only insulin preparation given intravenously. Regular insulin is given 30 to 60 minutes before a meal to achieve optimal results. Other forms of insulin are given on different schedules.

Insulin is injected into the arms, thighs, abdomen, or buttocks. Sites of insulin injection are rotated to prevent **lipodystrophy** (atrophy of subcutaneous fat), a problem that can interfere with the absorption of insulin from the injection site. Lipodystrophy appears as a slight dimpling or pitting of the subcutaneous fat. Because absorption rates vary at the different sites, with the abdomen having the most rapid rate of absorption, followed by the upper arm, thigh, and buttocks, some health care providers recommend rotating the injection sites within one specific area, rather than rotating areas. Localized allergic reactions, signs of inflammation, or other skin changes must be reported to the health care provider as soon as possible because a different type of insulin may be necessary. Patients who give their own injections need to be taught how to rotate sites (Key Concepts Box 30-2).

In addition to injection by syringe and needle, the insulin pump (Fig. 30-2) is used by some patients, such as a pregnant woman with diabetes with early long-term complications and those with, or candidates for, renal transplantation. This system uses only regular insulin, is battery-powered, and requires insertion of a needle into subcutaneous tissue. The amount of insulin injected can be adjusted according to blood glucose monitoring, which is usually performed four to eight times per day.

Blood glucose levels are monitored often in patients with diabetes (Key Concepts 30-2). The health care provider may order blood glucose levels to be tested before meals, after meals, and at bedtime. Less frequent monitoring may be performed if the patient's glucose levels are well controlled. The **glucometer** is a device used to monitor blood glucose levels. Patients must be taught to monitor their blood glucose levels at home.

KEY CONCEPTS

30-2   Key Points for Rotating Insulin Injection Sites

- Site rotation is crucial to prevent injury to the skin and fatty tissue. The following sites are acceptable for injection:
  - Upper arms, outer portion
  - Stomach, except for a 2-in. margin around the umbilicus (belly button)
  - Back, right, and left sides just below the waist
  - Upper thighs, both front and side
- To rotate sites, you should do the following:
  - Note the site of your last injection.
  - Place the side of your thumb at the old site and measure across its width—approximately 1 in.
  - Select a site on the other side of your thumb for the next injection
  - Repeat the procedure for each subsequent 10 to 15 injections and then move to another area

A patient with newly diagnosed diabetes often has many concerns regarding the diagnosis. For some, initially coping with diabetes and the methods required for controlling the disorder create many problems. They may have concerns or fears about giving themselves an injection, having to follow a diet, weight control, the complications associated with diabetes, and changes in eating times and habits. An effective education program helps relieve some of this anxiety.

FACT CHECK

30-6   What is diabetic ketoacidosis?
30-7   Why is it important for patients taking insulin to rotate injection sites?

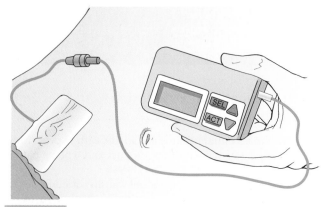

FIGURE 30-2   MiniMed insulin pump is attached to the patient.

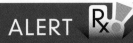

Educating the Patient and Family about Insulin

Noncompliance is a problem in some patients with diabetes, making patient and family teaching vital to the proper management of diabetes. Patients may occasionally lapse in their adherence to the prescribed diet, such as around holidays or other special occasions. This slip may not cause a problem if it is brief and not excessive, as long as the patient immediately returns to the prescribed regimen. However, some patients frequently stray from the prescribed regimen, take extra insulin to cover dietary indiscretions, fast for several days before follow-up blood glucose determinations, and engage in other dangerous behaviors. Although some patients can be convinced that failure to adhere to the prescribed therapeutic regimen is detrimental to their health, others continue to deviate from the prescribed regimen until serious complications develop. Every effort is made to stress the importance of adherence to the prescribed treatment during all office or clinic visits.

The patient's self-monitoring of blood glucose levels using a glucometer is important. The patient must learn to obtain a small sample of blood from the finger and use the device. Printed instructions and illustrations are supplied with the device and must be reviewed with the patient. Following are key points about insulin the patient and family members should know.

- Use the home test method recommended by your health care provider for blood glucose. Review the instructions included with the glucometer, including the technique for collecting the specimen, interpreting your test results, the number of times per day to test your blood, and a record of test results.
- Your health care provider will review your dosage of insulin and teach you how to calculate it. It is very important to use only the recommended type, source, and brand name of insulin. Do not change brands unless your health care provider approves, and keep a spare vial on hand.
- Keep your insulin at room temperature, away from heat and direct sunlight, and dispose the vial within 1 month of first puncturing. Store vials not in use in the refrigerator.
- Be certain to purchase the same brand and needle size each time.
- Your health care provider will teach you how to hold the syringe, how to withdraw insulin from the vial, how to measure the insulin in the syringe using the syringe scale, how to mix insulin in the same syringe (when appropriate), how to eliminate air in the syringe and needle, and what to do if the syringe or needle is contaminated.
- Your health care provider will teach you how to use an injection pen if the insulin you are using is available in a pen and you choose to use it instead of vials and syringes.
- Your insulin needs may change if you become ill, especially with vomiting or fever and during periods of stress or emotional disturbances. Contact your health care provider if these situations occur.
- It is important that you follow the prescribed diet, especially the calories allowed and the permissible food exchanges. Planning daily menus and establishing meal schedules are an important part of your care, as are selecting food from a restaurant menu, reading food labels, and the proper use of artificial sweeteners.
- It is important to carry an extra supply of insulin and a prescription for needles and syringes. Your health care provider will explain how to store insulin when traveling, to protect needles and syringes from theft, and the importance of discussing travel plans (especially foreign travel) before departing.
- Your health care provider will explain the signs and symptoms of hypoglycemia and hyperglycemia, what foods or fluids you should use to terminate a hypoglycemic reaction, and the importance of notifying your health care provider immediately if either reaction occurs.
- Good skin and foot care, personal cleanliness, frequent dental checkups, and routine eye examinations are an important part of treating your diabetes.
- Follow your health care provider's recommendations regarding physical activity.
- Notify your health care provider if you have an increase in blood glucose levels, if you become pregnant, if you have an occurrence of antidiabetic or hyperglycemic episodes, or if you have an illness, infection, or diarrhea (your insulin dosage may require adjustment). Tell your health care provider about any new problems (e.g., leg ulcers, numbness of the extremities, significant weight gain or loss).
- Wear identification, such as a medical alert tag, to inform medical personnel and others that you use insulin to control the disease

Antidiabetic Drugs

Antidiabetic drugs are used to treat patients with type 2 diabetes that is not controlled by diet and exercise alone. These drugs are not effective for treating type 1 diabetes. Eight types of antidiabetic drugs are currently in use:

- Sulfonylureas (chlorpropamide, glimepiride, glipizide, glyburide, tolazamide, tolbutamide)
- Biguanides (metformin)
- α-Glucosidase inhibitors (acarbose, miglitol)
- Meglitinides (nateglinide, repaglinide)
- Thiazolidinediones (pioglitazone, rosiglitazone)
- Amylin analogs (pramlintide)
- Dipeptidyl peptidase-4 inhibitor (linagliptin, saxagliptin, sitagliptin)
- Glucagon-like peptide 1 receptor agonist (exenatide, liraglutide)

Actions of Antidiabetic Drugs

Sulfonylureas

Sulfonylureas appear to lower blood glucose by stimulating the β-cells of the pancreas to release insulin. The sulfonylureas are not effective if the β-cells of the pancreas are unable to release a sufficient amount of insulin to meet a patient's needs. The first-generation sulfonylureas (e.g., chlorpropamide, tolazamide, and tolbutamide) are not commonly used today because they have a long duration of action and a higher incidence of adverse reactions and are more likely to react with other drugs. More commonly used sulfonylureas are the second- and third-generation drugs, such as glimepiride (Amaryl), glipizide (Glucotrol), and glyburide (DiaBeta, Glynase).

Biguanides

Metformin (Glucophage), currently the only biguanide, acts by reducing hepatic glucose production and increasing insulin sensitivity in muscle and fat cells. The liver normally releases glucose by detecting the level of circulating insulin. When insulin levels are high, glucose is available in the blood and the liver produces little or no glucose. When insulin levels are low, there is little circulating glucose, so the liver produces more glucose. In type 2 diabetes, the liver may not detect levels of glucose in the blood and, instead of regulating glucose production, releases glucose despite blood sugar levels. Metformin sensitizes the liver to circulating insulin levels and reduces hepatic glucose production.

α-Glucosidase Inhibitors

The α-glucosidase inhibitors, acarbose (Precose) and miglitol (Glyset), lower blood sugar by delaying the digestion of carbohydrates and absorption of carbohydrates in the intestine.

Meglitinides

Like the sulfonylureas, the meglitinides act to lower blood glucose levels by stimulating the release of insulin from the pancreas. This action depends on the ability of the β-cell in the pancreas to produce some insulin. Examples of the meglitinides include nateglinide (Starlix) and repaglinide (Prandin).

Thiazolidinediones

The thiazolidinediones, also called glitazones, decrease insulin resistance and increase insulin sensitivity by modifying several processes, with the end result being decreasing hepatic glucogenesis (formation of glucose from glycogen) and increasing insulin-dependent muscle glucose uptake. Examples of the thiazolidinediones are rosiglitazone (Avandia) and pioglitazone (Actos).

Amylin Analogs

The only amylin analog currently available is pramlintide (Symlin). Amylin is found in the body and is located in the secretory granules with insulin and secreted with insulin by the pancreas. Through several mechanisms, amylin affects the rate of postprandial glucose. If the body's β-cells are not secreting insulin, then they are not secreting amylin. The amylin analogs act like amylin in the body and produce several effects that aid in diabetes management. Pramlintide

reduces the rate at which food is released from the stomach after eating. It also decreases secretion of glucagon after a meal in patients using insulin. Finally, it produces a feeling of satiety that results in decreased caloric intake and possibly in weight loss.

Dipeptidyl Peptidase-4 Inhibitors

Dipeptidyl peptidase-4 is an enzyme in the body that breaks down incretin hormones, which results in increased levels of active incretin. The dipeptidyl peptidase-4 inhibitors prevent the metabolism of the incretin hormones. The result of increased incretin hormones is an increase in insulin secretion and a decrease in glucagon secretion. The three dipeptidyl peptidase-4 inhibitors are linagliptin (Tradjenta), saxagliptin (Onglyza) and sitagliptin (Januvia).

Glucagon-Like Peptide 1 Receptor Agonists

Glucagon-like peptide 1 is an incretin. The glucagon-like peptide 1 receptor agonists act on the same receptor in the body as the natural incretin hormone. The result of activating this receptor is an increase in insulin production and secretion from the pancreas in response to increased glucose levels. In addition, glucagon secretion is inhibited during periods of hyperglycemia. Finally, gastric emptying is delayed, which prolongs the time it takes for glucose to appear in circulation after eating. Exenatide (Byetta) and liraglutide (Victoza) are the two glucagon-like peptide 1 receptor agonists available.

FACT CHECK

30-8	What are the types of antidiabetic drugs?
30-9	Which two types of antidiabetics lower blood glucose by stimulating the pancreas to release insulin?
30-10	What two types of antidiabetic drugs affect the incretin hormones?

Uses of Antidiabetic Drugs

The antidiabetic drugs are of value only in the treatment of patients with type 2 diabetes whose condition cannot be controlled by diet alone. These drugs may also be used with insulin in the management of some patients with diabetes mellitus. Use of an antidiabetic drug with insulin may decrease the required insulin dosage in some individuals. Two antidiabetic drugs with different actions (e.g., sulfonylurea and metformin) may also be used together when one antidiabetic drug and diet do not control blood glucose levels in type 2 diabetes mellitus. A number of combination products are available and are listed in Table 30-3.

Adverse Reactions of Antidiabetic Drugs

Sulfonylureas

Adverse reactions seen with the sulfonylureas include hypoglycemia, nausea, vomiting, epigastric discomfort, and heartburn. Many, but not all, of them also cause anorexia, headache, and diarrhea. Often, these can be eliminated by reducing the

TABLE 30-3 Antidiabetic Combination Products for Type 2 Diabetes

Generic Name	Trade Name	Dosage Form	Pregnancy Category
glipizide/metformin	Metaglip, generic	Tablets: 2.5/250 mg, 2.5/500 mg	C
glyburide/metformin	Glucovance, generic	Tablets: 1.25/250 mg, 2.5/500 mg, 5/500 mg	B
pioglitazone/glimepiride	Duetact	Tablets: 30/2 mg, 30/4 mg	C
pioglitazone/metformin	ActoPlus Met, ActoPlus Met XR	Tablets: 15/500 mg, 15/850 mg ER tabs: 15/1000 mg, 30/1000 mg	C
repaglinide/metformin	PrandiMet	Tablets: 1/500 mg, 2/500 mg	C
rosiglitazone/glimepiride	Avandaryl	Tablets: 4/1 mg, 4/2 mg, 4/4 mg, 8/2 mg	C
rosiglitazone/metformin	Avandamet	Tablets: 2/500 mg, 2/1000 mg, 4/500 mg, 4/1000 mg	C
saxagliptin/metformin	Kombiglyze XR	ER tabs: 5/500 mg, 2.5/1000 mg, 5/1000 mg	B
sitagliptin/metformin	Janumet	Tablets: 50/500 mg, 50/1000 mg	B

dosage or by giving the drug in divided doses. If these reactions become severe, then the health care provider may try another antidiabetic drug or discontinue the use of these drugs. If the drug therapy is discontinued, then it may be necessary to control the diabetes with insulin.

Biguanides

Adverse reactions associated with the biguanide (metformin) include asthenia, headache, and gastrointestinal upset (such as abdominal bloating, nausea, cramping, diarrhea, flatulence, vomiting, indigestion). These adverse reactions are self-limiting and can be reduced if a patient is started on a low dose and the dosage increases slowly, and if the drug is taken with meals. Hypoglycemia rarely occurs when metformin is used alone.

Lactic acidosis (buildup of lactic acid in the blood) may also occur with metformin use. Although lactic acidosis is a rare adverse reaction, it is serious and can be fatal. Lactic acidosis occurs mainly in patients with kidney dysfunction. Symptoms of lactic acidosis include malaise (vague feeling of bodily discomfort), abdominal pain, rapid respirations, shortness of breath, and muscular pain. In some patients, vitamin B_{12} levels are decreased. This can be reversed with vitamin B_{12} supplements or with discontinuation of the drug therapy. Because weight loss can occur, metformin is sometimes recommended for obese patients or patients with insulin-resistant diabetes.

α-Glucosidase Inhibitors

Because the α-glucosidase inhibitors, acarbose or miglitol, increase the transit time of food in the digestive tract, gastrointestinal disturbances may occur. The most common adverse reactions are bloating and flatulence. Other adverse reactions such as abdominal pain and diarrhea can occur. Although most antidiabetic drugs produce hypoglycemia, acarbose and miglitol, when used alone, do not cause hypoglycemia.

Meglitinides

Adverse reactions of the meglitinides include upper respiratory infection, back pain, and hypoglycemia. Nateglinide may also cause flu symptoms and dizziness. Repaglinide may also cause headache, nausea, diarrhea, and arthralgia.

Thiazolidinediones

Adverse reactions of the thiazolidinediones include aggravated diabetes mellitus, upper respiratory infections, sinusitis, headache, pharyngitis, myalgia, diarrhea, and back pain. When used alone, rosiglitazone and pioglitazone rarely cause hypoglycemia. However, patients receiving these drugs in combination with insulin or other hypoglycemics (e.g., sulfonylureas) are at greater risk for hypoglycemia. A reduction in the dosage of insulin or the sulfonylurea may be required to prevent episodes of hypoglycemia. In some patients, thiazolidinediones may cause or exacerbate congestive heart failure.

Amylin Analogs

Adverse reactions of the amylin analogs include headache, nausea, anorexia, and vomiting. In addition, they can cause hypoglycemia.

Dipeptidyl Peptidase-4 Inhibitors

Adverse reactions of the dipeptidyl peptidase-4 inhibitors include nasopharyngitis and hypoglycemia. In addition, saxagliptin and sitagliptin both cause headache, upper respiratory tract infections, and headache.

Glucagon-Like Peptide 1 Receptor Agonist

Adverse reactions to the glucagon-like peptide 1 receptor agonists include nausea, vomiting, diarrhea, constipation, dizziness, and hypoglycemia. Since these medications are administered subcutaneously, injection-site reactions are also possible.

FACT CHECK

30-11   What potentially fatal adverse reaction can occur with metformin use?

30-12   What are the most common adverse reactions associated with the α-glucosidase inhibitors?

Contraindications, Precautions, and Interactions of Antidiabetic Drugs

- Antidiabetic drugs are contraindicated in patients with a known hypersensitivity, diabetic ketoacidosis, severe infection, or severe endocrine disease.

Sulfonylureas

- The first-generation sulfonylureas (chlorpropamide, tolazamide, and tolbutamide) are contraindicated in patients with coronary artery disease or liver or renal dysfunction.
- Other sulfonylureas are used cautiously in patients with impaired liver function because liver dysfunction can prolong the drug's effect. In addition, the sulfonylureas are used cautiously in patients with renal impairment and severe cardiovascular disease.
- There is a risk for cross-sensitivity with the sulfonylureas and the sulfonamides.
- The sulfonylureas may have an increased hypoglycemic effect when administered with the anticoagulants, chloramphenicol, clofibrate, fluconazole, histamine H_2 antagonists, methyldopa, MAOIs, salicylates, sulfonamides, and tricyclic antidepressants.
- The hypoglycemic effect of the sulfonylureas may be decreased when the agents are administered with β-blockers, calcium channel blockers, cholestyramine, corticosteroids, estrogens, hydantoins, isoniazid, oral contraceptives, phenothiazines, thiazide diuretics, and thyroid agents.

Biguanides

- Metformin is contraindicated in patients with heart failure, renal disease, hypersensitivity to metformin, and acute or chronic metabolic acidosis, including ketoacidosis. The drug is also contraindicated in patients older than age 80 and during lactation.
- The drug is used cautiously during surgery. Metformin use is temporarily discontinued for surgical procedures. The drug therapy is restarted when a patient's oral intake has been resumed and renal function is normal.
- There is a risk of acute renal failure when iodinated contrast material used for radiological studies is administered with metformin. Metformin therapy is stopped for 48 hours before and after radiological studies using iodinated material.
- Alcohol, amiloride, digoxin, morphine, procainamide, quinidine, quinine, ranitidine, triamterene, trimethoprim, vancomycin, cimetidine, and furosemide all increase the risk of hypoglycemia.
- There is an increased risk of lactic acidosis when metformin is administered with the glucocorticoids.

α-Glucosidase Inhibitors

- The α-glucosidase inhibitors are contraindicated in patients with a hypersensitivity to the drug and in those with diabetic ketoacidosis, cirrhosis, inflammatory bowel disease, colonic ulceration, partial intestinal obstruction or predisposition to intestinal obstruction, or chronic intestinal diseases.
- Acarbose and miglitol are used cautiously in patients with renal impairment or preexisting gastrointestinal problems such as irritable bowel syndrome and Crohn disease.
- Digestive enzymes may reduce the effect of miglitol.
- The effects of acarbose may increase when administered with the loop or thiazide diuretics, glucocorticoids, oral contraceptives, calcium channel blockers, phenytoin, thyroid drugs, or the phenothiazines.
- Miglitol may decrease absorption of ranitidine and propranolol.

Meglitinides

- These drugs are contraindicated in patients with hypersensitivity to the drug, type 1 diabetes, and diabetic ketoacidosis.
- These drugs are used cautiously in patients with liver or kidney disease. Certain drugs, such as NSAIDs, salicylates, MAOIs, and β-adrenergic blocking drugs, may potentiate the hypoglycemic action of the meglitinides.
- Drugs such as the thiazides, corticosteroids, thyroid drugs, and sympathomimetics may decrease the hypoglycemic action of these drugs. A patient receiving one or more of these drugs along with an antidiabetic drug must be closely monitored.

Thiazolidinediones

- The thiazolidinediones are contraindicated in patients with a known hypersensitivity to any component of the drug and in patients with severe heart failure.
- The thiazolidinediones are used cautiously in patients with edema, cardiovascular disease, and liver or kidney disease.
- These drugs may alter the effects of oral contraceptives.

Amylin Analogs

- Pramlintide is contraindicated in patients with a known hypersensitivity to any component of the drug and in patients with diagnosed gastroparesis or hypoglycemia unawareness.
- Pramlintide should not be combined with drugs that alter GI motility, such as anticholinergics, or drugs that inhibit absorption of nutrients, such as α-glucosidase inhibitors.

Dipeptidyl Peptidase-4 Inhibitors

- Dipeptidyl peptidase-4 inhibitors are contraindicated in patients with a history of hypersensitivity to any component of the drug.
- Combination with insulin secretagogues, such as sulfonylureas, may result in hypoglycemia.
- Rifampin decreases the effectiveness of the dipeptidyl peptidase-4 inhibitors.

- Antacids that contain aluminum and magnesium salts and simethicone inhibits the absorption of saxagliptin.
- Coadministration with other antidiabetics may affect the blood levels of saxagliptin and sitagliptin. Dosages may need to be adjusted.
- Saxagliptin's blood levels are increased with coadministration of simvastatin, medications that inhibit cytochrome P-450, and diltiazem. Dosage adjustment may be necessary.
- Sitagliptin blood levels are increased by cyclosporine.
- Sitagliptin causes an increase in the blood levels of digoxin, which may require a dosage adjustment.
- Monitor patients on sitagliptin for pancreatitis.

Glucagon-Like Peptide 1 Receptor Agonist

- Glucagon-like peptide 1 receptor agonists are contraindicated in patients with a history of hypersensitivity to any component of the drug.
- Liraglutide is contraindicated in patients with a history or a family history of medullary thyroid carcinoma and in patients with multiple endocrine neoplasia type 2.
- Patients should be monitored for pancreatitis after drug therapy has been initiated.
- Exenatide interacts with acetaminophen, digoxin, lovastatin, oral antibiotics, and oral contraceptives when coadministered. Liraglutide interacts with acetaminophen, atorvastatin, digoxin, and griseofulvin. Dosage administration should be separated by taking these drugs 1 hour before or 4 hours after exenatide.
- The risk of hypoglycemia is increased when these drugs are combined with other antidiabetic drugs.
- Exenatide increases blood levels of warfarin when coadministered. PT times should be closely monitored and the warfarin dose may need to be adjusted.

Patient Management Issues with Antidiabetic Drugs

Patients are observed every 2 to 4 hours for symptoms of hypoglycemia, particularly during the initial therapy or after a change in dosage. If both an antidiabetic drug and insulin or two antidiabetic drugs are given, then the patient is observed more frequently for hypoglycemic episodes during the initial period of combination therapy. If the patient is receiving only an antidiabetic drug and a hypoglycemic reaction occurs, it is often (but not always) less intense than if it occurred with insulin administration.

When some patients learn that diet and a drug can help them manage their diabetes, they have a tendency to discount the seriousness of the disorder. The importance of following the prescribed treatment regimen should be emphasized.

There is no fixed dosage for the treatment of diabetes. The drug regimen is individualized on the basis of the effectiveness and tolerance of the drug(s) used and the maximum recommended dose of the drug(s).

Sulfonylureas

Chlorpropamide, tolazamide, and tolbutamide are given with food to prevent gastrointestinal upset. However, because food delays absorption, glipizide is given 30 minutes before a meal. Glyburide is administered with breakfast or with the first main

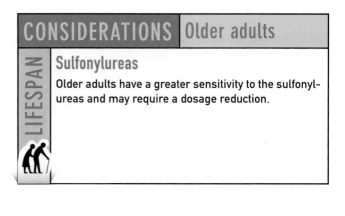

ALERT

Stabilizing Blood Glucose Levels
Exposure to stress, such as infection, fever, surgery, or trauma, may cause a loss of control of blood glucose levels in patients who have been stabilized with antidiabetic drugs. Should this occur, the health care provider might discontinue use of the drug and administer insulin.

meal of the day. Glimepiride is give once daily with breakfast or with the first main meal of the day.

After a patient has been taking sulfonylureas for a period of time, a condition called secondary failure may occur. **Secondary failure** occurs when the sulfonylurea loses its effectiveness. When a patient who has a history of good diabetes management has a gradual increase in blood sugar levels, secondary failure may be the cause. This increase in blood glucose levels can be caused by an increase in the severity of the diabetes or a decreased response to the drug. When secondary failure occurs, the health care provider may prescribe another sulfonylurea or add an antidiabetic drug such as metformin to the drug regimen.

Biguanides

Metformin is given two to three times per day with meals. If a patient has not experienced a response in 4 weeks using the maximum dose of metformin, then the health care provider may add a sulfonylurea while continuing metformin at the maximum dose. The extended release formulations are administered once daily with the evening meal.

α-Glucosidase Inhibitors

Acarbose and miglitol are given three times per day with the first bite of the meal because food increases absorption. Some patients begin therapy with a lower dose once daily to minimize gastrointestinal effects such as abdominal discomfort, flatulence, and diarrhea. The dose is then gradually increased to three times daily.

Meglitinides

Repaglinide is usually taken 15 minutes before meals but can be taken immediately or up to 30 minutes before the meal. Nateglinide is taken up to 30 minutes before meals.

CONSIDERATIONS Older adults

LIFESPAN

Sulfonylureas
Older adults have a greater sensitivity to the sulfonylureas and may require a dosage reduction.

Thiazolidinediones

The thiazolidinediones, pioglitazone and rosiglitazone, are given with or without meals. If the dose is missed at the usual meal, then the drug is taken at the next meal. Once the drug is taken, the meal should not be delayed. Delay of a meal for as little as 30 minutes can cause hypoglycemia.

Amylin Analogs

Pramlintide is to be given subcutaneously immediately prior to major meals. The dose can be increased once the patient has not experienced nausea for 3 days. Once the target dose of pramlintide has been reached, then the insulin dose can be adjusted for optimal glycemic control.

Injection sites should be rotated. The injection site should be distinct from the site where insulin is being injected. Pramlintide cannot be mixed with insulin for injecting.

Dipeptidyl Peptidase-4 Inhibitors

These drugs can be taken with or without food and without regard to meals.

Glucagon-Like Peptide 1 Receptor Agonist

Liraglutide is administered subcutaneously once daily. It can be administered any time of the day without regard to meals. Exenatide is administered subcutaneously twice daily within 60 minutes before the morning and evening meal or the two major meals of the day. It should not be administered after a meal. The doses should be 6 hours or more apart. Both drugs should be administered in the abdomen, thigh, or upper arm.

FACT CHECK

30-13   What is secondary failure?
30-14   Which type of the antidiabetic drugs used to treat type 2 diabetes is injected subcutaneously?

Educating the Patient and Family about Antidiabetic Drugs

Patients taking an antidiabetic drug may fail to comply with the prescribed treatment regimen because of the erroneous belief that not having to take insulin means that their disease is not serious. A patient may also mistakenly conclude that strict adherence to the recommended dietary plan is not

---

ALERT Rx

α-Glucosidase Inhibitors and Hypoglycemia
When hypoglycemia occurs in a patient taking an α-glucosidase inhibitor (e.g., acarbose or miglitol), the patient is given an oral form of glucose, such as glucose tablets or dextrose, rather than sugar (sucrose). Absorption of sugar is blocked by acarbose or miglitol.

CONSIDERATIONS | Older adults

LIFESPAN

Hypoglycemia

Although elderly patients taking an antidiabetic drug are particularly susceptible to hypoglycemic reactions, these reactions may be difficult to detect in the elderly. The health care provider should be notified if blood sugar levels are elevated or if ketones are present in the urine.

---

required. The patient needs to understand that control of their diabetes is just as important as for patients requiring insulin and that control is achieved only when they adhere to the prescribed treatment regimen.

Although taking an antidiabetic drug is less complicated than self-administration of insulin, a patient with diabetes who is taking one of these drugs needs a thorough explanation of the management of the disease. Following are key points about antidiabetic drugs the patient and family members should know:

- Take the drug exactly as directed on the container, for example, with food or 30 minutes before a meal.
- To control your diabetes, follow exactly the diet and drug regimen prescribed by your health care provider.
- The drug prescribed for you is not oral insulin and cannot be substituted for insulin.
- Never stop taking this drug or increase or decrease the dose unless told to do so by your health care provider.
- Take the drug at the same time or times each day.
- Eat meals at approximately the same time each day. Erratic meal hours or skipped meals may cause you to have difficulty in controlling diabetes with this drug.
- Avoid alcohol, dieting, commercial weight-loss products, and strenuous exercise programs unless your health care provider has approved.
- Test your blood for glucose and urine for ketones as directed by your health care provider. Keep a record of your test results and bring this record to each visit to your health care provider.
- Maintain good foot and skin care and have routine eye and dental examinations for the early detection of any complications that may occur.
- Perform moderate exercise; avoid strenuous exercise and erratic periods of exercise.
- Wear identification, such as a medical alert tag, to inform medical personnel and others of your diabetes and the drug or drugs you currently use to treat the disease.
- Notify your health care provider if you experience any of the following: episodes of hypoglycemia, apparent symptoms of hyperglycemia, elevated blood glucose levels, positive results of urine tests for glucose or ketone bodies, or pregnancy. Also notify your health care provider of any serious illness not requiring hospitalization.
- Know the symptoms of hypoglycemia and hyperglycemia and your health care provider's recommended method for terminating a hypoglycemic reaction.

- Metformin: there is a risk of lactic acidosis when you use this drug. Discontinue the drug therapy and notify your health care provider immediately if you experience any of the following: respiratory distress, muscular aches, unusual difficulty sleeping, unexplained malaise, or nonspecific abdominal distress.
- α-Glucosidase Inhibitors: these drugs do not generally cause hypoglycemia. However, if sulfonylureas or insulin are used in combination with acarbose or miglitol, your blood sugar levels can be lowered enough to cause symptoms or even life-threatening hypoglycemia. Have a ready source of glucose to treat symptoms of low blood sugar when taking insulin or a sulfonylurea with these drugs.
- Meglitinides: if you skip a meal, do not take the drug. Similarly, if you add a meal, add a dose of the drug for that meal.

Chapter Review

KEY POINTS

- Diabetes mellitus is a chronic disorder characterized either by insufficient insulin production in the β-cells of the pancreas or by cellular resistance to insulin. Insulin insufficiency results in elevated blood glucose levels, or hyperglycemia, and may cause other serious health conditions.
- Insulin and the antidiabetic drugs, along with diet and exercise, are the cornerstones of treatment for diabetes mellitus. They are used to prevent episodes of hypoglycemia and to normalize carbohydrate metabolism.
- Patients with type 1 diabetes produce insulin in insufficient amounts and therefore must have insulin supplementation to survive. Symptoms include hyperglycemia, polydipsia, polyphagia, polyuria, and weight loss. Treatment of type 1 diabetes is difficult and requires a strict regimen that typically includes a carefully calculated diet, planned physical activity, home glucose testing several times per day, and multiple daily insulin injections.
- Insulin preparations may be classified as rapid-acting, short-acting, intermediate-acting, or long-acting.
- The two major adverse reactions seen with insulin administration are hypoglycemia (low blood glucose or sugar) and hyperglycemia (elevated blood glucose or sugar). Insulin is contraindicated in patients with hypersensitivity to any ingredient of the product or when a patient is hypoglycemic and is used cautiously in patients with liver or kidney disease and during pregnancy and lactation.
- Drugs used to elevate glucose levels in patients experiencing hypoglycemia include diazoxide, glucose, and glucagon.
- Type 2 diabetes involves either a decreased production of insulin by the β-cells of the pancreas or a decreased sensitivity of the cells to insulin, making the cells insulin resistant. Risk factors include obesity, older age, family history of diabetes, history of gestational diabetes, impaired glucose tolerance, minimal or no physical activity, and race/ethnicity.
- The antidiabetic drugs are of value only in the treatment of patients with type 2 diabetes whose condition cannot be controlled by diet alone. Both insulin and an antidiabetic may be prescribed, but use of an antidiabetic drug with insulin may decrease the insulin dosage in some patients. Two antidiabetic drugs may also be used together when one antidiabetic drug and diet do not control blood glucose levels in type 2 diabetes mellitus.
- The antidiabetic drugs are contraindicated in patients with a known hypersensitivity, diabetic ketoacidosis, severe infection, or severe endocrine disease.

CRITICAL THINKING CASE STUDY
CASE 1
Type 2 Diabetes

Mr. Goddard, age 78 years, was recently diagnosed with type 2 diabetes, and his health care provider has prescribed an antidiabetic drug. Mr. Goddard says his friend with diabetes takes insulin and he wonders why insulin was not prescribed for him.

1. What explanation should be given to Mr. Goddard's initial question?
   a. Antidiabetics are used to treat patients with type 2 diabetes because insulin is used only for type 1 diabetes.
   b. Insulin is sometimes used for type 2 diabetes, but Mr. Goddard's case may not require it.
   c. Older patients are more responsive to antidiabetics than to insulin.
   d. Both a and c
2. As a patient with newly diagnosed disease, Mr. Goddard requires instruction on which of the following topics?
   a. Diet
   b. Diet and exercise
   c. Diet, exercise, and stress reduction
   d. Diet, exercise, stress reduction, and alcohol intake
3. Mr. Goddard has been prescribed metformin 500 mg twice daily. He cannot remember anything else about how to take it. What should you tell him?

CASE 2
Type 1 Diabetes

Ms. May has been diagnosed with type 1 diabetes. She is 15 years old. Her physician has prescribed an insulin regimen for her.

1. How is insulin administered?
   a. Intradermally
   b. Subcutaneously
   c. Intramuscularly

    d.   Intravenously
2.   Where are insulin injections given?
    a.   Upper arms, outer portion
    b.   Stomach, except for a 2-in. margin around the umbilicus (belly button)
    c.   Back, right, and left sides just below the waist
    d.   All of the above
3.   Ms. May will need to be informed about monitoring parameters. What should you tell her?

Review Questions

MULTIPLE CHOICE

1.   Which of the following would most likely terminate a hypoglycemic reaction?
    a.   Regular insulin
    b.   pH insulin
    c.   Orange juice
    d.   Crackers and milk
2.   What are the adverse effects of meglitinides?
    a.   Photophobia
    b.   Aches in legs, shortness of breath
    c.   Skin rashes, urinary frequency
    d.   Headache, back pain
3.   Which of the following symptoms indicate a possible hyperglycemic reaction?
    a.   Fatigue, weakness, confusion
    b.   Pale skin, elevated temperature
    c.   Thirst, abdominal pain, nausea
    d.   Rapid, shallow respirations, headache, nervousness
4.   First-generation sulfonylureas are contraindicated in patients with known hypersensitivity and in those with
    a.   coronary artery disease
    b.   liver dysfunction
    c.   renal dysfunction
    d.   all of the above
5.   Because elderly patients have a greater sensitivity to the sulfonylureas, they may require
    a.   administration of insulin
    b.   administration of a second oral antidiabetic
    c.   an increased dosage
    d.   a reduced dosage
6.   How should acarbose be taken?
    a.   Before meals
    b.   After meals
    c.   With the first bite of the meal
    d.   With or without food
7.   When should sitagliptin be taken?
    a.   Before meals
    b.   After meals
    c.   With the first bit of the meal
    d.   With or without food

MATCHING

Match each drug on the left with the correct classification on the right.

_____ 8. pramlintide	a.	sulfonylurea
_____ 9. linagliptin	b.	biguanide
_____ 10. exenatide	c.	a-glucosidase inhibitor
_____ 11. metformin	d.	meglitinides
_____ 12. glipizide	e.	thiazolidinediones
_____ 13. repaglinide	f.	amylin analog
_____ 14. acarbose	g.	dipeptidyl peptidase-4 inhibitor
_____ 15. pioglitazone	h.	glucagon-like peptide 1 receptor agonist

Match the generic drug name on the left with the correct brand name on the right.

_____ 16. nateglinide	a.	Byetta
_____ 17. metformin	b.	Symlin
_____ 18. insulin glargine	c.	Januvia
_____ 19. rosiglitazone	d.	Starlix
_____ 20. insulin glulisine	e.	Precose
_____ 21. glyburide	f.	Lantus
_____ 22. exenatide	g.	Apidra
_____ 23. acarbose	h.	Glynase
_____ 24. pramlintide	i.	Avandia
_____ 25. sitagliptin	j.	Glucophage

TRUE OR FALSE

_____ 26.   In patients receiving oral hypoglycemic drugs, hypoglycemic reactions may be less intense than reactions seen with insulin administration.

_____ 27.   The effects of oral contraceptives may be altered by rosiglitazone and pioglitazone.

_____ 28.   Many patients can control type 1 diabetes with diet, exercise, and antidiabetic medication.

_____ 29.   A patient undergoing a surgical procedure would have to temporarily discontinue metformin use.

_____ 30.   Insulin dosage for type 1 diabetes is standardized for all patients.

_____ 31.   A patient who is taking acarbose or miglitol would be given glucose tablets when hypoglycemia occurs.

_____ 32.   Amylin affects the rate of postprandial glucose.

FILL IN THE BLANKS

33.   Oral contraceptives _____ the hypoglycemic effect of insulin.
34.   Hyperglycemia has a _____ onset and results in a blood glucose level of _____.
35.   _____ _____ is a potentially life-threatening deficiency of insulin that results in dangerously _____ levels of glucose in the blood.
36.   Patients taking antidiabetic drugs may need to test their blood for _____ and urine for _____.

37. If iodinated contrast material used for radiological studies is administered with _____, a patient would be at risk for acute renal failure.

38. Insulin should be kept at room temperature, away from _____ and direct sunlight, and the vial should be disposed of within _____ month of first puncturing.

39. The glucagon-like peptide 1 receptor agonists act on the same receptor in the body as the natural incretin hormone, which results in a(n) _____ in insulin production and secretion from the pancreas in response to increased glucose levels.

SHORT ANSWERS

40. Compare and contrast the symptoms of hypoglycemia and hyperglycemia.

41. How do pregnancy and delivery affect insulin requirements?

42. Lactic acidosis can occur with metformin use. What are the symptoms? What would you advise a patient who is experiencing these symptoms to do?

43. Why is it important for patients taking antidiabetic drugs to eat meals at roughly the same time each day?

Web Activities

1. Go to the American Diabetes Association Web site (http://www.diabetes.org) and conduct a search for "diabetes statistics." What is the total prevalence of diabetes? What race and ethnic differences are found in the prevalence of diabetes?

2. On the same Web site, search for the "Diabetes Risk Test." Using the flow chart, take the risk test and calculate your score. Although this is a simple assessment, this score can help you understand your own risk.

SUMMARY DRUG TABLE   Insulin Preparations
(left, Types of Insulin; right, trade)

Comprehensive Summary Drug Tables, including uses, adverses effects, dosages, and pregnancy classifications, are provided on the companion website, http:// thePoint.lww.com/PharmacologyHP2e

Rapid-Acting Insulins	
insulin lispro (insulin analog) *in'-soo-lin lye'-spror*	Humalog (Rx), Humalog Mix 50/50, Humalog Mix 75/25
insulin aspart solution (insulin analog) *in'-soo-lin as'-part*	NovoLog (Rx)
insulin glulisine *in'-soo-lin gloo-lis'-een*	Apidra (Rx), Apidra OptiClik, Apidra SoloStar
Short-Acting Insulins	
insulin injection (regular) *in'-soo-lin*	Humulin R (OTC), Novolin R (OTC), Novolin R InnoLet, Novolin R PenFill
Intermediate-Acting Insulin	
isophane insulin suspension (NPH)	Humulin N Pen (OTC), Novolin N (OTC), Novolin N Innolet, Novolin N PenFill
Long-Acting Insulins	
insulin detemir	Levemir
insulin glargine solution *in'-soo-lin glar'-jeen*	Levemir FlexPen Lantus (Rx), Lantus OptiClik, Lantus SoloStar
Mixed Insulins	
70% isophane insulin suspension (NPH) and 30% insulin injections (regular)	Humulin 70/30 (OTC), Novolin 70/30 (OTC)
50% isophane insulin suspension (NPH) and 30% insulin injection (regular)	Humulin 50/50
70% insulin aspart protamine suspension and 30% insulin aspart solution	Novolog 70/30 (Rx)
High-Potency Insulin	
insulin injection concentrated	Humulin R U-500 (Rx)

SUMMARY DRUG TABLE   Glucose Elevating Agents
(left, generic; right, trade)

Comprehensive Summary Drug Tables, including uses, adverses effects, dosages, and pregnancy classifications, are provided on the companion website, http:// thePoint.lww.com/PharmacologyHP2e

diazoxide *die-aze-ox'-ide*	Proglycem
glucose *gloo'-kose*	Glutose (OTC), Insta-Glucose, Insulin Reaction Dex4 Glucose, BD Glucose
glucagon *glue-kuh-gahn*	GlucaGen, Glucagon Emergency

SUMMARY DRUG TABLE   Antidiabetic Drugs
(left, generic; right, trade)

Comprehensive Summary Drug Tables, including uses, adverses effects, dosages, and pregnancy classifications, are provided on the companion website, http:// thePoint.lww.com/PharmacologyHP2e

Sulfonylureas	
chlorpropamide *klor-proe'-pa-mide*	*generic*
glimepiride *glye-meh'-per-ide*	Amaryl, *generic*
glipizide *glip'-i-zide*	Glucotrol, Glucotrol XL, *generic*
glyburide (glibenclamide) *glye-byoor-ide*	DiaBeta, Glynase, *generic*
tolazamide *tole-az'-a-mide*	*generic*
tolbutamide *tole-byoo'-ta-mide*	*generic*
Biguanide	
metformin *met-for'-min*	Fortamet, Glucophage, Glucophage XR, Glumetza, Riomet, *generic*
α-Glucosidase Inhibitors	
acarbose *aye-kar'-bose*	Precose
miglitol *mi'-gli-tole*	Glyset
Meglitinides	
nateglinide *nah-teg'-lah-nyde*	Starlix, *generic*
repaglinide *re-pag'-lah-nyd*	Prandin
Thiazolidinediones	
pioglitazone HCl *pie-oh-glit'-ah-zohn*	Actos
rosiglitazone maleate *roh-zee-glit'-ah-zohn*	Avandia
Amylin Analog	
pramlintide *pram'-lin-tide*	Symlin
Dipeptidyl Peptidase-4 Inhibitor	
linagliptin	Tradjenta
saxagliptin *sax-a-glip'-tin*	Onglyza
sitagliptin *sit-a-glip'-tin*	Januvia
Glucagon-Like Peptide 1 Receptor Agonist	
exenatide *ex-en'-a-tide*	Byetta
liraglutide *lir-a-gloo'-tide*	Victoza

31

Pituitary and Adrenocortical Hormones

CHAPTER OBJECTIVES

On completion of this chapter, students will be able to:

1. Define the chapter's key terms.
2. Identify the hormones of the anterior pituitary.
3. Discuss the timing of growth hormone use.
4. Identify the hormones of the posterior pituitary.
5. Explain the multiple functions of glucocorticoids within the body.
6. Identify clinically significant interactions between glucocorticoids and select drugs.
7. Discuss the different needs of patient education for short-term, alternate-day, and long-term or high-dose glucocorticoid therapy.
8. Describe the general drug actions, uses, adverse reactions, contraindications, precautions, and interactions of pituitary and adrenocortical hormones.
9. Discuss important points to keep in mind when educating the patient or family members about the use of pituitary and adrenocortical hormones.

KEY TERMS

adrenal insufficiency—a critical deficiency of the mineralocorticoids and the glucocorticoids that requires immediate treatment

corticosteroids—the collective name for the glucocorticoids and mineralocorticoids, hormones secreted by the adrenal cortex and essential to life

cryptorchism—failure of the testes to descend into the scrotum

Cushing syndrome—a disease caused by the overproduction of endogenous glucocorticoids

diabetes insipidus—a disease resulting from the failure of the posterior pituitary to secrete vasopressin or from surgical removal of the pituitary

CHAPTER OVERVIEW

Drug classes covered in this chapter are:

- Anterior pituitary hormones
- Posterior pituitary hormones
- Adrenocortical hormones

Drugs by classification are listed on page 326.

thePOINT RESOURCES

- Comprehensive Summary Drug Tables
- Lippincott's Interactive Tutorials: Drugs Affecting the Endocrine System
- Interactive Practice and Review
- Monographs of Most Commonly Prescribed Drugs

glucocorticoids—a hormone essential to life produced by the adrenal cortex

gonadotropins—hormones that promote growth and function of the gonads

hyperstimulation syndrome—sudden ovarian enlargement with accumulation of serous fluid in the peritoneal cavity

mineralocorticoids—a hormone essential to life produced by the adrenal cortex

somatotropic hormone—a growth hormone secreted by the anterior pituitary

---

The pituitary gland lies deep within the cranial vault, connected to the brain by the infundibular stalk (a downward extension of the floor of the third ventricle) and protected by an indentation of the sphenoid bone called the sella turcica (see Fig. 31-1). It is a small, gray, rounded structure with two parts:

- Anterior pituitary (adenohypophysis)
- Posterior pituitary (neurohypophysis)

The pituitary gland secretes hormones that regulate growth, metabolism, the reproductive cycle, electrolyte balance, and water retention or loss. Because this gland secretes so many hormones that regulate numerous vital processes, it is often referred to as the "master gland." The hormones secreted by the anterior and posterior pituitary and the organs influenced by these hormones are shown in Figure 31-2.

Anterior Pituitary Hormones

The hormones of the anterior pituitary include

- Follicle-stimulating hormone
- Luteinizing hormone
- Growth hormone
- Adrenocorticotropic hormone
- Thyroid-stimulating hormone and prolactin

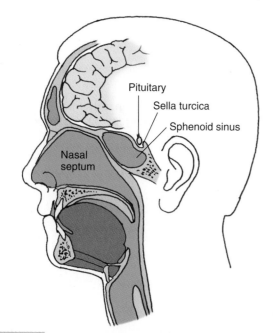

FIGURE 31-1 Location of the pituitary gland.

This chapter discusses follicle-stimulating hormone, luteinizing hormone, growth hormone, and adrenocorticotropic hormone. Follicle-stimulating hormone and luteinizing hormone are called **gonadotropins** because they influence the gonads (the organs of reproduction). Growth hormone, also called somatotropin, contributes to the growth of the body during childhood, especially the growth of muscles and bones. Adrenocorticotropic hormone is produced by the anterior pituitary and stimulates the adrenal cortex to secrete glucocorticoids and mineralocorticoids, which are collectively called the corticosteroids. The anterior pituitary hormone, thyroid-stimulating hormone, is discussed in Chapter 32. Prolactin, which is also secreted by the anterior pituitary, stimulates the production of breast milk in the postpartum patient. Additional functions of prolactin are not well understood. Prolactin is the only anterior pituitary hormone that is not used medically.

> ## FACT CHECK
> **31-1** Which hormones are secreted by the anterior pituitary gland?

GONADOTROPINS

The gonadotropins (follicle-stimulating hormone and luteinizing hormone) influence the secretion of sex hormones, the development of secondary sex characteristics, and the reproductive cycle in both men and women. The gonadotropins discussed in this chapter include menotropins, follitropins, clomiphene, and chorionic gonadotropin.

Actions of Gonadotropins

Menotropins (Menopur) and urofollitropin (Bravelle) are purified preparations of the gonadotropins extracted from the urine of postmenopausal women and induce ovulation and pregnancy. In men, menotropins and some of the follitropins induce the production of sperm. The follitropins stimulate growth of the follicle in the ovary in women who have healthy ovaries. Follitropin alfa and beta are hormones that are identical to FSH found in the body.

Clomiphene (Clomid) is a synthetic nonsteroidal compound that binds to estrogen receptors, decreasing the number of available estrogen receptors and causing the anterior pituitary to increase secretion of follicle-stimulating hormone and luteinizing hormone. Chorionic gonadotropin

Pituitary Gland

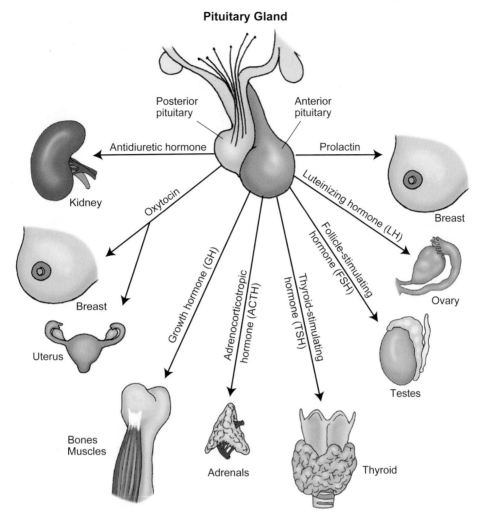

FIGURE 31-2 The pituitary gland and the hormones secreted by the anterior pituitary and the posterior pituitary.

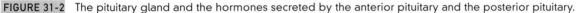

is extracted from human placentas. The actions of chorionic gonadotropin are identical to those of the pituitary luteinizing hormone.

Uses of Gonadotropins

Menotropins are used to induce ovulation and pregnancy in anovulatory (failure to produce an ovum or failure to ovulate) women. Menotropins are also used with human chorionic gonadotropin in women to stimulate multiple follicles for in vitro fertilization. In men, menotropins are used to induce the production of sperm (spermatogenesis). Follitropin alfa and beta are used to induce ovulation and pregnancy in anovulatory women. They are also used to develop multiple follicles for in vitro fertilization. In men, they are used to induce spermatogenesis. Urofollitropin is used to induce ovulation in women with polycystic ovarian disease and to stimulate multiple follicular development in ovulatory women for in vitro fertilization. Lutropin is used with follitropin alfa in the initial treatment cycle.

Clomiphene and chorionic gonadotropin are both used to induce ovulation in anovulatory (nonovulating) women. Chorionic gonadotropin is also used for the treatment of

prepubertal **cryptorchism** (failure of the testes to descend into the scrotum) and in men to treat selected cases of hypogonadotropic hypogonadism (inadequate secretion of gonadal hormones).

FACT CHECK

31-2 Which hormones are gonadotropins?
31-3 What do gonadotropins influence?

Adverse Reactions of Gonadotropins

The adverse reactions of the menotropins include headache, abdominal enlargement, cramps and/or fullness, abdominal pain, nausea, and ovarian hyperstimulation. Urofollitropin may result in mild to moderate ovarian enlargement, abdominal discomfort, nausea, headache, hot flashes, and irritation at the injection site. The follitropins may result in enlarged abdomen, abdominal pain, breast pain in women, flatulence, and nausea.

Administration of clomiphene may result in vasomotor flushes (like the hot flashes of menopause), abdominal discomfort, ovarian enlargement, blurred vision, nausea, vomiting, and nervousness. Chorionic gonadotropin may result in headache, irritability, restlessness, fatigue, edema, and precocious puberty (when given for cryptorchism).

Contraindications, Precautions, and Interactions of Gonadotropins

- The gonadotropins are contraindicated in patients who have a known hypersensitivity to any component of the drug.
- The gonadotropins are contraindicated in patients with high gonadotropin levels, thyroid dysfunction, adrenal dysfunction, abnormal bleeding, ovarian cysts, or those with an organic intracranial lesion.
- Chorionic gonadotropin, choriogonadotropin alfa, clomiphene, follitropins, lutropin, menotropins, and urofollitropin are all contraindicated during pregnancy.
- Clomiphene is contraindicated in patients with liver disease, abnormal bleeding of undetermined origin, or ovarian cysts.
- Chorionic gonadotropin is contraindicated in patients with precocious puberty, prostatic cancer, or androgen-dependent neoplasm.
- Clomiphene and chorionic gonadotropin are used cautiously in patients with epilepsy, migraine headaches, asthma, cardiac or renal dysfunction, and during lactation. There are no clinically significant known interactions with the gonadotropins.
- Serious pulmonary and vascular complications have been reported with follitropins. Patients should be monitored closely.
- Multiple births are possible with gonadotropin use.

Patient Management Issues with Gonadotropins

These drugs are almost always administered on an outpatient basis. Before prescribing any one of these drugs, the health care provider will take a thorough medical history and perform a physical examination. Additional laboratory and diagnostic tests for ovarian function and tubal patency may also be performed. A pelvic examination may be performed to rule out ovarian enlargement, pregnancy, or uterine problems. Female patients taking gonadotropins are usually examined by the

KEY CONCEPTS

31-1 Hyperstimulation Syndrome

Some female patients may experience hyperstimulation syndrome, which is sudden ovarian enlargement with accumulation of serous fluid in the peritoneal cavity. The patient may also experience pain. This syndrome usually develops quickly over a period of 3 to 4 days and requires hospitalization and discontinuation of the drug therapy. Abdominal pain and distention are indicators that hyperstimulation syndrome may be developing.

ALERT Rx

Clomiphene

If a patient reports visual disturbances, then the drug is discontinued and the health care provider should be notified. An examination by an ophthalmologist is usually required.

health care provider every other day during treatment and at 2-week intervals to detect excessive ovarian stimulation, called **hyperstimulation syndrome** (Key Concepts 31-1).

Gonadotropin injections are given in the health care provider's office or clinic. These drugs are administered intramuscularly or subcutaneously because they are destroyed in the gastrointestinal tract. Urofollitropin may cause pain and irritation at the injection site, and sites should be rotated and previous sites examined for redness and irritation.

Educating the Patient and Family about Gonadotropins

Patients taking gonadotropins should keep all health care provider appointments, and adverse reactions should be reported. Following are key points about gonadotropins that the patient and family members should know.

Menotropins and Follitropins

- Before beginning therapy, be aware of the possibility of multiple births and birth defects. Discuss any concerns or questions you may have with your health care provider.
- It is a good idea to use a calendar to track your treatment schedule and ovulation.
- Report bloating, abdominal pain, flushing, breast tenderness, and pain at the injection site to your health care provider.

Clomiphene

- Take the drug as prescribed (5 days) and do not stop taking the drug before the course of therapy is finished unless told to do so by your health care provider.
- Notify your health care provider if you experience bloating, stomach or pelvic pain, jaundice, blurred vision, hot flashes, breast discomfort, headache, nausea, or vomiting.
- If ovulation has not occurred after the first course, then a second or third course of therapy may be used. If the drug is not successful after three regimens, then the therapy may be considered unsuccessful and the drug is discontinued.

GROWTH HORMONE

Growth hormone, also called **somatotropic hormone**, is secreted by the anterior pituitary. This hormone regulates the growth of the individual until early adulthood or the time when the person no longer gains height.

Actions of Growth Hormone

Growth hormone is available as the synthetic products somatrem (Protropin) and somatropin (Humatrope). Both are recombinant DNA products, are identical to human growth hormone, and produce skeletal growth in children.

Uses of Growth Hormone

These drugs are administered to children who have not grown because of a deficiency of pituitary growth hormone. They must be used before closure of bone epiphyses. Bone epiphyses are the ends of bones, separated from the main bone but joined to its cartilage, that allow for growth or lengthening of the bone. Growth hormone is ineffective in patients with closed epiphyses because when the epiphyses close, growth (in height) can no longer occur.

Adverse Reactions of Growth Hormone

These hormones cause few adverse reactions when administered as directed. Antibodies to somatropin may develop in a small number of patients, resulting in a failure of the drug to produce growth in the child. Some patients may experience hypothyroidism or insulin resistance. Swelling, joint pain, and muscle pain may also occur.

Contraindications, Precautions, and Interactions of Growth Hormone

- Somatropin is contraindicated in patients with known hypersensitivity to somatropin or sensitivity to benzyl alcohol, and those with epiphyseal closure or underlying cranial lesions.
- The drug is used cautiously in patients with thyroid disease or diabetes.
- Excessive amounts of glucocorticoids may decrease response to somatropin.

Patient Management Issues with Growth Hormone

A thorough physical examination and laboratory and diagnostic tests are performed before a child is accepted into a growth program. Before therapy is started, a patient's vital signs, height, and weight are recorded.

Children may increase their growth rate from 3.5 to 4 cm per year before treatment to 8 to 10 cm per year during the first year of treatment. Each time the child visits the health care provider's office or clinic (usually every 3–6 months), the child's height and weight are measured and recorded to evaluate the response to therapy. Bone age is monitored periodically. The bone age monitors bone growth and detects epiphyseal closure, at which time therapy must be stopped.

Periodic testing of growth hormone levels, glucose tolerance, and thyroid functioning may be performed at intervals during treatment.

Educating the Patient and Family about Growth Hormone

When the patient is receiving growth hormone, the health care provider discusses in detail the therapeutic regimen for increasing growth (height) with the child's parents or guardians. If the drug is to be given at bedtime (which most closely adheres to the body's natural release of the hormone), the parents are instructed on the proper technique to administer the injections. The parents are encouraged to keep all clinic or office visits. The child may experience sudden growth and an increase in appetite, and it is important for the parents to understand these possibilities. The parents are asked to report lack of growth, symptoms of diabetes (e.g., increased hunger, increased thirst, or frequent voiding), or symptoms of hypothyroidism (e.g., fatigue, dry skin, or intolerance to cold).

FACT CHECK

31-4 Why is the timing of growth hormone therapy in children important?

ADRENOCORTICOTROPIC HORMONE: CORTICOTROPIN

Actions of Corticotropin

Corticotropin is an anterior pituitary hormone that stimulates the adrenal cortex to produce and secrete adrenocortical hormones, primarily the glucocorticoids. Cosyntropin is a synthetic version of corticotropin.

Uses of Corticotropin

Corticotropin and cosyntropin are used for diagnostic testing of adrenocortical function. Corticotropin may also be used for the management of acute exacerbations of multiple sclerosis, nonsuppurative thyroiditis, and hypercalcemia associated with cancer. It is also used as an anti-inflammatory and immunosuppressant drug when conventional glucocorticoid therapy has not been effective (see Uses of Glucocorticoids).

Adverse Reactions of Corticotropin

Because ACTH stimulates the release of glucocorticoids from the adrenal gland, adverse reactions of this hormone are similar to those seen with the glucocorticoids (see Adverse Reactions of Glucocorticoids) and affect many body systems. The most common adverse reactions are listed below:

- **Allergic:** especially in patients with allergic responses to proteins manifesting as dizziness, nausea and vomiting, shock, skin reactions
- **Cardiovascular:** hypertension, necrotizing angiitis, congestive heart failure

- **CNS:** convulsions, increased intracranial pressure with papilledema, pseudotumor cerebri (usually after treatment), headache, vertigo
- **Dermatologic:** impaired wound healing, thin fragile skin, petechiae and ecchymoses, facial erythema, increased sweating, suppression of skin test reactions, acne, hyperpigmentation
- **Electrolyte disturbances:** sodium retention, fluid retention, potassium loss, hypokalemic alkalosis, calcium loss
- **Endocrine:** menstrual irregularities; development of cushingoid state; suppression of growth in children; secondary adrenocortical and pituitary unresponsiveness, particularly in times of stress, as in trauma, surgery, or illness; decreased carbohydrate tolerance; manifestations of latent diabetes mellitus; increased requirements for insulin or oral hypoglycemic agents in diabetics; hirsutism
- **GI:** peptic ulcer with possible perforation and hemorrhage, pancreatitis, abdominal distention, ulcerative esophagitis
- **Metabolic:** negative nitrogen balance caused by protein catabolism
- **Ophthalmic:** posterior subcapsular cataracts, increased intraocular pressure, glaucoma with possible damage to optic nerve, exophthalmos
- **Miscellaneous:** abscess, loss of stimulatory effect resulting from prolonged use of ACTH (antibodies to it may develop)

Contraindications, Precautions, and Interactions of Corticotropin

- Corticotropin is contraindicated in patients with adrenocortical insufficiency or hyperfunction, scleroderma, osteoporosis, recent surgery, history of current peptic ulcer, CHF, systemic fungal infections, ocular herpes simplex, scleroderma, or hypertension.
- Corticotropin is contraindicated in patients with a sensitivity to pork or pork products.
- Patients taking corticotropin also should avoid any vaccinations with live virus.
- Corticotropin is used cautiously in patients with diabetes, diverticulosis, renal insufficiencies, myasthenia gravis, tuberculosis (may reactivate the disease), hypothyroidism, cirrhosis, nonspecific ulcerative colitis, heart failure, seizures, or febrile infections.

CONSIDERATIONS Infants & Children

LIFESPAN

Corticotropin Use

Corticotropin is used cautiously in children because it can inhibit skeletal growth. If the drug is used, it should be given intermittently and the child should be observed carefully.

- Corticotropin is used cautiously in children because it can inhibit skeletal growth.
- When amphotericin B or diuretics are administered with corticotropin, the potential for hypokalemia is increased.
- There may be an increased need for insulin or oral antidiabetic drugs in a patient with diabetes who is taking corticotropin.
- There is a decreased effect of corticotropin when the agent is administered with a barbiturate.
- Profound muscular depression is possible when corticotropin is administered with an anticholinesterase drug.
- Live virus vaccines taken while taking corticotropin may potentiate virus replication, increase the vaccine's adverse reaction, and decrease the patient's antibody response to the vaccine.

Patient Management Issues with Corticotropin

Corticotropin may mask signs of infection, including fungal or viral eye infections. Any symptoms of sore throat, cough, fever, malaise, sores that do not heal, or redness or irritation of the eyes should be reported. The patient may have a decreased resistance and inability to localize infection. The patient's skin should be observed daily for localized signs of infection, especially at injection sites or intravenous access sites. Visitors are monitored to protect the patient against those with infectious illness.

Corticotropin can also cause alterations in the psyche. Any evidence of behavior change, such as mental depression, insomnia, euphoria, mood swings, or nervousness must be reported. Anxiety is decreased with understanding of the therapeutic regimen.

Patients with diabetes may require a dosage adjustment of their insulin or oral hypoglycemic medication.

The physician should be notified if the patient experiences a headache, seizure, abdominal pain, muscle weakness, or marked fluid retention.

Educating the Patient and Family about Corticotropin

Following are key points about corticotropin that the patient and family members should know:

- Report any adverse reactions to your health care provider.
- Avoid contact with those who have an infection because your resistance to infection may be decreased.
- Report any symptoms of infection immediately (e.g., sore throat, fever, cough, or sores that do not heal).
- Patients with diabetes: Monitor your blood glucose (if you are performing self-monitoring) or urine closely, and notify your health care provider if glucose appears in the urine or the blood glucose level increases significantly. An increase in the dosage of the oral antidiabetic drug or insulin may be needed.
- Notify your health care provider of a marked weight gain, swelling in the extremities, muscle weakness, persistent headache, visual disturbances, or behavior change.

Posterior Pituitary Hormones

The posterior pituitary gland produces two hormones: vasopressin (antidiuretic hormone) and oxytocin (see Chapter 34). Posterior pituitary hormones are summarized in the Summary Drug Table: Anterior and Posterior Pituitary Hormones.

VASOPRESSIN

Actions of Vasopressin

Vasopressin (Pitressin Synthetic) and its derivative desmopressin (DDAVP) regulate the reabsorption of water by the kidneys. The pituitary secretes vasopressin when body fluids must be conserved. An example of this mechanism may be seen when a patient has severe vomiting and diarrhea with little or no fluid intake. When this and similar conditions are present, the posterior pituitary releases the hormone vasopressin, water in the kidneys is reabsorbed into the blood (i.e., conserved), and the urine becomes concentrated. Vasopressin exhibits its greatest activity on the renal tubular epithelium, where it promotes water resorption and smooth muscle contraction throughout the vascular bed. Vasopressin has some vasopressor activity.

Uses of Vasopressin

Vasopressin and its derivatives are used in the treatment of **diabetes insipidus**, a disease resulting from the failure of the pituitary to secrete vasopressin or from surgical removal of the pituitary. Diabetes insipidus is characterized by marked increase in urination (as much as 10 L in 24 hours) and excessive thirst. Treatment with vasopressin therapy replaces the hormone in the body and restores normal urination and thirst. Vasopressin may also be used for the prevention and treatment of postoperative abdominal distention and to dispel gas interfering with abdominal x-rays.

Adverse Reactions of Vasopressin

Local or systemic hypersensitivity reactions may occur in some patients receiving vasopressin. Tremor, sweating, vertigo, nausea, vomiting, abdominal cramps, and water intoxication (overdosage, toxicity) may also occur.

The adverse reactions of vasopressin, such as skin blanching, abdominal cramps, and nausea, may be decreased by administering the agent with one or two glasses of water. If these adverse reactions occur, the patient should be told that these reactions are not serious and should disappear within a few minutes.

Contraindications, Precautions, and Interactions of Vasopressin

- Vasopressin is contraindicated in patients with chronic renal failure, increased blood urea nitrogen, or an allergy to beef or pork proteins.
- Vasopressin is used cautiously in patients with a history of seizures, migraine headaches, asthma, congestive heart failure, or vascular disease (may precipitate angina or myocardial infarction) and in those with perioperative polyuria.
- The antidiuretic effects of vasopressin may be decreased when the agent is taken with the following drugs: lithium, heparin, norepinephrine, or alcohol. The antidiuretic effect may be increased when the drug is used with carbamazepine, clofibrate, or fludrocortisone.

Patient Management Issues with Vasopressin

Before administering the first dose of vasopressin for the management of diabetes insipidus, the patient's blood pressure, pulse, respiratory rate, and weight are measured. Serum electrolyte levels and other laboratory tests may be ordered.

Before administering vasopressin to relieve abdominal distention, the patient's blood pressure, pulse, and respiratory rate are taken, and the patient's abdominal girth is measured and recorded.

Vasopressin may be given intramuscularly or subcutaneously to treat diabetes insipidus. The injection solution may also be administered intranasally on cotton pledgets or by nasal spray or dropper. The health care provider instructs the patient about intranasal administration. To prevent or relieve abdominal distension, it may be given intramuscularly.

Desmopressin may be given orally, intranasally, subcutaneously, or intravenously. The oral dose must be individualized for each patient and adjusted according to the patient's response to therapy. When the drug is administered nasally, a nasal tube is used for administration.

Managing Fluid Volume

The symptoms of diabetes insipidus include the voiding of a large volume of urine at frequent intervals during the day and throughout the night. Accompanied by frequent urination is the need to drink large volumes of fluid because these patients are continually thirsty. Patients must be supplied with large amounts of drinking water. When the patient has limited ability to move about, water should be readily available. Until controlled by a drug, the symptoms of frequent urination and excessive thirst may cause a great deal of anxiety. The patient should be reassured that with the proper drug therapy, these symptoms will most likely be reduced or eliminated.

Educating the Patient and Family about Vasopressin

Patients should be reminded of the importance of adhering to their prescribed treatment program. Following are key points about vasopressin that the patient and family members should know:

- Drink one or two glasses of water immediately before taking the drug.
- Measure the amount of fluids you drink each day.
- Measure the amount of urine passed at each voiding, and then total the amount for each 24-hour period.
- Do not drink alcohol while taking these drugs.
- Rotate injection sites for parenteral administration.
- Contact your primary health care provider immediately if you experience any of the following: a significant increase or decrease in urinary output, abdominal cramps, blanching of the skin, nausea, signs of inflammation or infection at the injection sites, confusion, headache, or drowsiness.
- Wear a medical alert tag identifying the diabetes insipidus and your drug regimen.

FACT CHECK

31-8   A serious adverse reaction of vasopressin is water intoxication. What are its symptoms?

Adrenocortical Hormones

The adrenal gland lies on the superior surface of each kidney. It is a double organ composed of an outer cortex and an inner medulla. In response to adrenocorticotropic hormone secreted by the anterior pituitary, the adrenal cortex secretes several hormones (the glucocorticoids, the mineralocorticoids, and small amounts of sex hormones).

This section of the chapter discusses the hormones produced by the adrenal cortex or the adrenocortical hormones, which are the **glucocorticoids** and **mineralocorticoids.** These hormones are essential to life and influence many organs and structures of the body. The glucocorticoids and mineralocorticoids are collectively called **corticosteroids**.

FACT CHECK

31-9   Where is the adrenal cortex located?
31-10   Which hormones are produced by the adrenal cortex?

GLUCOCORTICOIDS

Actions of Glucocorticoids

The glucocorticoids influence or regulate functions such as the immune response, the regulation of glucose, fat and protein metabolism, and control of the anti-inflammatory response. Table 31-1 describes the activity of the glucocorticoids within the body.

The glucocorticoids enter target cells and bind to receptors, initiating many complex reactions in the body. Some of these actions are considered undesirable, depending on the indication for which these drugs are being used. Examples of the glucocorticoids include cortisone, hydrocortisone, prednisone, prednisolone, and triamcinolone.

Uses of Glucocorticoids

The glucocorticoids are used as replacement therapy for adrenocortical insufficiency and to treat allergic reactions, collagen diseases (e.g., systemic lupus erythematosus), dermatologic conditions, rheumatic disorders, shock, and other conditions listed below. The anti-inflammatory activity of these hormones makes them valuable as anti-inflammatories and as immunosuppressants to suppress inflammation and modify the immune response.

- **Endocrine disorders:** primary or secondary adrenal cortical insufficiency, congenital adrenal hyperplasia, nonsuppressive thyroiditis, hypercalcemia associated with cancer
- **Rheumatic disorders:** short-term management of acute ankylosing spondylitis, acute and subacute bursitis, acute nonspecific tenosynovitis, acute gouty arthritis,

TABLE 31-1 Activity of Glucocorticoids in the Body

Function within the Body	Description of Bodily Activity
Anti-inflammatory	Stabilizes lysosomal membrane and prevents the release of proteolytic enzymes released during the inflammatory process
Regulation of blood pressure	Potentiates vasoconstrictor action of norepinephrine. Without glucocorticoids, the vasoconstricting action is decreased and blood pressure falls.
Metabolism of carbohydrates and protein	Facilitates the breakdown of protein in the muscle, leading to increased plasma amino acid levels. Increases activity of enzymes necessary for glucogenesis, producing hyperglycemia, which can aggravate diabetes, precipitate latent diabetes, and cause insulin resistance
Metabolism of fat	A complex phenomena that promotes the use of fat for energy (a positive effect) and permits fat stores to accumulate in the body, causing buffalo hump and moon-shaped or round face (a negative effect)
Interference with the immune response	Decreases the production of lymphocytes and eosinophils in the blood by causing atrophy of the thymus gland; blocks the release of cytokines, resulting in a decreased performance of T and B monocytes in the immune response (this action, coupled with the anti-inflammatory action, makes the corticosteroids useful in delaying organ rejection in patients with transplants)
Stress	As a protective mechanism, the corticosteroids are released during periods of stress (e.g., injury or surgery). The release of epinephrine or norepinephrine by the adrenal medulla during stress has a synergistic effect along with the corticosteroids.
Central nervous system disturbances	Affects mood and possibly causes neuronal or brain excitability, causing euphoria, anxiety, depression, psychosis, and an increase in motor activity in some individuals

psoriatic arthritis, rheumatoid arthritis, posttraumatic osteoarthritis, synovitis of osteoarthritis, epicondylitis
- **Collagen diseases:** lupus erythematosus, acute rheumatic carditis, systemic dermatomyositis
- **Dermatologic diseases:** pemphigus, bullous dermatitis herpetiformis, severe erythema multiforme (Stevens-Johnson syndrome), exfoliative dermatitis, mycosis fungoides, severe psoriasis, severe seborrheic dermatitis, angioedema, urticaria, various skin disorders, such as lichen planus or keloids
- **Allergic states:** control of severe or incapacitating allergic conditions not controlled by other methods, bronchial asthma (including status asthmaticus), contact dermatitis, atopic dermatitis, serum sickness, drug hypersensitivity reactions
- **Ophthalmic diseases:** severe acute and chronic allergic and inflammatory processes, keratitis, allergic corneal marginal ulcers, herpes zoster of the eye, iritis, iridocyclitis, chorioretinitis, diffuse posterior uveitis, optic neuritis, sympathetic ophthalmia, anterior segment inflammation
- **Respiratory diseases:** sarcoidosis, berylliosis, fulminating or disseminating pulmonary tuberculosis, aspiration pneumonia
- **Hematologic disorders:** idiopathic or secondary thrombocytopenic purpura, hemolytic anemia, red blood cell anemia, congenital hypoplastic anemia
- **Neoplastic diseases:** leukemia, lymphomas
- **Edematous states:** to induce diuresis or remission of proteinuria in the nephrotic state
- **Gastrointestinal diseases:** during critical period of ulcerative colitis, regional enteritis, intractable sprue
- **Nervous system:** acute exacerbations of multiple sclerosis

Adverse Reactions of Glucocorticoids

The adverse reactions of glucocorticoids are listed below. Long- or short-term high-dose therapy may also produce many of the signs and symptoms seen with **Cushing syndrome** (Key Concepts 31-2).

- **Fluid and electrolyte disturbances:** sodium and fluid retention, congestive heart failure in susceptible patients, potassium loss, hypokalemic alkalosis, hypertension, hypocalcemia, hypotension or shock-like reactions, metabolic alkalosis, hypocalcemia
- **Musculoskeletal:** muscle weakness, loss of muscle mass, tendon rupture, osteoporosis, aseptic necrosis of femoral and humoral heads, spontaneous fractures, steroid myopathy

KEY CONCEPTS

31-2 Cushing Syndrome

Cushing syndrome is a disease caused by the overproduction of endogenous glucocorticoids. Some of the signs and symptoms of this Cushing-like (or cushingoid) state include a "buffalo" hump (a hump on the back of the neck), moon face, oily skin and acne, osteoporosis, purple striae on the abdomen and hips, skin pigmentation, and weight gain. When a serious disease or disorder is being treated, it is often necessary to allow these effects to occur because therapy with these drugs is absolutely necessary.

- **Cardiovascular:** thromboembolism or fat embolism, thrombophlebitis, necrotizing angiitis, syncopal episodes, cardiac arrhythmias, aggravation of hypertension, myocardial rupture in patients who have recently experienced an MI
- **Gastrointestinal:** pancreatitis, abdominal distention, ulcerative esophagitis, nausea, increased appetite and weight gain, possible peptic ulcer with perforation, hemorrhage, vomiting, perforation of small and large intestines particularly in patients with inflammatory bowel disease
- **Dermatologic:** impaired wound healing, thin fragile skin, petechiae, ecchymoses, erythema, increased sweating, suppression of skin test reactions, subcutaneous fat atrophy, purpura, striae, hyperpigmentation, hirsutism, acneiform eruptions, urticaria, angioneurotic edema, lupus erythematosus–like lesions, allergic dermatitis, perineal irritation, urticaria, angioneurotic edema
- **Neurologic:** convulsions, increased intracranial pressure with papilledema (usually after treatment is discontinued), vertigo, headache, neuritis or paresthesia, steroid psychosis, aggravation of preexisting psychiatric disorders
- **Endocrine:** amenorrhea, postmenopausal bleeding, other menstrual irregularities, development of cushingoid state, suppression of growth in children, secondary adrenocortical and pituitary unresponsive (particularly in times of stress), increased sweating, decreased carbohydrate tolerance, manifestation of latent diabetes

ALERT Rx

Ending Glucocorticoid Therapy
At no time should glucocorticoid therapy be discontinued suddenly. When administration of a glucocorticoid extends beyond 5 days and the drug therapy is to be discontinued, the dosage must be tapered off over several days. In some instances, it may be necessary to taper the dose over 7 to 10 or more days. Abrupt discontinuation of glucocorticoid therapy usually results in acute adrenal insufficiency, which, if not recognized in time, can result in death. Tapering the dosage allows normal adrenal function to return gradually, preventing adrenal insufficiency.

mellitus, increased requirements for insulin or oral hypoglycemic agents (in diabetics), hyperglycemia, glycosuria, hirsutism
- **Ophthalmic:** posterior subcapsular cataracts, increased intraocular pressure, glaucoma, exophthalmos
- **Metabolic:** negative nitrogen balance (caused by protein catabolism)
- **Others:** anaphylactoid or hypersensitivity reactions, aggravation of existing infections, masking of infections, malaise, fatigue, leukocytosis, insomnia, increase or decrease in sperm motility and number
- When administered as an intra-articular injection, the patient may experience osteonecrosis, tendon rupture, skin atrophy, infection, facial flushing, postinjection flare, and hypersensitivity.
- When administered as an intraspinal injection, the patient may experience meningitis, adhesive arachnoiditis, and conus medullaris syndrome.

Contraindications, Precautions, and Interactions of Glucocorticoids

- The glucocorticoids are contraindicated in patients with serious infections, such as tuberculosis and fungal and antibiotic-resistant infections. The glucocorticoids are administered with caution to patients with renal or hepatic disease, hypothyroidism, ulcerative colitis, diverticulitis, peptic ulcer disease, inflammatory bowel disease, hypertension, osteoporosis, convulsive disorders, or diabetes.
- The glucocorticoids should be used with caution during pregnancy and lactation.
- Many drug interactions may occur with the glucocorticoids. Table 31-2 identifies select clinically significant interactions.

ALERT Rx

Adrenal Insufficiency
Administration of the glucocorticoids poses the threat of **adrenal insufficiency** (particularly if the alternate-day therapy is not prescribed). Administration of glucocorticoids several times per day and during a short time (as little as 5–10 days) results in shutting off the pituitary release of adrenocorticotropic hormone because there are always high levels of the glucocorticoids in the plasma (caused by the body's own glucocorticoid production plus the administration of a glucocorticoid drug). Ultimately, the pituitary atrophies and ceases to release adrenocorticotropic hormone. Without adrenocorticotropic hormone, the adrenals fail to manufacture and release (endogenous) glucocorticoids. When this happens, the patient has acute adrenal insufficiency, which is a life-threatening situation until corrected with the administration of an exogenous glucocorticoid. Symptoms of adrenal insufficiency include fever, myalgia, arthralgia, malaise, anorexia, nausea, orthostatic hypotension, dizziness, fainting, dyspnea, and hypoglycemia. Situations producing stress (e.g., trauma, surgery, severe illness) may precipitate the need for an increase in dosage of the corticosteroids until the crisis situation is resolved.

FACT CHECK
31-11 What is adrenal insufficiency?
31-12 When are glucocorticoids contraindicated?

TABLE 31-2   Select Drug Interactions of Glucocorticoids

Precipitant Drug	Object Drug	Description
Barbiturates	Corticosteroids	Decreased pharmacologic effects of the corticosteroid may be observed.
Cholestyramine	Hydrocortisone	The effects of hydrocortisone may be decreased.
Contraceptives, oral	Corticosteroids	Corticosteroid concentration may be increased and clearance decreased.
Estrogens	Corticosteroids	Corticosteroid clearance may be decreased.
Hydantoin	Corticosteroids	Corticosteroid clearance may be increased, resulting in reduced therapeutic effects.
Ketoconazole	Corticosteroids	Corticosteroid clearance may be decreased.
Rifampin	Corticosteroids	Corticosteroid clearance may be increased, resulting in decreased therapeutic effects.
Corticosteroids	Anticholinesterases	Anticholinesterase effects may be antagonized in myasthenia gravis.
Corticosteroids	Anticoagulants, oral	Anticoagulant dose requirements may be reduced; corticosteroids may decrease the anticoagulant action.
Corticosteroids	Digitalis glycosides	Coadministration may enhance the possibility of digitalis toxicity associated with hypokalemia.
Corticosteroids	Isoniazid	Isoniazid serum concentrations may be decreased.
Corticosteroids	Potassium-depleting diuretics	Hypokalemia may occur.
Corticosteroids	Salicylates	Corticosteroids will reduce serum salicylate levels and may decrease their effectiveness.
Corticosteroids	Somatrem	Growth-promoting effect of somatrem may be inhibited.
Corticosteroids	Theophyllines	Alterations in the pharmacologic activity of either agent may occur.

MINERALOCORTICOIDS

Actions of Mineralocorticoids

The mineralocorticoids consist of aldosterone and desoxy-corticosterone, which play an important role in conserving sodium and increasing the excretion of potassium. Because of these activities, the mineralocorticoids are important in controlling salt and water balance. Aldosterone is the more potent of these two hormones. Deficiencies of the mineralocorticoids result in a loss of sodium and water and a retention of potassium. Fludrocortisone (Florinef) has both glucocorticoid and mineralocorticoid activity and is the only currently available mineralocorticoid drug.

Uses of Mineralocorticoids

Fludrocortisone is used for replacement therapy for primary and secondary adrenocortical deficiency. Even though this drug has both mineralocorticoid and glucocorticoid activity, it is used only for its mineralocorticoid effects.

Adverse Reactions of Mineralocorticoids

Adverse reactions may occur if the dosage is too high or prolonged, or if withdrawal is too rapid. Administration of fludrocortisone may cause edema, hypertension, congestive heart failure, enlargement of the heart, increased sweating,

or allergic skin rash. Additional adverse reactions include hypokalemia, muscular weakness, headache, and hypersensitivity reactions. Because this drug has glucocorticoid and mineralocorticoid activity and is often given with a glucocorticoid, adverse reactions of the glucocorticoid must be closely monitored as well.

Fluid and electrolyte imbalances, particularly excess fluid volume, are common with corticosteroid therapy. If signs of electrolyte imbalance or glucocorticoid drug effects occur, then the health care provider should be notified. Dietary adjustments are made for the increased loss of potassium and the retention of sodium if necessary. Consultation with a dietitian may be indicated.

Contraindications, Precautions, and Interactions of Mineralocorticoids

- Fludrocortisone is contraindicated in patients with hypersensitivity to fludrocortisone and those with systemic fungal infections.
- Fludrocortisone is used cautiously in patients with Addison disease or infection and during pregnancy and lactation.
- Fludrocortisone decreases the effects of the barbiturates, hydantoins, and rifampin.
- There is a decrease in serum levels of the salicylates when those agents are administered with fludrocortisone.

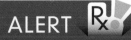

ALERT

Missing a Glucocorticoid Dosage

A glucocorticoid dosage must never be omitted. If the patient cannot take the drug orally because of nausea or vomiting, then the health care provider must be notified immediately because the drug needs to be given parenterally. Patients who are receiving nothing by mouth for any reason must have parenteral glucocorticoid.

FACT CHECK

31-13 High-dose therapy with glucocorticoids may produce a cushingoid state. What are the signs and symptoms?

31-14 What is the result of mineralocorticoid deficiency?

Patient Management Issues with Glucocorticoids and Mineralocorticoids

Because these drugs are used to treat a great many diseases and conditions, an evaluation of drug response is based on the patient's diagnosis and the signs and symptoms of disease.

Adverse effects of the mineralocorticoid or glucocorticoid, particularly signs of electrolyte imbalance, such as hypocalcemia, hypokalemia, and hypernatremia (see Chapter 25), are closely monitored. The patient's mental status is monitored for any change, especially if there is a history of depression or other psychiatric problems, or if high doses of the drug are being given. The patient is also monitored for signs of an infection, which may be masked by glucocorticoid therapy. Patients receiving long-term glucocorticoid therapy, especially those allowed limited activity, should be observed for signs of compression fractures of the vertebrae and pathologic fractures of the long bones. If the patient reports back or bone pain, then the health care provider should be notified. The blood of patients without diabetes is checked weekly for glucose levels because glucocorticoids may aggravate latent diabetes. Those with diabetes must be checked more frequently.

When administering fludrocortisone, the patient's blood pressure is monitored at frequent intervals. Hypotension may

CONSIDERATIONS Older adults

LIFESPAN

Corticosteroid Use

Corticosteroids are administered with caution in older adults because they are more likely to have preexisting conditions, such as congestive heart failure, hypertension, osteoporosis, or arthritis, that may be worsened by the use of such agents. Older adults are monitored for exacerbation of existing conditions during corticosteroid therapy. In addition, lower dosages may be needed because of the effects of aging, such as decreased muscle mass, renal function, and plasma volume.

indicate insufficient dosage. Edema, particularly swelling of the feet and hands, is closely monitored. The lungs are auscultated for adventitious sounds (e.g., rales or crackles).

Alternate-Day Therapy

An alternate-day therapy with glucocorticoid is used in the treatment of diseases and disorders requiring long-term therapy, especially arthritic disorders. This regimen involves giving twice the daily dose of the glucocorticoid every other day. The purpose of alternate-day administration is to provide the patient requiring long-term glucocorticoid therapy with the beneficial effects of the drug while minimizing certain undesirable reactions (see Adverse Reactions of Glucocorticoids).

Plasma levels of the endogenous adrenocortical hormones vary throughout the day and nighttime hours. They are normally higher between 2.00 AM and approximately 8.00 AM and lower between 4.00 PM and midnight. When plasma levels are lower, the anterior pituitary releases adrenocorticotropic hormone, which in turn stimulates the adrenal cortex to manufacture and release glucocorticoids. When plasma levels are high, the pituitary gland does not release adrenocorticotropic hormone. The response of the pituitary to high or low plasma levels of glucocorticoids and the resulting release or nonrelease of adrenocorticotropic hormone is an example of the feedback mechanism, which may also be seen in other glands of the body, such as the thyroid gland. The feedback mechanism is how the body maintains most hormones at relatively constant levels within the bloodstream. When the hormone concentration falls, the rate of production of that hormone increases. Likewise, when the hormone level becomes too high, the body decreases production of that hormone.

Administration of a short-acting glucocorticoid on alternate days and before 9.00 AM, when glucocorticoid plasma levels are still relatively high, does not affect the release of adrenocorticotropic hormone later in the day, yet it gives the patient the benefit of exogenous glucocorticoid therapy.

Patients with Diabetes

Patients with diabetes who are receiving a glucocorticoid may require frequent adjustment of their insulin or oral hypoglycemic drug dosage. Blood glucose levels are monitored several times daily or as prescribed by the health care provider. If the patient's blood glucose levels increase or if the urine is positive for glucose or ketones, then the health care provider should be notified. Some patients may have latent (hidden) diabetes. In these cases, the corticosteroid may precipitate hyperglycemia. Therefore, all patients, those with diabetes and those without, should have frequent checks of blood glucose levels.

Educating the Patient and Family about Glucocorticoid and Mineralocorticoid Therapy

Following are key points about glucocorticoid and mineralocorticoid therapy that the patient and family members should know:

- These drugs may cause gastrointestinal upset. To decrease gastrointestinal effects, take the oral drug with meals or snacks.
- Take antacids between meals to help prevent peptic ulcer.

Short-Term Glucocorticoid Therapy

- Take the drug exactly as directed on the prescription container. Do not increase, decrease, or omit a dose unless advised to do so by your health care provider.
- Take single daily doses before 9.00 AM.
- Follow the instructions for tapering the dose because they are extremely important.
- If the problem does not improve, then contact your health care provider.

Alternate-Day Oral Glucocorticoid Therapy

- Take this drug before 9.00 AM once every other day. Use a calendar or some other method to identify the days of each week to take the drug.
- Do not stop taking the drug unless advised to do so by your health care provider.
- If the problem becomes worse, especially on the days the drug is not taken, then contact your health care provider.

Most of the information below may also apply to alternate-day therapy, especially when higher doses are used and therapy extends over many months.

Long-Term or High-Dose Glucocorticoid Therapy

- Do not miss a dose of this drug or increase or decrease the dosage except on the advice of your health care provider.
- Inform your other health care providers, dentists, and all medical personnel that you are taking this drug. Wear a medical alert tag or other form of identification to alert medical personnel of your long-term therapy with a glucocorticoid.
- Do not take any nonprescription drug unless your health care provider has approved its use.
- Do not take live virus vaccinations (e.g., smallpox) because of the risk of a lack of antibody response. This does not include patients receiving the corticosteroids as replacement therapy.
- Whenever possible, avoid exposure to infections. Contact your health care provider if minor cuts or abrasions fail to heal or if you experience persistent joint swelling or tenderness, fever, sore throat, upper respiratory infection, or other signs of infection.
- If you cannot take this drug orally for any reason or if you have diarrhea, then contact your health care provider immediately. If you are unable to contact your health care provider before the next dose is due, then go to the nearest hospital emergency department (preferably where the original treatment was started or where your health care provider is on the hospital staff) because the drug has to be given by injection.
- Weigh yourself weekly. If you experience significant weight gain or swelling of the extremities, then contact your health care provider.
- Remember that dietary recommendations made by the health care provider are an important part of the therapy and must be followed.
- Follow the health care provider's recommendations regarding periodic eye examinations and laboratory tests.

Intra-Articular or Intralesional Administrations

- Do not overuse the injected joint, even if the pain is gone.
- Follow your health care provider's instructions concerning rest and exercise.

Mineralocorticoid (Fludrocortisone) Therapy

- Take the drug as directed. Do not increase or decrease the dosage except as instructed to do so by your health care provider.
- Do not stop using the drug abruptly.
- Inform your health care provider if you experience the following adverse reactions: edema, muscle weakness, weight gain, anorexia, swelling of the extremities, dizziness, severe headache, or shortness of breath.
- Carry patient identification, such as a medical alert tag, so that medical personnel will know your drug therapy during an emergency situation.
- Keep follow-up appointments to determine if a dosage adjustment is necessary.

Chapter Review

KEY POINTS

- The pituitary gland secretes hormones that regulate growth, metabolism, the reproductive cycle, electrolyte balance, and water retention or loss. The hormones of the anterior pituitary include follicle-stimulating hormone, luteinizing hormone, growth hormone, adrenocorticotropic hormone, thyroid-stimulating hormone, and prolactin.
- The gonadotropins (follicle-stimulating hormone and luteinizing hormone) influence the secretion of sex hormones, development of secondary sex characteristics, and the reproductive cycle in both men and women. These include menotropins, follitropins, clomiphene, and chorionic gonadotropin.
- Menotropins and follitropins induce ovulation and pregnancy. In men, menotropins are used to induce the production of sperm (spermatogenesis). Multiple births and birth defects have been reported with the use of both menotropins and follitropins.
- The actions of chorionic gonadotropin are identical to those of the pituitary luteinizing hormone. Clomiphene and chorionic gonadotropin are both used to induce ovulation in anovulatory women. Chorionic gonadotropin is also used for the treatment of prepubertal cryptorchism and in men to treat selected cases of hypogonadotropic hypogonadism.

- Growth hormone is secreted by the anterior pituitary and regulates the growth of the individual until early adulthood. Growth hormone is available as the synthetic product somatropin and is administered to children who have not grown because of a deficiency of pituitary growth hormone. The drug must be used before closure of bone epiphyses in order to be effective.

- Corticotropin is an anterior pituitary hormone that stimulates the adrenal cortex to produce and secrete adrenocortical hormones, primarily glucocorticoids. It is used for diagnostic testing of adrenocortical function. It may also be used for the management of acute exacerbations of multiple sclerosis, nonsuppurative thyroiditis, or hypercalcemia associated with cancer, and as an anti-inflammatory and immunosuppressant drug when conventional glucocorticoid therapy has not been effective. Adverse reactions may affect many body systems.

- Vasopressin, a posterior pituitary gland hormone, and its derivatives regulate the resorption of water by the kidneys and are used in the treatment of diabetes insipidus. Vasopressin may also be used for the prevention and treatment of postoperative abdominal distention and to dispel gas interfering with abdominal x-rays. Water intoxication (fluid overload) is a serious adverse reaction that may occur with vasopressin use.

- The adrenal cortex secretes several hormones (the glucocorticoids, the mineralocorticoids, and small amounts of sex hormones). The glucocorticoids and mineralocorticoids are collectively called corticosteroids.

- The glucocorticoids influence or regulate functions such as the immune response system, the regulation of glucose, fat and protein metabolism, and control of the anti-inflammatory response. The glucocorticoids are used as replacement therapy for adrenocortical insufficiency and to treat allergic reactions, collagen diseases, dermatologic conditions, rheumatic disorders, shock, and other conditions. Because of their anti-inflammatory activity, they are valuable as anti-inflammatories and as immunosuppressants to suppress inflammation and modify the immune response. High-dose therapy may produce many of the signs and symptoms seen with Cushing syndrome.

- The mineralocorticoids aldosterone and desoxycorticosterone play an important role in conserving sodium and increasing the excretion of potassium and are important in controlling salt and water balance. Deficiencies of the mineralocorticoids result in a loss of sodium and water and a retention of potassium. Fludrocortisone (Florinef) has both glucocorticoid and mineralocorticoid activity and is the only currently available mineralocorticoid drug.

CRITICAL THINKING CASE STUDY
CASE 1
Clomiphene Therapy

Judy Cowan, age 28 years, has been prescribed clomiphene to induce ovulation and pregnancy. Judy is very anxious and wants desperately to become pregnant. Her husband, Jim, has come to the clinic with her.

1. Before beginning treatment with clomiphene, the health care provider would want to determine if Judy has
   a. liver disease
   b. ovarian cysts
   c. abnormal bleeding of unknown cause
   d. all of the above
2. Adverse reactions to clomiphene include
   a. ovarian enlargements
   b. vasomotor flushes
   c. abdominal discomfort
   d. all of the above
3. How is clomiphene usually taken?

CASE 2
Contact Dermatitis

Mr. Barnes was working in his yard last weekend and was exposed to poison ivy. At the time, he did not realize what it was until he had a red, itchy rash all over his forearms. His physician has prescribed a methylprednisolone dosepak.

1. How should Mr. Barnes take methylprednisolone with regard to food?
   a. With food because it may upset his stomach
   b. Without food because food slows absorption
   c. With or without food because it does not have any GI adverse reactions
   d. At least 1 hour before or 2 hours after food because food will prevent absorption
2. While taking methylprednisolone, Mr. Barnes should be monitored for
   a. electrolyte imbalance
   b. mental status changes
   c. signs of infection
   d. all of the above
3. The dosepak requires that Mr. Barnes take 6 tablets the first day, gradually tapering down by one tablet every day until the dosepak is complete. He asks you why the drug is dosed this way. What should you tell him?

Review Questions

MULTIPLE CHOICE

1. Somatotropic hormone is
   a. secreted by the anterior pituitary
   b. secreted by the posterior pituitary
   c. used for diabetes insipidus
   d. used for prepubertal cryptorchism
2. Vasopressin is contraindicated in patients with all of the following conditions EXCEPT
   a. chronic renal failure
   b. increased blood urea nitrogen
   c. systemic fungal infections
   d. allergy to beef or pork proteins
3. Which of the following drugs would likely be prescribed for a patient experiencing ovulatory failure?
   a. clomiphene
   b. somatropin
   c. menotropins
   d. vasopressin

4. What are the adverse reactions of glucocorticoids?
   a. Increased appetite and weight gain
   b. Impaired wound healing
   c. Fluid and electrolyte disturbances
   d. All of the above

5. Which of the following occurs when corticosteroids are administered with salicylates?
   a. Serum salicylate levels are increased.
   b. Serum salicylate levels are reduced.
   c. Salicylate toxicity will occur.
   d. None of the above

6. Which of the following adverse reactions would lead the health care provider to suspect cushingoid appearance in a patient taking a corticosteroid?
   a. Moon face
   b. Kyphosis, periorbital edema
   c. Dry skin
   d. Exophthalmos

MATCHING

Match the drug on the left with the correct category on the right.

_____ 7. vasopressin	a.	Anterior pituitary hormone
_____ 8. betamethasone	b.	Posterior pituitary hormone
_____ 9. clomiphene	c.	Glucocorticoid
_____ 10. fludrocortisone	d.	Mineralocorticoid

Match the generic name on the left with the correct trade name on the right.

_____ 11. methylprednisolone	a.	Celestone
_____ 12. clomiphene	b.	DDAVP
_____ 13. betamethasone	c.	Acthar HP
_____ 14. corticotropin	d.	Pitressin Synthetic
_____ 15. desmopressin	e.	Menopur
_____ 16. menotropins	f.	Medrol
_____ 17. budesonide	g.	Clomid
_____ 18. vasopressin	h.	Entocort EC

TRUE OR FALSE

_____ 19. Patients receiving vasopressin should be instructed to drink one or two glasses of water immediately before taking the drug.

_____ 20. Chorionic gonadotropin is used to stimulate spermatogenesis.

_____ 21. Patients with diabetes who are taking a glucocorticoid may require frequent dosage adjustments of their insulin or oral hypoglycemic drug.

_____ 22. Patients taking clomiphene may experience vasomotor flushes similar to menopausal hot flashes.

_____ 23. A patient with diabetes insipidus would have decreased urination and excessive thirst.

_____ 24. Fludrocortisone is contraindicated in patients with systemic fungal infections.

FILL IN THE BLANKS

25. Growth hormone is contraindicated in patients with _____ closure.

26. Follicle-stimulating hormone and _____ hormone are called _____, which influence the secretion of sex hormones, development of secondary sex characteristics, and the male and female reproductive cycle.

27. A patient with polycystic ovarian disease would likely be prescribed _____ to induce ovulation.

28. A patient whose testes have failed to descend into the scrotum would likely be treated with _____ _____.

29. Patients on long-term _____ therapy should be instructed to weigh themselves _____ and to contact the health care provider if they experience significant weight gain or edema.

30. _____ and _____ are used to treat diabetes insipidus.

SHORT ANSWERS

31. Why should glucocorticoid therapy NOT be discontinued abruptly?

32. Why is growth hormone ineffective in patients with closed epiphyses?

33. What are the symptoms that indicate hyperstimulation syndrome may be developing?

34. Why are corticosteroids used with caution in older adults?

35. What key instructions are needed for patients taking parenteral vasopressin?

36. Why are menotropins, urofollitropin, and chorionic gonadotropin administered intramuscularly?

Web Activities

1. Go to the MedlinePlus Web site (http://www.nlm.nih.gov/medlineplus/) and conduct a search for "ovarian hyperstimulation syndrome" or "OHSS." What are the causes of OHSS?

2. Go to the Mayo Clinic Web site (www.mayoclinic.com) and conduct a search on human growth hormone. Does human growth hormone slow aging? For an adult with a growth hormone deficiency, what are the benefits of growth hormone injections?

SUMMARY DRUG TABLE Anterior and Posterior Pituitary Hormones (left, generic; right, trade)

Comprehensive Summary Drug Tables, including uses, adverses effects, dosages, and pregnancy classifications, are provided on the companion website, http://thePoint.lww.com/PharmacologyHP2e

Anterior Pituitary Hormones	
human chorionic gonadotropin (hCG) *go-nad'-oh-tro-pin*	Novarel, Pregnyl, *generic*
choriogonadotropin alfa	Ovidrel
clomiphene citrate *klo'-mi-feen*	Clomid, Serophene, *generic*
corticotropin (ACTH) *kor-ti-ko-trop'-in*	Acthar HP
cosyntropin *koe-sin-troe'-pin*	Cortrosyn, *generic*
follitropin alfa *foe-li-tro'-pin al'-fa*	Gonal-f, Gonal-f RFF, Gonal-f RFF Pen
follitropin beta *foe-li-tro'-pin bay'-ta*	Follistim AQ
lutropin alfa *loo'-troe-pin al'-fa*	Luveris
menotropins *men-oh-troe'-pins*	Menopur, Repronex
somatropin *soe-ma-tro'-pin*	Genotropin, Genotropin MiniQuick, Humatrope, Norditropin, Norditropin FlexPro, Norditropin FlexPro Pen, Nutropin, Nutropin AQ, Nutropin AQ Pen, Omnitrope, Saizen, Saizen Click Easy, Serostim, Tev-Tropin, Zorbtive
urofollitropin *your-oh-fahl-ih-troe'-pin*	Bravelle
Posterior Pituitary Hormones	
desmopressin acetate *des-moe-press'-in*	DDAVP, DDAVP Rhinal Tube, Desmopressin Ace Rhinal Tube, Desmopressin Ace Spray Refrig, Minirin, Stimate, *generic*
vasopressin *vay-soe-press'-in*	Pitressin Synthetic, *generic*

SUMMARY DRUG TABLE Adrenocortical Hormones: Glucocorticoids and Mineralocorticoids (left, generic; right, trade)

Comprehensive Summary Drug Tables, including uses, adverses effects, dosages, and pregnancy classifications, are provided on the companion website, http://thePoint.lww.com/PharmacologyHP2e

Glucocorticoids	
betamethasone *bay-ta-meth'-a-zone*	Oral: Celestone Topical: Beta-Val, Luxiq, *generic*
betamethasone sodium phosphate/betamethasone acetate	Celestone Soluspan
budesonide *bue-des'-oh-nide*	Entocort EC (oral), Pulmicort (inhalation), Rhinocort Aqua (nasal)
cortisone *kor'-ti-sone*	*generic*
dexamethasone *dex-a-meth'-a-sone*	Oral: Baycadron, Dexamethasone Intensol, DexPak, *generic* Injection: *generic* Ophthalmic: Maxidex, *generic* Intraocular: Ozurdex
hydrocortisone (cortisol) *hye-droe-kor-ti-zone*	Oral: *generic* Topical: many trade names, *generic* (Rx and OTC) Rectal: many trade names, *generic* Injection: Solu-Cortef Enema: Cortenema, Colocort, *generic*
methylprednisolone *meth-ill-pred-niss'-oh-lone*	Oral: Medrol, *generic* Injection: A-Methapred, Depo-Medrol, Solu-Medrol, *generic*
prednisolone *pred-niss'-oh-lone*	Oral: AsmaPred Plus, Millipred, Orapred, Pediapred, Prelone, Veripred, *generic* Ophthalmic: Pred Forte, Pred Mild, Prelone, *generic*
prednisone *pred'-ni-sone*	Prednisone Intensol, Sterapred, Sterapred DS, *generic*
triamcinolone *trye-am-sin'-oh-lone*	Injection: Aristospan, Kenalog, *generic* Topical: Kenalog, Triderm, *generic* Nasal: Nasacort AQ Oral paste: Oralone Intraocular: Triesence
Mineralocorticoid	
fludrocortisone acetate *floo-droe-kor-te-sone*	*generic*

32

Thyroid and Antithyroid Drugs

CHAPTER OBJECTIVES

On completion of this chapter, students will be able to:

1. Define the chapter's key terms.
2. Describe the general drug actions, uses, adverse reactions, contraindications, precautions, and interactions of thyroid and antithyroid drugs.
3. Compare and contrast the signs and symptoms of hypothyroidism and hyperthyroidism.
4. Discuss important points to keep in mind when educating the patient or family members about the use of thyroid and antithyroid drugs.

KEY TERMS

euthyroid—a normal thyroid
goiter—enlargement of the thyroid gland
hyperthyroidism—an increase in the amount of thyroid hormones secreted
hypothyroidism—a decrease in the amount of thyroid hormones secreted
iodism—excessive amounts of iodine in the body
myxedema—a severe hypothyroidism manifested by a variety of symptoms
thyroid storm—a severe form of hyperthyroidism, also known as thyrotoxicosis
thyrotoxicosis—a severe form of hyperthyroidism, also known as thyroid storm
thyroxine—a hormone manufactured and secreted by the thyroid gland
triiodothyronine—a hormone manufactured and secreted by the thyroid gland

CHAPTER OVERVIEW

Drug classes covered in this chapter are:

- Thyroid hormones
- Antithyroid drugs

Drugs by classification are listed on page 334.

thePOINT RESOURCES

- Comprehensive Summary Drug Tables
- Lippincott's Interactive Tutorials: Drugs Affecting the Endocrine System
- Interactive Practice and Review
- Monographs of Most Commonly Prescribed Drugs

The thyroid gland is located in the neck in front of the trachea. This highly vascular gland manufactures and secretes two hormones: **thyroxine** and **triiodothyronine**. Iodine is essential for the manufacture of both of these hormones. The activity of the thyroid gland is regulated by thyroid-stimulating hormone (TSH), produced by the anterior pituitary gland (see Figure 31-1). When the level of circulating thyroid hormones decreases, the anterior pituitary secretes TSH, which then activates the cells of the thyroid to release stored thyroid hormones. This is an example of the feedback mechanism.

Two diseases are related to the hormone-producing activity of the thyroid gland:

- **Hypothyroidism:** a decrease in the amount of thyroid hormones manufactured and secreted
- **Hyperthyroidism:** an increase in the amount of thyroid hormones manufactured and secreted

The signs and symptoms of hypothyroidism and hyperthyroidism are given in Table 32-1. A severe form of hyperthyroidism, called **thyrotoxicosis** or **thyroid storm**, is characterized by high fever, extreme tachycardia, and altered mental status. Thyroid hormones are used to treat hypothyroidism, and antithyroid drugs and radioactive iodine are used to treat hyperthyroidism.

FACT CHECK

32-1 Which two hormones are secreted by the thyroid gland?

32-2 What are the two most common thyroid disorders?

Thyroid Hormones

Thyroid hormones used in medicine include both the natural and synthetic hormones. Synthetic hormones are generally preferred because they are more uniform in potency than the natural hormones obtained from animals. Thyroid hormones are listed in the Summary Drug Table: Thyroid and Antithyroid Drugs.

Actions of Thyroid Hormones

The thyroid hormones influence every organ and tissue of the body. These hormones are principally concerned with increasing the metabolic rate of tissues, which results in increases in the heart and respiratory rate, body temperature, cardiac output, oxygen consumption, and the metabolism of fats, proteins, and carbohydrates. The exact mechanisms by which the thyroid hormones exert their influence on body organs and tissues are not well understood.

Uses of Thyroid Hormones

Thyroid hormones are used as replacement therapy when the patient is hypothyroid. By supplementing the decreased endogenous thyroid production and secretion with exogenous thyroid hormones, an attempt is made to create a **euthyroid** (normal thyroid) state. Levothyroxine (Synthroid) is the drug of choice for hypothyroidism because it is relatively inexpensive, requires once-per-day dosages, and has a more uniform potency than other thyroid hormone replacement drugs.

Myxedema is a severe hypothyroidism manifested by lethargy, apathy, memory impairment, emotional changes, slow speech, deep coarse voice, thick dry skin, cold intolerance, slow pulse, constipation, weight gain, and absence of menses.

Thyroid hormones are also used in the treatment or prevention of various types of euthyroid **goiters** (enlargement of the thyroid gland), including thyroid nodules, subacute or chronic lymphocytic thyroiditis (Hashimoto), and multinodular goiter, and in the management of thyroid cancer. The hormone may be used with the antithyroid drugs to treat thyrotoxicosis. Thyroid hormones also may be used as a diagnostic measure to differentiate suspected hyperthyroidism from euthyroidism.

Adverse Reactions of Thyroid Hormones

During initial therapy, the most common adverse reactions seen are signs of overdose and hyperthyroidism (see Table 32-1). Adverse reactions other than symptoms of hyperthyroidism are rare.

TABLE 32-1   Signs and Symptoms of Thyroid Dysfunction

Body System or Function	Hypothyroidism	Hyperthyroidism
Metabolism	Decreased with anorexia, intolerance to cold, low body temperature, weight gain despite anorexia	Increased with increased appetite, intolerance to heat, elevated body temperature, weight loss despite increased appetite
Cardiovascular	Bradycardia, moderate hypotension	Tachycardia, moderate hypertension
Central nervous system	Lethargy, sleepiness, depression, fatigue	Nervousness, anxiety, insomnia, tremors
Skin, skin structures	Pale, cool, dry skin; face appears puffy; coarse hair; thick and hard nails	Flushed, warm, moist skin
Ovarian function	Heavy menses, may be unable to conceive, loss of fetus possible	Irregular or scant menses
Testicular function	Low sperm count	Low sperm count

Contraindications, Precautions, and Interactions of Thyroid Hormones

- Thyroid hormones are contraindicated in patients with a known hypersensitivity to any or all constituents of the drug, after a recent myocardial infarction (heart attack), or in patients with thyrotoxicosis (severe hypothyroidism). When hypothyroidism is a cause or contributing factor to myocardial infarction or heart disease, the health care provider may prescribe small doses of thyroid hormone.
- These drugs are used cautiously in patients with Addison disease and during lactation.
- When administered with cholestyramine or colestipol, there is a decreased absorption of the oral thyroid preparations. These drugs should not be administered within 4 to 6 hours of the thyroid hormones.
- When administered with an oral anticoagulant, there is an increased risk of bleeding; it may be advantageous to decrease the dosage of the anticoagulant.
- There is a decreased effectiveness of the digitalis preparation if taken with a thyroid preparation.
- Thyroid hormone replacement therapy in patients with diabetes may increase the intensity of the symptoms or the diabetes. A patient with diabetes is monitored during thyroid hormone replacement therapy for signs of hyperglycemia (see Chapter 30), and the health care provider should be notified if this problem occurs.
- Patients with cardiovascular disease are closely monitored while taking thyroid hormones. The development of chest pain or worsening of cardiovascular disease should be reported to the health care provider immediately because the patient may require a reduction in dosage.

Patient Management Issues with Thyroid Hormones

Before therapy starts, the patient's vital signs, weight, and history are obtained. A general physical assessment is performed to determine the signs of hypothyroidism.

Thyroid hormones are administered once per day, early in the morning and preferably before breakfast. An empty stomach increases the absorption of the oral preparation. Levothyroxine also can be given intravenously or intramuscularly and is prepared for administration immediately before use.

The dosage is individualized for the patient. The dose of thyroid hormones must be carefully adjusted according to the patient's hormone requirements. Several upward or downward dosage adjustments are often made until the optimal therapeutic dosage is reached and the patient becomes euthyroid (Key Concepts 32-1).

Some patients may have anxiety related to the symptoms of their disorder, as well as concern about relief of their symptoms. A patient should be reassured that although relief may not be immediate, symptoms should begin to decrease or disappear in a few weeks.

Educating the Patient and Family about Thyroid Hormones

Following are key points about thyroid hormone therapy the patient and family members should know:

- Replacement therapy is for life, with the exception of transient hypothyroidism seen in those with thyroiditis. Therefore, it is important to maintain the dosage as prescribed by your health care provider: Do not increase, decrease, or skip a dose unless advised to do so.
- Take this drug in the morning, preferably before breakfast, unless advised by your health care provider to take it at a different time of day.
- Notify your health care provider if you experience any of the following: headache, nervousness, palpitations, diarrhea, excessive sweating, heat intolerance, chest pain, increased pulse rate, or any unusual physical change or event.
- The dosage of this drug may require periodic adjustments; this is normal. Dosage changes are based on your response to therapy and thyroid function tests.
- Therapy needs to be evaluated at periodic intervals, which may vary from every 2 weeks at the beginning of therapy to every 6 to 12 months once your symptoms are controlled. Periodic thyroid function tests are needed.

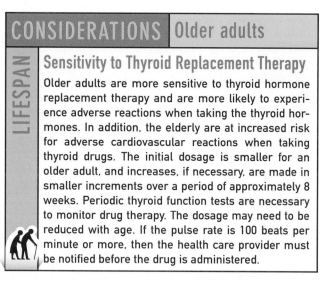

LIFESPAN

CONSIDERATIONS Older adults

Sensitivity to Thyroid Replacement Therapy

Older adults are more sensitive to thyroid hormone replacement therapy and are more likely to experience adverse reactions when taking the thyroid hormones. In addition, the elderly are at increased risk for adverse cardiovascular reactions when taking thyroid drugs. The initial dosage is smaller for an older adult, and increases, if necessary, are made in smaller increments over a period of approximately 8 weeks. Periodic thyroid function tests are necessary to monitor drug therapy. The dosage may need to be reduced with age. If the pulse rate is 100 beats per minute or more, then the health care provider must be notified before the drug is administered.

- Weigh yourself weekly and report any significant weight gain or loss to your health care provider.
- Do not change from one brand of this drug to another without consulting your health care provider.

FACT CHECK

32-3   What is the drug of choice for treating hypothyroidism?

Antithyroid Drugs

Antithyroid drugs or thyroid antagonists are used to treat hyperthyroidism. In addition to the antithyroid drugs, hyperthyroidism may be treated by the administration of strong iodine solutions, use of radioactive iodine (^{131}I), or by surgical removal of some or almost all of the thyroid gland (subtotal thyroidectomy).

Actions of Antithyroid Drugs

Antithyroid drugs inhibit the manufacture of thyroid hormones. They do not affect existing thyroid hormones that are circulating in the blood or stored in the thyroid gland. For this reason, the therapeutic effects of the antithyroid drugs may

LIFESPAN

CONSIDERATIONS Older adults

Hypothyroidism

The symptoms of hypothyroidism may be confused with symptoms associated with aging, such as depression, cold intolerance, weight gain, confusion, or unsteady gait. The presence of these symptoms should be thoroughly evaluated and documented in the preadministration assessment and periodically throughout therapy.

not be observed for 3 to 4 weeks. Antithyroid drugs are listed in the Summary Drug Table: Thyroid and Antithyroid Drugs.

Strong iodide solutions act by decreasing the vascularity of the thyroid gland by rapidly inhibiting the release of the thyroid hormones. Radioactive iodine is distributed within the cellular fluid and excreted. The radioactive isotope accumulates in the cells of the thyroid gland, where destruction of thyroid cells occurs without damaging other cells throughout the body.

Uses of Antithyroid Drugs

Methimazole (Tapazole) and propylthiouracil (PTU) are used for the medical management of hyperthyroidism. Not all patients respond adequately to antithyroid drugs; therefore, a thyroidectomy (removal of the thyroid gland) may be necessary. Antithyroid drugs may be administered before surgery to temporarily return a patient to a euthyroid state. When used for this reason, the vascularity of the thyroid gland is reduced, and the tendency to bleed excessively during and immediately after surgery is decreased.

Strong iodine solution, also known as Lugol solution, is potassium iodide. It may be given orally with methimazole or PTU to prepare the patient for thyroid surgery. Iodine solutions are also used for rapid treatment of hyperthyroidism because they can decrease symptoms in 2 to 7 days. Radioactive iodine (^{131}I) may be used for treatment of hyperthyroidism and selected cases of cancer of the thyroid.

Adverse Reactions of Antithyroid Drugs

Methimazole

The most serious adverse reaction associated with methimazole is agranulocytosis (decrease in the number of white blood cells, e.g., neutrophils, basophils, and eosinophils). Reactions observed with agranulocytosis include hay fever, sore throat, skin rash, fever, or headache. Other major reactions include granulocytopenia, thrombocytopenia, aplastic anemia, hypoprothrombinemia, and hepatitis. Minor reactions, such as nausea, vomiting, epigastric distress, and paresthesias, also may occur.

Propylthiouracil

The major adverse reactions of PTU are not as common as the more minor adverse reactions. Major adverse reactions include erythema nodosum, exfoliative dermatitis, aplastic anemia, hypoprothrombinemia and bleeding, and hepatitis. The minor, but more common, adverse reactions include drowsiness, headache, hair loss, and epigastric distress.

Strong Iodine Solutions

Reactions that may occur with strong iodine solution include symptoms of **iodism** (excessive amounts of iodine in the body), which are a metallic taste in the mouth, swelling and soreness of the parotid glands, burning of the mouth and throat, sore teeth and gums, symptoms of a head cold, and occasionally gastrointestinal upset. Allergy to iodine may occur and can be serious. Symptoms of iodine allergy include swelling of parts of the face and body, fever, joint pains, and sometimes difficulty in breathing. Difficulty breathing requires immediate medical attention.

Radioactive Iodine (^{131}I)

Reactions after administration of ^{131}I include sore throat, swelling in the neck, nausea, vomiting, cough, and pain on swallowing. Other reactions include bone marrow depression, anemia, leukopenia, thrombocytopenia, and tachycardia.

Contraindications, Precautions, and Interactions of Antithyroid Drugs

- The antithyroid drugs are contraindicated in patients with a known hypersensitivity to them or any constituent of the drug.
- Methimazole and PTU are contraindicated during lactation.
- Radioactive iodine is contraindicated during pregnancy (pregnancy category X) and lactation.
- Methimazole and PTU are used with extreme caution during pregnancy because they can cause hypothyroidism in the fetus. However, if an antithyroid drug is necessary during pregnancy or lactation, PTU is often prescribed. In many pregnant women, thyroid dysfunction diminishes as the pregnancy proceeds, making a dosage reduction possible.
- Methimazole and PTU are used cautiously in patients older than age 40, because there is an increased risk of agranulocytosis, and in patients with a decrease in bone marrow reserve (e.g., after radiation therapy for cancer).
- An additive bone marrow depression occurs when methimazole or PTU is administered with other bone marrow depressants, such as the antineoplastic drugs, or with radiation therapy.
- When methimazole is administered with digitalis, there is an increased effectiveness of the digitalis and increased risk of toxicity.
- There is an additive effect of PTU when the drug is administered with lithium, potassium iodide, or sodium iodide.
- When iodine products are administered with lithium products, synergistic hypothyroid activity is likely to occur.

ALERT ℞

Agranulocytosis

Agranulocytosis (a decrease or lack of granulocytes, a type of white blood cell) is potentially the most serious adverse reaction to methimazole and PTU. The patient must be protected from individuals with infectious disease because if agranulocytosis is present, the patient is at increased risk for contracting any infection, particularly an upper respiratory infection. The patient should be monitored for signs of infection. The health care provider should be notified if fever, sore throat, rash, headache, hay fever, yellow discoloration of the skin, or vomiting occurs.

FACT CHECK

32-4 Which drugs are used to treat hyperthyroidism?
32-5 What is the most serious adverse reaction of methimazole?

Patient Management Issues with Antithyroid Drugs

Before therapy with an antithyroid drug begins, the patient is assessed, including a history of the symptoms of hyperthyroidism (see Table 32-1), vital signs, and weight. If the patient is prescribed an iodine solution, then a careful allergy history, particularly to iodine or seafood (which contains iodine), is included.

During therapy, the patient is monitored for adverse drug effects. With short-term therapy before surgery, adverse drug reactions are usually minimal. Long-term therapy is usually on an outpatient basis. Relief of symptoms, as well as signs or symptoms indicating an adverse reaction related to the blood cells, such as fever, sore throat, easy bruising or bleeding, fever, cough, or any other signs of infection, is monitored. As the patient becomes euthyroid, signs and symptoms of hyperthyroidism become less obvious. The patient is monitored for signs of thyroid storm (high fever, extreme tachycardia, and altered mental status), which can occur in patients whose hyperthyroidism is inadequately treated.

A patient with an enlarged thyroid gland may have difficulty swallowing the tablet. In this case, strong iodine solution may be prescribed. It is measured in drops, which are added to water or fruit juice. This drug has a strong, salty taste. The patient is allowed to experiment with various types of fruit juices to determine which one best disguises the taste of the drug. Iodine solutions should be drunk through a straw because they may cause tooth discoloration.

The health care provider gives radioactive iodine orally as a single dose. The effects of iodides are evident within 24 hours, with maximum effects attained after 10 to 15 days of continuous therapy. If the patient is hospitalized, then radiation safety precautions identified by the hospital's department of nuclear medicine are followed.

Once a euthyroid state is achieved, the health care provider may add a thyroid hormone to the therapeutic regimen to prevent or treat hypothyroidism, which may develop slowly during long-term antithyroid drug therapy or after administration of ^{131}I.

A patient with hyperthyroidism is likely to have cardiac symptoms such as tachycardia or palpitations. Propranolol, an adrenergic blocking drug (see Chapter 12), may be prescribed by the health care provider as adjunctive treatment for several weeks until the therapeutic effects of the antithyroid drug occur.

Educating the Patient and Family about Antithyroid Drugs

Following are key points about antithyroid drugs the patient and family members should know.

Methimazole and Propylthiouracil

- Take these drugs at regular intervals around the clock (e.g., q8h) unless directed otherwise by your health care provider.
- Do not take these drugs in larger doses or more frequently than as directed on the prescription container.
- Notify your health care provider promptly if you experience any of the following: sore throat, fever, cough, easy bleeding or bruising, headache, or a general feeling of malaise.
- Record your weight twice per week and notify your health care provider if you have any sudden weight gain or loss. (Note: Your health care provider may also want you to monitor your pulse rate. If so, then your health care provider will show you the proper technique and how to record the pulse rate. Bring the record to your health care provider's office or clinic.)
- Avoid the use of nonprescription drugs unless your health care provider has approved the use of a specific drug.

Strong Iodine Solution

- Dilute the solution with water or fruit juice. Fruit juice often disguises the strong, salty taste more than water. Experiment with the types of fruit juice that best reduces the unpleasant taste of this drug. Drink iodine solutions through a straw to avoid tooth discoloration.
- Discontinue the use of this drug and notify your health care provider if you experience any of the following: skin rash, metallic taste in the mouth, swelling and soreness in front of the ears, sore teeth and gums, severe gastrointestinal distress, or symptoms of a head cold.

Radioactive Iodine

- Follow the directions of the department of nuclear medicine regarding precautions to be taken. (Note: In some instances, the dosage is small, and no special precautions may be necessary.)
- Thyroid hormone replacement therapy may be necessary if hypothyroidism develops.
- Follow-up evaluations of the thyroid gland and the effectiveness of treatment with this drug are necessary.

FACT CHECK

32-6   How should strong iodide be dosed and administered?

Chapter Review

KEY POINTS

- The thyroid gland secretes thyroxin and triiodothyronine. Two diseases related to the hormone-producing activity of the thyroid gland are hypothyroidism and hyperthyroidism.
- Signs and symptoms of hypothyroidism include decreased metabolism, bradycardia, lethargy and sleepiness, dry skin, coarse hair, thick nails, heavy menses, or decreased testicular function. Signs and symptoms of hyperthyroidism include increased metabolism, tachycardia, nervousness and insomnia, moist skin, and irregular or scant menses.
- Thyroid hormones used in medicine include both natural and synthetic hormones. The synthetic hormones are generally preferred because they are more uniform in potency than are the natural hormones obtained from animals.
- Thyroid hormones increase the metabolic rate of tissues, which results in increases in the heart and respiratory rate, body temperature, cardiac output, oxygen consumption, and the metabolism of fats, proteins, and carbohydrates. Thyroid hormones are used as replacement therapy when the patient is hypothyroid. The most common adverse reactions seen are signs of overdose and hyperthyroidism; other adverse reactions are rare.
- Antithyroid drugs or thyroid antagonists are used to treat hyperthyroidism. Hyperthyroidism may also be treated by the administration of strong iodine solutions, use of radioactive iodine (^{131}I), or by surgical removal of some or almost all of the thyroid gland (subtotal thyroidectomy).
- Antithyroid drugs inhibit the manufacture of thyroid hormones. Methimazole (Tapazole) and PTU are used for the medical management of hyperthyroidism. The most common adverse reaction of methimazole is agranulocytosis. The most common adverse reactions of PTU are erythema nodosum, other skin disorders, aplastic anemia, hypoprothrombinemia and hepatitis.
- Strong iodide solutions act by decreasing the vascularity of the thyroid gland by rapidly inhibiting the release of the thyroid hormones. Strong iodine solution, also known as Lugol solution, may be given orally with methimazole or PTU to prepare for thyroid surgery. Iodine solutions are also used for rapid treatment of hyperthyroidism. Reactions to strong iodine solution include symptoms of iodism, such as a metallic taste in the mouth, swelling and soreness of the parotid glands, burning of the mouth and throat, sore teeth and gums, symptoms of a head cold, and occasionally gastrointestinal upset. Iodine allergy can be serious.
- Radioactive iodine (^{131}I) may be used for treatment of hyperthyroidism and selected cases of cancer of the thyroid. Reactions to ^{131}I include sore throat, swelling in the neck, nausea, vomiting, cough, and pain on swallowing.

CRITICAL THINKING CASE STUDY

Hypothyroidism

Ms. Hedrick has been diagnosed with hypothyroidism. Her physician has prescribed levothyroxine 100 mcg daily.

1. What adverse reactions should Ms. Hedrick expect while taking levothyroxine?
   a. Bradycardia
   b. Palpitations
   c. Agranulocytosis
   d. Aplastic anemia
2. When should Ms. Hedrick take levothyroxine?
   a. In the morning
   b. With lunch
   c. In the evening
   d. Right before bedtime
3. If the dose is inadequate, Ms. Hedrick might experience symptoms of hypothyroidism. What should you tell her to watch for?

Review Questions

MULTIPLE CHOICE

1. What adverse reaction is most likely to occur in the early days of therapy in a patient taking a thyroid hormone?
   a. Signs of congestive heart failure
   b. Signs of hyperthyroidism
   c. Signs of hypothyroidism
   d. Signs of euthyroidism
2. The patient is informed that therapy with a thyroid hormone may not produce a full therapeutic response for
   a. 24 hours
   b. 2 or 3 days
   c. several weeks or more
   d. 8 to 12 months
3. Symptoms of myxedema include
   a. lethargy, cold intolerance
   b. tachycardia, heat intolerance
   c. weight loss, insomnia
   d. all of the above
4. Which of the following statements made by a patient would indicate to the health care provider that the patient is experiencing an adverse reaction to radioactive iodine?
   a. "I am sleepy most of the day."
   b. "I am unable to sleep at night."
   c. "My throat hurts when I swallow."
   d. "My body aches all over."

MATCHING

Match the generic name on the left with the trade name on the right.

_____ 5. methimazole   a. Cytomel
_____ 6. radioactive iodine (^{131}I)   b. Armour Thyroid
_____ 7. strong iodide   c. Thyrolar
_____ 8. levothyroxine   d. Hicon
_____ 9. liothyronine   e. Synthroid
_____ 10. liotrix   f. Lugol solution
_____ 11. thyroid desiccated   g. Tapazole

TRUE OR FALSE

_____ 12. A patient with euthyroid would likely be prescribed methimazole.
_____ 13. Patients with hypothyroidism must take thyroid replacement hormones for life.
_____ 14. Thyroid hormones are Pregnancy Category A but are used cautiously during lactation.
_____ 15. Propylthiouracil (PTU) is usually taken in divided doses at 4-hour intervals.

FILL IN THE BLANKS

16. Symptoms of _____ _____ include fever, joint pains, face and body swelling, dysphagia, and shortness of breath.
17. _____ is a severe form of hyperthyroidism characterized by high fever, extreme tachycardia, and altered mental status.
18. When methimazole is administered with digitalis, there is a(n) _____ effectiveness of digitalis and increased risk of _____.
19. Strong iodine solution should be discontinued and the health care provider notified if the patient experiences a(n) _____ taste in the mouth.

SHORT ANSWERS

20. What are the symptoms of agranulocytosis?
21. What interactions may occur when thyroid hormones are administered with oral anticoagulants or digitalis preparations?
22. A patient taking strong iodine solution complains about the drug's taste. What would you recommend?
23. Why is levothyroxine the drug of choice for hypothyroidism?

Web Activities

1. Go to the Mayo Clinic Web site (www.mayoclinic.com) and search for "hypothyroidism diet." Is there such a thing as a hypothyroidism diet? What foods can impair the absorption of synthetic thyroid hormones?
2. On the same Web site, conduct a search on "Graves disease." What are the causes and risk factors of Graves disease?

SUMMARY DRUG TABLE Thyroid and Antithyroid Drugs (left, generic; right, trade)

Comprehensive Summary Drug Tables, including uses, adverses effects, dosages, and pregnancy classifications, are provided on the companion website, http://thePoint.lww.com/PharmacologyHP2e

Thyroid Hormones		Antithyroid Preparations	
levothyroxine sodium (T$_4$) *lee-voe-thye-rox'-een*	Levothroid, Levoxyl, Synthroid, Tirosint, Unithroid, Unithroid Direct, *generic*	methimazole *meth-im'-a-zole*	Northyx, Tapazole, *generic*
liothyronine sodium (T$_3$) *lye'-oh-thye'-roe-neen*	Cytomel, Triostat, *generic*	propylthiouracil (PTU) *proe-pill-thye-oh-yoor'-a-sill*	*generic*
liotrix *lye'-oh-triks*	Thyrolar	radioactive iodine (^{131}I)	Hicon, *generic*
thyroid desiccated *thye'-roid*	Armour Thyroid, Nature-Thyroid, Westhroid	potassium iodide, strong iodide solution *eye'-oh-dine*	Iosat, Lugol solution, Pima, SSKI, ThyroSafe, ThyroShield, *generic*

33

Male and Female Hormones and Drugs for Erectile Dysfunction

CHAPTER OBJECTIVES

On completion of this chapter, students will be able to:

1. Define the chapter's key terms.

2. Describe the general drug actions, uses, adverse reactions, contraindications, precautions, and interactions of male and female hormones.

3. Discuss important points to keep in mind when educating the patient or family members about the use of male and female hormones.

4. Explain the differences between the different types of oral contraceptives.

5. Compare and contrast the signs of estrogen and progestin excess and deficiency.

6. Discuss the general drug actions, uses, and common adverse reactions of drugs used to treat erectile dysfunction.

7. Explain how to properly take or use drugs used to treat erectile dysfunction.

8. Explain the actions, use, and dosage of drugs for emergency contraception.

KEY TERMS

androgens—hormones that stimulate activity of the accessory male sex organs
estradiol—the most potent of the three endogenous estrogens
estriol—one of three endogenous estrogens
estrogens—female hormones influenced by the anterior pituitary gland
estrone—one of three endogenous estrogens
priapism—prolonged erection accompanied by pain and tenderness
progesterone—female hormones influenced by the anterior pituitary gland
progestins—natural or synthetic substances that cause changes similar to those of progesterone
testosterone—the most potent naturally occurring androgen
virilization—acquisition of male sexual characteristics by a woman

CHAPTER OVERVIEW

Drug classes covered in this chapter are:

- Male hormones
- Erectile dysfunction drugs
- Female hormones

Drugs by classification are listed on pages 351-352.

thePOINT RESOURCES

- Comprehensive Summary Drug Tables
- Lippincott's Interactive Tutorials: Drugs Affecting the Endocrine System
- Interactive Practice and Review
- Monographs of Most Commonly Prescribed Drugs

Male Hormones

Male and female hormones play a vital role in the development and maintenance of secondary sex characteristics and are necessary for human reproduction. Although the body naturally produces hormones, a male or female hormone is used in the treatment of certain disorders, such as inoperable breast cancer, male hypogonadism, or male or female hormone deficiency. Hormones also are used as contraceptives and for treating the symptoms of menopause. (see Chapter 41 for more information.)

Male Hormones

Male hormones—**testosterone** (the most potent naturally occurring androgen) and its derivatives—are collectively called **androgens.** Androgen secretion is under the influence of the anterior pituitary gland. Small amounts of male and female hormones are also produced by the adrenal cortex. The anabolic steroids are closely related to the androgen testosterone and have both androgenic and anabolic (stimulate cellular growth and repair) activity. Androgen hormone inhibitors inhibit the conversion of testosterone into a potent androgen.

Actions of Male Hormones

Androgens

The male hormone testosterone and its derivatives activate reproductive potential in adolescent boys. From puberty onward, androgens continue to aid in the development and maintenance of secondary sex characteristics: facial hair, deep voice, body hair, body fat distribution, and muscle development. Testosterone also stimulates the growth of the accessory sex organs (penis, testes, vas deferens, prostate) at the time of puberty (Fig. 33-1). The androgens also promote tissue-building processes (anabolism) and reverse tissue-depleting processes (catabolism). Examples of androgens are fluoxymesterone (Androxy), methyltestosterone (Android, Testred), and testosterone. Additional examples of androgens are given in the Summary Drug Table: Male Hormones.

> ## FACT CHECK
>
> 33-1   What are the male hormones?

Anabolic Steroids

The anabolic steroids are synthetic drugs chemically related to the androgens. Like androgens, they promote tissue-building processes. Given in normal doses, they have a minimal effect on the accessory sex organs and secondary sex characteristics. Examples of anabolic steroids are given in the Summary Drug Table: Male Hormones.

Androgen Hormone Inhibitor

The androgen hormone inhibitor finasteride (Proscar) is a synthetic compound drug that inhibits the conversion of testosterone into the potent androgen 5α-dihydrotestosterone (DHT). The development of the prostate gland depends on α-DHT. The lowering of serum levels of α-DHT reduces the effect of this hormone on the prostate gland, resulting in a decrease in the size of the gland and the symptoms associated with prostatic gland enlargement.

Dutasteride (Avodart) inhibits the conversion of testosterone to 5α-DHT, which is responsible for the initial development and later enlargement of the prostate gland.

Uses of Male Hormones

Androgens

In male patients, androgen therapy may be given as replacement therapy for testosterone deficiency. Deficiency states in male patients, such as hypogonadism (failure of the testes to develop), selected cases of delayed puberty, and the development of testosterone deficiency after puberty may be treated with androgens. A transdermal testosterone system may be used for replacement therapy when endogenous testosterone is deficient or absent.

In female patients, androgen therapy may be used as part of the treatment for inoperable metastatic breast carcinoma in women who are 1 to 5 years past menopause. In addition, some breast carcinomas in women are "hormone-dependent" tumors; in other words, the female hormone, estrogen, influences their growth and spread. Administration of an androgen to patients with this type of malignant breast tumor counteracts the effect of estrogen on these tumors. Androgens may also be administered to premenopausal women with metastatic breast carcinoma that is believed to be hormone-dependent and whose tumor growth and spread have been slowed after an oophorectomy (removal of the ovaries).

Anabolic Steroids

The uses of the various anabolic steroids include management of anemia of renal insufficiency, control of metastatic breast cancer in women, and promotion of weight gain in those with weight loss after surgery, trauma, or infections.

Androgen Hormone Inhibitor

Finasteride (Proscar) and dutasteride (Avodart) are used in the treatment of the symptoms associated with benign prostatic hypertrophy (Fig. 33-2), such as difficulty starting the urinary stream, frequent passage of small amounts of urine, and having to urinate during the night (nocturia). Several months of therapy may be required before a significant

> ## ALERT Rx
>
> ### Anabolic Steroid Abuse
>
> The use of anabolic steroids to promote an increase in muscle mass and strength is a serious problem. Anabolic steroids are not intended for this use. Unfortunately, deaths in young, healthy individuals have been directly attributed to this use of these drugs. The illegal use of anabolic steroids to increase muscle mass should be discouraged.

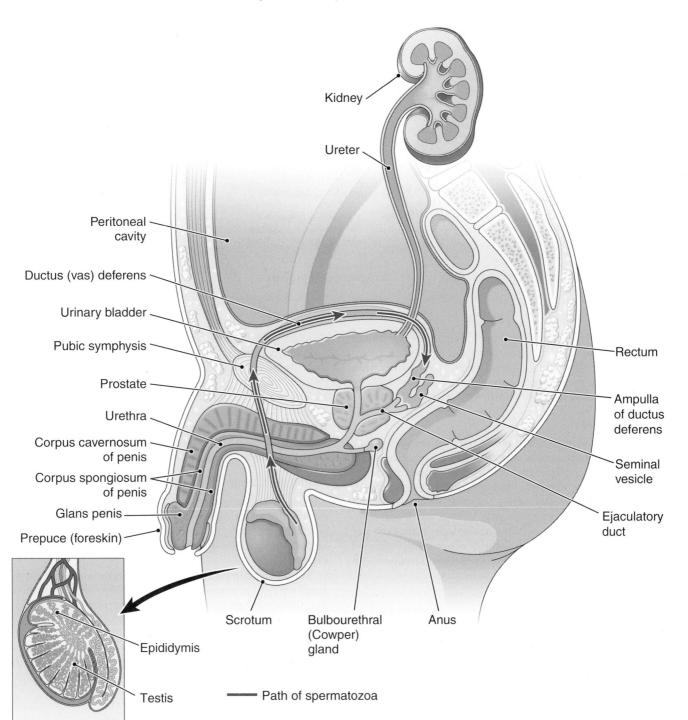

FIGURE 33-1 Male reproductive system. Organs of the urinary system are also shown.

improvement occurs and the symptoms decrease. Finasteride is also used for the prevention of male pattern baldness in men with early signs of hair loss under the trade name Propecia.

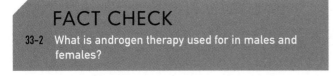

FACT CHECK

33-2 What is androgen therapy used for in males and females?

Adverse Reactions of Male Hormones

Androgens

In men, administration of an androgen may result in breast enlargement (gynecomastia), testicular atrophy, inhibition of testicular function, impotence, enlargement of the penis, nausea, jaundice, headache, anxiety, male pattern baldness, acne, and depression. Fluid and electrolyte imbalances, which include sodium, water, chloride, potassium, calcium, and phosphate retention, may also occur.

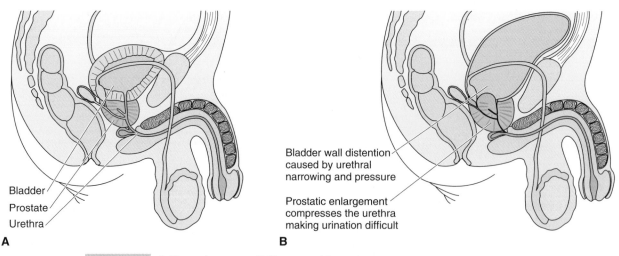

Bladder
Prostate
Urethra

A

Bladder wall distention
caused by urethral
narrowing and pressure

Prostatic enlargement
compresses the urethra
making urination difficult

B

FIGURE 33-2   A. Normal prostate. B. Hypertrophic prostate.

In women receiving an androgen preparation for breast carcinoma, the most common adverse reactions are amenorrhea, other menstrual irregularities, and **virilization** (acquisition of male sexual characteristics by a woman). See Key Concepts 33-1 for more information about virilization.

Anabolic Steroids

Virilization in women is the most common reaction associated with anabolic steroids, especially when higher doses are used. Acne occurs frequently in all age groups and both sexes. Nausea, vomiting, diarrhea, fluid and electrolyte imbalances (the same as for the androgens), testicular atrophy, jaundice, anorexia, and muscle cramps may also occur. Blood-filled cysts of the liver and sometimes the spleen, malignant and benign liver tumors, an increased risk of atherosclerosis, and mental changes are the most serious adverse reactions with prolonged use.

KEY CONCEPTS

33-1   Virilization and Long-Term Use of Androgens

With long-term administration of androgens, a female patient may experience mild to moderate masculine changes, including facial hair, a deepening of the voice, and enlargement of the clitoris. Male pattern baldness, patchy hair loss, skin pigmentation, and acne may also occur. Although these adverse effects are not life threatening, they often are distressing and add to the patient's discomfort and anxiety. These problems may be easy to identify, but they are not always easy to solve. If hair loss occurs, then the wearing of a wig can be suggested. Mild skin pigmentation may be covered with makeup, but severe and widespread pigmented areas and acne are often difficult to conceal.

Many serious adverse drug reactions occur in healthy individuals using anabolic steroids. There is some indication that prolonged high-dose use has resulted in psychological and possibly physical addiction, and some individuals have required treatment in drug abuse centers. Severe mental changes, such as uncontrolled rage, severe depression, suicidal tendencies, malignant and benign liver tumors, aggressive behavior, increased risk of atherosclerosis, inability to concentrate, and personality changes are common.

Androgen Hormone Inhibitor

Adverse reactions with finasteride usually are mild and do not require discontinuing use of the drug. Adverse reactions, when they occur, are related to the sexual drive and include impotence, decreased libido, and a decreased volume of ejaculate.

The most common adverse reactions associated with dutasteride include impotence, decreased libido, breast disorders that include breast enlargement and tenderness, and ejaculation disorders.

FACT CHECK

33-3   What are the adverse reactions of anabolic steroids?

Contraindications, Precautions, and Interactions of Male Hormones

Androgens

- The androgens are contraindicated in patients with a known hypersensitivity, liver disorders, or serious cardiac disease, and in men with prostate gland disorders (e.g., prostate carcinoma and prostate enlargement).
- The androgens are classified as pregnancy category X drugs and should not be administered during pregnancy and lactation.
- When the androgens are administered with anticoagulants, the anticoagulant effect may be increased.

Anabolic Steroids

- Anabolic steroids are contraindicated in patients with a known hypersensitivity, liver disorders, or serious cardiac disease, and in men with prostate gland disorders (e.g., prostate carcinoma or prostate enlargement).
- The anabolic steroids are classified as pregnancy category X drugs and should not be administered during pregnancy and lactation.
- Anabolic steroids are contraindicated for use to enhance physical appearance or athletic performance.
- When the anabolic steroids are administered with anticoagulants, the anticoagulant effect may be increased.
- Administration of methyltestosterone with imipramine may cause a paranoid response in some patients.
- The anabolic steroids may increase the hypoglycemic action when administered with the sulfonylureas.

Androgen Hormone Inhibitor

- Finasteride and dutasteride are contraindicated in patients with hypersensitivity to the drug or any component of the drug, in women who are pregnant or women who may potentially be pregnant, and during lactation.
- These drugs are used cautiously in patients with liver function impairment.

Patient Management Issues with Male Hormones

Androgens

In most instances, androgens are administered to men on an outpatient basis. Before and during therapy, the health care provider may order electrolyte studies because these drugs can cause fluid and electrolyte imbalances. For example, sodium and water retention may occur with both androgens and anabolic steroids, causing the patient to become edematous. Other electrolyte imbalances, such as hypercalcemia, may also occur. Signs of fluid and electrolyte disturbances should be closely monitored (see Chapter 45 for signs and symptoms of electrolyte disturbance).

Anabolic Steroids

The patient's physical and nutritional status are recorded before therapy is started, including the patient's weight, blood pressure, pulse, and respiratory rate. Baseline laboratory studies may include a complete blood count, hepatic function tests, and serum electrolytes and serum lipid levels.

CONSIDERATIONS Older adults

LIFESPAN

Older Men and Steroid Treatment

Older men treated with steroids are at increased risk for prostate enlargement and prostate cancer.

CONSIDERATIONS Older adults

LIFESPAN

Sodium and Water Retention

Older adults with cardiac problems or kidney disease are at increased risk for sodium and water retention when taking an androgen or anabolic steroid.

A daily comparison is made of the patient's pre-administration weight with current weights. The presence of puffy eyelids and dependent swelling of the hands or feet (if the patient can walk) or the sacral area (if the patient is unable to walk) should be reported to the health care provider. Daily fluid intake and output are monitored to calculate fluid balance.

If the androgen is to be administered as a buccal tablet, then the patient is warned not to swallow the tablet but to allow it to dissolve in the mouth. The patient should not smoke or drink water until the tablet is dissolved. Oral and parenteral androgens are often taken or given by injection on an outpatient basis. When given by injection, the injection is administered deep intramuscularly into the gluteal muscle. Oral testosterone is given with or before meals to decrease gastric upset.

When the testosterone transdermal system is prescribed, the system is placed on clean, dry skin of the back, abdomen, upper arms, or thighs. It should not be applied to the scrotum. The selected site should not have prolonged pressure during sleep or sitting. The sites should be rotated, and the same site should not be used again for 7 days. After removing the protective release liner, the patch should immediately be pressed onto the skin, making sure there is good contact with the skin, especially around the edges.

When these drugs are given to female patients with inoperable breast carcinoma, the patient's current status (physical, emotional, and nutritional) is carefully monitored and recorded in the patient's chart. Baseline laboratory tests may include a complete blood count, hepatic function tests, serum electrolytes, and serum and urinary calcium levels.

When the androgens are administered to a patient with diabetes, blood glucose measurements should be performed frequently because glucose tolerance may be altered. Adjustments may need to be made in insulin dosage, oral antidiabetic drugs, or diet. The patient is monitored for signs for hypoglycemia and hyperglycemia (see Chapter 30).

Androgen Hormone Inhibitors

The patient is questioned at length about symptoms of benign prostatic hypertrophy, such as frequency of voiding during the day and night and difficulty starting the urinary stream.

Educating the Patient and Family about Male Hormones

Following are key points about androgens, anabolic steroids, and androgen hormone inhibitors that the patient and family members should know:

ANDROGENS

- Notify your health care provider if you experience any of the following: nausea, vomiting, swelling of the legs, or jaundice. Women should report any signs of virilization.
- Oral tablets: Take with food or a snack to avoid gastrointestinal upset.
- Buccal tablets: Place the tablet between your cheek and molars and allow it to dissolve in your mouth. Do not smoke or drink water until the tablet is dissolved.
- Testosterone transdermal system: Apply the patch according to the directions supplied with the product. Be sure your skin is clean and dry and the placement area is free of hair. Do not store the patch outside the pouch or use a damaged patch. Discard the patch folded together in household trash in a safe manner to prevent ingestion by children or pets.

ANABOLIC STEROIDS

- These drugs may cause nausea and gastrointestinal upset. Take this drug with food or meals.
- Keep all health care provider visits because close monitoring of your therapy is essential.
- Female patients: Notify your health care provider if you experience signs of virilization.

ANDROGEN HORMONE INHIBITOR

- Take this drug without regard to meals.
- Inform your health care provider immediately if your sexual partner is or may become pregnant because additional measures such as discontinuing the drug or use of a condom may be necessary.

FACT CHECK

33-4   What are the contraindications of androgens and anabolic steroids?

Erectile Dysfunction Drugs

Erectile dysfunction, also known as impotence, is the inability to achieve and maintain an erection that is sufficient for intercourse. Although occasional impotence is not a cause for concern, an ongoing problem with erectile dysfunction can put stress on a relationship and result in decreased self-confidence for men. The cause of erectile dysfunction can be physical or psychological in nature. Examples of erectile dysfunction drugs are given in the Summary Drug Table: Drugs for Erectile Dysfunction.

COMPLEMENTARY & ALTERNATIVE MEDICINE

Saw Palmetto

The herb saw palmetto is used to treat benign prostatic hypertrophy. It is thought to increase the flow of urine and reduce urinary frequency and the sleep interruption associated with it. The only known adverse effect of this herb is upset stomach.

Actions of Erectile Dysfunction Drugs

Two types of drugs are used to treat erectile dysfunction. The phosphodiesterase 5 (PDE5) inhibitors include sildenafil (Viagra), tadalafil (Cialis), and vardenafil (Levitra). They work by causing smooth muscle relaxation in the penis, which allows for increased blood flow to the area resulting in an erection.

Alprostadil (Caverject) is a prostaglandin. It is also a smooth muscle relaxant, which acts on the smooth muscles in the penis. It works by relaxing the smooth muscle and dilating the cavernosal arteries found in the penis.

Uses of Erectile Dysfunction Drugs

The PDE5 inhibitors are used to treat erectile dysfunction. However, they are also used for primary arterial hypertension. It should be noted that the trade names differ based on the drugs use.

Alprostadil is used to treat erectile dysfunction by either intracavernosal injection or urogenital insertion. As a pediatric injection, it is also used to treat patent ductus arteriosus so surgery can be performed in neonates.

Adverse Reactions of Erectile Dysfunction Drugs

The most common adverse reactions of PDE5 inhibitors are headache and impairment of color discrimination, specifically blue/green.

The most common adverse reactions of alprostadil are directly related to the route of administration. Penile pain is the most common and is associated with both dosage forms.

Contraindications, Precautions, and Interactions of Erectile Dysfunction Drugs

- The PDE5 inhibitors are contraindicated in patients with a known hypersensitivity to the drug and those currently taking nitrates.
- Alprostadil is contraindicated in patients with a known hypersensitivity to the drug or other prostaglandins.
- Erectile dysfunction drugs are contraindicated in patients with a condition that might predispose them to **priapism** (prolonged erection accompanied by pain and tenderness), anatomical deformations of the penis, and penile implants.

- Erectile dysfunction drugs are contraindicated in men for whom sexual activity is not advised or is contraindicated due to an underlying cardiovascular issue.
- Alprostadil is intended for use only in adult men.
- Alprostadil may increase bleeding in patients taking anticoagulants.
- These drugs should be used with caution in patients who currently take anticoagulants, α-adrenergic blockers, or medications for hypertension.

Patient Management Issues with Erectile Dysfunction Drugs

Patients taking either PDE5 inhibitors or alprostadil should seek medical attention if they experience a prolonged erection (greater than 4 hours) or priapism.

Phosphodiesterase 5 Inhibitors

Patients taking a PDE5 inhibitor should seek medical attention immediately if they lose vision in one or both eyes or have a sudden decrease or loss of hearing.

Alprostadil

Alprostadil comes in an injection or a urethral pellet; both will cause pain upon administration. The patient must be trained on proper insertion of the urethral pellet or on proper preparation of the injectable forms and injection technique.

Educating the Patient and Family about Erectile Dysfunction Drugs

Patients taking PDE5 inhibitors or alprostadil should be informed that neither of these drugs protects against sexually transmitted diseases. Following are key points about PDE5 inhibitors and alprostadil that the patient and family members should know:

Phosphodiesterase 5 Inhibitors

- Note that these drugs have no effect in the absence of sexual stimulation.
- Be aware that excessive consumption of alcohol can result in signs and symptoms of orthostatic hypotension.
- Take these drugs approximately 60 minutes before intercourse; they may be taken with or without food.
- Use the orally disintegrating tablets immediately after removing them from the blister package.
- Do not take these drugs more than once a day.

Alprostadil

- Store the injection in the freezer or refrigerator. Once refrigerated, the ampule must be used within 7 days. It cannot be refrozen. The ampule is designed for only one use and should be discarded.
- Store the sterile powder at or below 24°C (77°F). It should not be frozen. After reconstitution, it must be used within 24 hours.
- Store the dual-chamber system at room temperature. After mixing, it should be used within 24 hours.

- Use the proper preparation and injection technique to prevent needle breakage.
- Use the proper insertion technique for the urethral pellet.
- This drug should produce an erection in 5 to 20 minutes, and it should last for approximately an hour. Do not use alprostadil more than three times a week and ensure that there is at least 24 hours between uses.

FACT CHECK

33-5   How do the PDE5 inhibitors work to treat erectile dysfunction?

33-6   How is alprostadil administered?

Female Hormones

The two endogenous (produced by the body) female hormones are the **estrogens** and **progesterone**. Like androgens, their production is under the influence of the anterior pituitary gland. The endogenous estrogens are **estradiol**, **estrone**, and **estriol**. The most potent of these three estrogens is estradiol. Examples of estrogens used as drugs include estropipate (Ortho-Est) and estradiol (Estrace).

There are natural and synthetic progesterones, which are collectively called **progestins**. Examples of progestins used as drugs include medroxyprogesterone (Provera) and norethindrone (Aygestin). Examples of estrogens and progestins are given in the Summary Drug Table: Female Hormones.

Actions of Female Hormones

Estrogens

The estrogens are secreted by the ovarian follicle and in smaller amounts by the adrenal cortex. Estrogens are important in the development and maintenance of the female reproductive system (Fig. 33-3) and the primary and secondary sex characteristics. At puberty, they promote growth and development of the vagina, uterus, fallopian tubes, and breasts. They also affect the release of pituitary gonadotropins.

Other actions of estrogen include fluid retention, protein anabolism, thinning of the cervical mucus, and the inhibition or facilitation of ovulation. Estrogens contribute to the conservation of calcium and phosphorus, the growth of pubic and axillary hair, and pigmentation of the breast nipples and genitals. Estrogens also stimulate contraction of the fallopian tubes (which promotes movement of the ovum), modify the physical and chemical properties of the cervical mucus, and restore the endometrium after menstruation.

Progestins

Progesterone is secreted by the corpus luteum, by the placenta, and in small amounts by the adrenal cortex. Progesterone and its derivatives (i.e., the progestins) transform the proliferative endometrium into a secretory endometrium. Progestins are necessary for the development of the placenta and inhibit the secretion of pituitary gonadotropins, which in turn prevents maturation of the ovarian follicle and ovulation. The synthetic

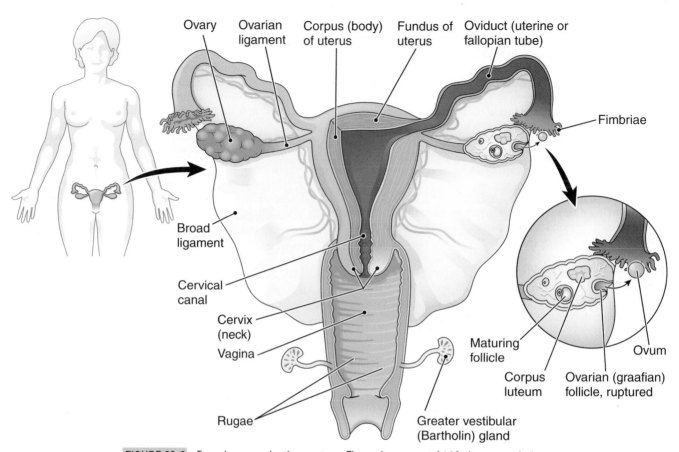

FIGURE 33-3 Female reproductive system. The enlargement (*right*) shows ovulation.

progestins are usually preferred for medical use because of the decreased effectiveness of progesterone when administered orally.

Uses of Female Hormones

Estrogens

Estrogen is most commonly used in combination with progesterones as contraceptives or as hormone replacement therapy in postmenopausal women. The estrogens are used to relieve moderate to severe vasomotor symptoms of menopause (flushing, sweating), female hypogonadism, atrophic vaginitis (orally and intravaginally), osteoporosis in women past menopause, palliative treatment for advanced prostatic carcinoma, and selected cases of inoperable breast carcinoma. The estradiol transdermal system is used as estrogen replacement therapy for moderate to severe vasomotor symptoms associated with menopause, for female hypogonadism, after removal of the ovaries in premenopausal women (female castration), for primary ovarian failure, and in the prevention of osteoporosis.

Estrogen is given intramuscularly or intravenously to treat uterine bleeding caused by hormonal imbalance. When estrogen is used to treat menopausal symptoms in a woman with an intact uterus, concurrent use of progestin is recommended to decrease the risk of endometrial cancer. After a hysterectomy, estrogen alone may be used for estrogen replacement therapy.

The estrogens, in combination with a progestin, are also used as oral contraceptives (Table 33-1). The use of estrogens in the treatment of carcinoma is discussed in Chapter 41.

Progestins

The progestins are used in the treatment of amenorrhea, endometriosis, and functional uterine bleeding. Progestins are also used as oral contraceptives, either alone or in combination with an estrogen (see Table 33-1).

Contraceptive Hormones

Estrogens and progestins (combination oral contraceptives) are used as oral contraceptives. There are four types of estrogen and progestin combination oral contraceptives: monophasic, biphasic, triphasic, and 4-phasic. The monophasic oral contraceptives provide a fixed dose of estrogen and progestin throughout the cycle. The biphasic, triphasic, and 4-phasic oral contraceptives deliver hormones similar to the levels naturally produced by the body (Table 33-1). The oral contraceptives have changed a great deal since their introduction in the 1960s. Today, the levels of hormones provide lower dosages of hormones compared with the older formulations while retaining the same degree of effectiveness (>99% when used as prescribed).

TABLE 33-1   Oral and Miscellaneous Contraceptive Products Systems

Generic Name	Trade Name
Monophasic Oral Contraceptives	
50 mcg ethinyl estradiol acetate, 1 mg norethindrone	Ovcon-50
50 mcg ethinyl estradiol, 1 mg ethynodiol diacetate	Zovia 1/50E
50 mcg ethinyl estradiol, 0.5 mg norgestrel	Ovral
35 mcg ethinyl estradiol, 1 mg norethindrone	Necon 1/35, Norinyl l+35, Nortrel 1/35, Ortho-Novum 1/35
35 mcg ethinyl estradiol, 0.5 mg norethindrone	Brevicon, Modicon, Necon 0.5/35, Notrel 0.5/35
35 mcg ethinyl estradiol, 0.4 mg norethindrone	Ovcon-35, Femcon FE, Valziva, Zenchent
35 mcg ethinyl estradiol, 0.25 mg norgestimate	Ortho-Cyclen, MonoNessa, Previfem, Sprintec
35 mcg ethinyl estradiol, 1 mg ethynodiol diacetate	Zovia 1/35 E, Kelnor 1/35
30 mcg ethinyl estradiol, 3 mg drospirenone	Ocella, Safyral, Yasmin
30 mcg ethinyl estradiol, 1.5 mg norethindrone acetate	Loestrin, 21 1.5/30, Loestrin Fe 1.5/30, Microgestin Fe 1.5/30, Junel 21 Day 1.5/30, Junel Fe 1.5/30
30 mcg ethinyl estradiol, 0.3 mg norgestrel	Lo/Ovral, Low-Ogestrel, Cryselle
30 mcg ethinyl estradiol, 0.15 mg desogestrel	Apri, Desogen, Ortho-Cept, Reclipsen
30 mcg ethinyl estradiol, 0.15 mg levonorgestrel	Levora, Nordette-28, Portia, Jolessa, Quasense, Seasonale
20 mcg ethinyl estradiol, 3 mg drospirenone	Beyaz, Gianvi, YAZ
20 mcg ethinyl estradiol, 0.09 mg levonorgestrel	Lybrel
20 mcg ethinyl estradiol, 1 mg norethindrone acetate	Loestrin 21 1/20, Loestrin Fe 1/20, Junel 21 Day 1/20, Junel Fe 1/20, Microgestin Fe 1/20, Loestrin 24 Fe
20 mcg ethinyl estradiol, 0.1 mg levonorgestrel	Alesse, Aviane, Lessina, Lutera, Sronyx,
50 mcg mestranol, 1 mg norethindrone	Necon 1/50, Norinyl 1+50, Ortho-Novum 1/50
30 mcg ethinyl estradiol, 0.15 mg desogestrel	Solia
Biphasic Oral Contraceptives	
Phase one: 35 mcg ethinyl estradiol, 0.5 mg norethindrone Phase two: 35 mcg ethinyl estradiol, 1 mg norethindrone	Necon 10/11, Ortho-Novum 10/11
Phase one: 20 mcg ethinyl estradiol, 0.15 mg desogestrel Phase two: 10 mcg ethinyl estradiol	Azurette, Kariva, Mircette
Phase one: 20 mcg ethinyl estradiol, 0.1 mg levonorgestrel Phase two: 10 mcg ethinyl estradiol	LoSeasonique
Phase one: 30 mcg ethinyl estradiol, 0.15 mg levonorgestrel Phase two: 10 mcg ethinyl estradiol	Seasonique
Triphasic Oral Contraceptives	
Phase one: 35 mcg ethinyl estradiol, 0.5 mg norethindrone Phase two: 35 mcg ethinyl estradiol, 1 mg norethindrone Phase three: 35 mcg ethinyl estradiol, 0.5 mg norethindrone	Tri-Norinyl, Aranelle, Leena
Phase one: 35 mcg ethinyl estradiol, 0.5 mg norethindrone Phase two: 35 mcg ethinyl estradiol, 0.75 mg norethindrone Phase three: 35 mcg ethinyl estradiol, 1 mg norethindrone	Ortho-Novum 7/7/7, Necon 7/7/7
Phase one: 30 mcg ethinyl estradiol, 0.05 mg levonorgestrel Phase two: 40 mcg ethinyl estradiol, 0.075 mg levonorgestrel Phase three: 30 mcg ethinyl estradiol, 0.125 mg levonorgestrel	Triphasil, Trivora, Enpresse

(continued)

TABLE 33-1   Oral and Miscellaneous Contraceptive Products Systems *(continued)*

Generic Name	Trade Name
Phase one: 35 mcg ethinyl estradiol, 0.18 mg norgestimate Phase two: 35 mcg ethinyl estradiol, 0.215 mg norgestimate Phase three: 35 mcg ethinyl estradiol, 0.25 mg norgestimate	Ortho Tri-Cyclen, Tri-Previfem, TriNessa, Tri-Sprintec
Phase one: 25 mcg ethinyl estradiol, 0.18 mg norgestimate Phase two: 25 mcg ethinyl estradiol, 0.215 mg norgestimate Phase three: 25 mcg ethinyl estradiol, 0.25 mg norgestimate	Ortho Tri-Cyclen Lo
Phase one: 1 mg norethindrone acetate, 20 mcg ethinyl estradiol Phase two: 30 mcg ethinyl estradiol, 1 mg norethindrone acetate Phase three: 35 mcg ethinyl estradiol, 1 mg norethindrone acetate	Estrostep 21, Estrostep Fe, Tilia Fe, Tri-Legest, Tri-Legest Fe
Phase one: 25 mcg ethinyl estradiol, 0.1 mg desogestrel Phase two: 25 mcg ethinyl estradiol, 0.125 mg norgestimate Phase three: 25 mcg ethinyl estradiol, 0.15 mg norgestimate	Cyclessa, Cesia Velivet
Phase one: 25 mcg ethinyl estradiol, 0.1 mg desogestrel Phase two: 25 mcg ethinyl estradiol, 0.125 mg desogestrel Phase three: 25 mcg ethinyl estradiol, 0.15 mg desogestrel	Caziant
4-Phasic	
Phase one: 3 mg estradiol valerate Phase two: 2 mg estradiol valerate, 2 mg dienogest Phase three: 2 mg estradiol valerate, 3 mg dienogest Phase four: 1 mg estradiol valerate	Natazia
Progestin-Only Contraceptives	
0.35 mg norethindrone	Camila, Errin, Heather, Jolivette, Nor-QD, Nora-BE, Ortho Micronor
Miscellaneous Contraceptive Systems	
etonogestrel implant etonogestrel/ethinyl estradiol vaginal ring levonorgestrel vaginal insert norelgestromine/ethinyl estradiol transdermal	Implanon NuvaRing Mirena Ortho Evra
Emergency Contraception	
Levonorgestrel	Next Choice, Plan B, Plan B One-Step, generic
Ulipristal	Ella

KEY CONCEPTS

33-2 Health Benefits of Contraceptive Hormones

Taking contraceptive hormones provides other health benefits besides contraception, such as regulating the menstrual cycle and decreased blood loss and lowering the incidence of iron deficiency anemia and dysmenorrhea. Health benefits related to the inhibition of ovulation include a decrease in ovarian cysts and ectopic pregnancies. In addition, there is a decrease in fibrocystic breast disease, acute pelvic inflammatory disease, endometrial cancer, ovarian cancer, maintenance of bone density, and symptoms related to endometriosis in women taking contraceptive hormones. Newer combination contraceptives such as norgestimate and ethinyl estradiol combinations found in Ortho Tri-Cyclen have been shown to help reduce moderate acne and maintain clear skin in women 15 years of age or older (who menstruate, want contraception, and have no response to topical antiacne medications).

Taking contraceptive hormones also provides health benefits not related to contraception, as discussed in Key Concepts 33-2.

FACT CHECK

33-7 What are the two endogenous female hormones?
33-8 What are the most common uses of estrogens and progestins?

Adverse Reactions of Female Hormones

Estrogens

Administration of estrogens by any route may result in many adverse reactions, although the incidence and intensity of these reactions vary. Some of the adverse reactions of estrogens include

- Central nervous system: headache, migraine, dizziness, mental depression
- Dermatologic: chloasma (pigmentation of the skin) or melasma (discoloration of the skin), which may continue when use of the drug is discontinued
- Gastrointestinal: nausea, vomiting, abdominal cramps, dermatitis, pruritus
- Genitourinary: breakthrough bleeding, withdrawal bleeding, spotting, change in menstrual flow, dysmenorrhea, premenstrual-like syndrome, amenorrhea, vaginal candidiasis, cervical erosion, vaginitis
- Local: pain at injection site, sterile abscess, redness, and irritation at the application site with transdermal system
- Ophthalmic: steepening of corneal curvature, intolerance to contact lenses
- Miscellaneous: edema, changes in libido, reduced carbohydrate tolerance, venous thromboembolism, pulmonary embolism, increase or decrease in weight, skeletal pain, and breast pain, enlargement, and tenderness

Warnings associated with the administration of estrogen include an increased risk of endometrial cancer, gallbladder disease, hypertension, hepatic adenoma (a benign tumor of the liver), cardiovascular disease, increased risk of thromboembolic disease, and hypercalcemia in those with breast cancer and bone metastases.

In addition to experiencing physical effects, some patients taking these drugs may also experience anxiety. For example, a woman taking female hormones may have concerns about long-term therapy with these drugs. Although there are dangers associated with long-term use of female hormones, many of these adverse reactions are rare. When the health care provider monitors a patient closely, the dangers associated with long-term use are often minimal. Male patients with inoperable prostatic carcinoma also may have concerns about taking a female hormone. The patient needs to be reassured that the dosage is carefully regulated and that feminizing effects, if they occur at all, are usually minimal.

Progestins

Administration of the progestins by any route may result in many adverse reactions, although the incidence and intensity of these reactions varies. Progestin may result in breakthrough bleeding, spotting, change in the menstrual flow, amenorrhea, breast tenderness, edema, weight increase or decrease, acne, chloasma or melasma, and mental

TABLE 33-2 Estrogen and Progestin: Excess and Deficiency

Hormone*	Signs of Excess	Signs of Deficiency
estrogen	Nausea, bloating, cervical mucorrhea (increased cervical discharge), polyposis (numerous polyps), melasma (discoloration of the skin), hypertension, migraine headache, breast fullness or tenderness, edema	Early or midcycle breakthrough bleeding, increased spotting, hypomenorrhea
progestin	Increased appetite, weight gain, tiredness, fatigue, hypomenorrhea, acne, oily scalp, hair loss, hirsutism (excessive growth of hair), depression, monilial vaginitis, breast regression	Late breakthrough bleeding, amenorrhea, hypermenorrhea

*Hormonal balance is achieved by adjusting the estrogen/progestin dosage. Oral contraceptives have different amounts of progestin and estrogen varying the estrogenic and progestational activity in each product.

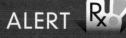

Sodium and Water Retention

Sodium and water retention may occur during female hormone therapy. Any swelling of the hands, ankles, or feet should be reported to the health care provider. A hospitalized patient is weighed daily, an accurate record of the intake and output is kept, walking is encouraged, and the patient is encouraged to eat a diet low in sodium (if prescribed by the health care provider).

depression. The use of medroxyprogesterone acetate contraceptive injection may result in the same adverse reactions as those of any progestin.

Contraceptive Hormones

When estrogen/progestin combinations are used as oral contraceptives, the adverse reactions of the estrogens and the progestins may occur. These drugs may cause adverse reactions that vary depending on their estrogen or progestin content. Table 33-2 identifies the symptoms of estrogen and progestin excess or deficiency. Adjusting the estrogen progestin balance or dosage can minimize the adverse effects.

Contraindications, Precautions, and Interactions of Female Hormones

Estrogens

- Estrogen therapy is contraindicated in patients with a known hypersensitivity, breast cancer (except for metastatic disease), estrogen-dependent neoplasms, undiagnosed abnormal genital bleeding, known or suspected pregnancy (pregnancy category X), or thromboembolic disorders.

ALERT Rx

Thromboembolic Effects

There is an increased risk of postoperative thromboembolic complications in women taking oral contraceptives. If possible, the drug is discontinued at least 4 weeks before a surgical procedure associated with thromboembolism or during prolonged immobilization. The patient is monitored for signs of thromboembolic effects, such as pain, swelling, tenderness in the extremities, headache, chest pain, and blurred vision. These adverse effects should be reported to the health care provider. Patients with previous venous insufficiency, who are on bed rest for other medical reasons, or who smoke are at increased risk for thromboembolic effects. The patient is encouraged to elevate the lower extremities when sitting, if possible, and to exercise the lower extremities by walking.

- Estrogens are used cautiously in patients with gallbladder disease, hypercalcemia (may lead to severe hypercalcemia in patients with breast cancer and bone metastasis), cardiovascular disease, or liver impairment.
- The effects of oral anticoagulants may be decreased when administered with an estrogen.
- When an estrogen is combined with a tricyclic antidepressant, there is an increased risk of toxicity of the antidepressant.
- Barbiturates or rifampin may decrease estrogen blood levels, increasing the risk for breakthrough bleeding.
- When an estrogen is administered concurrently with a hydantoin, breakthrough bleeding, spotting, and pregnancy may occur. A loss of seizure control has also been reported.
- Cigarette smoking increases the risk for cardiovascular complications.

Progestins

- The progestins are contraindicated in patients with a known hypersensitivity, thromboembolic disorders, cerebral hemorrhage, impaired liver function, or cancer of the breast or genital organs.
- Both the estrogens and progestins are classified as pregnancy category X drugs and are contraindicated during pregnancy.
- The progestins are used cautiously in patients with a history of migraine headaches, epilepsy, asthma, or cardiac or renal impairment.
- The effects of the progestins are decreased when administered with an anticonvulsant, barbiturate, or rifampin.
- Administration of a penicillin or tetracycline with an oral contraceptive decreases the effects of the oral contraceptive.

Contraceptive Hormones

See the preceding sections on "Contraindications, Precautions, and Interactions" of estrogens and progestins for information regarding the combination oral contraceptives. The warnings associated with the use of oral contraceptives are the same as those for estrogens and progestins and include cigarette smoking, which increases the risk of cardiovascular side effects, such as venous and arterial thromboembolism, myocardial infarction, and thrombotic and hemorrhagic stroke. Also reported with oral contraceptive use are hepatic adenomas and tumors, visual disturbances, gallbladder disease, hypertension, and fetal abnormalities.

Patient Management Issues with Female Hormones

Before administering an estrogen or progestin, a complete patient health history is obtained including menstrual history, which includes the menarche (age of onset of first menstruation), menstrual pattern, and any changes in the menstrual pattern (including a menopause history when applicable). In patients prescribed an estrogen (including oral contraceptives), a history of thrombophlebitis or other vascular disorders, smoking history, and a history of liver diseases are included. Vital signs are taken. The health care provider usually performs a breast and pelvic examination and a Pap smear test before starting therapy. Liver function tests may be ordered.

If the male or female patient is being treated for a malignancy, then the patient's physical status and mental status are evaluated. The health care provider may also order laboratory tests, such as serum electrolytes and liver function tests.

At each office visit, the patient's vital signs and weight are recorded, along with any adverse drug effects and the result of drug therapy. If the patient is receiving an estrogen for the symptoms of menopause, then her original symptoms are compared with the symptoms she is currently experiencing, if any. A steady weight gain or loss is also noted. A periodic physical examination is performed by the health care provider and may include a pelvic examination, breast examination, Pap smear test, and laboratory tests. A patient with a prostatic or breast carcinoma usually requires more frequent evaluations of response to drug therapy.

In patients with breast carcinoma or prostatic carcinoma, signs indicating a response to therapy are monitored, such as relief of pain, an increased appetite, or feeling of well-being. With prostatic carcinoma, the response to therapy may be rapid, but with breast carcinoma, the response is usually slow.

With the estrogens, it is important to monitor for breakthrough bleeding. If breakthrough bleeding occurs with either estrogen or progestin, then the patient should notify the health care provider. A dosage change may be necessary.

Gastrointestinal upsets, such as nausea, vomiting, abdominal cramps, and bloating, may also occur. Nausea usually decreases or subsides within 1 to 2 months of therapy. However, until that time, the discomfort may lessen if the drug is taken with food. If nausea is continual, then frequent small meals may help. If nausea and vomiting persist, then an antiemetic may be prescribed. Bloating may be lessened with light to moderate exercise or by limiting fluid intake with meals.

A patient with diabetes who is taking female hormones must be carefully monitored. The health care provider should be notified if blood glucose levels are elevated or the urine is positive for glucose or ketone bodies because a change in the dosage of insulin or the oral hypoglycemic drug may be required. See Chapter 30 for how to manage hypoglycemic and hyperglycemic episodes.

Estrogens

Oral estrogens are administered with food or immediately after eating to reduce gastrointestinal upset. When estrogens are given vaginally for atrophic vaginitis, the patient is given instructions on proper use.

Contraceptive Hormones

The oral contraceptives are often taken on a 21-day regimen, with the first tablet taken on the first Sunday after menses begins. After 21 days, then next 7 days are skipped, and then the cycle is begun again. Some regimens contain seven placebo tablets for the "off days" for easier management. Some oral contraceptives are taken on a 24-day regimen, with only 4 days "off." Others have extended regimens in which pills are taken for several months at a time, such as Seasonique

ALERT Rx

Frequency of Medroxyprogesterone Acetate Intramuscular Injections

With an interval greater than 14 weeks between intramuscular injections, the health care provider must be certain that the patient is not pregnant before administering the next injection.

or LoSeasonique. The extended regimen oral contraceptives decrease the number of menstrual cycles from monthly to quarterly. Oral contraceptives with "Fe" in the trade name usually have an iron supplement in the tablets designed for "off" days. Beyaz contains a daily dose of folate.

Medroxyprogesterone Acetate Contraceptive Injection

Medroxyprogesterone acetate (Depo-Provera), a synthetic progestin used in the treatment of abnormal uterine bleeding and secondary amenorrhea, is also used as a contraceptive. This drug is given intramuscularly every 3 months, with the initial dosage given within the first 5 days of menstruation or within 5 days postpartum.

Educating the Patient and Family about Female Hormones

Each oral contraceptive product has detailed patient instruction sheets regarding starting oral contraceptive therapy, including instructions for missed doses. All instructions are discussed with the patient. The patient is given a thorough explanation of the dose regimen and adverse reactions that may occur. Patients taking oral contraceptives are reminded that skipping a dose could result in pregnancy.

The health care provider usually performs periodic examinations, including laboratory tests, a pelvic examination, or a Pap smear test. The patient is encouraged to keep all appointments for follow-up evaluation of therapy. Following are key points about female hormones the patient and family members should know:

Estrogens and Progestins

- A patient package insert comes with the drug. Read the information carefully. If you have any questions about this information, discuss them with your health care provider.
- If you experience gastrointestinal upset, take the drug with food.
- Notify your health care provider if you experience any of the following: pain in the legs or groin area, sharp chest pain or sudden shortness of breath, lumps in the breast, sudden severe headache, dizziness or fainting, vision or speech disturbances, weakness or numbness in the arms or legs, severe abdominal pain, depression, or yellowing of the skin or eyes.

- If you think you may be pregnant or you experience abnormal vaginal bleeding, stop taking the drug and contact your health care provider immediately.
- If you have diabetes, check your blood glucose daily, or more often. Contact your health care provider if your blood glucose is elevated. An elevated blood glucose level may require a change in diabetic therapy (insulin, oral hypoglycemic drug) or diet; your health care provider must make these changes.

Oral Contraceptives

- A patient package insert comes with the drug. Read the information carefully. Begin the first dose as directed in the package insert or as directed by your health care provider. If you have any questions about this information, discuss them with your health care provider.
- To obtain a maximum effect, take this drug as prescribed and at intervals not exceeding once every 24 hours. An oral contraceptive is best taken with the evening meal or at bedtime. The effectiveness of this drug depends on following the prescribed dosage schedule. Failure to comply with the dosage schedule may result in a pregnancy.
- Use an additional method of birth control (as recommended by your health care provider) until after the first week in the initial cycle.
- If you miss one day's dose, take the missed dose as soon as remembered or take 2 tablets the next day. If you miss 2 days, take 2 tablets for the next 2 days and continue on with the normal dosing schedule. However, another form of birth control must be used until the cycle is completed and a new cycle is begun. If you miss 3 days in a row or more, discontinue use of the drug and use another form of birth control until a new cycle can begin. Before restarting the dosage regimen, make sure a pregnancy did not result from the break in the dosage regimen.
- If you have any questions regarding what to do about a missed dose, discuss the procedure with your health care provider.
- Do not smoke and avoid exposure to second-hand smoke while taking these drugs; cigarette smoking during estrogen therapy may increase the risk of cardiovascular effects.
- Report adverse reactions such as fluid retention or edema of the extremities; weight gain; pain, swelling, or tenderness in the legs; blurred vision; chest pain; yellowed skin or eyes; dark urine; or abnormal vaginal bleeding.
- While taking these drugs, periodic examinations by your health care provider and laboratory tests are necessary.

Estradiol Transdermal System

- Alora, Estraderm, and Vivelle-Dot are applied twice per week; Climara and Menostar are applied every 7 days.
- Apply the patch immediately after opening the pouch, with the adhesive side down. Apply to clean, dry skin of your trunk (not breast or waistline), buttocks, abdomen, upper inner thigh, or upper arm. (Do not apply to breasts or a site exposed to sunlight.) The area should not be oily or irritated.
- Press the patch firmly in place with the palm of your hand for approximately 10 seconds. Rotate the application site with at least 1-week intervals between applications to a particular site.
- Avoid areas that may be exposed to rubbing or where your clothing may rub the system off or loosen the edges.
- Remove the old patch before applying a new one unless your health care provider directs otherwise. Rotate application sites to prevent skin irritation.
- Follow the directions of your health care provider regarding application of the patch (e.g., continuous 3-week use followed by 1 week off, changed weekly, or applied twice weekly).
- If the patch falls off, then reapply it or apply a new patch. Continue the original treatment schedule.

Intravaginal Application

- Use the applicator correctly. Refer to the package insert for the correct procedure. The applicator is marked with the correct dosage and accompanies the drug when purchased.
- Wash the applicator after each use in warm water with a mild soap and rinse it well.
- Stay in a recumbent position for at least 30 minutes after instillation.
- Use a sanitary napkin or panty liner to protect your clothing if necessary.

COMPLEMENTARY & ALTERNATIVE MEDICINE

Black Cohosh

The herb black cohosh is popular as an alternative to hormone alternative replacement therapy, which may increase the woman's risk of serious illness, including cancer, depression, and high blood pressure. When taken orally, black cohosh may reduce physical menopausal symptoms, including night sweats, hot flashes, headaches, heart palpitations, dizziness, vaginal atrophy, and tinnitus. It may also improve the regularity of menstrual cycles and reduce the psychological symptoms associated with menopause, including insomnia, nervousness, irritability, and depression.

The primary adverse effect of black cohosh is nausea, and other possible effects include dizziness, headache, impaired vision, and vomiting. Pregnant women should not take black cohosh.

Women taking hormone alternative replacement therapy should consult with their health care provider before taking black cohosh.

- Do not double the dosage if you miss a dose. Instead, skip the dose and resume treatment the next day.
- When using the vaginal ring, press the ring into an oval and insert it into the upper third of the vaginal vault.

FACT CHECK

33-9 When taking a history for patients prescribed an estrogen, what key information must be included?

Emergency Contraception

Emergency contraception is used when unprotected intercourse occurs to prevent pregnancy. The emergency contraception medications available contain a progestin. The progestin prevents ovulation and thickens the cervical mucus, which prevents implantation. Emergency contraception should not be used as routine contraception. Emergency contraception products do not protect against sexually transmitted diseases.

There are currently two emergency contraceptives available. The most widely known contains levonorgestrel and is available under the trade names Next Choice, Plan B, and Plan B One-Step. These products are available over the counter for patients 17 years of age and older. For patients under 17, a prescription is required. Next Choice and Plan B contain two 0.75 levonorgestrel tablets. The first tablet should be taken within 72 hours of unprotected intercourse, and the second tablet taken 12 hours after the first tablet. Plan B One-Step contains one 1.5 mg tablet that should be taken as soon as possible within 72 hours after unprotected intercourse. Next Choice and Plan B could be taken as a single dose (two tablets at one time) like Plan B One-Step. Research is currently being conducted to determine if the window of opportunity for use extends beyond 72 hours after unprotected intercourse. Levonorgestrel is not effective if implantation has already begun and will not cause an abortion.

The other emergency contraceptive currently available is ulipristal, marketed under the trade name Ella. Ulipristal is a progesterone agonist/antagonist. It also works by delaying or preventing ovulation, but it likely also prevents implantation. Prior to taking, a pregnancy test should be used. If negative, then the patient should take one 30 mg tablet as soon as possible within 5 days (120 hours) of unprotected intercourse. Ulipristal is classified as FDA pregnancy category X. It is not indicated for termination of an existing pregnancy. These drugs are listed in Table 33-1.

FACT CHECK

33-10 How is levonorgestrel available and how is it to be taken?

Chapter Review

KEY POINTS

- Male and female hormones aid in development and maintenance of secondary sex characteristics and are necessary for human reproduction.
- A male or female hormone may be used to treat certain disorders, such as inoperable breast cancer, male hypogonadism, or a male or female hormone deficiency, and are used as contraceptives and for treating the symptoms of menopause.
- Testosterone, the most potent naturally occurring androgen, and its derivatives are called androgens. Testosterone and its derivatives activate the reproductive potential in adolescent boys and stimulate the growth of accessory sex organs at the time of puberty. The androgens also promote tissue-building processes anabolism and reverse tissue-depleting processes catabolism.
- In female patients, androgen therapy may be used as part of the treatment for inoperable metastatic breast carcinoma in postmenopausal women. Androgens may also be given to premenopausal women with metastatic breast carcinoma that is believed to be hormone-dependent and whose tumor growth and spread have been slowed after an oophorectomy.
- Anabolic steroids, synthetic drugs chemically related to the androgens, promote tissue-building processes. They are used to treat anemia of renal insufficiency, to control metastatic breast cancer in women, and to promote weight gain in those with weight loss after surgery, trauma, or infections.

- Virilization in women is the most common reaction associated with anabolic steroids, especially with higher doses. Abuse of anabolic steroids for muscle tissue development is a growing problem and should be discouraged.
- Androgen hormone inhibitors are synthetic compound drugs that inhibit the conversion of testosterone into the potent androgen 5-DHT. Finasteride and dutasteride are used to treat the symptoms of prostatic hypertrophy and for the prevention of male pattern baldness in men with early signs of hair loss.
- The PDE5 inhibitors are used to treat erectile dysfunction. These drugs are taken approximately 60 minutes prior to intercourse. The most common adverse reaction is headache.
- Alprostadil is available for erectile dysfunction. It is available as an intercavernosal injection and a urogenital pellet. Each dosage form requires the patient be educated on proper preparation and delivery of the dosage form. The most common adverse reaction is penile pain.
- The two female hormones are the estrogens and progesterone. The endogenous estrogens are estradiol, estrone, and estriol. Natural and synthetic progesterones are collectively called progestins.
- Estrogens are important in the development and maintenance of the female reproductive system and the primary and secondary sex characteristics. Other actions include fluid retention, protein anabolism, thinning of the cervical mucus, and the inhibition or facilitation of ovulation. Estrogen is most commonly used in combi-

nation with progesterones as contraceptives or as hormone replacement therapy in postmenopausal women.

- Estrogens have many adverse reactions. Warnings include an increased risk of endometrial cancer, gallbladder disease, hypertension, hepatic adenoma, cardiovascular disease, increased risk of thromboembolic disease, and hypercalcemia in those with breast cancer and bone metastases.
- Progestins are necessary for the development of the placenta and inhibit the secretion of pituitary gonadotropins, which in turn prevents maturation of the ovarian follicle and ovulation. The synthetic progestins are usually used medically because of the decreased effectiveness of progesterone when administered orally. The progestins are used in the treatment of amenorrhea, endometriosis, and functional uterine bleeding. Progestins are also used as oral contraceptives, either alone or in combination with an estrogen.
- Progestins have many adverse reactions, including breakthrough bleeding, spotting, change in the menstrual flow, amenorrhea, breast tenderness, edema, weight increase or decrease, acne, chloasma or melasma, and mental depression.
- Estrogens and progestins are used combined as oral contraceptives. Contraceptive hormones provide health benefits not related to contraception, such as regulating the menstrual cycle and decreasing blood loss, iron deficiency anemia, and dysmenorrhea. When estrogen/progestin combinations are used as oral contraceptives, the adverse reactions of both may occur.
- Two emergency contraceptive products are available. Levonorgestrel is a progestin that is available over the counter for patients 17 years of age and older but requires a prescription for those under 17. It will not terminate an existing pregnancy. Ulipristal is a progesterone agonist/antagonist. It is available by prescription only. It is rated at FDA pregnancy category X. It is not indicated for termination of an existing pregnancy.

CRITICAL THINKING CASE STUDY
CASE STUDY 1
Menopause

1. Ms. Hess has been experiencing symptoms of menopause. She went to her gynecologist and was given a prescription for Climara Pro. Climara Pro contains
   a. an estrogen
   b. a progestin
   c. an anabolic steroid
   d. both an estrogen and a progestin
2. How often should Ms. Hess apply the patch?
   a. Once daily
   b. Once weekly
   c. Twice weekly
   d. Every 3 days (72 hours)
3. Ms. Hess tells you that one of her friends takes a tablet called Prempro. She asks if Prempro treats the same symptoms as Climara Pro. What should you tell her?

CASE STUDY 2
Erectile Dysfunction

At his monthly checkup, Mr. Rabb confides in you that he is having a little trouble lately "in bed." He mentions that he has seen commercials about some products that might help him. You suggest that he ask the health care provider about the products available for erectile dysfunction. His physician prescribes Levitra.

1. How should he take Levitra?
   a. Once daily in the morning
   b. Once daily with dinner
   c. 15 minutes before sexual activity
   d. 60 minutes before sexual activity
2. Which medication should vardenafil not be combined with?
   a. Nitroglycerin
   b. Aspirin
   c. Acetaminophen
   d. Cetirizine
3. Mr. Rabb is concerned that if he takes the medication as prescribed that it might work before he wants it to. What should you tell him?

Review Questions

MULTIPLE CHOICE

1. When teaching the patient who is taking an oral contraceptive for the first time, the health care provider emphasizes the importance of taking
   a. two tablets per day at the first sign of ovulation
   b. the drug with the evening meal or at bedtime
   c. the drug early in the morning before arising
   d. the drug each day for 20 days beginning on the first of the month
2. Actions of androgens include all of the following EXCEPT
   a. reverse tissue-depleting processes
   b. promote tissue-building processes
   c. inhibit secretion of pituitary gonadotropins
   d. growth of accessory sex organs
3. Which of the following male hormones may cause GI upset?
   a. Oxandrolone
   b. Fluoxymesterone
   c. Nandrolone decanoate
   d. All of the above
4. All of the following are estrogens EXCEPT
   a. ethinyl estradiol
   b. estradiol
   c. estradone
   d. estrone

MATCHING

Match the medication on the left with the category on the right.

_____ 5. oxandrolone	a. PDE5 inhibitor
_____ 6. estradiol	b. Anabolic steroid
_____ 7. medroxyprogesterone	c. Estrogen
_____ 8. finasteride	d. Progestin
_____ 9. sildenafil	e. Androgen
_____ 10. testosterone	f. Androgen hormone inhibitor

Match the generic name on the left with the trade name on the right.

_____	11. medroxyprogesterone	a.	Cialis
_____	12. fluoxymesterone	b.	Viagra
_____	13. oxandrolone	c.	Climara
_____	14. synthetic conjugates estrogens, A	d.	Premarin
_____	15. dutasteride	e.	Estrace
_____	16. estradiol	f.	Depo-Provera
_____	17. conjugated estrogens	g.	Avodart
_____	18. estradiol, transdermal patch	h.	Cenestin
_____	19. tadalafil	i.	Oxandrin
_____	20. sildenafil	j.	Androxy

TRUE OR FALSE

_____ 21. Progestins may be administered to counteract the effect of estrogen on hormone-dependent tumors in women with breast carcinoma.

_____ 22. Androgens are commonly used in men with prostate carcinoma and prostate enlargement.

_____ 23. Use of anabolic steroids to enhance physical appearance or athletic performance is contraindicated.

_____ 24. Increased spotting and hypomenorrhea are signs of estrogen deficiency.

_____ 25. The PDE5 inhibitors should not be combined with nitrates, such as nitroglycerin.

FILL IN THE BLANKS

26. Administration of a penicillin or _____ with an oral contraceptive decreases the effects of the oral contraceptive.

27. Signs of progestin deficiency include late breakthrough bleeding, amenorrhea, or _____.

28. A patient taking the androgen hormone inhibitor _____ may experience impotence and decreased _____.

29. Two anabolic steroids used for anemia are _____ and _____.

30. The most common adverse reaction of the PDE5 inhibitors is _____ .

SHORT ANSWERS

31. Taking oral contraceptives has health benefits unrelated to contraception. What are some of these benefits?

32. Older male patients treated with steroids are at increased risk for which disorders?

33. When giving instructions to a patient taking estrogens or progestins, what should you advise her to do if she thinks she may be pregnant?

34. What are the most common adverse reactions for women taking an androgen preparation for breast carcinoma?

35. How do the emergency contraceptive products prevent pregnancy?

Web Activities

1. Go to The National Institute on Drug Abuse Web site (http://www.steroidabuse.org) and find the information titled "NIDA for Teens—Anabolic Steroids." Read the information about the use of anabolic steroids among adolescents and write a paragraph summarizing that information.

2. Go to the National Kidney and Urologic Diseases Information Clearinghouse (http://kidney.niddk.nih. gov) Web site and conduct a search for "erectile dysfunction." What is the prevalence of erectile dysfunction in the USA? How does an erection occur? How is ED treated?

SUMMARY DRUG TABLE Male Hormones (left, generic; right, trade)

Comprehensive Summary Drug Tables, including uses, adverses effects, dosages, and pregnancy classifications, are provided on the companion website, http://thePoint.lww. com/PharmacologyHP2e

Androgens	
fluoxymesterone *floo-oxi-mes'-te-rone*	Androxy (CIII)
methyltestosterone *meth-ill-tess-toss'-ter-one*	Android (CIII), Testred
testosterone buccal *tess-toss'-ter-one*	Striant
testosterone implant	Testopel
testosterone transdermal	Androderm, AndroGel, Axiron, First-Testosterone, Fortesta, Testim, First-Testosterone
testosterone cypionate (in oil)	Depo- Testosterone, *generic*
testosterone enanthate	Delatestryl, *generic*
danazol *da'-na-zole*	*generic*

Anabolic Steroids	
oxymetholone *oks-i-meth'-oh-lone*	Anadrol-50 (CIII)
oxandrolone *oks-an-droe-lone*	Oxandrin (CIII), *generic*
Androgen Hormone Inhibitor	
dutasteride *doo-tas'-teer-ide*	Avodart
finasteride *fin-as'-teh-ride*	Propecia, Proscar, *generic*

SUMMARY DRUG TABLE Female Hormones (left, generic; right, trade)

Comprehensive Summary Drug Tables, including uses, adverses effects, dosages, and pregnancy classifications, are provided on the companion website, http://thePoint.lww.com/PharmacologyHP2e

Estrogens	
conjugated estrogens, vaginal *es'-troe-jenz*	Premarin Vaginal
conjugated estrogen, injection	Premarin
conjugated estrogen, oral	Premarin
esterified estrogens	Menest
estradiol, oral *ess-troe-dye'-ole*	Estrace, Femtrace, *generic*
estradiol cypionate in oil *ess-troe-dye'-ole sip-ee-oh-nate*	Depo-Estradiol
estradiol transdermal patch *ess-troe-dye-ole*	Alora, Climara, Estraderm, FemPatch, Menostar Vivelle, Vivelle-Dot, *generic*
estradiol transdermal patch	Alora, Estraderm, Vivelle-Dot, Climara, Menostar
estradiol transdermal	Divigel, Elestrin, EstroGel, Estrasorb, Evamist
estradiol vaginal ring	Estring, Femring
estradiol vaginal tablet	Vagifem
estradiol vaginal cream	Estrace
estradiol valerate in oil *ess-troc-dye'-ole val-eh-rate*	Delestrogen, *generic*
estropipate *ess-troe-pi'-pate*	Ogen, Ortho-Est, *generic*
synthetic conjugated estrogens, A	Cenestin
synthetic conjugated estrogens, B	Enjuvia

Progestins	
hydroxyprogesterone caproate *hi-drox-ee-pro-jess'- te-rone cap-row'-ate*	Makena
medroxyprogesterone acetate *me-droks'-ee-proe-jes'-te-rone*	Depo-Provera, Provera, *generic*
megestrol acetate *me-jess'-troll*	Megace ES, Megace Oral, *generic*
norethindrone acetate, *nor-eth-in-drone*	Aygestin, *generic*
progesterone vaginal *proe-jess'-te-rone*	Crinone, Endometrin, First Progesterone-VGS, Prochieve
progesterone oral	Prometrium
progesterone injection	*generic*

Combination Products	
estrogens and progestin, combination, oral	Prempro, Premphase, Angeliq, Femhrt, Jinteli, Activella, Mimvey, Prefest, estradiol and norethindrone acetate, *generic*
estrogen and progestin, combination, transdermal	Climara Pro, CombiPatch
estrogen and androgen, combination, oral	Covaryx, Covaryx H.S., Estratest, Estratest H.S., esterified estrogens and methyltestosterone, *generic*

SUMMARY DRUG TABLE Erectile Dysfunction
(left, generic; right, trade)

Comprehensive Summary Drug Tables, including uses, adverses effects, dosages, and pregnancy classifications, are provided on the companion website, http://thePoint.lww.com/PharmacologyHP2e

phosphodiesterase 5 inhibitors sildenafil *sil-den'-a-fil*	Revatio, Viagra
tadalafil *tah-da'-la-fil*	Adcirca, Cialis
vardenafil *var-den'-a-fil*	Levitra, Staxyn

Drugs	
alprostadil, intracavernosal *al-pros'-ta-dill*	Caverject, Caverject Impulse, Edex
alprostadil, urogenital *al-pros'-ta-dill*	Muse

34

Uterine Drugs

CHAPTER OBJECTIVES

On completion of this chapter, students will be able to:

1. Define the chapter's key terms.
2. Compare and contrast the different uses of the oxytocic drugs.
3. Describe the general drug actions, uses, adverse reactions, contraindications, precautions, and interactions of drugs acting on the uterus.
4. Discuss important points to keep in mind when educating the patient or family members about the use of drugs acting on the uterus.

KEY TERMS

ergotism—an overdose of ergonovine characterized by necrosis of the extremities due to contraction of the peripheral vascular bed
oxytocic drugs—used before birth to induce uterine contractions similar to those of normal labor
oxytocin—an endogenous hormone produced by the posterior pituitary gland
uterine atony—marked relaxation of the uterine muscle

CHAPTER OVERVIEW

Drug classes covered in this chapter are:

- Oxytocic drugs

Drugs by classification are listed on page 359.

thePOINT RESOURCES

- Comprehensive Summary Drug Tables
- Lippincott's Interactive Tutorials: Drugs Affecting the Endocrine System
- Interactive Practice and Review
- Monographs of Most Commonly Prescribed Drugs

Drug therapy is often beneficial during labor and delivery to promote the well-being of a mother and her fetus. Depending on a patient's need, drugs may be used to stimulate or intensify uterine contractions. This chapter discusses the oxytocic drugs. Specific drugs are listed in the Summary Drug Table: Drugs Acting on the Uterus.

Oxytocic Drugs

Oxytocic drugs are used before birth to induce uterine contractions similar to those of normal labor. These drugs are desirable when early vaginal delivery is in the best interest of a mother and her fetus. They are also used to cause an abortion and to control postpartum vaginal hemorrhage. When applied cervically, they can initiate or continue cervical ripening for delivery.

An oxytocic drug is one that stimulates the uterus. Included in this group of drugs are ergonovine, methylergonovine (Methergine), oxytocin (Pitocin), carboprost (Hemabate), dinoprostone (Cervidil), and mifepristone (Mifeprex).

Actions of Oxytocic Drugs

Oxytocin

Oxytocin is an endogenous hormone produced by the posterior pituitary gland (see Chapter 31). This hormone has uterine-stimulating properties, especially on a pregnant uterus. As pregnancy progresses, the sensitivity of the uterus to oxytocin increases, reaching a peak sensitivity immediately before the birth of the infant. This sensitivity enables oxytocic drugs to exert their full therapeutic effect on the uterus

to produce the desired results (Fig. 34-1). Oxytocin also has antidiuretic and vasopressor effects. The exact mechanism of oxytocin in normal labor and medically induced labor is not well understood.

Ergonovine and Methylergonovine

Ergonovine and methylergonovine increase the strength, duration, and frequency of uterine contractions and decrease the incidence of uterine bleeding.

Carboprost

Carboprost is similar to naturally occurring prostaglandin $F_{2-\alpha}$. It stimulates uterine smooth muscle, resulting in contractions.

Dinoprostone

Dinoprostone is a synthetic preparation of prostaglandin E_2, which is a naturally occurring prostaglandin. Dinoprostone induces uterine contractions by stimulating the smooth muscle of the uterus. As an insert, it promotes cervical ripening by acting directly on the local receptors and relaxing the smooth muscles of the cervix.

Mifepristone

Mifepristone was once widely known as RU-486. It is a synthetic steroid that has both antiprogesterone as well as antiglucocorticoid activity. Depending on when it is given, mifepristone has different actions. If given within 72 hours of unprotected intercourse, it prevents implantation and acts like the emergency contraceptives discussed in Chapter 33. In abortion, it acts as an antagonist of progesterone and inhibits the support of the endometrium. It also increases the synthesis

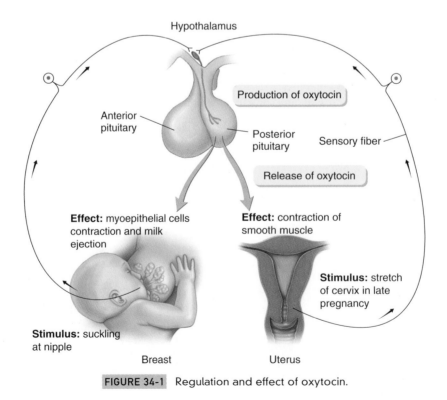

FIGURE 34-1 Regulation and effect of oxytocin.

and decreases the metabolism of prostaglandins. Eventually, this will result in menstrual bleeding and termination of the pregnancy. It also acts to ripen the cervix.

Uses of Oxytocic Drugs

Oxytocin

Oxytocin is administered intravenously for starting or improving labor contractions to obtain an early vaginal delivery of the fetus. An early vaginal delivery may be advisable when there are fetal or maternal problems, for example, a mother with diabetes and a large fetus, Rh blood–type problems, premature rupture of the membranes, uterine inertia, and eclampsia or preeclampsia. Oxytocin may also be used in the management of inevitable or incomplete abortion. Oxytocin is given intramuscularly during the third stage of labor (after the birth occurs and before the placenta is expelled) to produce uterine contractions and control postpartum bleeding and hemorrhage.

Ergonovine and Methylergonovine

Ergonovine and methylergonovine are given after the delivery of the placenta and are used to prevent postpartum and postabortal hemorrhage caused by **uterine atony** (marked relaxation of the uterine muscle).

Carboprost

Carboprost is used to terminate a pregnancy between gestational week 13 and 20. It is also used for postpartum uterine hemorrhage.

Dinoprostone

As a suppository, dinoprostone is used to terminate a pregnancy from the 12th through the 20th gestation weeks. It is used to evacuate the uterine contents in the event of a missed abortion or intrauterine fetal death up to 28 gestational weeks. As a cervical gel and vaginal insert, it is used to ripen the cervix.

Mifepristone

Mifepristone is used in combination with misoprostol (Chapter 28) to terminate an intrauterine pregnancy through day 49 of pregnancy.

FACT CHECK

34-1 What is oxytocin used for?
34-2 What are ergonovine and methylergonovine used for?
34-3 Which of the oxytocic drugs are used to terminate a pregnancy?

Adverse Reactions of Oxytocic Drugs

Oxytocin

Oxytocin may cause fetal bradycardia, uterine rupture, uterine hypertonicity (extreme tension of the uterine muscle), nausea, vomiting, cardiac arrhythmias, and anaphylactic reactions. Serious water intoxication (fluid volume excess) may occur, particularly when the drug is administered by continu-

KEY CONCEPTS

34-1 Managing Adverse Effects of Oxytocin

If contractions are frequent, prolonged, or excessive, then the oxytocin infusion is stopped to prevent fetal anoxia or trauma to the uterus. Excessive stimulation of the uterus can cause uterine hypertonicity and possible uterine rupture. The patient is placed on her side and given supplemental oxygen. The effects of the drug diminish rapidly because oxytocin is short acting.

When oxytocin is administered intravenously, there is a danger of fluid volume excess (water intoxication) because oxytocin has an antidiuretic effect. Fluid intake and output are measured. In some instances, hourly measurements of the output are necessary. The patient is monitored for signs of fluid overload (see Chapter 45). If any of these signs or symptoms is noted, then the oxytocin infusion should be immediately discontinued.

ous infusion and a patient is receiving fluids by mouth (Key Concepts 34-1).

Ergonovine and Methylergonovine

The adverse reactions of ergonovine include nausea, vomiting, elevated blood pressure, and ergotism. **Ergotism** (overdosage of ergonovine) is manifested by chest pain, muscle cramps or pain, weakness, numbness or tingling of the extremities, and an increased blood pressure. Methylergonovine most commonly causes nausea and vomiting. In some instances, hypertension associated with seizure or headache may occur. In severe cases, these symptoms are followed by hypotension, respiratory depression, hypothermia, gangrene of the fingers and toes, convulsions, hallucinations, and coma.

Carboprost

Carboprost causes vomiting, diarrhea, nausea, temperature elevation, and flushing. Occasionally, endometriosis can occur. It is also possible to retain bits of the placenta or for the patient to experience excessive uterine bleeding.

Dinoprostone

The adverse effects of dinoprostone are different depending on the dosage form. The suppository may cause vomiting, temperature elevations, diarrhea, nausea, headache, shivering

ALERT

Ergonovine and Calcium Deficiency

In some patients who are calcium deficient, the uterus may not respond to ergonovine. The lack of response should immediately be reported to the health care provider. Administration of calcium by intravenous injection usually restores the drug response.

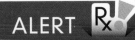

ALERT

Ergotism
Symptoms of ergotism that must be reported immediately include coolness, numbness, and tingling of the extremities; muscle cramps or pain; tachycardia or bradycardia; and chest pain. If these reactions occur, then they must immediately be reported to the health care provider because use of the drug must be discontinued.

and chills, and a drop in diastolic blood pressure. The gel may result in uterine contractile abnormalities, gastrointestinal (GI) disturbances, and fetal heart rate abnormalities. The insert may cause uterine hyperstimulation with or without fetal distress or fetal distress without uterine hyperstimulation. It is important for the fetus to be monitored during the use of dinoprostone.

Mifepristone

Mifepristone may cause dizziness, fatigue, headache, abdominal cramping or pain, diarrhea, nausea, vomiting, and back pain.

FACT CHECK

34-4   Why is water intoxication likely to occur with IV oxytocin administration?

34-5   What is ergotism, and what are the symptoms associated with it?

Contraindications, Precautions, and Interactions of Oxytocics

Oxytocin

- Oxytocin is contraindicated in patients with known hypersensitivity, cephalopelvic disproportion (the fetal head is too large to travel through the mother's pelvis), an unfavorable fetal position or presentation, obstetric emergencies, fetal distress when delivery is not imminent, severe toxemia (preeclampsia, eclampsia), hypertonic uterus, total placenta previa, or while inducing labor when vaginal delivery is contraindicated.
- Oxytocin is not ordinarily a risk to the fetus when administered as indicated.
- When oxytocin is administered with a vasopressor, severe hypertension may occur.

Ergonovine and Methylergonovine

- Ergonovine is contraindicated in those with a known hypersensitivity, in patients with hypertension, and before the delivery of the placenta.
- Ergonovine is used cautiously in patients with heart disease, obliterative vascular disease, or liver or kidney disease and in lactating women.
- Ergonovine is contraindicated with serotonin-receptor agonists, vasoconstrictors, beta-blockers, antiangina

drugs, antiretrovirals, SSRIs, SNRIs, and inhibitors of CYP3A4.
- Ergonovine and methylergonovine should not be coadministered with each other or other ergot alkaloids.
- Methylergonovine is contraindicated in patients with a known hypersensitivity, hypertension, or preeclampsia.
- Methylergonovine should not be used to induce labor.
- Methylergonovine is used cautiously in patients with renal or hepatic impairment.
- When methylergonovine is administered concurrently with vasopressors or to patients who are heavy cigarette smokers, excessive vasoconstriction may occur.

Carboprost

- Carboprost is contraindicated in patients with a known hypersensitivity to dinoprostone or prostaglandins and in those with acute pelvic inflammatory disease and active cardiac, pulmonary, renal, or hepatic disease.
- Carboprost should be used with caution in patients with a history of hypotension.
- Carboprost should not be used with other oxytocic drugs.

Dinoprostone

- Dinoprostone is contraindicated in patients with a known hypersensitivity to dinoprostone or prostaglandins and in those with acute pelvic inflammatory disease and active cardiac, pulmonary, renal, or hepatic disease.
- The cervical gel and vaginal insert are contraindicated in patients in whom prolonged contractions of the uterus are considered inappropriate.
- The vaginal insert is contraindicated in patients in whom delivery is not imminent and there is suspected or definite evidence of fetal distress and unexplained vaginal bleeding.
- Dinoprostone should not be combined with other oxytocic therapy.

Mifepristone

- Mifepristone and misoprostol should not be used to terminate a pregnancy if the pregnancy is confirmed or suspected to be ectopic, the patient has an undiagnosed adnexal mass, or the patient has an IUD in place. They should not be used in patients with chronic adrenal failure, concurrent long-term corticosteroid use, hemorrhagic disorders, concurrent anticoagulant therapy, or a history of allergy to mifepristone, misoprostol, or prostaglandins.
- Mifepristone is metabolized by cytochrome P450 3A4 and will interact with any other medication that induces or inhibits this enzyme.

Patient Management Issues with Oxytocics

Oxytocin

The patient's blood pressure, pulse, and respiratory rate are measured every 5 to 10 minutes after the drug is administered. Excessive bleeding should be immediately reported to the health care provider.

ALERT Rx

Oxytocin

All patients receiving intravenous oxytocin must be constantly observed to identify any complications. The health care provider should be immediately available at all times.

ALERT Rx

Oxytocic Drugs and Hyperstimulation of the Uterus

Hyperstimulation of the uterus during labor may lead to uterine tetany (cramping) with marked impairment of the uteroplacental blood flow, uterine rupture, cervical rupture, amniotic fluid embolism, and trauma to the infant. Overstimulation of the uterus is dangerous to both the fetus and the mother and may occur in a uterus that is hypersensitive to oxytocin even when the drug is administered properly.

An electronic infusion device is used to control the infusion rate of oxytocin. The strength, frequency, and duration of contractions and the fetal heart rate are monitored closely.

Ergonovine and Methylergonovine

When ergonovine and methylergonovine are administered after delivery, the patient's vital signs are monitored every 4 hours. The character and amount of vaginal bleeding are noted. The patient may report abdominal cramping with the use of these drugs. If cramping is moderately severe to severe, then the health care provider should be notified because it may be necessary to discontinue use of the drug.

Ergonovine is usually given during the third stage of labor after the placenta has been delivered. It is usually administered intramuscularly, but in emergencies when quicker response is needed, the drug may be administered intravenously.

Methylergonovine is usually given intramuscularly at the time of the delivery of the anterior shoulder or after the delivery of the placenta. The drug is not usually given intravenously because it may produce sudden hypertension and stroke. If the drug is given intravenously, then it is administered slowly over a period of 1 minute or more with close monitoring of the patient's blood pressure.

Carboprost

Carboprost should only be administered in a hospital that can provide immediate intensive medical as well as surgical care.

Dinoprostone

The suppository will be inserted high into the vagina. The physician will determine if additional dosing and at what interval it is necessary for the cervical gel. After the vaginal insert has been put in place, the patient must remain in a supine position for 2 hours. After the 2 hours, the patient may move around.

Mifepristone

The patient should have a follow-up visit approximately 14 days after the dose of mifepristone to ensure that the pregnancy has been successfully terminated. The patient must follow the treatment schedule and keep follow-up appointments. Vaginal bleeding and cramping will occur. Heavy prolonged bleeding does not indicate that a complete abortion has occurred. If the treatment fails, there is risk of fetal malformation, and a surgical termination of the pregnancy may be necessary. The patient can get pregnant after the termination and even prior to menses returning.

FACT CHECK

34-6 Does heavy and prolonged bleeding after use of mifepristone signify that an abortion has occurred?

34-7 What are the complications in the event of a treatment failure with mifepristone?

Educating the Patient and Family about Oxytocic Drugs

The treatment regimen is explained to the patient and family (when appropriate), and the patient is instructed to report any adverse reactions. These drugs will cause vaginal bleeding or uterine cramping. If the medication is being taken to end a pregnancy, the patient should understand that prolonged heavy bleeding is not proof of a complete abortion, and they should keep follow-up appointments.

Chapter Review

KEY POINTS

- Oxytocic drugs are used to induce uterine contractions similar to those of normal labor when early vaginal delivery is in the best interest of a mother and her fetus.
- Oxytocin, an endogenous hormone produced by the posterior pituitary gland, has uterine-stimulating properties, especially on a pregnant uterus. Oxytocin is administered intravenously for starting or improving labor contractions to obtain an early vaginal delivery of the fetus.
- Oxytocin may cause fetal bradycardia, uterine rupture, uterine hypertonicity, nausea, vomiting, cardiac arrhythmias, anaphylactic reactions, and serious water intoxication. When oxytocin is administered intravenously, there is a danger of a fluid volume excess (water intoxication). If contractions are frequent, prolonged, or excessive, the infusion is stopped to prevent fetal anoxia or trauma to the uterus.
- Ergonovine and methylergonovine both increase the strength, duration, and frequency of uterine contractions and decrease the incidence of uterine bleeding.
- Carboprost is used to terminate a pregnancy and to treat postpartum uterine hemorrhage.
- Dinoprostone is similar to prostaglandin E2. It is available in several dosage forms. The suppository is used to terminate a pregnancy and to cause evacuation of uterine contents. The cervical gel and insert are used to ripen the cervix for delivery.
- Mifeprisone is used in combination with misoprostol to terminate a pregnancy.

CRITICAL THINKING CASE STUDY

Labor Induction

Judith Watson, 28 years old, is admitted to the obstetric unit and is to receive oxytocin to induce labor. This is her first child, and she is extremely anxious.

1. What information should Ms. Watson's health care provider share with her?
   a. Oxytocin is administered intravenously to start or improve labor contractions.
   b. Oxytocin is administered intramuscularly to speed up labor contractions.
   c. Oxytocin is administered to slow contractions.
   d. It is not advisable to share any information with Ms. Watson regarding oxytocin.
2. What patient management issues arise with oxytocin?
   a. Patients receiving intravenous oxytocin must be under constant observation to watch for complications.
   b. To minimize hypotension, the patient is placed in a left lateral position unless the health care provider orders a different position.
   c. Overstimulation of the uterus is healthy for both the fetus and the mother.
   d. All of the above

3. Ms. Watson feels mild nausea as a result of the oxytocin. How should the health care provider respond?
   a. The drug should be immediately discontinued.
   b. The dosage of oxytocin should be doubled.
   c. Mifepristone should be used instead of oxytocin.
   d. Reassure Ms. Watson that this is normal and that it will pass soon after the drug wears off.
4. Ms. Watson tells you about her friend who received oxytocin after delivering her baby. She asks you why this drug would be given after delivery. What should you tell her?

Review Questions

MULTIPLE CHOICE

1. Which of the following symptoms would indicate that the patient is experiencing an adverse reaction to carboprost?
   a. Nervousness, tremor, anxiety
   b. Vomiting, diarrhea, temperature elevation
   c. Hypokalemia
   d. Headache, bradycardia
2. A patient receiving oxytocin to induce labor would be administered the drug
   a. intravenously
   b. intramuscularly
   c. either intravenously or intramuscularly
   d. none of the above
3. Contraindications of methylergonovine include all of the following EXCEPT
   a. preeclampsia
   b. hypersensitivity
   c. bronchial asthma
   d. hypertension
4. Which of the following adverse reactions is most indicative of ergotism?
   a. Numbness, tingling of the extremities
   b. Headache, blurred vision
   c. Tachycardia and cardiac arrhythmia
   d. Diaphoresis, increased respiration

MATCHING

Match the generic drug name on the left with the trade name on the right.

_____ 5. carboprost   a. Mifeprex
_____ 6. dinoprost   b. Pitocin
_____ 7. methylergonovine   c. Hemabate
_____ 8. mifepristone   d. Cervidil
_____ 9. oxytocin   e. Methergine

TRUE OR FALSE

_____ 10. Patients receiving methylergonovine may experience abdominal cramping.

_____ 11. Chills, a drop in diastolic blood pressure, and GI effects are common adverse reactions of dinoprostone.

_____ 12. The uterus becomes less sensitive to oxytocin as the pregnancy progresses.

_____ 13. Dinoprostone is used vaginally as an insert or a gel to ripen the cervix for delivery.

FILL IN THE BLANKS

14. Carboprost stimulates uterine _____ muscle, resulting in contractions.

15. Ergotism (overdosage of ergonovine) is manifested by chest pain, muscle cramps or pain, weakness, numbness or tingling of the _____, and an increased blood pressure.

16. Oxytocic drugs _____ the uterus and _____ the strength and frequency of uterine contractions.

17. Some patients with _____ deficiency may not respond to ergonovine.

SHORT ANSWERS

18. What may happen if hyperstimulation of the uterus occurs during labor?

19. What conditions may require use of oxytocin for an early vaginal delivery?

20. What is oxytocin, and where is it produced in the body?

21. What is the dosage regimen for mifepristone?

Web Activities

1. Go to the Mayo Clinic Web site (www.mayoclinic.com) and conduct a search on labor and delivery. What are the stages of labor?

2. On the same Web site, conduct a search for "inducing labor." What are the risks of inducing labor?

SUMMARY DRUG TABLE Drugs Acting on the Uterus
(left, generic; right, trade)

Comprehensive Summary Drug Tables, including uses, adverses effects, dosages, and pregnancy classifications, are provided on the companion website, http://thePoint.lww.com/PharmacologyHP2e

Oxytocics	
carboprost tromethamine _kar'-boe-prost tro-meth'-a-meen_	Hemabate
dinoprostone (prostaglandin E$_2$) _dye-noe-prost'-one_	Cervidil, Prepidil, Prostin E2
ergonovine maleate _er-goe-noe'-veen_	_generic_
methylergonovine maleate _meth-ill-er-goe noe'-veen_	Methergine, _generic_
mifepristone _mi-fe'-pris-tone_	Mifeprex
oxytocin (parenteral) _ox-i-toe'-sin_	Pitocin, _generic_

IX

ANTI-INFECTIVE DRUGS

35

Antibacterial Drugs

CHAPTER OBJECTIVES

On completion of this chapter, students will be able to:

1. Define the chapter's key terms.
2. Describe the difference between bacteriostatic and bactericidal.
3. Explain the need for culture and sensitivity tests.
4. Describe how to manage a burn.
5. Describe the different classes of penicillins.
6. Explain the differences between the generations of cephalosporins.
7. For each class of anti-infective, describe the general drug actions and uses.
8. Identify common adverse reactions for each class of anti-infective.
9. Describe the signs and symptoms of common adverse reactions seen with many of the anti-infectives, such as Stevens–Johnson syndrome or pseudomembranous colitis. Identify common adverse reactions for each class of anti-infective.
10. Identify common contraindications, precautions, and interactions for each class of anti-infective.
11. Discuss important points to keep in mind when educating the patient or family members about the use of antibacterial drugs.

KEY TERMS

anaphylactic shock—a severe form of hypersensitivity reaction
antibacterial—active against bacteria
anti-infective—another word for antibacterial; drugs used to treat infections and bacteria
bacterial resistance—ability of bacteria to produce substances that inactivate or destroy impact of a drug
bactericidal—an agent or drug that destroys bacteria

CHAPTER OVERVIEW

Drug classes covered in this chapter are:

- Sulfonamides
- Penicillins
- Cephalosporins
- Tetracyclines, Macrolides, and Lincosamides
- Fluoroquinolones and Aminoglycosides

Drugs by classification are listed on pages 381-382.

thePOINT RESOURCES

- Comprehensive Summary Drug Tables
- Lippincott's Interactive Tutorials: Drugs Used to Treat Infections
- Interactive Practice and Review
- Monographs of Most Commonly Prescribed Drugs

bacteriostatic—drugs that slow or retard the multiplication of bacteria

bowel prep—the use of drugs preoperatively to reduce the number of bacteria normally present in the intestine

cross-allergenicity—allergy to drugs in the same or related group

cross-sensitivity—synonymous with cross-allergenicity

culture and sensitivity tests—culturing performed to grow bacteria along with tests of their sensitivity to specific drugs

hypersensitivity—allergic

nonpathogenic—not disease causing

normal flora—nonpathogenic microorganisms within or on the body

pathogen—any virus, microorganism, or other substance that causes disease

penicillinase—an enzyme that inactivates penicillin

prophylaxis—prevention

pseudomembranous colitis—a common bacterial superinfection

Stevens–Johnson syndrome—serious allergic reaction to a drug, which initially exhibits reactions easily confused with less severe disorders

superinfection—an overgrowth of bacterial or fungal microorganisms not affected by the antibiotic being used for treatment

---

Antibacterial drugs are drugs that are active against bacteria. Another term that may be used to describe the general action of these drugs is **anti-infective** because they are used to treat infections caused by certain bacteria. We commonly refer to these drugs as antibiotics. This chapter provides information on the sulfonamides, penicillins, cephalosporins, tetracyclines, macrolides, lincosamides, fluoroquinolones, and aminoglycosides, all used for bacterial infections. In order to determine which of these antibacterial drugs will be most effective in treating a specific infection, **culture and sensitivity tests** are performed (Key Concepts 35-1).

Sulfonamides

The sulfonamides (sulfa) drugs were the first antibiotic drugs developed that effectively treated infections. Although the use of sulfonamides has declined after the introduction of more effective anti-infectives, such as the penicillins and other antibiotics, these drugs still remain important for the treatment of certain types of infections. Sulfadiazine, sulfisoxazole, and sulfamethoxazole are examples of sulfonamide preparations. Sulfadiazine is available as a single-ingredient product. Sulfisoxazole is combined with erythromycin ethylsuccinate. Sulfamethoxazole is combined with trimethoprim. In addition, mafenide and silver sulfadiazine are also sulfonamides. They are used topically to treat burns. Sulfasalazine, which was discussed in Chapter 29, is also a sulfonamide.

Actions of Sulfonamides

Sulfonamides are primarily **bacteriostatic**, which means they slow or retard the multiplication of bacteria. This bacteriostatic activity is caused by sulfonamide antagonism to para-aminobenzoic acid, a substance that some, but not all, bacteria need to multiply. Once the rate of bacterial multiplication is slowed, the body's own defense mechanisms (white blood cells) are able to rid the body of the invading microorganisms and therefore control the infection.

Uses of Sulfonamides

Sulfonamides are often used to control urinary tract infections caused by certain bacteria such as *Escherichia coli*, *Staphylococcus aureus*, and *Klebsiella enterobacter*. Sulfadiazine is also used to treat other types of infections including malaria, meningococcal meningitis, rheumatic fever, and others. The combination products, trimethoprim/sulfamethoxazole and erythromycin ethylsuccinate/sulfisoxazole, are used to treat otitis media. Mafenide (Sulfamylon) and silver sulfadiazine (Silvadene) are topical sulfonamides also used in the treatment of partial-thickness and full-thickness burns (Box 35-1).

KEY CONCEPTS

35-1 Identifying the Appropriate Antibacterial Drug

To determine if a specific type of bacteria is sensitive to a particular antibacterial drug, culture and sensitivity tests are performed. A culture is performed by placing infectious material obtained from areas such as the skin, respiratory tract, and blood on a culture plate that contains a special growing medium. This growing medium is "food" for the bacteria. After a specified time, the bacteria are examined under a microscope and identified. The sensitivity test involves placing the infectious material on a separate culture plate and then placing small disks impregnated with various antibiotics over the area. After a specified time, the culture plate is examined. If there is little or no growth around a disk, then the bacteria are considered sensitive to that particular antibiotic. Therefore, this antibiotic will control the infection (Fig. 35-1). If there is considerable growth around the disk, the bacteria are considered resistant to that particular antibiotic, and this antibiotic will not control the infection.

After a culture and sensitivity test is performed, the strain of microorganisms causing the infection is known, and the antibiotic to which these microorganisms are sensitive and resistant is identified. The health care provider then selects the antibiotic to which the microorganism is sensitive because that is the antibiotic that will be effective in the treatment of the infection.

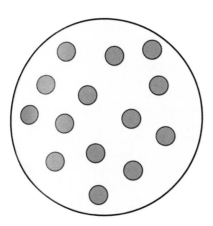

A. Culture plate with small disks containing various antibiotics.

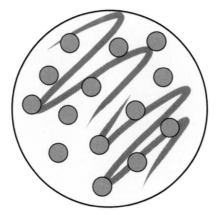

B. Infectious material is spread on the culture plate.

C. After a specific time, the culture plate is inspected. If there is little or no growth around a disk, the bacteria is said to be sensitive to that antibiotic. That antibiotic is considered a drug that will control the infection.

FIGURE 35-1   Action of penicillin.

Adverse Reactions of Sulfonamides

Sulfonamides can cause a variety of adverse reactions. Some of these are serious or potentially serious; others are mild. The following hematologic changes may occur during sulfonamide therapy:

- Agranulocytosis: decrease in or lack of granulocytes, a type of white blood cell
- Thrombocytopenia: decrease in the number of platelets
- Aplastic anemia: anemia caused by deficient red blood cell production in the bone marrow
- Leukopenia: decrease in the number of white blood cells

These are examples of serious adverse reactions. If any of these occurs, then discontinuation of sulfonamide therapy may be required.

Anorexia (loss of appetite) is an example of a mild adverse reaction. Unless it becomes severe and pronounced weight loss occurs, it may not be necessary to discontinue sulfonamide therapy.

Various types of **hypersensitivity** (allergic) reactions may occur during sulfonamide therapy, including Stevens–Johnson syndrome, urticaria (hives), pruritus (itching), and generalized skin eruptions (Key Concepts 35-2). **Stevens–Johnson syndrome** is manifested by fever, cough, muscular aches and pains, and headache, all of which are signs and symptoms of many other disorders. However, the appearance of lesions on the skin, mucous membranes, eyes, and other organs are diagnostically significant and may be the first conclusive signs of this syndrome. Any of these symptoms must be reported to the health care provider immediately.

Other adverse reactions that may occur during therapy include nausea, vomiting, diarrhea, abdominal pain, chills,

BOX 35.1

Managing Burns

When mafenide or silver sulfadiazine is used in the treatment of burns, the treatment regimen is outlined by the health care provider or the personnel in the burn treatment unit. There are various burn treatment regimens, such as debridement (removal of burned or dead tissue from the burned site), special dressings, and cleansing of the burned area. The use of a specific treatment regimen often depends on the extent of the burned area, the degree of the burns, and the physical condition and age of the patient. Other concurrent problems, such as lung damage caused by smoke or heat or physical injuries that occurred at the time of the burn injury, also may influence the treatment regimen.

The surface of the skin is cleaned and debris removed before each application of mafenide or silver sulfadiazine is applied with a sterile gloved hand. The drug is applied approximately one-sixteenth of an inch thick; thicker application is not recommended. The patient is kept away from any draft of air because even the slightest movement of air across the burned area can cause pain. The patient should be warned that stinging or burning might be felt during, and for a short time after, application of mafenide. Some burning also may be noted with the application of silver sulfadiazine.

KEY CONCEPTS

35-2 Managing Adverse Reactions of Antibacterials

Patients taking any of the antibacterial drugs are observed for adverse reactions, especially an allergic reaction (see Chapter 1). If one or more adverse reactions should occur, then the next dose of the drug is withheld and the health care provider should be notified.

fever, and stomatitis (inflammation of the mouth). In some instances, these may be mild. Other times, they may cause serious problems requiring discontinuation of the drug.

Crystalluria (crystals in the urine) may occur during use of a sulfonamide, although this problem occurs less frequently with some of the newer sulfonamide preparations. Increasing fluid intake during sulfonamide therapy can often prevent this potentially serious problem.

The most frequent adverse reaction seen with the application of mafenide is a burning sensation or pain when the drug is applied to the skin. Other possible allergic reactions include rash, itching, edema, and urticaria. Burning, rash, and itching may also occur with silver sulfadiazine. It may be difficult to distinguish between an adverse reaction caused by the use of mafenide or silver sulfadiazine and reactions that may occur from the severe burn injury or from other agents used at the same time for the management of the burns.

FACT CHECK

35-3 What hematologic changes may occur during sulfonamide therapy?

35-4 What are the signs and symptoms of Stevens–Johnson syndrome?

ALERT ℞

Stevens–Johnson Syndrome

Stevens–Johnson syndrome is a serious and sometimes fatal hypersensitivity reaction. Lesions on the skin and mucous membranes are a diagnostically important symptom of this syndrome. The lesions appear as red wheals or blisters, often starting on the face, in the mouth, or on the lips, neck, and extremities. This syndrome, which also may occur with the use of other types of drugs, can be fatal. The health care provider must be alerted and the next dose of the drug withheld. In addition, care must be exercised to prevent injury to the involved areas.

Contraindications, Precautions, and Interactions of Sulfonamides

- Sulfonamides are contraindicated in patients with known hypersensitivity, during lactation, and in children younger than 2 years old.
- Sulfonamides are not used near the end (at term) of pregnancy. If a sulfonamide is given near the end of pregnancy, then significant blood levels of the drug may occur, causing jaundice or hemolytic anemia in the neonate.
- Sulfonamides are not used for infections caused by group A beta-hemolytic streptococci because the sulfonamides have not been shown to be effective in preventing complications, such as rheumatic fever or glomerulonephritis.
- Sulfonamides are used with caution in patients with kidney or liver impairment or bronchial asthma.
- These drugs are given with caution to patients with allergies.
- When a sulfonamide is taken with an oral anticoagulant, the action of the anticoagulant may be enhanced.
- The risk of bone marrow suppression may be increased when a sulfonamide is administered with methotrexate.
- When a sulfonamide is administered with a hydantoin, the serum hydantoin level may be increased.
- Sulfonamides may inhibit the (hepatic) metabolism of the oral hypoglycemic drugs tolbutamide (Orinase) and chlorpropamide (Diabinese). This would increase the possibility of a hypoglycemic reaction.

Patient Management Issues with Sulfonamides

Temperature, pulse, respiratory rate, and blood pressure should be assessed every 4 hours or as ordered by the health care provider. If fever is present and the patient's temperature suddenly increases or if the temperature was normal and suddenly increases, then the health care provider should be contacted immediately.

When a sulfonamide is used for a burn, the burned areas are inspected every 1 to 2 hours because some treatment regimens require keeping the affected areas covered with the mafenide or silver sulfadiazine ointment at all times. Any adverse reactions should be reported immediately to the health care provider.

ALERT ℞

Fluid Intake and Output with Sulfonamide Use

Patients taking sulfonamide need to maintain adequate fluid intake and output. Patients should be encouraged to increase fluid intake to 2000 mL or more per day to prevent crystalluria and stone formation in the genitourinary tract, as well as to aid in the removal of microorganisms from the urinary tract. The health care provider should be notified if the patient's urinary output decreases or the patient fails to increase his or her oral intake.

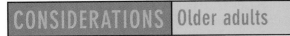

CONSIDERATIONS Older adults

LIFESPAN

Sulfonamides

Because kidney impairment is common in older adults, sulfonamides should be given with great caution. There is an increased danger of sulfonamides causing additional renal damage when renal impairment is already present. An increase of fluid intake up to 2000 mL (if the older adult can tolerate this amount) decreases the risk of crystals and stones forming in the urinary tract.

A patient receiving a sulfonamide drug almost always has an active infection. Some patients may be receiving one of these drugs to prevent an infection (prophylaxis) or as part of the management of a disease such as ulcerative colitis.

Unless the health care provider orders otherwise, sulfonamides are given to the patient when the stomach is empty, usually 1 hour before or 2 hours after meals. The patient should be instructed to drink a full glass of water when taking an oral sulfonamide and to drink at least eight large glasses of water each day until therapy is finished.

Educating the Patient and Family about Sulfonamides

When a sulfonamide is prescribed for an infection, some outpatients have a tendency to discontinue the drug once their symptoms have been relieved. The importance of completing the prescribed course of therapy to be sure all microorganisms causing the infection are eradicated is emphasized. Failure to complete a course of therapy may result in a recurrence of the infection. Following are key points about sulfonamides the patient and family members should know:

- Take the drug as prescribed by your health care provider.
- Take the drug on an empty stomach either 1 hour before or 2 hours after a meal.
- Take the drug with a full glass of water. Do not increase or decrease the time between doses except as directed by your health care provider.
- Complete the full course of therapy. Do not discontinue this drug even though the symptoms of the infection have disappeared (unless advised to do so by your health care provider).
- Drink at least 8 to 10 8-oz glasses of fluid every day.
- Prolonged exposure to sunlight may result in skin reactions similar to a severe sunburn (photosensitivity reactions). When going outside, cover exposed areas of your skin or apply a protective sunscreen to exposed areas.
- Notify your health care provider immediately if you experience any of the following: fever, skin rash or other skin problems, nausea, vomiting, unusual bleeding or bruising, sore throat, or extreme fatigue.
- Keep all follow-up appointments to ensure your infection is controlled.

FACT CHECK

35-5 What is crystalluria and how can it be prevented?
35-6 How should sulfonamides be taken with regard to meals?

Penicillins

The development of the sulfonamide antibiotics was a breakthrough in the treatment of bacterial infections. Since that time, there has been a quest to develop new and more effective antibiotic drugs. Sir Arthur Fleming discovered the antibacterial properties of natural penicillins in 1928 while he was performing research on influenza. Ten years later, British scientists studied the effects of natural penicillins on disease-causing microorganisms. After 1941, natural penicillins were used clinically for the treatment of infections. Although used for more than 70 years, the penicillins are still an important and effective group of antibiotics for the treatment of susceptible **pathogens** (disease-causing microorganisms).

There are four groups of penicillins: natural penicillins, penicillinase-resistant penicillins, aminopenicillins, and the extended-spectrum penicillins. See the Summary Drug Table: Penicillins for a more complete listing of the penicillins. Following are examples of the various groups:

- Natural penicillins: penicillin G and penicillin V
- Penicillinase-resistant penicillin: dicloxacillin, nafcillin, oxacillin
- Aminopenicillins: ampicillin, amoxicillin
- Extended-spectrum penicillins: piperacillin, ticarcillin

Drug Resistance

Because natural penicillins have been used for many years, drug-resistant strains of microorganisms have developed, making the natural penicillins less effective than some of the newer antibiotics for treating a broad range of infections. **Bacterial resistance** is the ability of bacteria to produce substances that inactivate or destroy an anti-infective drug. One example of bacterial resistance is the ability of certain bacteria to produce **penicillinase**, an enzyme that inactivates penicillin. Penicillinase-resistant penicillins were developed to combat this problem.

Natural penicillins also have a fairly narrow spectrum of activity, which means that they are effective against only a few strains of bacteria. Newer penicillins have been developed to combat this problem. These penicillins are a result of chemical treatment of a biologic precursor to penicillin. Because of their chemical modifications, they are more slowly excreted by the kidneys and, thus, have a somewhat wider spectrum of antibacterial activity. Penicillin β-lactamase inhibitor combinations are a type of penicillin that has a wider spectrum of antibacterial activity. Certain bacteria have developed the ability to produce enzymes called β-lactamases, which can destroy a component of the penicillin called the β-lactam ring. Fortunately, chemicals were discovered that inhibit the activity of these enzymes. Three examples of these β-lactamase inhibitors are clavulanic acid, sulbactam, and tazobactam. When these chemicals are used alone, they have little antimicrobial activity. However, when combined with certain penicillins, they extend the spectrum of penicillin's antibacterial activity. The β-lactamase inhibitors bind with penicillin and protect penicillin from destruction.

Actions of Penicillins

Penicillins have the same type of action against bacteria. Penicillins prevent bacteria from using a substance that is necessary for the maintenance of the bacteria's outer cell wall. Unable to use this substance for cell wall maintenance, the bacteria swell, rupture, assume unusual shapes, and finally die (Fig. 35-2).

Penicillins may be **bactericidal** (destroy bacteria) or bacteriostatic (slow or retard the multiplication of bacteria). They are bactericidal against sensitive microorganisms (i.e., those microorganisms that will be affected by penicillin), provided there is an adequate concentration (blood level) of penicillin in the body. An inadequate concentration (or inadequate blood level) of penicillin may produce bacteriostatic activity, which may or may not control the infection.

Uses of Penicillins

Infectious Disease

Natural and semisynthetic penicillins are used in the treatment of bacterial infections caused by susceptible microorganisms. Penicillins may be used to treat infections such as urinary tract infections, septicemia, meningitis, intra-abdominal infection, gonorrhea, syphilis, pneumonia, and other respiratory infections. Examples of infectious microorganisms (bacteria) that may respond to penicillin therapy include gonococci, staphylococci, streptococci, and pneumococci. Culture and sensitivity tests are performed whenever possible to determine which penicillin will best control an infection caused by a specific strain of bacteria. A penicillinase-resistant penicillin is used as initial therapy for any suspected staphylococcal infection until culture and sensitivity results are known.

Prophylaxis

Penicillin is of no value in the treatment of viral or fungal infections. However, health care providers occasionally prescribe penicillin as **prophylaxis** (prevention) against a potential secondary bacterial infection that can occur in a patient with a viral infection. In these situations, the viral infection has weakened the body's defenses and the person is susceptible to other infections, particularly a bacterial infection. Penicillin also may be prescribed as prophylaxis for a potential infection in high-risk individuals, such as those with a history of rheumatic fever. Penicillin is taken several hours or, in some instances, days before and after an operative procedure, such as dental, oral, or upper respiratory tract procedures that can result in bacteria entering the bloodstream. Taking penicillin before and after the procedure will usually prevent a bacterial infection in these high-risk patients. Penicillin also may be given prophylactically on a continuing basis to those with rheumatic fever and chronic ear infections.

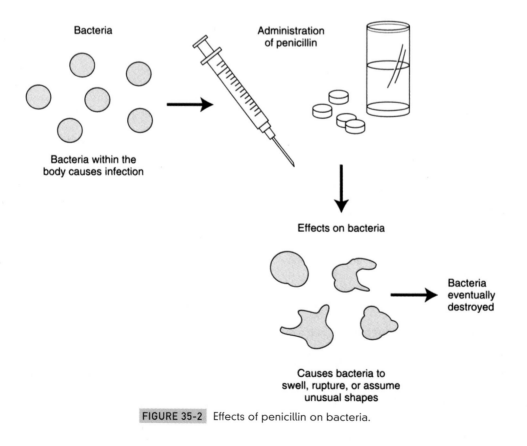

FIGURE 35-2　Effects of penicillin on bacteria.

FACT CHECK

35-7 What are examples of bacteria that may respond to penicillin therapy?

35-8 What are two main uses of penicillins?

Adverse Reactions of Penicillins

Common adverse reactions include mild nausea, vomiting, diarrhea, sore tongue or mouth, fever, and pain at injection site. Penicillin can stimulate a hypersensitivity (allergic) reaction within the body. Another adverse reaction that may be seen with penicillin, as well as with almost all antibiotics, is a **superinfection** (a secondary infection that occurs during antibiotic treatment).

Other adverse reactions associated with penicillin are hematopoietic changes such as anemia, thrombocytopenia (low platelet count), leukopenia (low white blood cell count), and bone marrow depression. When penicillin is given orally, glossitis (inflammation of the tongue), stomatitis (inflammation of the mouth), dry mouth, gastritis, nausea, vomiting, diarrhea, and abdominal pain occur. Some patients may experience a black hairy tongue while taking penicillin. When penicillin is given intramuscularly, there may be pain at the injection site. Irritation of the vein and phlebitis (inflammation of a vein) may occur with intravenous use.

Hypersensitivity Reactions

A hypersensitivity (or allergic) reaction to a drug occurs in some patients, especially those with a history of allergy to many substances. Signs and symptoms of a hypersensitivity to penicillin are highlighted in the Signs and Symptoms box. **Anaphylactic shock,** which is a severe form of hypersensitivity reaction, also can occur (see Chapter 1). Anaphylactic shock occurs more frequently after parenteral use but can occur with oral use. This reaction is likely to be immediate and severe in susceptible patients. Signs of anaphylactic shock include severe hypotension, loss of consciousness, and acute respiratory distress. If not immediately treated, anaphylactic shock can be fatal.

Once a patient is allergic to one type of penicillin, he or she is most likely allergic to all penicillins. Those allergic to penicillin also have a higher incidence of allergy to the cephalosporins, which are discussed later in this chapter. Allergy to drugs in the same or related groups is called **cross-sensitivity** or **cross-allergenicity**.

Superinfections

Antibiotics can disrupt the **normal flora** (nonpathogenic microorganisms within the body), causing a superinfection. This new infection is "superimposed" on the original infection. The destruction of large numbers of **nonpathogenic** bacteria (normal flora) by the antibiotic alters the chemical environment. This allows uncontrolled growth of bacteria or fungal microorganisms, which are not affected by the antibiotic being used. A superinfection may occur with the use of any antibiotic, especially when these drugs are given for a long time or when repeated courses of therapy are necessary. A superinfection can develop rapidly and is potentially serious or life-threatening. Bacterial superinfections are commonly seen with the use of the oral penicillins and occur in the bowel. **Pseudomembranous colitis** is a common bacterial superinfection.

Fungal superinfections commonly occur in the vagina, mouth, and anal and genital areas. Candidiasis or moniliasis is a common type of fungal superinfection. Candidiasis or moniliasis may occur because of an overgrowth of the yeastlike fungi that usually exist in small numbers in the vagina. The multiplication rate of these microorganisms is normally slowed and kept under control because of the presence of a strain of bacteria (*Döderlein bacillus*) in the vagina. If penicillin therapy destroys these normal microorganisms of the vagina, the fungi are now uncontrolled, multiply at a rapid rate, and cause symptoms of a fungal infection called candidiasis (or moniliasis). The Signs and Symptoms box provides more information on bacterial and fungal superinfections.

FACT CHECK

35-9 What are two common types of superinfections?

35-10 What are the signs and symptoms of C. *difficile* infection?

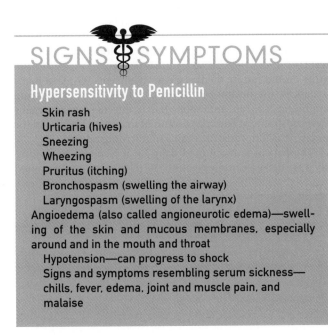

SIGNS ✚ SYMPTOMS

Hypersensitivity to Penicillin

Skin rash
Urticaria (hives)
Sneezing
Wheezing
Pruritus (itching)
Bronchospasm (swelling the airway)
Laryngospasm (swelling of the larynx)
Angioedema (also called angioneurotic edema)—swelling of the skin and mucous membranes, especially around and in the mouth and throat
Hypotension—can progress to shock
Signs and symptoms resembling serum sickness—chills, fever, edema, joint and muscle pain, and malaise

CONSIDERATIONS | Infants & Children

LIFESPAN

Candida Fungal Superinfections

Children taking antibiotics may experience Candida fungal superinfections (commonly called thrush), which may occur in the mouth and around the anal and genital areas. These require antifungal therapy, and patients should be referred to the health care provider. If the diet permits, yogurt, buttermilk, or acidophilus capsules may be taken to reduce the risk of fungal superinfections.

SIGNS SYMPTOMS

Superinfection

Patients taking any antibacterial drugs who experience any of the following signs and symptoms should immediately contact their health care provider:

Signs and symptoms of bacterial superinfection:
- Diarrhea, possibly severe with visible blood and mucus
- Rectal bleeding
- Fever
- Abdominal cramps

Signs and symptoms of fungal superinfection:
- Scaly, reddened, papular rash commonly in the breast folds, at the axillae, groin, or umbilicus
- White or yellow vaginal discharge
- Localized redness, inflammation, and excoriation, particularly inside the mouth, in the groin, or skin folds of the anogenital area
- Anal or vaginal itching
- Creamy white lace-like patches on the tongue, mouth, or throat
- Burning sensation in the mouth or throat

Contraindications, Precautions, and Interactions of Penicillins

- Penicillins are contraindicated in patients with a history of hypersensitivity to penicillin
- Penicillins should be used cautiously in patients with renal disease, during lactation (may cause diarrhea or candidiasis in the infant), and in those with a history of allergies. Any indication of sensitivity is reason for caution.
- The drug is also used with caution in patients with asthma, renal disease, bleeding disorders, and gastrointestinal disease.
- Some penicillins may interfere with the effectiveness of birth control pills that contain estrogen. An alternative form of birth control should be used while on the penicillin and continued until a new birth control pack is started.
- There is potential for cross-sensitivity with cephalosporins. The penicillins should be used cautiously in patients who have a documented cephalosporin allergy, especially to a first- or second-generation cephalosporin.
- There is a decreased effectiveness of the penicillin when it is administered with the tetracyclines.

ALERT ℞

Pseudomembranous Colitis
Pseudomembranous colitis may occur after 4 to 9 days of treatment with penicillin or as long as 6 weeks after the drug is discontinued.

CONSIDERATIONS | Older adults

LIFESPAN

Penicillin Use

Older adults who are debilitated, chronically ill, or taking penicillin for an extended period of time are more likely to have a superinfection. Pseudomembranous colitis is one type of a bacterial superinfection. This potentially life-threatening problem develops because of an overgrowth of the microorganism *Clostridium difficile*. This organism produces a toxin that affects the lining of the colon. Signs and symptoms include severe diarrhea with visible blood and mucus, fever, and abdominal cramps. This adverse reaction usually requires immediate discontinuation of the antibiotic. Mild cases may respond to drug discontinuation. Moderate to severe cases may require treatment with intravenous fluids and electrolytes, protein supplementation, and oral vancomycin (Vancocin).

- Large doses of penicillin can increase bleeding risks of patients taking anticoagulant agents.
- Some reports indicate that when oral penicillins are administered with beta-adrenergic blocking drugs (see Chapter 12), the patient may be at increased risk for an anaphylactic reaction.
- Absorption of most penicillins is affected by food. In general, penicillins should be given 1 hour before or 2 hours after meals.

Patient Management Issues with Penicillins

Before the first dose of penicillin, the patient's general health history is reviewed. If the patient has a history of allergy, particularly a drug allergy, then this must be explored to ensure the patient is not allergic to penicillin or a cephalosporin.

The patient's infected area is assessed when possible. Any signs and symptoms related to the patient's infection, such as color and type of drainage from a wound, pain, redness and inflammation, color of sputum, elevated body temperature or presence of an odor are noted. A culture and sensitivity test is almost always ordered. The results of a culture and sensitivity test take several days because time is needed for the bacteria to grow on the culture media (see Key Concepts 35-1). In many instances, the health care provider selects a broad-spectrum antibiotic (i.e., an antibiotic that is effective against many types or strains of bacteria) for initial treatment because of the many penicillin-resistant strains of microorganisms.

The patient is monitored daily for a response to therapy, such as a decrease in temperature, the relief of symptoms caused

ALERT ℞

Intramuscular Use of Penicillin
A patient who has been given penicillin intramuscularly in the outpatient setting is asked to wait in the area for at least 30 minutes. Anaphylactic reactions are most likely to occur within 30 minutes after injection.

by the infection (such as pain or discomfort), an increase in appetite, and a change in the appearance or amount of drainage (when originally present). Once an infection is controlled, patients often look better and even state that they feel better. The health care provider should be notified if signs and symptoms of the infection appear to worsen.

Additional culture and sensitivity tests may be performed during therapy because microorganisms causing the infection may become resistant to penicillin, or a superinfection may occur.

Educating the Patient and Family about Penicillins

Some patients do not adhere to the prescribed drug regimen for a variety of reasons, such as failure to comprehend the prescribed regimen or failure to understand the importance of continued and uninterrupted therapy. The drug regimen is carefully explained, and the importance of continued and uninterrupted therapy is stressed when the patient is educated about their prescription. Following are key points about penicillins the patient or family members should know:

Prophylaxis (Prevention)

- Take the drug as prescribed until your health care provider discontinues therapy.

Infection

- Complete the full course of therapy. Do not stop taking the drug, even if your symptoms have disappeared, unless directed to do so by your health care provider.
- Take the drug at the prescribed times of day because it is important to keep an adequate amount of the drug in your body throughout the entire 24 hours of each day.

Penicillin (Oral)

- Take the drug on an empty stomach either 1 hour before or 2 hours after meals (exceptions: penicillin V and amoxicillin).
- Take each dose with a full glass of water.
- To reduce the risk of superinfection, eat yogurt, drink buttermilk, or take acidophilus capsules.
- Notify your health care provider immediately if you experience any of the following: skin rash; hives (urticaria); severe diarrhea; vaginal or anal itching; sore mouth; black, furry tongue; sores in the mouth; swelling around the mouth or eyes; breathing difficulty; or gastrointestinal disturbances such as nausea, vomiting, and diarrhea. Do not take the next dose of the drug until you discuss the problem with your health care provider.

Oral Suspensions

- Make note of storage requirements; most will require refrigeration. Drugs that are kept refrigerated lose their potency when kept at room temperature, so return the drug to the refrigerator immediately after pouring the dose. Shake the drug well before pouring. A small amount of the drug may be left after the last dose is

ALERT ℞

Hypersensitivity Reaction

The patient should be closely observed for a hypersensitivity reaction, which may occur any time during therapy with the penicillins. If it should occur, then the health care provider should be contacted immediately and the drug withheld until the patient is seen by the health care provider. Treatment of minor hypersensitivity reactions may include use of an antihistamine such as Benadryl (for a rash or itching). Major hypersensitivity reactions, such as bronchospasm, laryngospasm, hypotension, and angioneurotic edema, require immediate treatment with drugs such as epinephrine, cortisone, or an intravenous antihistamine. When respiratory difficulty occurs, a tracheostomy may need to be performed.

Adequate blood levels of the drug must be maintained for the drug to be effective. Accidental omission or delay of a dose results in decreased blood levels, which will reduce the effectiveness of the antibiotic. Oral penicillins should be given on an empty stomach, 1 hour before or 2 hours after a meal. Penicillin V and amoxicillin may be given without regard to meals.

When penicillin is administered intramuscularly, the patient may feel a stinging or burning sensation at the time the drug is injected into the muscle. Discomfort at the time of injection occurs because the drug is irritating to the tissues. Previous areas used for injection are checked for continued redness, soreness, or other problems. The health care provider should be informed if injection areas appear red or the patient reports pain in the area.

The use of oral penicillin may result in a fungal superinfection in the oral cavity. With impaired oral mucous membranes will be varying degrees of inflamed oral mucous membranes, swollen and red tongue, swollen gums, and pain in the mouth and throat. To detect this problem early, the patient's mouth is inspected daily for evidence of glossitis, sore tongue, ulceration, or a black, furry tongue. The mouth and gums are inspected often, and frequent mouth care is given with a nonirritating solution. A soft-bristled toothbrush is used when brushing is needed. A nonirritating soft diet may be required. Dietary intake is monitored to assure the patient is receiving adequate nutrition. Antifungal agents and/or local anesthetics are sometimes recommended to soothe the irritated membranes.

taken. Discard any remaining drug because the drug (in suspension form) begins to lose its potency after 7 to 14 days. The discard date should be noted on the medication bottle.

- Women prescribed ampicillin and penicillin V who take birth control pills containing estrogen should use additional contraception measures.
- Never give this drug to another individual, even if their symptoms appear the same as your symptoms.
- Notify your health care provider if the symptoms of your infection do not improve or if your condition becomes worse.
- If you are taking penicillin as prevention, you may feel well even though you need the long-term antibiotic therapy. Avoid any temptation to skip one or more doses or to stop taking the drug for an extended time. Never skip doses or stop therapy unless told to do so by your health care provider.

FACT CHECK

35-11   Penicillins should be used with caution in patients with a history of hypersensitivity to penicillin and which other drug?

35-12   What should a woman taking an oral contraceptive containing estrogen be told prior to starting penicillin therapy?

Cephalosporins

The effectiveness of penicillin in the treatment of infections prompted research directed toward finding new antibiotics with a wider range of antibacterial activity. Cephalosporins are a valuable group of drugs that are effective in the treatment of almost all of the strains of bacteria affected by the penicillins, as well as some strains of bacteria that have become resistant to penicillin. Cephalosporins are structurally and chemically related to penicillin.

Cephalosporins are divided into first-, second-, third-, fourth-, and fifth-generation drugs (Key Concepts 35-3). Particular cephalosporins also may be differentiated within each group according to the microorganisms that are sensitive to them. Generally, progression from the first-generation to the second-generation and then to the third-generation drugs shows an increase in the sensitivity of gram-negative microorganisms

KEY CONCEPTS

35-3   Generations of Cephalosporins

First: cefadroxil, cefazolin, cephalexin
Second: cefaclor, cefotetan, cefoxitin, cefprozil, cefuroxime
Third: cefdinir, cefditoren, cefixime, cefotaxime, cefpodoxime, ceftazidime, ceftibuten, ceftizoxime, ceftriaxone
Fourth: cefepime
Fifth: ceftaroline

and a decrease in the sensitivity of gram-positive microorganisms. For example, a first-generation cephalosporin would have more use against gram-positive microorganisms than would a third-generation cephalosporin. This scheme of classification is becoming less clearly defined as newer drugs are introduced. For a complete listing, see the Summary Drug Table: Cephalosporins.

Actions of Cephalosporins

Cephalosporins affect the bacterial cell wall, making it defective and unstable. This action is similar to the action of penicillin. Cephalosporins are usually bactericidal (capable of destroying bacteria).

Uses of Cephalosporins

Cephalosporins are used in the treatment of infections caused by susceptible microorganisms. Examples of microorganisms that may be susceptible to cephalosporins include streptococci, staphylococci, citrobacters, gonococci, shigella, and clostridia. Culture and sensitivity tests are performed whenever possible to determine which antibiotic, including a cephalosporin, can best control an infection caused by a specific strain of bacteria. Pharyngitis, tonsillitis, otitis media, lower respiratory infections, urinary tract infections, septicemia, and gonorrhea are examples of the types of infections that may be treated with the cephalosporins.

Cephalosporins also may be used before, during, or after surgery to prevent infection in patients having surgery on a contaminated or potentially contaminated area, such as the gastrointestinal tract or vagina. In some instances, a specific drug may be recommended for postoperative prophylactic use only.

FACT CHECK

35-13   What is the difference between a first-generation and a third-generation cephalosporin?

35-14   How do cephalosporins act against bacteria?

Adverse Reactions of Cephalosporins

The most common adverse reactions of cephalosporins are gastrointestinal disturbances, such as nausea, vomiting, and diarrhea.

Hypersensitivity (allergic) reactions may occur with use of the cephalosporins and range from mild to life-threatening. Mild hypersensitivity reactions include pruritus, urticaria, and skin rashes. More serious hypersensitivity reactions include Stevens–Johnson syndrome, liver or kidney dysfunction, aplastic anemia (anemia caused by deficient red blood cell production), and epidermal necrolysis (death of the epidermal layer of the skin).

Because of the close relation of the cephalosporins to penicillin, a patient allergic to penicillin also may be allergic to the cephalosporins. This cross-sensitivity seems to be more common with first- and second-generation cephalosporins and in patients with a true allergy to penicillin. Patients should be questioned on the nature and type of allergic reaction to either penicillin or a cephalosporin prior to anti-infective therapy being initiated.

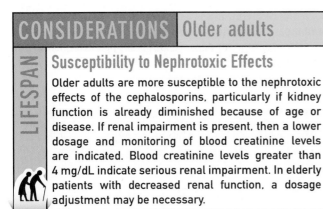

ALERT

Nephrotoxicity and Cephalosporins
Nephrotoxicity may occur with the use of these drugs. Early signs of this adverse reaction may become apparent by a decrease in urine output. Fluid intake and output are monitored and the health care provider notified if the output is less than 500 mL/day. Any changes in the fluid intake-to-output ratio or in the appearance of the urine may indicate nephrotoxicity. These findings should be reported to the health care provider promptly.

Other adverse reactions that may be seen with cephalosporin use are headache, dizziness, nephrotoxicity (damage to the kidneys), malaise, heartburn, and fever. Intramuscular use often results in pain, tenderness, and inflammation at the injection site. Intravenous use has resulted in thrombophlebitis and phlebitis.

Therapy with cephalosporins may result in a bacterial or fungal superinfection. Diarrhea may be an indication of pseudomembranous colitis, which is one type of bacterial superinfection.

Rare cases of hemolytic anemia, including fatalities, have been reported with cephalosporins. The patient should be monitored for anemia. If a patient experiences anemia within 2 to 3 weeks after the start of cephalosporin therapy, then drug-induced anemia should be considered. If hemolytic anemia is suspected, then the health care provider will discontinue the drug therapy. The patient may require blood transfusions to correct the anemia. Frequent hematological studies may be required.

Contraindications, Precautions, and Interactions of Cephalosporins

- Cephalosporins should not be used if the patient has a history of allergies to cephalosporins.
- Cephalosporins should be used cautiously in patients with renal or hepatic impairment and in patients with bleeding disorders.
- Safety of cephalosporin use has not been established in lactation.

CONSIDERATIONS | Older adults

LIFESPAN

Susceptibility to Nephrotoxic Effects
Older adults are more susceptible to the nephrotoxic effects of the cephalosporins, particularly if kidney function is already diminished because of age or disease. If renal impairment is present, then a lower dosage and monitoring of blood creatinine levels are indicated. Blood creatinine levels greater than 4 mg/dL indicate serious renal impairment. In elderly patients with decreased renal function, a dosage adjustment may be necessary.

- The risk of nephrotoxicity increases when cephalosporins are used with the aminoglycosides.
- The risk for bleeding increases when cephalosporins are taken with oral anticoagulants.
- A disulfiram-like reaction may occur if alcohol is consumed within 72 hours after cephalosporin use. Symptoms of a disulfiram-like reaction include flushing, throbbing in the head and neck, respiratory difficulty, vomiting, sweating, chest pain, and hypotension. Severe reactions may cause arrhythmias and unconsciousness.

Patient Management Issues with Cephalosporins

Patients with a history of an allergy to penicillin may also be allergic to a cephalosporin even though they have never received one of these drugs. If an allergy to either of these drug groups is suspected, then the health care provider is informed of this before the first dose of the drug is given. Liver and kidney function tests may be ordered.

The patient is monitored for a decrease in fever, the relief of symptoms caused by the infection (e.g., pain or discomfort), an increase in appetite, and a change in the appearance or amount of drainage (when originally present). The health care provider is notified if symptoms of the infection appear to worsen. The patient's skin is checked regularly for rash and the patient monitored for any loose stools or diarrhea.

Patients must be questioned about a possible allergy to cephalosporins or the penicillins before taking the first dose, even when an accurate drug history has been taken. If a patient has a history of possible cephalosporin or penicillin allergy, the health care provider is notified.

Cephalosporins are taken around the clock to provide adequate blood levels. Most cephalosporins may be taken with food to prevent gastric upset. The absorption of oral cefuroxime and cefpodoxime is increased when given with food. However, if the patient experiences gastrointestinal upset, the drug can be taken with food. Oral suspensions should be shaken well before taken.

Educating the Patient and Family about Cephalosporins

Following are key points about cephalosporins the patient and family members should know:

- Complete the full course of therapy. Do not stop the drug even if your symptoms disappear unless directed to do so by your health care provider.
- Take the drug at the prescribed times of day because it is important to keep an adequate amount of drug in your body at all times through each day.
- Take each dose with food or milk if you have stomach upset after taking the drug.
- Do not drink alcoholic beverages when taking the cephalosporins and for 3 days after completing the course of therapy because severe reactions may occur.
- Notify your health care provider immediately if you experience any of the following: vomiting, skin rash, hives (urticaria), severe diarrhea, vaginal or anal itching, sores in the mouth, swelling around the mouth or eyes, breathing difficulty, or stomach disturbances such

as nausea, vomiting, and diarrhea. Do not take the next dose of the drug until you discuss the problem with your health care provider.

- Never give this drug to another person, even if their symptoms seem the same as yours.
- Notify your health care provider if the symptoms of your infection do not improve or if your condition becomes worse.

Oral Suspensions

- Make note of storage requirements; most will require refrigeration. Drugs that are kept refrigerated lose their potency when kept at room temperature, so return the drug to the refrigerator immediately after pouring the dose. Shake the drug well before pouring. A small amount of the drug may be left after the last dose is taken. Discard any remaining drug because the drug (in suspension form) begins to lose its potency after 7 to 14 days. The discard date should be noted on the medication bottle.

FACT CHECK

35-15   Serious hypersensitivity reactions may occur with cephalosporin use. What are they?
35-16   Why are cephalosporins and other anti-infectives taken around the clock?

Tetracyclines, Macrolides, and Lincosamides

This section discusses three groups of broad-spectrum antibiotics: the tetracyclines, the macrolides, and the lincosamides. Examples of the tetracyclines include demeclocycline (Declomycin), doxycycline (Vibramycin), minocycline (Minocin), and tetracycline. Examples of the macrolides include azithromycin (Zithromax), clarithromycin (Biaxin), and erythromycin. The lincosamides include clindamycin (Cleocin) and lincomycin (Lincocin). The Summary Drug Table: Tetracyclines, Macrolides, and Lincosamides lists these types of broad-spectrum antibiotics.

Actions of Tetracyclines, Macrolides, and Lincosamides

Tetracyclines

Tetracyclines are a group of anti-infectives composed of natural and semisynthetic compounds. Tetracyclines exert their effect by inhibiting bacterial protein synthesis, which is a process necessary for reproduction of the microorganism. The ultimate effect of this action is that the bacteria are either destroyed or their multiplication rate is slowed. Tetracyclines are bacteriostatic (capable of slowing or retarding the multiplication of bacteria), whereas the macrolides and lincosamides may be bacteriostatic or bactericidal (capable of destroying bacteria).

Macrolides

Macrolides are effective against a wide variety of pathogenic organisms, particularly infections of the respiratory and genital tract. Macrolides are bacteriostatic or bactericidal in susceptible bacteria. The drugs act by binding to cell membranes and causing changes in protein function.

Lincosamides

Lincosamides are effective against many gram-positive organisms, such as streptococci and staphylococci. Lincosamides act by inhibiting protein synthesis in susceptible bacteria, causing death.

Uses of Tetracyclines, Macrolides, and Lincosamides

Tetracyclines

Tetracyclines are useful in select infections when the organism shows sensitivity to them, such as in cholera, Rocky Mountain spotted fever, and typhus. These antibiotics are effective in the treatment of infections caused by a wide range of gram-negative and gram-positive microorganisms. Tetracyclines are used for infections caused by Rickettsiae (Rocky Mountain spotted fever, typhus fever, and tick fevers). Tetracyclines are also used in situations in which penicillin is contraindicated, in the treatment of intestinal amebiasis, and in some skin and soft tissue infections. Oral tetracyclines are used in the treatment of uncomplicated urethral, endocervical, or rectal infections caused by *Chlamydia trachomatis* and as adjunctive treatment in severe acne. Tetracycline in combination with metronidazole and bismuth subsalicylate is useful in treating *Helicobacter pylori* (bacteria in the stomach that can cause peptic ulcer). (See Table 28-2 for information on agents used to treat *H. pylori*.)

Macrolides

These antibiotics are effective in the treatment of infections caused by a wide range of gram-negative and gram-positive microorganisms. In addition, the drugs are used to treat acne vulgaris and skin infections, in conjunction with sulfonamides to treat upper respiratory infections caused by *Haemophilus influenzae*, and as prophylaxis before dental or other procedures in patients allergic to penicillin.

Lincosamides

Because of their high potential for toxicity, lincosamides are usually used only for the treatment of serious infections in which penicillin or erythromycin (a macrolide) is not effective. These antibiotics are effective in the treatment of infections caused by a wide range of gram-negative and gram-positive microorganisms. Lincosamides are used for the more serious infections and may be used in conjunction with other antibiotics.

FACT CHECK

35-17   How do tetracyclines act?
35-18   Why are lincosamides usually used only for the treatment of serious infections in which penicillin or erythromycin (a macrolide) is not effective?

Adverse Reactions of Tetracyclines, Macrolides, and Lincosamides

Tetracyclines

Gastrointestinal reactions that may occur during tetracycline use include nausea, vomiting, diarrhea, epigastric distress, stomatitis, and sore throat. Skin rashes also may occur. A photosensitivity (phototoxic) reaction may occur with these drugs, manifested by an exaggerated sunburn reaction when the skin is exposed to sunlight even for brief periods. Demeclocycline seems to cause the most serious photosensitivity reaction, whereas minocycline is least likely to cause this reaction.

Tetracyclines are not given to children younger than 9 years of age unless their use is absolutely necessary because these drugs may cause permanent yellow-gray-brown discoloration of the teeth. The use of the tetracyclines, especially prolonged or repeated therapy, may result in bacterial or fungal overgrowth of nonsusceptible organisms.

Macrolides

Most of the adverse reactions seen with the use of azithromycin and clarithromycin are related to the gastrointestinal tract and include nausea, vomiting, diarrhea, and abdominal pain. Abdominal cramping, nausea, vomiting, diarrhea, and allergic reactions have been reported with the use of erythromycin. However, there appears to be a low incidence of adverse reactions associated with normal oral doses of erythromycin. As with almost all antibacterial drugs, pseudomembranous colitis may occur ranging in severity from mild to life-threatening.

Lincosamides

Abdominal pain, esophagitis, nausea, vomiting, diarrhea, skin rash, and blood dyscrasias may occur with the use of lincosamides. These drugs also can cause pseudomembranous colitis, which may range from mild to very severe. Discontinuing the drug may relieve mild symptoms of pseudomembranous colitis.

Contraindications, Precautions, and Interactions of Tetracyclines, Macrolides, and Lincosamides

Tetracyclines

- Tetracyclines are contraindicated in patients with hypersensitivity, during pregnancy because of the possibility of toxic effects to the developing fetus, during lactation, and in children younger than 9 years (may cause permanent discoloration of the teeth).
- Tetracyclines are used cautiously in patients with renal function impairment. Larger doses can be extremely damaging to the liver.
- Antacids containing aluminum, zinc, magnesium, or bismuth salts or foods high in calcium impair absorption of tetracyclines.
- Dairy products should be consumed either 1 hour before or 2 hours after tetracycline.
- When taken with oral anticoagulants, an increase in the effects of the anticoagulant may occur.
- When tetracyclines are given to women using oral contraceptives, a decrease in the effect of the oral contraceptive

may occur. This may result in breakthrough bleeding or pregnancy.
- When digoxin is used with a tetracycline, there is an increased risk for digitalis toxicity (see Chapter 18). The effects of this could last for months after tetracycline use is discontinued.
- Tetracyclines may reduce insulin requirements. Blood glucose levels should be monitored frequently during tetracycline therapy.

Macrolides

- These drugs are contraindicated in patients with hypersensitivity and patients with preexisting liver disease.
- These drugs are used cautiously during lactation.
- Because azithromycin and erythromycin are primarily eliminated from the body by the liver, these drugs should be used with great caution in patients with liver dysfunction.
- There is a decreased gastrointestinal absorption of the macrolides when administered with kaolin, aluminum salts, or magaldrate.
- Use of macrolides increases serum levels of digoxin and increases the effects of anticoagulants.
- Use of antacids decreases the absorption of most macrolides.
- Macrolides should not be taken with clindamycin, lincomycin, or chloramphenicol; a decrease in the therapeutic activity of the macrolides can occur.
- Concurrent use of macrolides with theophylline may increase serum theophylline levels.

Lincosamides

- Lincosamides are contraindicated in patients with hypersensitivity, those with minor bacterial or viral infections, and during lactation and infancy.
- These drugs are used with caution in patients with a history of gastrointestinal disorders, renal disease, or liver impairment.
- The neuromuscular blocking action of the lincosamides poses a danger to patients with myasthenia gravis (an autoimmune disease manifested by extreme weakness and exhaustion of the muscles).
- When kaolin or aluminum is used with lincosamides, the absorption of the lincosamide is decreased.
- When lincosamides are used with the neuromuscular blocking drugs (drugs that are used as adjuncts to anesthetic drugs that cause paralysis of the respiratory system), the action of the neuromuscular blocking drug is enhanced, possibly leading to severe and profound respiratory depression.

Patient Management Issues with Tetracyclines, Macrolides, and Lincosamides

To help track the patient's progress, the patient's signs and symptoms of infection are identified and recorded before the drug is initially taken. Signs and symptoms may vary and often depend on the organ or system involved and whether the infection is external or internal. Examples of some of the signs and symptoms of an infection in various areas of the body are pain, drainage, redness, changes in the appearance of sputum, general malaise, chills and fever, cough, and swelling.

A thorough allergy history is taken, especially a history of drug allergies. Some antibiotics have a higher incidence of hypersensitivity reactions in those with a history of allergy to drugs or other substances.

The patient's vital signs are taken before the first dose of the antibiotic is given. The health care provider may order culture and sensitivity tests, and these should also be performed before the first dose of the drug is given. Other laboratory tests such as renal and hepatic function tests, complete blood count, and urinalysis may also be ordered.

When an antibiotic is ordered for the prevention of a secondary infection (prophylaxis), the patient is observed for signs and symptoms that may indicate the beginning of an infection despite the prophylactic use of the antibiotic. If signs and symptoms of an infection occur, then they must be reported to the health care provider.

Oral Use

Tetracyclines

Tetracyclines are given on an empty stomach and should not be taken with dairy products (milk or cheese). The exceptions are doxycycline (Vibramycin) and minocycline (Minocin), which may be taken with dairy products or food. All tetracyclines should be given with a full glass of water (240 mL).

Macrolides

Clarithromycin can be given without regard to meals. Clarithromycin may be taken with milk, if desired. Azithromycin tablets may be given without regard to meals. However, azithromycin suspension is taken 1 hour or more before a meal or 2 hours or more after a meal. Erythromycin is taken on an empty stomach (1 hour before or 2 hours after meals) and with 180 to 240 mL of water but may be taken with food if it upsets the stomach.

Lincosamides

Food impairs the absorption of lincomycin. The patient should not eat for 1 to 2 hours before and after taking lincomycin. Clindamycin may be given without regard to food.

ALERT ℞

Tetracyclines and Dairy Products

Tetracyclines should not be given along with dairy products (milk or cheese), antacids, laxatives, or products containing iron. When these drugs are prescribed, they are taken 2 hours before or after taking a tetracycline. Food or drugs containing calcium, magnesium, aluminum, or iron prevent the absorption of the tetracyclines if ingested concurrently.

Educating the Patient and Family about Tetracyclines, Macrolides, and Lincosamides

The patient and family must understand the prescribed therapeutic regimen. Often patients stop taking a prescribed drug because they feel better.

In easy-to-understand terms, the adverse reactions associated with the specific prescribed antibiotic should be explained to the patient. The patient should be told to contact the health care provider if any potentially serious adverse reactions occur, such as hypersensitivity reactions, moderate to severe diarrhea, sudden onset of chills and fever, sore throat, or sores in the mouth. The patient should report any signs of superinfection or diarrhea (see Box 35-2).

BOX 35.2
Aminoglycosides and Toxic Effects

Neurotoxicity

Patients should be carefully observed for symptoms such as numbness or tingling of the skin, circumoral paresthesia, peripheral paresthesia (numbness or tingling in the extremities), tremors, and muscle twitching or weakness. Any symptom of neurotoxicity should be immediately reported to the health care provider. Convulsions can occur if the drug is not discontinued.

Nephrotoxicity

The patient's intake and output are measured, and the health care provider is notified if the patient's output is less than 750 mL/day. A record is kept of the fluid intake and output as well as daily weight to assess hydration and renal function. Fluid intake is encouraged to 2000 mL/day (if the patient's condition permits). Any changes in the intake-to-output ratio or in the appearance of the urine may indicate nephrotoxicity. Such changes should be reported to the health care provider promptly. Daily laboratory tests (i.e., serum creatinine and blood urea nitrogen [BUN]) may be ordered to monitor renal function. Any elevation in the creatinine or BUN level is reported to the health care provider because an elevation may indicate renal dysfunction.

Ototoxicity

Auditory changes are irreversible, usually bilateral, and may be partial or total. The risk is greater in patients with renal impairment or those with preexisting hearing loss. Any problems with hearing should be reported to the health care provider because continued use could lead to permanent hearing loss. To detect ototoxicity, the patient's symptoms or comments related to hearing are carefully evaluated, such as a ringing or buzzing in the ears or difficulty hearing. If hearing problems do occur, then this problem should be reported to the health care provider immediately. To monitor for damage to the eighth cranial nerve, an evaluation of hearing may be performed by audiometry before and throughout the course of therapy.

Following are key points about tetracycline, macrolides, and lincosamides the patient and family members should know:

- Take the drug at the prescribed time intervals. These time intervals are important because a certain amount of the drug must be in your body at all times for the infection to be controlled.
- Do not increase or skip a dose unless advised to do so by your health care provider.
- Complete the entire course of treatment. Never stop the drug, except on the advice of your health care provider, before the course of treatment is completed even if symptoms improve or disappear. Failure to complete the prescribed course of treatment may result in a return of the infection.
- Take each dose with a full glass of water. Follow the directions given by your pharmacist regarding taking the drug on an empty stomach or with food.
- Notify your health care provider if symptoms of your infection become worse or there is no improvement in the original symptoms after approximately 5 days.
- Do not drink alcoholic beverages during therapy unless approved by your health care provider.
- If taking a tetracycline, avoid exposure to the sun or any type of tanning lamp or bed. When exposure to direct sunlight is unavoidable, completely cover your arms and legs and wear a wide-brimmed hat to protect your face and neck. Application of a sunscreen may or may not be effective. Therefore, consult your health care provider before using a sunscreen to prevent a photosensitivity reaction.
- Although some drugs may be taken with food or milk to minimize the risk for gastrointestinal upset, most tetracyclines, when given with foods containing calcium, such as dairy products, are not absorbed as well as when they are taken on an empty stomach. If you are taking tetracycline at home, take the drug on an empty stomach, 1 hour before or 2 hours after a meal.

In addition, you should avoid the following foods before or after taking the drug:

- Milk (whole, low-fat, skim, condensed, or evaporated)
- Cream (half-and-half, heavy, light)
- Sour cream
- Coffee creamers
- Creamy salad dressings
- Eggnog
- Milkshakes
- Cheese (natural and processed)
- Yogurt (regular, low-fat, or nonfat)
- Cottage cheese
- Ice cream
- Frozen custard
- Frozen yogurt
- Ice milk

FACT CHECK

35-19 Why are tetracyclines contraindicated in children under age 9?

35-20 What are the frequent adverse reactions of macrolides?

Fluoroquinolones and Aminoglycosides

As various microorganisms became resistant to antibiotics, researchers sought to develop more powerful drugs that would be effective against these resistant pathogens. The fluoroquinolones and aminoglycosides are two groups of broad-spectrum antibiotics that resulted from this research. The Summary Drug Table: Fluoroquinolones and Aminoglycosides lists the fluoroquinolones and aminoglycosides discussed in this chapter.

Actions of Fluoroquinolones and Aminoglycosides

Fluoroquinolones

Fluoroquinolones include ciprofloxacin (Cipro), gemifloxacin (Factive), levofloxacin (Levaquin), moxifloxacin (Avelox), norfloxacin (Noroxin), and ofloxacin (Floxin),

Fluoroquinolones exert their bactericidal (bacteria-destroying) effect by interfering with an enzyme (DNA gyrase) needed by bacteria for the synthesis of DNA. This interference prevents cell reproduction, leading to death of the bacteria.

Aminoglycosides

Aminoglycosides include amikacin, gentamicin (Garamycin), kanamycin, neomycin, paromomycin, streptomycin, and tobramycin, which exert their bactericidal effect by blocking a step in protein synthesis necessary for bacterial multiplication. They disrupt the functional ability of the bacterial cell membrane, causing cell death.

Uses of Fluoroquinolones and Aminoglycosides

Fluoroquinolones

Fluoroquinolones are used in the treatment of infections caused by susceptible microorganisms and are effective in the treatment of infections caused by gram-positive and gram-negative microorganisms. They are primarily used in the treatment of susceptible microorganisms in lower respiratory infections, infections of the skin, urinary tract infections, and sexually transmitted diseases. Ciprofloxacin, levofloxacin, moxifloxacin, and ofloxacin are available in ophthalmic forms for infections in the eyes.

Aminoglycosides

Aminoglycosides are used in the treatment of infections caused by susceptible microorganisms, and primarily in the treatment of infections caused by gram-negative microorganisms. Because oral aminoglycosides are poorly absorbed, they are useful for suppressing gastrointestinal bacteria. Oral aminoglycoside and neomycin is used preoperatively to reduce the number of bacteria normally present in the intestine **(bowel prep)**. A reduction in intestinal bacteria is thought to lessen the possibility of abdominal infection that may occur after surgery on the bowel.

Neomycin and paromomycin are used orally in the management of hepatic coma. In this disorder, liver failure results in an elevation of blood ammonia levels. By reducing the number of ammonia-forming bacteria in the intestines, blood ammonia levels may be lowered, thereby temporarily reducing some of the symptoms associated with this disorder.

Adverse Reactions of Fluoroquinolones and Aminoglycosides

Fluoroquinolones

Bacterial or fungal superinfections and pseudomembranous colitis may occur with the use of these drugs. The use of any drug may result in a hypersensitivity reaction, which can range from mild to severe and, in some cases, can be life-threatening. Mild hypersensitivity reactions may only require discontinuing the drug, whereas the more serious reactions require immediate treatment. (Chapter 1 discusses hypersensitivity reactions.)

More common adverse effects of these drugs include nausea, diarrhea, headache, abdominal pain or discomfort, and dizziness. A more serious adverse reaction seen with use of the fluoroquinolones is a photosensitivity reaction. This is manifested by an exaggerated sunburn reaction when the skin is exposed to the ultraviolet rays of sunlight or sunlamps.

Aminoglycosides

Aminoglycosides may cause nephrotoxicity (damage to the kidneys) and ototoxicity (damage to the organs of hearing). Signs and symptoms of nephrotoxicity may include protein in the urine (proteinuria), hematuria (blood in the urine), an elevated blood urea nitrogen level, decreased urine output, and an increase in the serum creatinine concentration. Nephrotoxicity is usually reversible once the drug is discontinued. Signs and symptoms of ototoxicity include tinnitus, dizziness, roaring in the ears, vertigo, and a mild to severe loss of hearing. If hearing loss occurs, then it is most often permanent. Ototoxicity may occur during drug therapy or even after the drug is discontinued. The short-term use of the oral aminoglycosides as a preparation for bowel surgery rarely causes these two adverse reactions.

Neurotoxicity (damage to the nervous system by a toxic substance) may also occur with aminoglycosides. Signs and symptoms of neurotoxicity include numbness, skin tingling, circumoral (around the mouth) paresthesia, peripheral paresthesia, tremors, muscle twitching, convulsions, muscle weakness, and neuromuscular blockade (acute muscular paralysis and apnea). Box 35-2 describes management of the potentially neurotoxic, nephrotoxic, and ototoxic effects of aminoglycosides.

Additional adverse reactions of aminoglycosides may include nausea, vomiting, anorexia, rash, and urticaria. When these drugs are given, individual drug references, such as the package insert, should be consulted for more specific adverse reactions.

As with the other anti-infectives, bacterial or fungal superinfections and pseudomembranous colitis may occur with the use of these drugs. The use of aminoglycosides may result in a hypersensitivity reaction, which can range from mild to severe and, in some cases, can be life threatening. Mild hypersensitivity reactions may only require discontinuing the drug, whereas more serious reactions require immediate treatment.

Contraindications, Precautions, and Interactions of Fluoroquinolones and Aminoglycosides

Fluoroquinolones

- Fluoroquinolones are contraindicated in patients with a history of hypersensitivity, and in children younger than 18 years. These drugs also are contraindicated in patients whose lifestyles do not allow for adherence to the precautions regarding photosensitivity.
- Fluoroquinolones are used cautiously in patients with renal impairment or a history of seizures, in geriatric patients, and in patients on dialysis.
- Concurrent use of fluoroquinolones with theophylline causes an increase in serum theophylline levels.
- When used concurrently with cimetidine, cimetidine may interfere with the elimination of fluoroquinolones.
- Use of fluoroquinolones with an oral anticoagulant may cause an increase in the effects of the oral coagulant.
- Taking fluoroquinolones with antacids, iron salts, or zinc will decrease absorption of fluoroquinolones.
- There is a risk of seizures if fluoroquinolones are given with the nonsteroidal anti-inflammatory drugs.
- There is a risk of severe cardiac arrhythmias when the fluoroquinolones, gatifloxacin and moxifloxacin, are used with drugs that increase the QT interval (e.g., quinidine, procainamide, amiodarone, and sotalol).

Aminoglycosides

- Aminoglycosides are contraindicated in patients with hypersensitivity and should not be given to patients requiring long-term therapy because of the potential for ototoxicity and nephrotoxicity. One exception is the use of streptomycin for long-term management of tuberculosis. These drugs are also contraindicated in patients with preexisting hearing loss, myasthenia gravis, Parkinsonism, and during lactation or pregnancy.
- Aminoglycosides are used cautiously in patients with renal failure (dosage adjustments may be necessary), in the elderly, and in patients with neuromuscular disorders.
- Use of an aminoglycoside with a cephalosporin may increase the risks of nephrotoxicity.
- When an aminoglycoside is used with a loop diuretic, there is an increased risk of ototoxicity (irreversible hearing loss).
- There is an increased risk of neuromuscular blockage (paralysis of the respiratory muscles) if an aminoglycoside is given soon after general anesthetics (neuromuscular junction blockers).

ALERT ℞

Respiratory Difficulties and Aminoglycosides

Neuromuscular blockade or respiratory paralysis may occur after aminoglycosides use. Therefore, any symptoms of respiratory difficulty must be reported immediately. If neuromuscular blockade occurs, then it may be reversed by the use of calcium salts, but mechanical ventilation may be required.

Patient Management Issues with Fluoroquinolones and Aminoglycosides

The health care provider may order culture and sensitivity tests, and the culture is obtained before the first dose of the drug is given. When an aminoglycoside is to be given, laboratory tests such as renal and hepatic function tests, complete blood count, and urinalysis also may be ordered.

When neomycin and paromomycin are given for hepatic coma, the patient's level of consciousness and ability to swallow must be evaluated. A thorough allergy history, vital signs, and signs and symptoms of infection are also noted before giving the drug.

When an aminoglycoside is being used, the patient's respiratory rate must be monitored because neuromuscular blockade can occur with these drugs. Any changes in the respiratory rate or rhythm are reported to the health care provider because immediate treatment may be necessary.

Fluoroquinolones

Patients who receive a fluoroquinolone are encouraged to increase their fluid intake. Norfloxacin and is given on an empty stomach (e.g., 1 hour before or 2 hours after meals). Ciprofloxacin can be given without regard to meals. However, the manufacturer recommends that the drug be given 2 hours after a meal. Moxifloxacin is given once per day for the period prescribed. If the patient is taking an antacid, then moxifloxacin should be administered 4 hours before or 8 hours after the antacid.

Ciprofloxacin, levofloxacin, and moxifloxacin are the only fluoroquinolones given intravenously. None of the fluoroquinolones is given intramuscularly.

Aminoglycosides

Oral aminoglycosides are usually given without regard to meals. With the exception of paromomycin and neomycin, all of the aminoglycoside drugs can be given intramuscularly, and the health care provider is notified of any persistent localized reaction of pain, redness, or extreme tenderness. With the exception of paromomycin, neomycin, and streptomycin, all of the aminoglycoside drugs can be given intravenously.

ALERT ℞

Hyperthermia

The infectious process in a patient is usually accompanied by an elevated temperature. When the patient is being treated for infection, vital signs, particularly the body temperature, must be monitored. As the anti-infective works to rid the body of the infectious organism, the patient's body temperature should return to normal. Vital signs (temperature, pulse, and respiration) are taken frequently to monitor the drug's effectiveness in eradicating the infectious process. The health care provider should be notified if the patient's temperature is greater than 101°F.

Educating the Patient and Family about Fluoroquinolones and Aminoglycosides

Carefully planned patient and family education is important to encourage compliance, relieve anxiety, and promote the desired result. The patient should be advised of the signs and symptoms of potentially serious adverse reactions, such as hypersensitivity reactions, moderate to severe diarrhea, sudden onset of chills and fever, sore throat, sores in the mouth, or extreme fatigue. The patient must understand the necessity of contacting the health care provider immediately if such symptoms occur. The patient should be cautioned against the use of alcoholic beverages during therapy unless approved by the health care provider. Following are key points about fluoroquinolones and aminoglycosides the patient and family members should know:

- Take the drug at the prescribed time intervals. These time intervals are important because a certain amount of the drug must be in your body at all times for the infection to be controlled.
- Drink six to eight large glasses of fluids while taking these drugs and take each dose with a full glass of water.
- Do not increase or omit the dose unless advised to do so by your health care provider.
- Complete the entire course of treatment. Do not stop the drug, except on the advice of your health care provider, before the course of treatment is complete, even if your symptoms improve or disappear. Failure to complete the prescribed course of treatment may result in a return of the infection.
- Follow the directions supplied with the prescription regarding taking the drug with meals or on an empty stomach. With a drug that must be taken on an empty stomach, take it 1 hour before or 2 hours after a meal.
- Notify your health care provider if your symptoms of the infection become worse or do not improve after 5 to 7 days of drug therapy.
- Avoid any exposure to sunlight or ultraviolet light (tanning beds, sunlamps) while taking this drug and for several weeks after completing the course of therapy. Wear sunblock, sunglasses, and protective clothing when exposed to sunlight.
- Avoid tasks requiring mental alertness until you know how you will respond to the drug.

Fluoroquinolones

- When taking a fluoroquinolone, report any signs of tendinitis, such as pain or soreness in your leg, shoulder, or back of your heel. Periodic applications of ice may help relieve the pain. Rest the involved area and avoid exercise.
- Do not take antacids or drugs containing calcium, iron, or zinc because these drugs will decrease absorption of fluoroquinolones.

Aminoglycosides

- Notify your health care provider if you experience any ringing in the ears or difficulty hearing, numbness or tingling around your mouth or in your extremities, or any change in your urinary pattern.
- When taking an aminoglycoside for preparation of the bowel before surgery, take the prescribed drug at the exact times indicated on the prescription container. Some bowel prep regimens are complex. For example, kanamycin prescribed for suppression of intestinal bacteria is taken orally every hour for 4 hours followed by 1 g every 6 hours for 36 to 72 hours.

> **FACT CHECK**
>
> 35-21   How do fluoroquinolones work?
> 35-22   What are three serious adverse reactions of aminoglycosides?

Chapter Review

KEY POINTS

- Culture and sensitivity tests are performed whenever possible to determine which antibacterial agent can best control an infection caused by a specific strain of bacteria.
- Sulfonamides are primarily bacteriostatic, which means they slow or retard the multiplication of bacteria. They are used to control urinary tract infections and to treat full and partial thickness burns. Burn treatment regimens may include debridement, special dressings, and cleansing of the burned area. Hematologic changes may occur during sulfonamide therapy, including agranulocytosis, thrombocytopenia, aplastic anemia, and leukopenia. Sulfonamides are contraindicated in patients with known hypersensitivity, during lactation, and in children younger than 2 years old. Penicillins may be used to treat infections such as urinary tract infections, septicemia, meningitis, intra-abdominal infection, gonorrhea, syphilis, pneumonia, and other respiratory infections. Health care providers occasionally prescribe penicillin as prophylaxis against a potential secondary bacterial infection that can occur in a patient with a viral infection. Common adverse reactions include mild nausea, vomiting, diarrhea, sore tongue or mouth, fever, and pain at injection site. Penicillins are contraindicated in patients with a history of hypersensitivity to penicillin and should be used cautiously in patients with renal disease, cephalosporin allergy, during pregnancy and lactation (may cause diarrhea or candidiasis in the infant), and in those with a history of allergies.
- Cephalosporins are effective in the treatment of almost all of the strains of bacteria affected by the penicillins, as well as some strains of bacteria that have become resistant to penicillin. Cephalosporins are usually bactericidal (capable of destroying bacteria) and are used to treat infections caused by susceptible microorganisms, including streptococci, staphylococci, citrobacters, gonococci, shigella, and clostridia. The most common adverse reactions of cephalosporins are gastrointestinal disturbances, such as nausea, vomiting, and diarrhea. Cephalosporins should not be used if the patient has a history of allergies to cephalosporins or penicillins and should be used cautiously in patients with renal or hepatic impairment and in patients with bleeding disorders.
- Tetracyclines are used in select infections when the organism shows sensitivity to them, such as in cholera, Rocky Mountain spotted fever, and typhus. Gastrointestinal reactions that may occur during tetracycline use include nausea, vomiting, diarrhea, epigastric distress, stomatitis, and sore throat. Skin rashes also may occur. Tetracyclines are contraindicated if the patient is known to be hypersensitive and during pregnancy.
- Macrolides are effective against a wide variety of pathogenic organisms, particularly infections of the respiratory and genital tract. Adverse reactions of azithromycin and clarithromycin are related to the gastrointestinal tract and include nausea, vomiting, diarrhea, and abdominal pain. These drugs are contraindicated in patients with hypersensitivity and patients with preexisting liver disease.
- Lincosamides, another group of anti-infectives, are effective against many gram-positive organisms, such as streptococci and staphylococci. Because of their high potential for toxicity, lincosamides are usually used only for the treatment of serious infections in which penicillin or erythromycin (a macrolide) is not effective. Abdominal pain, esophagitis, nausea, vomiting, diarrhea, skin rash, and blood dyscrasias may occur with lincosamides. Lincosamides are contraindicated in patients with hypersensitivity, those with minor bacterial or viral infections, and during lactation and infancy.
- Fluoroquinolones are primarily used in the treatment of susceptible microorganisms in lower respiratory infections, infections of the skin, urinary tract infections, and sexually transmitted diseases. Bacterial or fungal superinfections and pseudomembranous colitis may occur with the use of both of these drugs. Fluoroquinolones are contraindicated in patients with a history of hypersensitivity, in children younger than 18 years, and in pregnant women.
- Aminoglycosides are used in the treatment of infections caused by susceptible microorganisms, primarily gram-negative microorganisms. Aminoglycosides may cause nephrotoxicity or ototoxicity. Aminoglycosides are contraindicated in patients with hypersensitivity and should not be given to patients requiring long-term therapy because of the potential for ototoxicity and nephrotoxicity. One exception is the use of streptomycin for long-term management of tuberculosis.

- Stevens–Johnson syndrome, a hypersensitivity reaction, and pseudomembranous colitis, a bacterial superinfection, are common reactions that may occur with many of the antibacterial drugs.

CRITICAL THINKING CASE STUDY
CASE 1
Pneumonia

Ms. Bartlett, age 80, has been prescribed Biaxin (clarithromycin) for community-acquired pneumonia.

1. Ms. Bartlett is to take Biaxin 500 mg twice daily. Which of the following best describes how she should take the medication?
   a. One tablet with breakfast and one with dinner
   b. One tablet when she wakes up and one before bedtime
   c. One tablet in the morning and the second tablet 12 hours later
   d. It doesn't matter as long as she takes two tablets daily.

2. Ms. Bartlett asks about potential adverse reactions with this drug. You tell her that any of the following adverse reactions may occur EXCEPT
   a. abnormal taste
   b. diarrhea
   c. nausea
   d. photosensitivity

3. Ms. Bartlett calls the medical office seven days later and says that she feels much better. She doesn't think she needs the other 3 days worth of medication. What should you tell her?

CASE 2
Fluoroquinolone Therapy

Mr. Gee was diagnosed with infectious diarrhea upon returning from an international trip. His physician has prescribed ciprofloxacin 500 mg to be taken one tablet twice daily for 7 days.

1. Which of the following is not an adverse reaction likely to be seen with ciprofloxacin therapy?
   a. Nausea
   b. Headache
   c. Photosensitivity
   d. Taste disturbances

2. When should he take his ciprofloxacin?
   a. Without regard to meals
   b. 1 hour before breakfast and 1 hour before dinner
   c. 1 hour before breakfast and 2 hours after dinner
   d. 2 hours after breakfast and at bedtime

3. Mr. Gee regularly takes a multivitamin which contains iron and zinc. Can he take his multivitamin at the same time as his ciprofloxacin?

Review Questions

MULTIPLE CHOICE

1. Mr. Thomas, who is receiving oral penicillin, reports he has a sore mouth and shows you his bright red oral mucous membranes. The health care provider should be notified immediately because these symptoms may be caused by
   a. a vitamin C deficiency
   b. a superinfection
   c. dehydration
   d. poor oral hygiene

2. Common adverse reactions to cephalosporin include
   a. hypotension, dizziness, urticaria
   b. nausea, vomiting, diarrhea
   c. skin rash, constipation, headache
   d. bradycardia, pruritus, insomnia

3. A patient asks why her health care provider prescribed an antibiotic when she was told that she has a viral infection. The most correct response is that the antibiotic may be used to prevent a
   a. primary fungal infection
   b. repeat viral infection
   c. secondary bacterial infection
   d. breakdown of the immune system

4. Patients taking a fluoroquinolone are encouraged to
   a. nap 1 to 2 hours daily while taking the drug
   b. eat a high-protein diet
   c. increase their fluid intake
   d. avoid foods high in carbohydrates

5. All of the following drugs are aminoglycosides EXCEPT
   a. amikacin
   b. kanamycin
   c. ciprofloxacin
   d. tobramycin

6. When a tetracycline is prescribed, the patient should be advised to
   a. take the drug with food or milk
   b. avoid sun exposure
   c. note that urine may turn orange
   d. keep the drug refrigerated

7. Macrolides are contraindicated in patients with
   a. liver disease
   b. renal disease
   c. gastrointestinal disease
   d. bleeding disorders

8. Which of the following sulfonamides are used topically to treat burns?
   a. Sulfamethoxazole
   b. Sulfisoxazole
   c. Sulfasalazine
   d. Sulfadiazine

9. Hearing loss may occur in patients taking which of the following drug groups?
   a. Macrolides
   b. Aminoglycosides
   c. Lincosamides
   d. All of the above

10. During therapy with cefadroxil, the patient experiences a decrease in urine output. This may be an early sign of
    a. fungal infection
    b. colitis
    c. nephrotoxicity
    d. hepatotoxicity

MATCHING

Match the drug on the left with the correct classification on the right.

_____ 11. ciprofloxacin   a. Sulfonamide
_____ 12. clindamycin   b. Penicillin
_____ 13. cefaclor   c. Cephalosporin
_____ 14. gentamicin   d. Tetracycline
_____ 15. clarithromycin   e. Macrolide
_____ 16. doxycycline   f. Lincosamide
_____ 17. sulfadiazine   g. Fluoroquinolone
_____ 18. amoxicillin   h. Aminoglycoside

Match the generic name on the left with the correct brand name on the right.

_____ 19. trimethoprim/   a. Vantin
     sulfamethoxazole   b. Zithromax
_____ 20. piperacillin/   c. Augmentin
     tazobactam   d. Biaxin
_____ 21. cefexime   e. Cipro
_____ 22. penicillin G   f. Unasyn
_____ 23. doxycycline   g. Bactrim
_____ 24. ampicillin/sulbactam   h. Suprax
_____ 25. azithromycin   i. Pfizerpen-G
_____ 26. levofloxacin   j. Levaquin
_____ 27. cefpodoxime   k. Zosyn
_____ 28. ciprofloxacin   l. Vibramycin
_____ 29. amoxicillin/clavulanate
     potassium
_____ 30. clarithromycin

TRUE OR FALSE

_____ 31. Patients who are allergic to one type of penicillin are unlikely to be allergic to other types of penicillins.

_____ 32. The neuromuscular blocking action of lincosamides presents a danger to patients with muscular dystrophy.

_____ 33. Large doses of penicillin can increase bleeding risks of patients taking anticoagulants.

_____ 34. Hearing loss that results from treatment with an aminoglycoside is most often temporary.

_____ 35. Macrolides are used as prophylaxis before dental or other procedures in patients who are allergic to penicillin.

_____ 36. In patients taking almost any antibacterial drug, diarrhea with fever and abdominal cramps may indicate pseudomembranous colitis.

_____ 37. Sulfonamides can be described as either antibacterial or anti-infective agents.

_____ 38. Tetracyclines are pregnancy category B drugs.

_____ 39. Cephalosporins are structurally and chemically related to penicillins.

_____ 40. Mafenide is a sulfonamide that is used to treat patients with superficial burns.

FILL IN THE BLANKS

41. A disulfiram-like reaction, including flushing, head throbbing, and respiratory difficulty, may occur if _____ is consumed within72 hours after cephalosporin use.

42. Culture and sensitivity tests are performed to determine if a specific type of _____ are _____ to specific drugs.

43. Neomycin is a(n) _____ that is used preoperatively to reduce the number of bacteria normally present in the intestine.

44. Signs and symptoms of _____ to penicillin include urticaria, pruritus, bronchospasm, and laryngospasm.

45. Patients who are taking lincomycin should not eat for 1 to 2 hours before and after taking the drug because food impairs its _____.

46. A woman taking _____, a fluoroquinolone, may experience external genital pruritus as an adverse reaction.

47. Patients who are allergic to _____ are also more likely to be allergic to cephalosporins.

48. _____ are often prescribed to control urinary tract infections.

49. A patient with intestinal amebiasis would likely be treated with _____.

50. Macrolides _____ serum levels of digoxin and _____ the effects of anticoagulants.

SHORT ANSWERS

51. What is the difference between drugs that are bacteriostatic and bactericidal?

52. When educating the patient about antibacterial drugs, why should you emphasize the importance of finishing all of the medication?

53. What is an allergy to drugs in the same or related group called?

54. Neuromuscular blockade may occur after aminoglycoside use. How is it reversed?

55. What is Stevens–Johnson syndrome, and what is its diagnostically important symptom?

56. An elderly patient with renal impairment has been prescribed a cephalosporin. How would the patient's condition affect the dosage?

Web Activities

1. Go to the Mayo Clinic Web site (www.mayoclinic.com) and search for "antibiotic misuse." What are the consequences of antibiotic misuse? What can you do to safeguard the effectiveness of antibiotics?

2. Go to the Web site for the National Center for Complementary and Alternative Medicine (nccam.nih.gov). Conduct a search for "probiotics." What are the uses for health purposes of probiotics?

SUMMARY DRUG TABLE Penicillins (left, generic; right, trade)

Comprehensive Summary Drug Tables, including uses, adverses effects, dosages, and pregnancy classifications, are provided on the companion website, http:// thePoint.lww.com/PharmacologyHP2e

Natural Penicillins	
penicillin G (aqueous) *pen-i-sill'-in*	Pfizerpen-G, *generic*
penicillin G benzathine	Bicillin L-A
penicillin G procaine, IM	*generic*
penicillin V potassium	*generic*
Penicillinase-Resistant Penicillins	
dicloxacillin sodium *dye-klox-a-sill'-in*	*generic*
nafcillin sodium *naf-sill'-in*	*generic*
oxacillin sodium *oks-a-sil'-in*	Bactocill, *generic*
Aminopenicillins	
amoxicillin *a-mox-i-sill'-in*	Moxataq, *generic*
amoxicillin and clavulanate potassium *a-mox-i-sill'-in/klah-view-lan'-ate*	Augmentin, Augmentin XR, Augmentin ES-600 Amoclan, *generic*
ampicillin *am-pi-sil'-in*	*generic*
ampicillin sodium	*generic*
ampicillin/sulbactam *am-pi-sill'-in/sull-bak'-tam*	Unasyn, *generic*
Extended-Spectrum Penicillins	
piperacillin sodium *pi-per'-a-sil-in*	*generic*
piperacillin sodium and tazobactam sodium *pi-per-a-sill'-in/ tay-zoe-back'-tam*	Zosyn, *generic*
ticarcillin/clavulanate *tye-kar-sil'-in/klav-yoo-lan'-ate*	Timentin

SUMMARY DRUG TABLE Tetracyclines, Macrolides, and Lincosamides (left, generic; right, trade)

Comprehensive Summary Drug Tables, including uses, adverses effects, dosages, and pregnancy classifications, are provided on the companion website, http:// thePoint.lww.com/PharmacologyHP2e

Tetracyclines	
demeclocycline HCl, generic *deh-meh-kloe- sye'- kleen*	Declomycin, *generic*
doxycycline *dox-i-sye'-kleen*	Monohydrate: Adoxa, Monodox, OraceaVibramycin, generic Hyclate: Alodox, Doryx, Morgidox, Oraxyl, Periostat, Vibramycin, generic Calcium: Vibramycin
minocycline HCL *min-oh-sye'-kleen*	Arestin, Dynacin, Minocin, Solodyn, *generic*
tetracycline HCl *tet-ra-sye'-kleen*	*generic*
Macrolides	
azithromycin *ay-zi-thro-my'-cin*	Ophthalmic: AzaSite, Oral: Zithromax, Zithromax Tri-Pak, Zithromax Z-Pak Zmax, *generic Intravenous: Zithromax, generic*
clarithromycin *klar-ith-ro-my'-cin*	Biaxin, Biaxin XL, Biaxin XL Pac, *generic*
erythromycin base *er-ith-roe-my'-sin*	Ery-Tab, PCE, *generic*
erythromycin ethylsuccinate	EryPed, E.E.S., *generic*
erythromycin lactobionate	*generic*
er-ith-roe-mye'-sin erythromycin stearate	*Erythrocin stearate*
Lincosamides	
clindamycin *klin-da-my'-sin*	Cleocin,, *generic*
lincomycin *lin-koe-my'-sin*	Lincocin

SUMMARY DRUG TABLE Cephalosporins
(left, generic; right, trade)
Comprehensive Summary Drug Tables, including uses, adverses effects, dosages, and pregnancy classifications, are provided on the companion website, http://thePoint.lww.com/PharmacologyHP2e

First-Generation Cephalosporins	
cefadroxil *saf-a-drox'-ill*	*generic*
cefazolin sodium *sef-a'-zoe-lin*	*generic*
cephalexin *sef'-a-lex-in*	Keflex, *generic*

Second-Generation Cephalosporins	
cefaclor *sef'-a-klor*	*generic*
cefotetan *sef-oh-tee'-tan*	*generic*
cefoxitin *sef-ox'-i-tin*	*generic*
cefprozil *sef-proe'-zil*	*generic*
cefuroxime *sef-yoor-ox'-eem*	Ceftin, Zinacef, generic

Third-Generation Cephalosporins	
cefdinir *sef'-din-er*	Omnicef, *generic*
cefditoren pivoxil *sef-de-tor'-en*	Spectracef, *generic*
cefixime *sef-ix'-eem*	Suprax
cefotaxime sodium *sef-oh-taks'-eem*	Claforan, Claforan in D5W, *generic*
cefpodoxime *sef-poed-ox'-eem*	Vantin, *generic*
ceftazidime *sef'-tay-zi-deem*	Fortaz, Tazicef, *generic*
ceftibuten *sef-tye'-byoo-ten*	Cedax
ceftizoxime *sef-ti-zoks'-eem*	Cefizox
ceftriaxone *sef-try-ax'-on*	Rocephin, *generic*

Fourth-Generation Cephalosporins	
cefepime HC *sef'-e-pim*	Maxipime, *generic*

Fifth-Generation Cephalosporins	
ceftaroline fosamil	Teflaro

SUMMARY DRUG TABLE The Sulfonamides
(left, generic; right, trade)
Comprehensive Summary Drug Tables, including uses, adverses effects, dosages, and pregnancy classifications, are provided on the companion website, http://thePoint.lww.com/PharmacologyHP2e

Single Agents	
sulfadiazine *sul-fa-dye'-a-zeen*	*generic*

Combination Preparations	
trimethoprim (TMP) and sulfamethoxazole (SMZ) *trye-meth'-oh-prim;* *sul-fa-meth-ox'-a-zole*	Bactrim, Bactrim DS, Septra DS, Sulfatrim, *generic*
erythromycin ethylsuccinate/ sulfisoxazole *er-ith-roe-mye'-sin* *sul-fi-soks'-a-zole*	*generic*

Miscellaneous Sulfonamide Preparations	
mafenide acetate *meph'-a-nide*	Sulfamylon
silver sulfadiazine *sil'-ver sul-fa-dye'-a-zeen*	Silvadene, Thermazene, SSD, generic

SUMMARY DRUG TABLE Fluoroquinolones and Aminoglycosides (left, generic; right, trade)
Comprehensive Summary Drug Tables, including uses, adverses effects, dosages, and pregnancy classifications, are provided on the companion website, http://thePoint.lww.com/PharmacologyHP2e

Fluoroquinolones	
ciprofloxacin *si-proe-flox'-a-sin*	Cipro, ProQuin XR, generic (oral and IV) Cetraxal (otic), Ciloxan (ophthalmic)
gemifloxacin *je-mi-floks'-a-sin*	Factive
levofloxacin *lee-voe-flox'-a-sin*	Levaquin (Oral and IV), Quixin, *generic (ophthalmic)*
moxifloxacin *mocks-ah-flox'-a- sin*	Avelox (Oral and IV), Moxeza, Vigamox (ophthalmic)
norfloxacin *nor- flox'-a-sin*	Noroxin
ofloxacin *oe-flox'-a-sin*	Floxin Otic (otic), Ocuflox (ophthalmic), *generic* (oral)

Aminoglycosides	
amikacin sulfate *am-i-kay'-sin*	*generic*
gentamicin *jen-ta-mye'-sin*	*generic (injection)* Garamycin, Gentak, generic (ophthalmic)
kanamycin sulfate *kan-a-mye'-sin*	*generic*
neomycin sulfate *nee-o-mye'-sin*	*generic*
paromomycin *par-oh-moe-mye'-sin*	*generic*
streptomycin sulfate *strep-toe-mye'-sin*	*generic*
tobramycin *toe-bra-mye'-sin*	generic (injection) Tobi (inhalation) Tobrex, *generic (ophthalmic)*

36

Antimycobacterial Drugs

CHAPTER OBJECTIVES

On completion of this chapter, students will be able to:

1. Define the chapter's key terms.
2. Identify drugs that are used as first-line antitubercular agents.
3. Discuss the need for multidrug therapy to treat tuberculosis.
4. Describe the actions, uses, contraindications, precautions, and interactions of antitubercular drugs.
5. Describe the actions, uses, contraindications, precautions, and interactions of leprostatic drugs.
6. Discuss important points to keep in mind when educating the patient and family members about the use of antitubercular and leprostatic drug therapies.

KEY TERMS

anaphylactoid reaction—unusual or exaggerated allergic reaction
antitubercular drugs—drugs used to treat active cases of tuberculosis
leprosy—a chronic, communicable disease spread by prolonged intimate contact with an infected person
Mycobacterium leprae—the bacteria that cause leprosy
Mycobacterium tuberculosis—the bacteria that cause tuberculosis
tuberculosis—a disease caused by *M. tuberculosis*

CHAPTER OVERVIEW

Drug classes covered in this chapter are:

- Antitubercular drugs
- Leprostatic drugs

Drugs by classification are listed on page 391.

thePOINT RESOURCES

- Comprehensive Summary Drug Tables
- Lippincott's Interactive Tutorials: Drugs Used to Treat Infections
- Interactive Practice and Review
- Monographs of Most Commonly Prescribed Drugs

The antimycobacterial drugs are used to treat the infectious diseases tuberculosis and leprosy.

Tuberculosis is an infectious disease caused by the **Mycobacterium tuberculosis** bacillus. The disease is transmitted from one person to another by droplets dispersed in the air when an infected person coughs or sneezes. These droplet nuclei are released into the air and inhaled by noninfected persons (Fig. 36-1). Although tuberculosis primarily affects the lungs, other organs may also be affected. For example, if a person's immune system is poor, then the infection can spread from the lungs to other organs of the body. Extrapulmonary (outside of the lungs) tuberculosis is the term used to distinguish tuberculosis affecting the lungs from infection with the *M. tuberculosis* bacillus in other organs of the body. Organs that can be affected include the liver, kidneys, spleen, uterus, and bones. People with acquired immunodeficiency syndrome (AIDS) are at risk for tuberculosis because of their compromised immune systems. Tuberculosis responds well to long-term treatment with a combination of three or more antitubercular drugs.

Leprosy is a chronic, communicable disease spread by prolonged, intimate contact with an infected person. Peripheral nerves and skin are affected. Lesions may be confined to a few isolated areas or may be fairly widespread over the entire body. Leprostatic drugs generally control the disease and prevent complications.

Leprosy, also referred to as Hansen disease, is caused by the bacterium **Mycobacterium leprae.** Although rare in colder climates, this disease may occur in tropical and subtropical zones.

KEY CONCEPTS

36-1 Resistance to Antitubercular Drugs

Of increasing concern is the development of mutant strains of tuberculosis that are resistant to many of the antitubercular drugs currently in use. Bacterial resistance develops, sometimes rapidly, with the use of antitubercular drugs. Treatment is individualized and based on laboratory studies identifying the drugs to which the organism is susceptible. To slow the development of bacterial resistance, the CDC recommends the use of three or more drugs in initial therapy and retreatment (see Box 36-1). Using a combination of drugs slows the development of bacterial resistance. Tuberculosis caused by drug-resistant organisms should be considered in patients who have no response to therapy and in patients who have been treated in the past.

Antitubercular Drugs

Antitubercular drugs are used to treat active cases of tuberculosis and as a prophylactic to prevent the spread of tuberculosis. The drugs used to treat tuberculosis do not "cure" the disease, but they render the patient noninfectious to others. Antitubercular drugs are classified as primary and secondary drugs. Primary (first-line) drugs provide the foundation for treatment. Secondary (second-line) drugs are less effective and more toxic than primary drugs. These drugs are used in various combinations to treat tuberculosis. Sensitivity testing may be performed to determine the most effective combination treatment, especially in areas of the country showing resistance (Key Concepts 36-1). Second-line drugs are used to treat extrapulmonary tuberculosis or drug-resistant organisms. The primary antitubercular drugs are discussed in this section. Both first- and second-line antitubercular drugs are listed in the Summary Drug Table: Antitubercular Drugs. Table 36-1 lists common combination products.

Actions of Antitubercular Drugs

Most antitubercular drugs are bacteriostatic (slow or retard the growth of bacteria) against the *M. tuberculosis* bacillus. These

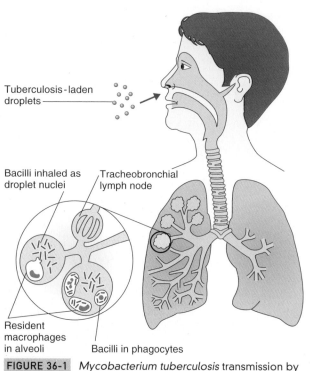

FIGURE 36-1 *Mycobacterium tuberculosis* transmission by inhalation of droplet nuclei.

Tuberculosis-laden droplets

Bacilli inhaled as droplet nuclei

Tracheobronchial lymph node

Resident macrophages in alveoli

Bacilli in phagocytes

TABLE 36-1   Isoniazid Combination Products

Drug	Form	Pregnancy Category
Rifater	Tablets	C
120 mg Rifampin		
50 mg Isoniazid		
300 mg Pyrazinamide		
IsonaRif, Rifamate	Capsules	C
300 mg Rifampin		
150 mg Isoniazid		

drugs usually act to inhibit bacterial cell wall synthesis, which slows the multiplication rate of the bacteria. Only isoniazid is bactericidal, with rifampin and streptomycin having some bactericidal activity.

Uses of Antitubercular Drugs

Antitubercular drugs are used in combination with other antitubercular drugs to treat active tuberculosis. Isoniazid is the only antitubercular drug used alone. Although isoniazid is used in combination with other drugs for the treatment of primary tuberculosis, a primary use is in preventive therapy (prophylaxis) against tuberculosis. For example, when a diagnosis of tuberculosis is present, family members of the infected individual must be given prophylactic treatment with isoniazid for 6 months to 1 year. Prophylactic uses for isoniazid include the following situations:

- Household members and other close associates of those with tuberculosis recently diagnosed
- Those whose tuberculin skin test has become positive in the past 2 years
- Those with positive skin tests whose radiographic findings indicate nonprogressive, healed, or quiescent (causing no symptoms) tubercular lesions
- Those at risk for tuberculosis (e.g., those with Hodgkin disease, severe diabetes mellitus, leukemia, and other serious illnesses and those receiving corticosteroids or drug therapy for a malignancy)
- All patients younger than 35 years (primarily children to age 7) who have a positive skin test
- Persons with AIDS or those who are positive for the human immunodeficiency virus (HIV) and have a positive tuberculosis skin test or a negative tuberculosis skin test but a history of a previous significant reaction to purified protein derivative (a skin test for tuberculosis)

Standard Treatment

The standard treatment of tuberculosis is divided into two phases: the initial phase followed by a continuing phase (Box 36-1). During the initial phase, drugs are used to kill the rapidly multiplying *M. tuberculosis* and to prevent drug resistance. The initial phase lasts approximately 2 months and the continuing phase approximately 4 months, with the total treatment regimen lasting for 6 to 9 months, depending on the patient's response to therapy.

The initial phase must contain three or more of the following drugs: isoniazid, rifampin, and pyrazinamide, along with either ethambutol or streptomycin. The Centers for Disease Control and Prevention (CDC) recommends treatment to begin as soon as possible after the diagnosis of tuberculosis. The treatment recommendation regimen is for the use of rifampin, isoniazid, ethambutol, and pyrazinamide for a minimum of 2 months (8 weeks), followed by rifampin and isoniazid for 4 months (18 weeks) in areas with a low incidence of tuberculosis (see Box 36-1).

Retreatment

At times, treatment fails because of noncompliance with the drug regimen or because of inadequate initial drug treatment. When treatment fails, retreatment is necessary. Retreatment

generally includes the use of four or more antitubercular drugs. Retreatment drug regimens most often consist of the secondary drugs ethionamide, aminosalicylic acid, cycloserine, and capreomycin. At times during retreatment, as many as seven or more drugs may be used, with the ineffective drugs discontinued when susceptibility test results are available.

BOX 36.1

Treatment Schedule for Tuberculosis Recommended by the CDC

Regimens for treating TB have an *initial phase* of 2 months, followed by a choice of several options for the *continuation phase* of either 4 or 7 months. Although basic TB regimens are broadly applicable, there are modifications that should be made under special circumstances (i.e., HIV infection, drug resistance, pregnancy, or treatment of children). Listed below are the basic regimens; please refer to *Treatment of Tuberculosis* for all options for the treatment of drug-susceptible TB.

Preferred Regimen	Alternative Regimen	Alternative Regimen
Initial Phase	Initial Phase	Initial Phase
Daily INH, RIF, PZA, and EMB* for 56 doses (8 wk)	Daily INH, RIF, PZA, and EMB* for 14 doses (2 wk), then twice weekly for 12 doses (6 wk)	Thrice-weekly INH, RIF, PZA, and EMB* for 24 doses (8 wk)
Continuation Phase	Continuation Phase	Continuation Phase
Daily INH and RIF for 126 doses (18 wk) Or Twice-weekly INH and RIF for 36 doses (18 wk)	Twice-weekly INH and RIF for 36 doses (18 wk)	Thrice-weekly INH and RIF for 54 doses (18 wk)

*EMB can be discontinued if drug susceptibility studies demonstrate susceptibility to first-line drugs.
INH, isoniazid; RIF, rifampin; EMB, ethambutol; PZA, pyrazinamide
Source: Centers for Disease Control and Prevention. Treatment of tuberculosis. *MMWR Morb Mortal Wkly Rep.* 2003;52 (No. RR-11). Retrieved from http://www.cdc.gov/tb/publications/factsheets/treatment/treatmentHIVnegative.htm.

FACT CHECK

36-1 What are the uses of antitubercular drugs?
36-2 Most antitubercular drugs are used in combination. Which is the only antitubercular drug to be prescribed alone?

Tuberculosis

Tuberculosis (TB) is one of the world's deadliest diseases:

- One-third of the world's population are infected with TB.
- Each year, over 9 million people around the world become sick with TB.
- Each year, there are almost 2 million TB-related deaths worldwide.
- TB is a leading killer of people who are HIV infected.

Source: Centers for Disease Control and Prevention

Adverse Reactions of Antitubercular Drugs

Ethambutol

Optic neuritis (a decrease in visual acuity and changes in color perception), which appears to be related to the dose given and the duration of treatment, has occurred in some patients receiving ethambutol. Usually, this adverse reaction disappears when the drug is discontinued. Other adverse reactions are dermatitis, pruritus, **anaphylactoid reaction** (an unusual or exaggerated allergic reaction), joint pain, anorexia, nausea, and vomiting.

Any changes in visual acuity or any visual changes should be promptly reported to the health care provider. Vision changes are usually reversible if the drug is discontinued as soon as symptoms appear. The patient may need help walking and with self-care activities if visual disturbances occur. Psychic disturbances may occur. If the patient appears depressed, withdrawn, and noncommunicative or has other personality changes, then the problem must be reported to the health care provider.

Isoniazid

The incidence of adverse reactions appears to be higher when larger doses of isoniazid are prescribed. Adverse reactions include hypersensitivity reactions, hematologic changes, jaundice, fever, skin eruptions, nausea, vomiting, and epigastric distress. Severe, and sometimes fatal, hepatitis has been associated with isoniazid therapy and may appear after many months of treatment. Peripheral neuropathy (numbness and tingling of the extremities) is the most common symptom of toxicity.

Because of the risk of hepatitis, patients must be carefully monitored at least monthly for any evidence of liver dysfunction. Patients should be told to report any of the following symptoms: anorexia, nausea, vomiting, fatigue, weakness, jaundice (yellowing of the skin or eyes), darkening of the urine, or numbness in the hands and feet.

Pyrazinamide

Hepatotoxicity is the principal adverse reaction of pyrazinamide use. Symptoms of hepatotoxicity may range from none (except for slightly abnormal hepatic function tests) to a more severe reaction such as jaundice. Nausea, vomiting, diarrhea, myalgia, and rashes also may occur.

Patients should have baseline liver functions tests to use as a comparison when monitoring liver function during pyrazinamide therapy. The patient should be closely monitored for symptoms of a decline in hepatic functioning (i.e., yellowing of the skin, malaise, liver tenderness, anorexia, or nausea). The health care provider may order periodic liver function tests. Hepatotoxicity appears to be dose related and may appear at any time during therapy.

Rifampin

Nausea, vomiting, epigastric distress, heartburn, fatigue, dizziness, rash, hematologic changes, and renal insufficiency may occur with rifampin. Rifampin may also cause a red-orange discoloration of body fluids, including urine, tears, saliva, sweat, and sputum. The patient is advised not to wear soft contact lenses during therapy because they may be permanently stained.

FACT CHECK

36-3 Patients receiving which antitubercular drug may experience optic neuritis?
36-4 Older adults are particularly susceptible to what adverse reaction associated with antitubercular therapy?

Contraindications, Precautions, and Interactions of Antitubercular Drugs

Ethambutol

- Ethambutol is contraindicated in patients with a history of hypersensitivity.
- Ethambutol is not recommended for children younger than 13 years.
- The drug is used with caution during lactation and in patients with hepatic and renal impairment.
- Because of the danger of optic neuritis, the drug is used cautiously in patients with diabetic retinopathy or cataracts.

CONSIDERATIONS | Older adults

LIFESPAN

Antitubercular Drug Use

Older adults are particularly susceptible to a potentially fatal hepatitis when taking isoniazid, especially if they consume alcohol on a regular basis. Two other antitubercular drugs, rifampin and pyrazinamide, can cause liver dysfunction in older adults. Careful observation and monitoring for signs of liver impairment are necessary (e.g., increased serum aspartate transaminase, increased serum alanine transferase, increased serum bilirubin, and jaundice).

Isoniazid

- Isoniazid is contraindicated in patients with a history of hypersensitivity.
- The drug is used with caution during lactation and in patients with liver or kidney impairment.
- Daily consumption of alcohol when taking isoniazid may result in a higher incidence of drug-related hepatitis.
- Aluminum salts may reduce the oral absorption of isoniazid.
- The action of the anticoagulants may be enhanced when taken with isoniazid.
- There is a possibility of increased serum levels of phenytoin with concurrent use of isoniazid. When isoniazid is taken with foods containing tyramine, such as aged cheese and meats, bananas, yeast products, and alcohol, an exaggerated sympathetic-type response can occur (e.g., hypertension, increased heart rate, palpitations).

Pyrazinamide

- Pyrazinamide is contraindicated in patients with a history of hypersensitivity and in patients with acute gout (a metabolic disorder resulting in increased levels of uric acid) and those with severe hepatic damage.
- The drug is used with caution during lactation, in patients with liver or kidney renal impairment, and during pregnancy.
- Pyrazinamide is used cautiously in patients infected with HIV, who may require longer treatment, and in patients with diabetes mellitus, in whom management is more difficult.
- Pyrazinamide decreases the effects of allopurinol, colchicines, and probenecid.

Rifampin

- Rifampin is contraindicated in patients with a history of hypersensitivity.
- The drug is used with caution during lactation and in patients with hepatic and renal impairment.
- Serum concentrations of digoxin may be decreased by rifampin.
- Isoniazid and rifampin used concurrently may result in a higher risk of hepatotoxicity than when either drug is used alone.
- The use of rifampin with an oral anticoagulant or oral hypoglycemic may decrease the effects of the anticoagulant or hypoglycemic drug.
- There is a decrease in the effect of the oral contraceptives, chloramphenicol, phenytoin, and verapamil when these agents are used concurrently with rifampin.

Patient Management Issues with Antitubercular Drugs

Once the diagnosis of tuberculosis is confirmed, the health care provider selects the drug that will best control the spread of the disease and make the patient noninfectious to others. Many laboratory and diagnostic tests may be necessary before starting antitubercular therapy, including radiographic studies, culture and sensitivity tests, and various types of laboratory

tests, such as a complete blood count. A family history and a history of contacts are included in the assessment if the patient has active tuberculosis.

Directly Observed Therapy

Because the antitubercular drugs must be taken for prolonged periods, compliance with the treatment regimen becomes a problem and increases the risk of the development of resistant strains of tuberculosis. To help prevent the problem of noncompliance, the patient may make periodic visits to the office of the health care provider or the health clinic, where the drug is taken in the presence of a health care worker. The patient is observed swallowing each dose of the medication regimen. In some cases, the antitubercular drug is given under observation in the patient's home, place of employment, or school. Directly observed therapy may occur daily or two to three times weekly, depending on the patient's health care regimen.

Treatment Regimens

Ethambutol

Ethambutol is given once every 24 hours at the same time each day with food to prevent gastric upset.

Isoniazid

Isoniazid is given to the patient whose stomach is empty, at least 1 hour before or 2 hours after meals. If gastrointestinal upset occurs, then the patient can take the drug with food. The patient is reminded to minimize alcohol consumption because of the increased risk of hepatitis. An alternative regimen of twice or three times per week is also available to increase compliance.

Pyrazinamide

This drug is given once per day with food to prevent gastric upset. An alternative regimen of twice-weekly dosing has been developed to promote patient compliance on an outpatient basis.

Rifampin

Rifampin is taken once daily on an empty stomach, at least 1 hour before or 2 hours after meals. Patients should be told that their urine, feces, saliva, sputum, sweat, and tears may be colored red-orange and that this is normal.

Educating the Patient and Family about Antitubercular Drugs

Antitubercular drugs are given for a long time, and careful patient and family education and close medical supervision are necessary. Noncompliance can be a problem whenever a disease or disorder requires long-term treatment. For this reason, the directly observed therapy method is preferred. The patient and family must understand that short-term therapy is of no value in treating this disease. Any statements the patient or family makes that suggest the patient may not be compliant should be reported to the health care provider.

The dosage schedule and adverse reactions associated with the prescribed antitubercular drug are reviewed with the patient and family. Following are key points the patient and family members should know:

- The results of your antitubercular therapy must be monitored at periodic intervals. Laboratory and diagnostic tests and visits to your health care provider's office or clinic are necessary.
- Take these drugs exactly as directed on the prescription container. Do not skip, increase, or decrease a dose unless advised to do so by your health care provider.
- Do not use nonprescription drugs, especially those containing aspirin, unless use is approved by your health care provider.
- Discuss alcoholic beverages with your health care provider. A limited amount of alcohol may be allowed, but excessive intake usually must be avoided.

Ethambutol

- Take this drug once per day at the same time each day. If you miss a dose, do not double the dose the next day. Notify your health care provider if you experience any changes in vision or a skin rash.

Isoniazid

- Take this drug 1 hour before or 2 hours after meals. However, if you experience gastric upset, take isoniazid with food.
- Notify your health care provider if you experience weakness, yellowing of your skin, loss of appetite, darkening of your urine, skin rashes, or numbness or tingling of your hands or feet.
- Avoid tyramine-containing foods, such as coffee, tea, colas, red wine, and certain dairy products; ask your health care provider for a list of foods not to eat.
- To prevent pyridoxine (vitamin B_6) deficiency, 6 to 50 mg of pyridoxine daily may be prescribed.

Pyrazinamide

- Notify your health care provider if you experience any of the following: nausea, vomiting, loss of appetite, fever, malaise, visual changes, yellow discoloration of your skin, or severe pain in your knees, feet, or wrists.

Rifampin

- Take the drug once daily on an empty stomach (1 hour before or 2 hours after meals).
- A red-brown or red-orange discoloration of tears, sputum, urine, or sweat may occur.
- Soft contact lenses may be permanently stained if you wear them while taking the drug. Talk to your eye doctor about wearing glasses during this time.
- Notify your health care provider if you experience any yellow discoloration of your skin, fever, chills, unusual bleeding or bruising, and skin rash or itching.

- If you are taking an oral contraceptive, check with your health care provider because reliability of the contraceptive may be affected.

> ### FACT CHECK
> **36-5** What is directly observed therapy for patients taking antitubercular drugs?
> **36-6** Which antitubercular agent may discolor the tears, sputum, urine, or sweat a red-brown or red-orange color that stains?

Leprostatic Drugs

Dapsone is the only drug currently approved to treat leprosy. It may be used in combination with rifampin or ethionamide in patients with bacteriologically negative tuberculoid and indeterminate disease or lepromatous and borderline lepromatous patients.

Actions and Uses of Leprostatic Drugs

Dapsone is bactericidal and bacteriostatic against *M. leprae*. The drug is used to treat leprosy and dermatitis herpetiformis, a chronic, inflammatory skin disease.

Adverse Reactions of Leprostatic Drugs

Use of dapsone may result in hemolysis (destruction of red blood cells), anemia, peripheral neuropathy, nausea, vomiting, anorexia, insomnia, and blurred vision.

Contraindications, Precautions, and Interactions of Leprostatic Drugs

- Dapsone is contraindicated during lactation.
- Dapsone is used with caution in patients with anemia, severe cardiopulmonary disease, and hepatic dysfunction.
- No significant drug–drug interactions are associated with the use of dapsone.

Patient Management Issues with Leprostatic Drugs

These drugs are often given on an outpatient basis. Treatment with a leprostatic drug may require many years. These patients are faced with long-term medical and drug therapy and possibly severe disfigurement.

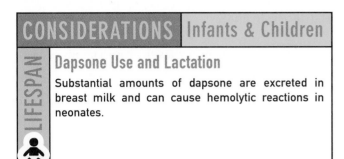

CONSIDERATIONS Infants & Children

LIFESPAN

Dapsone Use and Lactation

Substantial amounts of dapsone are excreted in breast milk and can cause hemolytic reactions in neonates.

Educating the Patient and Family about Leprostatic Drugs

Compliance can be a problem with the long-term treatment regimen. Depression or indifference may indicate treatment noncompliance. Patient education emphasizes the treatment regimen, the dosage schedule, possible adverse effects, and the importance of scheduled follow-up visits.

The patient should be told that changes in skin pigmentation might occur, ranging from red to brown-black. Skin discoloration may take months to years to reverse after use of the drug is discontinued.

Leprostatic drugs are given orally and with food to minimize gastric upset. Antitubercular drugs, such as rifampin, can be given concurrently during initial therapy to minimize bacterial resistance to the leprostatic drug.

FACT CHECK

36-7 What is the only drug currently available to treat leprosy?

36-8 Why is dapsone contraindicated during lactation?

Chapter Review

KEY POINTS

- Antitubercular drugs are used in combination with other antitubercular drugs to treat active tuberculosis.
- Optic neuritis, which appears to be related to the dose given and the duration of treatment, has occurred in some patients receiving ethambutol. Ethambutol is contraindicated in patients with a history of hypersensitivity. Ethambutol is not recommended for children younger than 13 years.
- With isoniazid use, the incidence of adverse reactions appears to be higher when larger doses are prescribed. Adverse reactions include hypersensitivity reactions, hematologic changes, jaundice, fever, skin eruptions, nausea, vomiting, and epigastric distress. Isoniazid is contraindicated in patients with a history of hypersensitivity.
- Hepatotoxicity is the principal adverse reaction seen with pyrazinamide use. Pyrazinamide is contraindicated in patients with a history of hypersensitivity or acute gout.
- Nausea, vomiting, epigastric distress, heartburn, fatigue, dizziness, rash, hematologic changes, and renal insufficiency may occur with rifampin. Rifampin is contraindicated in patients with a history of hypersensitivity. The drug is used with caution during lactation, in patients with hepatic and renal impairment, and during pregnancy.
- Dapsone is used to treat leprosy. Use of dapsone may result in hemolysis, nausea, vomiting, anorexia, and blurred vision. Dapsone is used with caution in patients with anemia, severe cardiopulmonary disease, or hepatic dysfunction and during pregnancy.

CRITICAL THINKING CASE STUDY

New Diagnosis of Tuberculosis

Mr. Hedrick is diagnosed with tuberculosis. His physician wants to initiate the preferred initial treatment regimen set forth by the CDC immediately.

1. Which of the following drugs would NOT be in the initial treatment regimen?
    a. rifampin
    b. isoniazid
    c. pyrazinamide
    d. streptomycin
2. How long will Mr. Hedrick be on the initial treatment regimen?
    a. 1 month
    b. 2 months
    c. 4 months
    d. 6 months
3. Mr. Hedrick wears contact lenses. What should he know about the adverse reactions of rifampin?

Review Questions

MULTIPLE CHOICE

1. All of the following are first-line antitubercular drugs EXCEPT
    a. cycloserine
    b. ethambutol
    c. rifampin
    d. streptomycin

2. What is the most common adverse reaction in patients receiving pyrazinamide?
    a. Optic neuritis
    b. Skin pigmentation
    c. Hepatotoxicity
    d. None of the above
3. Patients taking rifampin should be advised to take the drug
    a. with food
    b. 1 hour before or 2 hours after meals
    c. in the morning
    d. at bedtime
4. Which of the following hematologic changes may result from the use of dapsone?
    a. Hemolysis
    b. Leukopenia
    c. Decreased platelets
    d. Increased hematocrit

MATCHING

_____	5. ethambutol	a.	Trecator
_____	6. rifabutin	b.	Paser
_____	7. rifampin	c.	Seromycin
_____	8. rifapentine	d.	Rifadin
_____	9. aminosalicylate	e.	Mycobutin
_____	10. capreomycin	f.	Myambutol
_____	11. ethionamide	g.	Capastat sulfate
_____	12. cycloserine	h.	Priftin

TRUE OR FALSE

_____ 13. Dapsone is both bactericidal and bacteriostatic against *M. leprae.*

_____ 14. Use of antitubercular drugs will cure the disease.

_____ 15. Patients who wear soft contact lenses while taking rifampin may experience permanent staining of their lenses.

_____ 16. Dapsone is excreted in breast milk and can cause hemolytic reactions in nursing infants.

FILL IN THE BLANKS

17. _____ may be used prophylactically in patients who are younger than 35 years and have a positive skin test for _____.
18. Patients taking _____ should promptly report any vision changes to the health care provider.
19. _____ is used to treat leprosy and dermatitis herpetiformis.
20. Patients with acute gout and those with severe hepatic damage should not take _____.

SHORT ANSWERS

21. Why is compliance with the treatment regimen for antitubercular drugs often difficult for patients?
22. Patients taking isoniazid should be advised to report symptoms of hepatitis. What are these symptoms?
23. What are the CDC's recommendations for slowing the development of drug-resistant tuberculosis?
24. What is the preferred initial treatment regimen from the CDC for tuberculosis?

Web Activities

1. Go to the Centers for Disease Control and Prevention Web site (www.cdc.gov) and conduct a search for tuberculosis. What is the difference between latent TB infection and TB disease?
2. On the same Web site, conduct a search for leprosy or "Hansen Disease." Write a report on what you have learned about leprosy: incidence, transmission, treatment, and challenges.

SUMMARY DRUG TABLE Antitubercular Drugs
(left, generic; right, trade)

Comprehensive Summary Drug Tables, including uses, adverses effects, dosages, and pregnancy classifications, are provided on the companion website, http://thePoint.lww.com/PharmacologyHP2e

Primary (First-Line) Drugs	
ethambutol HCl (EMB) *eth-am'-byoo-tole*	Myambutol, *generic*
isoniazid (INH) *eye-soe-nye'-a-zid*	*generic*
pyrazinamide (PZA) *peer-a-zin'-a-mide*	*generic*
rifabutin *rif-ah-byou'-tin*	Mycobutin
rifampin (RIF) *rif-am'-pin*	Rifadin, *generic*
rifapentine *rif-a-pen'-teen*	Priftin
streptomycin *strep-toe-mye'-sin*	*generic*
Secondary (Second-Line Drugs)	
aminosalicylate *a-meen-oh-sal'-sa-late* (p-aminosalicylic acid; 4-aminosalicylic acid)	Paser
capreomycin sulfate *kap-ree-oh-mye'-sin*	Capastat Sulfate
ethionamide *e-thye-on-am'-ide*	Trecator
cycloserine *sye-kloe-ser'-een*	Seromycin, *generic*

SUMMARY DRUG TABLE Leprostatic Drugs
(left, generic; right, trade)

Comprehensive Summary Drug Tables, including uses, adverses effects, dosages, and pregnancy classifications, are provided on the companion website, http://thePoint.lww.com/PharmacologyHP2e

dapsone *dap'-sone*	Aczone (topical), *generic (oral)*

37

Antiviral, Antiretroviral, and Antifungal Drugs

CHAPTER OBJECTIVES

On completion of this chapter, students will be able to:

1. Define the chapter's key terms.
2. Compare and contrast common types of viruses.
3. Describe how antiviral drugs work.
4. Identify common adverse reactions for the antiviral drugs.
5. Describe how to take/use the antiviral drugs used to treat influenza.
6. Describe contraindications, precautions, and interactions of antiviral drugs.
7. Identify the six classes of antiretroviral drugs.
8. Identify common adverse reactions for the different classes of antiretroviral drugs.
9. Identify the actions, uses, contraindications, precautions, and interactions of antiretroviral drugs.
10. Identify the two types of fungal infections treated by antifungal drugs.
11. Compare and contrast the uses of antifungal drugs used systemically, topically, and vaginally.
12. Describe how adverse reactions of topical antifungals differ from those that may occur with use of systemic antifungals.
13. Describe the contraindications, precautions, and interactions of antifungal drugs.
14. Discuss important points to keep in mind when educating the patient or family members about the use of antiviral, antiretroviral, and antifungal drugs.

KEY TERMS

acquired immunodeficiency syndrome (AIDS)—syndrome of the immune system caused by an infection of HIV that is characterized by opportunistic infections
fungicidal—able to destroy fungi

CHAPTER OVERVIEW

Drug classes covered in this chapter are:

- Antiviral drugs
- Antiretroviral drugs
- Antifungal drugs

Drugs by classification are listed on pages 408-410.

thePOINT RESOURCES

- Comprehensive Summary Drug Tables
- Lippincott's Interactive Tutorials: Drugs Used to Treat Infections
- Interactive Practice and Review
- Monographs of Most Commonly Prescribed Drugs

fungistatic—able to slow or retard the multiplication of fungi

fungus—a colorless plant that lacks chlorophyll

human immunodeficiency virus (HIV)—a cytopathic retrovirus; human T-cell lymphotropic virus type III

mycotic infection—a superficial or deep infection caused by a fungi disease in humans that may be yeast-like or mold-like

onychomycosis—nail fungus condition

tinea corporis—ringworm

tinea cruris—jock itch

tinea pedis—athlete's foot

viral load—the blood level of HIV viral RNA; used for monitoring the course of AIDS

virus—infectious agent that lacks independent metabolism and cannot grow or reproduce without a living cell

---

Viruses and fungi can cause infection in humans. This chapter discusses antiviral, antiretroviral, and antifungal drugs.

Antiviral Drugs

More than 200 **viruses** have been identified that cause disease. Acute viruses, such as the common cold, have a rapid onset and quick recovery. Chronic viral infections, such as **acquired immunodeficiency syndrome (AIDS)**, have recurrent episodes of exacerbations (increases in severity of symptoms of the disease) and remissions (periods of partial or complete disappearance of the signs and symptoms). The viruses discussed in this chapter are described below.

Cytomegalovirus

Cytomegalovirus (CMV), a virus of the herpes family, is a common viral infection. Healthy individuals may become infected but have no symptoms. However, immunocompromised patients (such as those with HIV or cancer) may have the infection. Symptoms include malaise, fever, pneumonia, and superinfection. Infants may acquire the virus from the mother while in the uterus, resulting in learning disabilities and mental retardation. Cytomegalovirus can infect the eye, causing retinitis. Symptoms of CMV retinitis are blurred vision and decreased visual acuity. Visual impairment is irreversible and can lead to blindness if untreated.

Hepatitis

Hepatitis, which means inflammation of the liver, is a group of viral infections that attack the liver. Although there are five types, the most common are hepatitis A (HAV), hepatitis B (HBV), and hepatitis C (HCV). Viral hepatitis is the most common reason a patient would need a liver transplant and is also the leading cause of liver cancer. Hepatitis A is transmitted from the fecal to oral route by person-to-person contact or through contaminated food or water. Hepatitis B is transmitted from person to person via contaminated blood or body fluids that contain blood through either percutaneous or mucous membrane contact. Hepatitis C is the most common chronic bloodborne infection in the United States according to the CDC. It is transmitted through exposure to infected blood through a transfusion of unscreened blood or IV drug use. Hepatitis D is transmitted via skin or mucous membrane contact with contaminated blood. It can also be a coinfection with HBV or a superinfection in patients with HBV. Hepatitis E is transmitted by ingestion of fecal matter through contaminated food or water. Hepatitis Es is rare in the United States.

Herpes Simplex Virus

Herpes simplex virus (HSV) has two types: HSV-1, which causes oral, ocular, or facial infections, and HSV-2, which causes genital infection. However, either type can cause disease at either body site. HSV-1 causes painful vesicular lesions in the oral mucosa, face, or around the eyes. HSV-2, also called genital herpes, is usually transmitted by sexual contact and causes painful vesicular lesions on the mucous membranes of the genitalia. Vaginal lesions may appear as mucous patches with gray ulcerations. The patient may appear irritable, lethargic, and jaundiced and may have difficulty breathing or experience seizures. The lesions usually heal within 2 weeks. A severe systemic disease may develop in immunosuppressed patients.

Herpes Zoster

Herpes zoster (shingles) is caused by the varicella (chickenpox) virus. It is highly contagious. The virus causes chickenpox in children and is easily spread via the respiratory system. Recovery from childhood chickenpox results in the infection lying dormant in the nerve cells. The virus may become reactivated later in life as the older adult's immune system weakens or the individual becomes ill with other disorders. The lesions of herpes zoster appear as pustules along a sensory nerve route. Pain often continues for several months after the lesions have healed.

Influenza

Influenza, commonly called the flu, is an acute respiratory illness caused by influenza viruses A and B. Symptoms include fever, cough, sore throat, runny or stuffy nose, headache, muscle aches, and extreme fatigue. Most people recover within 1 to 2 weeks. Influenza may cause severe complications such as pneumonia in children, the elderly, and other vulnerable groups. The viruses causing influenza continually change over time, which enables them to evade the immune system of the host. These rapid changes in the most commonly circulating types of influenza virus necessitate annual changes in the composition of the "flu" vaccine.

Respiratory Syncytial Virus

Respiratory syncytial virus (RSV) infection is highly contagious and infects mostly children, causing bronchiolitis and pneumonia. Infants younger than 6 months are the most severely affected. In adults, RSV causes colds and bronchitis, with fever, cough, and nasal congestion. When RSV affects immunocompromised patients, the consequences can be severe and sometimes fatal.

Although viral infections are common, for many years, only a limited number of drugs were available for their treatment. Over the past decade, the number of antiviral drugs has increased significantly. Several of the antiviral drugs are discussed here in greater detail than others. These include acyclovir (Zovirax), amantadine (Symmetrel), oseltamivir (Tamiflu), ribavirin (Virazole), valacyclovir (Valtrex), and zanamivir (Relenza). The antiretrovirals are covered later in the chapter. The Summary Drug Table: Antiviral Drugs presents a more complete listing of the antiviral drugs currently in use.

Actions of Antiviral Drugs

Viruses can reproduce only within a living cell. A virus consists of either DNA or RNA surrounded by a protein shell. The virus can reproduce only when it uses the body's cellular material (Fig. 37-1). Most antiviral drugs act by inhibiting viral DNA or RNA replication in the virus, causing viral death.

Uses of Antiviral Drugs

Although infections caused by a virus are common, antiviral drugs have limited use because they are effective against only a small number of specific viral infections. General uses of the antiviral drugs include the treatment of

- Initial and recurrent mucosal and cutaneous herpes simplex virus 1 and 2 infections in immunocompromised patients, encephalitis, and herpes zoster
- Human immunodeficiency virus (combined with other drugs)
- Cytomegalovirus retinitis (inflammation of the retina of the eye)
- Genital herpes
- Influenza A respiratory tract illness
- Respiratory syncytial virus, a severe lower respiratory tract infection
- Viral herpes infections
- Hepatitis

FACT CHECK

37-1 What are the herpes viruses that are treated with antivirals?

37-2 How do most antiviral drugs act?

Adverse Reactions of Antiviral Drugs

Antiviral drugs are given systemically or as topical drugs. When used systemically, these drugs may be administered orally or intravenously. Rapid intravenous administration can result in crystalluria (presence of crystals in the urine). The most common adverse reactions when these drugs are administered systemically are gastrointestinal disturbances, such as nausea, vomiting, diarrhea, and anorexia. When administered topically, the antiviral drugs can cause transient burning, stinging, and pruritus at the application site.

Acyclovir

Acyclovir is used orally, topically, and parenterally (intravenously). When given intravenously, acyclovir can cause phlebitis, lethargy, confusion, tremors, skin rashes, nausea, and crystalluria. Adverse reactions when given orally include nausea, vomiting, diarrhea, headache, dizziness, and skin rashes. Topical use may cause transient burning, stinging, and pruritus.

Amantadine

Adverse reactions of amantadine include gastrointestinal upset with nausea and vomiting, anorexia, asthenia (weakness, loss of strength), constipation, depression, visual disturbances, psychosis, urinary retention, and orthostatic hypotension. The patient should be monitored for the occurrence of drowsiness, dizziness, light-headedness, or mood changes (irritability or mood change).

Oseltamivir

The most common adverse reactions in adults are fatigue, headache, diarrhea, nausea, and vomiting. In children, the most common adverse reactions are abdominal pain, diarrhea, vomiting, and otitis media.

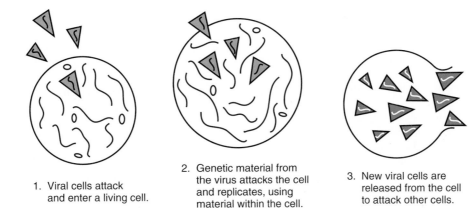

1. Viral cells attack and enter a living cell.

2. Genetic material from the virus attacks the cell and replicates, using material within the cell.

3. New viral cells are released from the cell to attack other cells.

FIGURE 37-1   1. Viral cells attack and enter a living cell. 2. Genetic material from the virus attacks the cell and replicates, using material within the cell. 3. New viral cells are released from the cell to attack other cells.

Ribavirin

Ribavirin is given by inhalation and can cause worsening of respiratory status, bacterial pneumonia, and bradycardia. Respiratory function should be monitored closely throughout therapy. Any worsening of respiratory function should be reported to the health care provider. Orally, ribavirin may cause hemolytic anemia, psychiatric reactions, GI disorders, and a flu-like syndrome.

Valacyclovir

The most common adverse reactions include headache, abdominal pain, and nausea.

Zanamivir

Common adverse effects include headache, fatigue, malaise, and cough. It can also cause nasal signs and symptoms and throat or tonsil discomfort. The most serious adverse reactions are related to respiratory effects and include severe bronchospasm that may lead to death. The risk is higher in patients with asthma or chronic obstructive pulmonary disease. A fast-acting bronchodilator should be on hand in case bronchospasm occurs. Zanamivir use should be discontinued and the health care provider notified promptly if respiratory symptoms worsen.

FACT CHECK

37-3 When used systemically, by which routes are antiviral drugs administered?

37-4 What adverse effect may occur with rapid intravenous administration of antiviral drugs?

Contraindications, Precautions, and Interactions of Antiviral Drugs

- All antiviral drugs are contraindicated in patients with previous hypersensitivity.
- The antiviral drugs are also contraindicated in patients with congestive heart failure, seizures, or renal disease, and during lactation.
- The antiviral drugs are given with caution in patients with renal impairment.
- Antivirals are used with caution in children and during lactation.

Acyclovir

- This drug is used cautiously in patients with preexisting neurologic, kidney, liver, respiratory, or fluid and electrolyte abnormalities.
- The drug is given with caution to patients with a history of seizures.
- Acyclovir is used cautiously during lactation.
- Incidences of extreme drowsiness have occurred when acyclovir is given with zidovudine.
- There is an increased risk of nephrotoxicity when acyclovir is administered with other nephrotoxic drugs.
- When administered with amphotericin B, the risk of nephrotoxicity is increased.
- Administration with probenecid causes a decrease in the renal excretion of acyclovir, prolonging the effects of acyclovir and increasing the risk of drug toxicity.

Amantadine

- Amantadine is used cautiously in patients with seizure disorders, psychiatric problems, kidney impairment, or cardiac disease.
- Amantadine is used cautiously during lactation.
- Concurrent use of antihistamines, phenothiazines, tricyclic antidepressants, disopyramide, and quinidine may increase the anticholinergic effects (dry mouth, blurred vision, constipation) of amantadine.

Oseltamivir

- Oseltamivir is contraindicated in patients with a hypersensitivity to oseltamivir.
- Oseltamivir should not be used in children less than 1 year old.
- Oseltamivir is only effective for the influenza viruses, types A and B, but not other viruses.
- Oseltamivir should not be used in immunocompromised patients.

Ribavirin

- Ribavirin may be teratogenic and embryotoxic and is contraindicated during pregnancy, in patients with chronic obstructive pulmonary disease, and during lactation.
- Ribavirin is used cautiously at all times during administration of the drug.
- Ribavirin may antagonize the antiviral action of zidovudine and potentiate the hematologic toxic effects of zidovudine.
- When ribavirin is used concurrently with digitalis, the risk of digitalis toxicity increases.

Valacyclovir

- Valacyclovir is contraindicated in patients with a hypersensitivity to valacyclovir or acyclovir.
- Valacyclovir should not be used in patients who are immunocompromised.
- Doses should be adjusted in the elderly and in patients with renal function impairment.
- Valacyclovir should be used with caution during lactation.

Zanamivir

- Zanamivir is used cautiously with pregnancy, lactation, asthma, chronic obstructive pulmonary disease, or other underlying respiratory diseases.
- Zanamivir contains lactose and should be used with caution in patients who are allergic or intolerant to lactose.
- No significant drug interactions have been reported with the use of zanamivir.

Patient Management Issues with Antiviral Drugs

Patients taking antiviral drugs may have a serious infection that causes a decrease in their natural defenses against disease. The patient's general state of health and resistance to infection are evaluated before using an antiviral drug.

The antiviral drugs may cause anorexia, nausea, or vomiting. These effects range from mild to severe. The patient may be able to tolerate small, frequent meals with soft, nonirritating foods if nausea is mild. Frequent sips of carbonated beverages or hot tea may be helpful for others. If the patient has severe nausea or is vomiting, then the health care provider should be notified.

Skin lesions are carefully monitored for worsening or improvement. Should the lesions not improve, the health care provider should be informed. When an antiviral drug is applied topically, gloves are used when applying it to avoid spreading the infection. These drugs may also cause a rash as an adverse reaction. Any rash should be reported to the health care provider. Depending on the patient's symptoms, vital signs may be monitored every 4 hours or as ordered by the health care provider.

Some patients with a viral infection are acutely ill. Others may experience fatigue, lethargy, dizziness, or weakness as an adverse reaction to the antiviral agent. These patients must be carefully monitored. Call lights are placed in a convenient place for the patient and are answered promptly. If fatigue, dizziness, or weakness is present, the patient may require help with walking or the activities of daily living. Activities should be planned so as to provide adequate rest periods.

When patients are immunosuppressed, they are at increased risk for bacterial or other infection. The patient should be protected from individuals with upper respiratory infections. All caregivers should use good handwashing technique.

Acyclovir

Treatment with acyclovir is begun as soon as symptoms of herpes simplex appear. The drug may be given topically, orally, or intravenously. The drug may be given orally, without regard to food. If gastrointestinal upset occurs, then acyclovir is given with food. Patients with a history of congestive heart failure may not be able to tolerate an increase in fluids, so they must be monitored closely to prevent fluid overload. Neurologic symptoms such as seizures may occur with the use of acyclovir. When used topically, a finger cot or glove is used to prevent spread of infection.

Amantadine

This drug is used for the prevention or treatment of respiratory tract illness caused by influenza A virus. Some patients are prescribed this drug to manage extrapyramidal effects caused by drugs used to treat parkinsonism (see Chapter 5). The capsules must be protected from moisture to prevent deterioration.

Oseltamivir

Oseltamivir therapy should be initiated as soon as possible after flu symptoms appear, but within 2 days. If used prophylactically, it should be initiated within 2 days of exposure. Oseltamivir is not a substitute for the annual flu vaccination.

Ribavirin

Ribavirin is taken by inhalation using a small-particle aerosol generator (SPAG-2 aerosol generator). It is also available as capsules that are taken by mouth.

Valacyclovir

Valacyclovir therapy should be initiated as soon as possible after onset of the herpes zoster rash or the tingling of a herpes labialis sore. Like acyclovir, valacyclovir is not a cure for genital herpes. Patients should take measures to prevent spreading the herpes virus.

Zanamivir

This drug is available as a powder blister for inhalation. The drug should be started within 2 days of onset of flu symptoms.

Educating the Patient and Family about Antiviral Drugs

When an antiviral drug is given orally, the dosage regimen is explained to the patient and family. The patient is instructed to take the drug exactly as directed and for the full course of therapy. If a dose is missed, then the patient should take it as soon as remembered but should not double the dose at the next dosage time. Any adverse reactions should be reported to the health care provider. The patient must understand that these drugs do not cure viral infections but should decrease symptoms and increase feelings of well-being.

Patients should report any symptoms of infection such as an elevated temperature (even a slight elevation), sore throat, difficulty breathing, weakness, or lethargy. The patient must be aware of possible signs of pancreatitis (nausea, vomiting, abdominal pain, jaundice [yellow discoloration of the skin or eyes]) and peripheral neuritis (tingling, burning, numbness, or pain in the hands or feet). Any indication of pancreatitis or peripheral neuritis should be reported at once.

Following are key points about antiviral drugs that the patient and family members should know.

Acyclovir

- This drug is not a cure for herpes simplex, but it will shorten the course of the disease and promote healing of the lesions.
- The drug will not prevent the spread of the disease to others.
- Do not apply the topical form more often than prescribed. Apply this drug with a finger cot or gloves and cover all lesions.
- Do not have sexual contact while lesions are present.
- Notify your health care provider if you experience burning, stinging, or itching, or if your rash worsens or becomes pronounced.

Amantadine

- Do not drive a car or perform work for which mental alertness is necessary until the effect of the drug is apparent because your vision and coordination can be affected.
- Rise slowly from a prone to a sitting position to decrease the possibility of light-headedness.
- Report changes such as nervousness, tremors, slurred speech, or depression.
- If you are on an alternate dosage schedule, then mark your calendar to designate the days the drug is to be taken.

Oseltamivir

- This drug is taken as soon as possible after the onset of flu symptoms.
- It is available as an oral suspension that should be stored in the refrigerator and is good for 10 days after reconstitution.

- Shake the suspension well before pouring.
- Take this drug with or without food.

Ribavirin

- This drug is taken through a SPAG. Report any worsening of your respiratory function, dizziness, confusion, or shortness of breath to your health care provider.
- Because this drug is a pregnancy category X drug, women of childbearing age should take care not to inhale the drug. When a child is taking the drug, the mother and other females of childbearing age in direct contact with the child should observe respiratory precautions.

Valacyclovir

- This drug is not a cure for herpes simplex, but it will shorten the course of the disease and promote healing of the lesions.
- The drug will not prevent the spread of the disease to others.
- Do not have sexual contact while lesions are present.
- Notify your health care provider if you experience burning, stinging, or itching, or if your rash worsens or becomes pronounced.

Zanamivir

- This drug is taken every 12 hours for 5 days using a Diskhaler delivery system. If you are also using a bronchodilator, then use the bronchodilator before the zanamivir if both are prescribed at the same time.
- The drug may cause dizziness. You should use caution if driving an automobile or operating dangerous machinery.
- Treatment with this drug does not decrease the risk of transmission of the "flu" to others.

FACT CHECK

37-5 What are the contraindications for all antiviral drugs?

37-6 Why must gloves be worn when applying a topical antiviral drug?

COMPLEMENTARY & ALTERNATIVE MEDICINE

Lemon Balm

For hundreds of years, the perennial herb lemon balm has been used for Graves disease and as a sedative, antispasmodic, and an antiviral agent. When used topically, lemon balm has antiviral activity against herpes simplex virus. No adverse reactions have been reported when lemon balm is used topically.

Antiretroviral Drugs

Human immunodeficiency virus (HIV), which causes AIDS, is a type of viral infection transmitted through an infected person's bodily secretions, such as blood or semen. HIV destroys the immune system, causing the body to develop opportunistic infections such as Kaposi sarcoma, *Pneumocystis jiroveci (formerly carinii)* pneumonia, or tuberculosis. Symptoms include chills and fever, night sweats, dry productive cough, dyspnea, lethargy, malaise, fatigue, weight loss, and diarrhea.

The drugs that are used to treat HIV are called antiretrovirals. The antiretrovirals are available in the following categories:

- Cellular chemokine receptor antagonists: maraviroc
- Fusion inhibitors (FIs): enfuvirtide
- Integrase inhibitors: raltegravir
- Nonnucleoside reverse transcriptase inhibitors (NNRTIs): delavirdine, efavirenz, etravirine, nevirapine
- Nucleoside/nucleotide analog reverse transcriptase inhibitors (NRTIs): abacavir, didanosine, emtricitabine, lamivudine, stavudine, telbivudine, tenofovir, zidovudine
- Protease inhibitors (PIs): atazanavir, darunavir, fosamprenavir, indinavir, nelfinavir, ritonavir, saquinavir, tipranavir
- Combinations products.

Figure 37-2 shows possible sites of intervention for several antiretroviral drugs.

Actions of Antiretroviral Drugs

- Cellular chemokine receptor antagonists (CCR5 antagonists) bind to the human chemokine receptor CCR5 on the cell membrane and prevent an interaction that is necessary for the HIV virus to enter the cell.
- Fusion inhibitors prevent the HIV virus from entering cells by inhibiting the fusion of the viral membrane with the cellular membrane.
- Integrase strand transfer inhibitors (INSTIs) prevent the activity of an HIV enzyme that is essential for viral replication. They prevent the HIV DNA from being inserted into the host cell, which prevents the formation of the HIV provirus. Without the provirus, the virus is unable to propagate.
- Nonnucleoside reverse transcriptase inhibitors bind to reverse transcriptase and block its actions. By blocking this enzyme, they prevent the RNA-dependent and DNA-dependent DNA polymerase activities necessary for viral replication.
- NRTIs inhibit the reverse transcriptase enzyme, which inhibits viral DNA growth.
- Protease inhibitors block the protease enzyme that is involved in the later stages of viral replication.

Uses of Antiretroviral Drugs

All of the antiretrovirals are used to decrease morbidity and mortality associated with HIV by preventing viral replication, also referred to as **viral load.** Current HIV treatment guidelines call for combination therapy (Box 37-1).

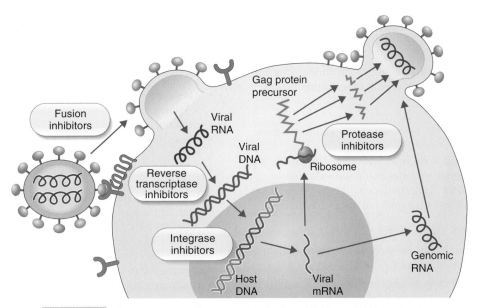

FIGURE 37-2 Possible sites of intervention in the inhibition of HIV replication.

Adverse Reactions of Antiretroviral Drugs

- Cellular chemokine receptor antagonists: The most common adverse reactions of maraviroc are hepatotoxicity, abdominal pain, cough, dizziness, musculoskeletal disorders, pyrexia, rash, upper respiratory tract infection, and orthostatic hypotension.
- Fusion inhibitors: The most common adverse reactions of enfuvirtide are local injection site reactions, increased bacterial pneumonia, and hypersensitivity reactions.
- Integrase inhibitors: The most common adverse reactions of raltegravir are diarrhea, headache, nausea, and pyrexia. Raltegravir may also cause muscle weakness and rhabdomyolysis.

- Nonnucleoside reverse transcriptase inhibitors: The most common adverse reactions associated with the NNRTIs are rash and increased liver enzymes. They all have the potential for causing a rash, but etravirine and nevirapine may cause Stevens–Johnson syndrome.
- Nucleoside/nucleotide analog reverse transcriptase inhibitors: The NNRTIs may cause a variety of different adverse reactions that are specific to the drug.
- Protease inhibitors: Common adverse reactions of the PIs include hyperglycemia, fat maldistribution, serum transaminase elevations, and hyperlipidemia.

BOX 37.1

HIV Treatment Guidelines

Acceptable regimens for treatment-naïve patients include NNRTI-based, PI-based, INSTI-based, or CCR5 antagonist–based regimens. The current preferred regimens for patients never before treated with antiretrovirals are
Nonnucleoside Reverse Transcriptase Inhibitor-Based Regimen
- efavirenz/tenofovir/emtricitabine
Protease Inhibitor-Based Regimen
- atazanavir/ritonavir + tenofovir/emtricitabine
- darunavir/ritonavir + tenofovir/emtricitabine
Integrase Strand Transfer Inhibitor-Based Regimen
- raltegravir + tenofovir/emtricitabine
Preferred Regimen for Pregnant Women
- lopinavir/ritonavir + zidovudine/lamivudine

Source: http://aidsinfo.nih.gov

Contraindications, Precautions, and Interactions of Antiretroviral Drugs

Cellular chemokine receptor antagonists:

- Maraviroc is contraindicated in patients with severe renal impairment or those with renal impairment who are taking CYP3A inhibitors or inducers.
- Maraviroc may cause hepatotoxicity and should be used with caution in patients with hepatitis or increased liver enzymes.
- This drug should be used with caution in patients at an increased risk of cardiovascular effects, and during lactation.
- Maraviroc may increase the risk of developing infections. Patients should see their health care provider if they exhibit symptoms of infection.
- This drug should be used with caution in patients with impaired renal function.
- Maraviroc interacts with any drugs that induce or inhibit CYP3A, such as clarithromycin, ketoconazole, carbamazepine, and other antiretrovirals.

Fusion inhibitors:

- Enfuvirtide is contraindicated in patients who are hypersensitive to the drug.
- Enfuvirtide should be used with caution during lactation.
- Enfuvirtide does not interact with other antiretrovirals.

Integrase inhibitors:

- These drugs should be used with caution during lactation.
- Raltegravir blood concentrations are increased by atazanavir, atazanavir/ritonavir, and omeprazole.
- Raltegravir blood concentrations are decreased by efavirenz, etravirine, rifampin, and tipranavir/ritonavir.

Nonnucleoside reverse transcriptase inhibitors:

- These drugs should not be used if the patient is hypersensitive to them or any of their ingredients.
- These drugs should be used with caution during lactation.
- These drugs have the potential for severe and possibly life-threatening skin reactions, including Stevens–Johnson syndrome.
- These drugs may cause hepatotoxicity and fat redistribution or accumulation of body fat.
- Delavirdine should not be coadministered with anticonvulsants, rifabutin, rifampin, ergot derivatives, HMG-CoA reductase inhibitors, pimozide, and sedative/hypnotics.
- Efavirenz, nevirapine, and rilpivirine interact with drugs that are metabolized by CYP3A4.

Nucleoside/nucleotide analog reverse transcriptase inhibitors:

- These drugs are contraindicated in patients who are hypersensitive to the active ingredients or any other component of the dosage form.
- These drugs may cause redistribution or accumulation of body fat, lactic acidosis, and hepatomegaly with steatosis.
- These drugs should be used with caution during lactation.
- Abacavir is contraindicated in patients with hepatic impairment.
- Abacavir interacts with ethanol and methadone.
- Didanosine should not be coadministered with allopurinol or ribavirin.
- Lamivudine should not be coadministered with zalcitabine.
- Lamivudine potentiates the effects of zidovudine.
- Stavudine should not be coadministered with zidovudine.
- Telbivudine may cause myopathy. Patients who are taking other drugs that may increase the risk of myopathy should be closely monitored for muscle pain, tenderness, or weakness.
- Telbivudine and interferon taken together may increase the risk of peripheral neuropathy.
- Tenofovir interacts with a number of medications including other antiretrovirals, nephrotoxic agents, NSAIDs, antivirals, and tacrolimus.
- Zidovudine should be used with caution in patients with bone marrow compromise. Zidovudine makes them more susceptible to infection and easy bruising.
- Zidovudine interacts with a number of medications including doxorubicin, fluconazole, ganciclovir, methadone, probenecid, valproic acid, and other antiretrovirals.

Protease inhibitors:

- These drugs should not be taken by patients who have a known hypersensitivity to them or any of their components.
- These drugs should be used with caution during lactation.
- These drugs may cause fat redistribution or accumulation.
- Patients with hemophilia may be at an increased risk for bleeding when taking these drugs.
- Atazanavir should be used with caution in patients with preexisting conduction system disease.
- Atazanavir interacts with drugs metabolized by cytochrome P450.
- Atazanavir should be taken 2 hours before or 1 hour after antacids.
- Darunavir, fosamprenavir, indinavir, nelfinavir, ritonavir, saquinavir, and tipranavir interact with drugs that induce or inhibit cytochrome P450.
- Saquinavir/ritonavir prolongs the PR interval. Patients with underlying abnormalities are at increased risk for conduction issues.
- Saquinavir/ritonavir causes QT prolongation.
- Tipranavir may cause hepatotoxicity and intracranial hemorrhage.

Patient Management Issues with Antiretroviral Drugs

Patients who have tested positive for the HIV infection should have a complete medical history and physical examination completed prior to beginning antiretroviral therapy. Laboratory tests that should be completed include, but are not limited to, HIV antibody test, CD4 T-cell count, plasma HIV RNA, complete blood count, fasting blood glucose, fasting lipid panel, and testing for hepatitis (A, B, and C).

Educating the Patient and Family about Antiretroviral Drugs

Following are key points about antiretroviral drugs that the patient and family members should know:

- Patients should understand that antiretroviral drugs are not a cure for disease.

ALERT Rx

Antiretrovirals for Human Immunodeficiency Virus
Patients receiving antiviral drugs for human immunodeficiency infections may continue to have opportunistic infections and other complications associated with the virus. All patients should be closely monitored for signs of infection such as fever (even low-grade fever), malaise, sore throat, or lethargy.

- The antiretrovirals also do not reduce the risk of transmitting HIV to others. Patients should be counseled on high-risk behaviors and how to prevent HIV transmission.
- Patients should take each medication exactly as prescribed, including whether it should be taken with or without food.
- Patients should not skip or alter doses or discontinue the medication without direction from their health care provider.

See the Facts About box for more information on HIV.

Antifungal Drugs

A **fungus** is a colorless plant that lacks chlorophyll. Fungi that cause disease in humans may be yeast-like or mold-like; the resulting infections are called **mycotic infections** or fungal infections. Fungal infections range from superficial skin infections to life-threatening systemic infections. Systemic fungal infections are serious infections that occur when fungi gain entrance into the interior of the body.

Mycotic (fungal) infections may be one of two types:

1. Superficial mycotic infections
2. Deep (systemic) mycotic infections

The superficial mycotic infections occur on the surface of, or just below, the skin or nails. Superficial infections include **tinea pedis** (athlete's foot), **tinea cruris** (jock itch), **tinea corporis** (ringworm), **onychomycosis** (nail fungus), and yeast infections, such as those caused by *Candida albicans*. Yeast infections or those caused by *C. albicans* affect women in the vulvovaginal area and can be difficult to control. Women who are at increased risk for vulvovaginal yeast infections include those who have diabetes, are pregnant, or are taking oral contraceptives, antibiotics, or corticosteroids.

Deep mycotic infections develop inside the body, such as in the lungs. Treatment for deep mycotic infections is often difficult and prolonged. The Summary Drug Table: Antifungal Drugs identifies drugs that are used to combat fungal infections.

Actions of Antifungal Drugs

Antifungal drugs may be **fungicidal** (able to destroy fungi) or **fungistatic** (able to slow or retard the multiplication of fungi). Amphotericin B (Amphotec), miconazole (Monistat), nystatin, and ketoconazole (Nizoral) are thought to have an effect on the cell membrane of the fungus, resulting in a fungicidal or fungistatic effect. The fungicidal or fungistatic effect of these drugs appears to be related to their concentration in body tissues. Fluconazole (Diflucan) has fungistatic activity that appears to result from the depletion of sterols (a group of substances related to fats) in the fungus cells.

Griseofulvin (Grifulvin-V, Gris-PEG) exerts its effect by being deposited in keratin precursor cells, which are then gradually lost (because of the constant shedding of top skin cells) and replaced by new, noninfected cells. The mode of action of flucytosine (Ancobon) is not clearly understood. Clotrimazole (Lotrimin AF, Mycelex-7) binds with phospholipids in the fungal cell membrane, increasing permeability of the cell and resulting in loss of intracellular components.

Uses of Antifungal Drugs

Antifungal drugs are used to treat superficial and deep fungal infections. The antifungal drugs specifically discussed in this chapter are amphotericin B, fluconazole, flucytosine, griseofulvin, ketoconazole, and miconazole. Miconazole is an antifungal drug used to treat vulvovaginal "yeast" infections and is representative of all of the vaginal antifungal agents. Fungal infections of the skin or mucous membranes may be treated with topical or vaginal preparations. Topical antifungal drugs and the vulvovaginal antifungal agents are listed in the Summary Drug Table: Antifungal Drugs.

Adverse Reactions of Antifungal Drugs

When topical antifungal drugs, such as clotrimazole, are applied to the skin or mucous membranes, few adverse reactions occur. On occasion, a local reaction, such as irritation or burning, may occur with topical use. The vulvovaginal antifungal drugs may cause local irritation, redness, stinging, or abdominal pain. Few adverse reactions occur with the use of the vulvovaginal antifungal drugs.

Amphotericin B

Amphotericin B is the most effective drug available for the treatment of most systemic fungal infections. Use often results in serious reactions, including fever, shaking, chills, headache, malaise, anorexia, joint and muscle pain, abnormal renal function or kidney damage, nausea, vomiting, and anemia. This drug is given parenterally, usually for a period of several months. Its use is reserved for serious and potentially life-threatening fungal infections. Some of these adverse reactions may be lessened by use of aspirin, antihistamines, or antiemetics.

Fluconazole

Use may result in nausea, vomiting, headache, diarrhea, abdominal pain, and skin rash. Abnormal liver function tests may occur and may require follow-up tests to determine if liver function has been affected.

Flucytosine

Use may result in nausea, vomiting, diarrhea, rash, anemia, leukopenia, and thrombocytopenia. Signs of renal impairment include elevated blood urea nitrogen and serum creatinine levels. Periodic renal function tests are usually performed during therapy.

Griseofulvin

Use may result in a hypersensitivity-like reaction that includes rash and urticaria. Nausea, vomiting, oral thrush, diarrhea, and headache also may occur.

Itraconazole

The most common adverse reactions are nausea, vomiting, and diarrhea. On occasion, severe hypokalemia (low potassium level) has occurred in patients receiving the drug on a daily basis. Hepatotoxicity is a possibility with itraconazole use.

Ketoconazole

This drug is usually well-tolerated, but nausea, vomiting, headache, dizziness, abdominal pain, and pruritus may occur. Most adverse reactions are mild and transient. On rare occasions, hepatic toxicity may occur, in which case the drug must be discontinued immediately. Periodic hepatic function tests are used to monitor for hepatic toxicity.

Miconazole

Use of miconazole for a vulvovaginal fungal infection may cause irritation, sensitization, or vulvovaginal burning. Skin irritation may result in redness, itching, burning, or skin fissures. Other adverse reactions with miconazole include cramping, nausea, and headache. Adverse reactions associated with topical use are usually not severe.

Contraindications, Precautions, and Interactions of Antifungal Drugs

Amphotericin B

- Amphotericin B is contraindicated in patients with a known hypersensitivity and during lactation.
- It is used cautiously in patients with renal dysfunction or electrolyte imbalances, and in combination with antineoplastic drugs (because it can cause severe bone marrow suppression).
- This drug is used during pregnancy only when the situation is life-threatening.
- When given with the corticosteroids, severe hypokalemia may occur.
- There may be an increased risk of digitalis toxicity if digoxin is administered concurrently with amphotericin B.
- Use with nephrotoxic drugs (e.g., aminoglycosides or cyclosporine) may increase the risk of nephrotoxicity in patients also taking amphotericin B.
- Amphotericin B decreases the effects of miconazole.
- Amphotericin B is given only under close supervision in the hospital setting.

Fluconazole

- Fluconazole is contraindicated in patients with known hypersensitivity.
- The drug is used cautiously in patients with renal impairment and during lactation.
- The drug is given during pregnancy only if the benefit of the drug clearly outweighs any possible risk to the infant.
- When fluconazole is taken with an oral hypoglycemic, there is an increased effect of the oral hypoglycemic.
- Fluconazole may decrease the metabolism of phenytoin and warfarin.

Flucytosine

- Flucytosine is contraindicated in patients with known hypersensitivity.

- Flucytosine is used cautiously in patients with bone marrow depression and with extreme caution in those with renal impairment.
- The drug is also used cautiously during lactation.
- When flucytosine and amphotericin B are taken concurrently, the risk of flucytosine toxicity is increased.

Griseofulvin

- Griseofulvin is contraindicated in patients with known hypersensitivity and in those with severe liver disease.
- This drug is used cautiously during lactation.
- It is used with caution when given concurrently with penicillin because of the possibility of cross-sensitivity.
- When griseofulvin is given with warfarin, the anticoagulant effect may be decreased.
- When used with a barbiturate, the effect of griseofulvin may be decreased.
- A decrease in the effects of an oral contraceptive may occur with griseofulvin therapy, causing breakthrough bleeding, pregnancy, or amenorrhea.
- Blood salicylate concentrations may be decreased when a salicylate is administered with griseofulvin.

Itraconazole

- Itraconazole is contraindicated in patients with a known hypersensitivity.
- The drug is used cautiously in patients with hepatitis, human immunodeficiency virus, or impaired liver function, and in pregnant women.
- In patients with hypochlorhydria, the absorption of itraconazole is decreased.
- Itraconazole elevates blood concentrations of digoxin and cyclosporine.
- Phenytoin decreases blood levels of itraconazole and alters the metabolism of phenytoin.
- Histamine antagonists, isoniazid, and rifampin decrease plasma levels of itraconazole.
- There is an increased anticoagulant effect when warfarin is used concurrently with itraconazole.

Ketoconazole

- Ketoconazole is contraindicated in patients with known hypersensitivity.
- Ketoconazole is used cautiously in patients with liver impairment and during pregnancy and lactation.
- The absorption of ketoconazole is impaired when the drug is taken with histamine antagonists and antacids.
- Ketoconazole enhances the anticoagulant effect of warfarin and causes an additive hepatotoxicity when given with other hepatotoxic drugs and alcohol.
- Use of ketoconazole with rifampin or isoniazid may decrease the blood levels of ketoconazole.

Miconazole

- Miconazole is contraindicated in patients with known hypersensitivity.
- The drug is given cautiously in cases of chronic or recurrent candidiasis.

- Recurrent or chronic candidiasis requires an evaluation for diabetes.
- The drug is used cautiously during pregnancy. If used during pregnancy, then a vaginal applicator may be contraindicated and manual insertion of the vaginal tablets preferred. Because small amounts of these drugs may be absorbed from the vagina, the drug is used during the first trimester only when essential.

FACT CHECK

37-10 Which drug works best for treating systemic fungal infections and what is its most serious adverse reaction?

37-11 Which antifungal drug *decreases* the anticoagulant effect of warfarin when given together? Which drugs *increase* warfarin's anticoagulant effects when given together?

Patient Management Issues with Antifungal Drugs

Careful observation of the patient is required every 2 to 4 hours for adverse drug reactions when the antifungal drug is given by the oral or parenteral route. When these drugs are applied topically to the skin, the area is inspected at the time of each application for localized skin reactions. When these drugs are administered vaginally, the patient is asked about any discomfort or other sensations experienced after insertion of the antifungal preparation. The patient's response to therapy should be monitored daily.

Periodic laboratory tests are usually ordered to monitor the patient's response to therapy and to detect toxic drug reactions. Serum creatinine levels and blood urea nitrogen levels are checked frequently during the course of therapy to monitor kidney function. If the blood urea nitrogen or the serum creatinine levels are excessive, then the health care provider may discontinue the drug therapy or reduce the dosage until kidney function improves.

Many fungal infections are associated with lesions that are at risk for infection. The patient is inspected for superficial fungal infections of the skin or skin structures (e.g., hair and nails). Any skin lesions, such as rough itchy patches, cracks between the toes, and sore and reddened areas are noted. The skin is checked for localized signs of infection (i.e., increased

KEY CONCEPTS

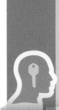

37-1   Issues with Prolonged Antifungal Therapy

Superficial and deep fungal infections respond slowly to antifungal therapy. Many patients experience anxiety and depression over the fact that therapy must continue for a prolonged time. The patient and family should be helped to understand that therapy must be continued until the infection is under control. In some cases, therapy may take weeks or months.

redness or swelling). Skin lesions are monitored daily. Gloves should be used when caring for open lesions to minimize autoinoculation or transmission of the disease.

Amphotericin B

Amphotericin B is taken daily or every other day over several months. The patient is often acutely ill with a life-threatening deep fungal infection. The intravenous infusion rate and the infusion site are checked frequently during use of the drug. This is especially important if the patient is restless or confused. On occasion, amphotericin B may be given as an oral solution for oral candidiasis. The patient is instructed to swish and hold the solution in the mouth for several minutes (or as long as possible) before swallowing.

Fluconazole

The drug may be taken orally or intravenously.

Flucytosine

Flucytosine is given orally. To decrease or prevent nausea and vomiting, the capsules may be taken a few at a time during a 15-minute period.

Griseofulvin

This drug is given orally. Prolonged therapy is usually needed to eliminate the fungus.

Itraconazole

This drug is given orally with food to increase absorption. When used intravenously, it is not diluted with any other diluent.

Ketoconazole

This drug is given with food to minimize gastrointestinal irritation. Antacids, anticholinergics, or histamine blockers should not be used until at least 2 hours after ketoconazole is given.

Miconazole

This drug is self-administered on an outpatient basis vaginally and topically. It is available as a buccal tablet by prescription. The buccal tablet is applied to the upper gum area once daily.

FACT CHECK

37-12 Why is it important for the patient and family to understand about the length of antifungal treatment?

Educating the Patient and Family about Antifungal Drugs

Following are key points about antifungal drugs that the patient and family members should know:

- Clean the involved area and apply the ointment or cream to your skin as directed by your health care provider.

- Do not increase or decrease the amount you use or how often you use the ointment or cream unless directed to do so by your health care provider.
- During treatment for a ringworm infection, keep your towels and facecloths separate from those of other family members to avoid the spread of the infection. Keep the affected area clean and dry.

Flucytosine

- You may experience nausea or vomiting with this drug. Reduce or eliminate these effects by taking a few capsules at a time during a 15-minute period. If your nausea, vomiting, or diarrhea persists, then notify your health care provider as soon as possible.

Griseofulvin

- Although you may not notice the beneficial effects for some time, take the drug for the full course of therapy. Avoid exposure to sunlight and sunlamps because an exaggerated skin reaction (which is similar to severe sunburn) may occur even after a brief exposure to ultraviolet light. Notify your health care provider if you experience fever, sore throat, or skin rash.

Ketoconazole

- Complete the full course of therapy as prescribed by your health care provider. Do not take this drug with an antacid. In addition, avoid the use of nonprescription drugs unless use of a specific drug is approved by your health care provider. This drug may produce headache, dizziness, and drowsiness. If you experience drowsiness or dizziness, then be cautious while driving or performing other hazardous tasks. Notify your health care provider if your abdominal pain, fever, or diarrhea becomes pronounced.

Itraconazole

- Take this drug with food. Therapy will continue for at least 3 months until the infection is controlled. Report unusual fatigue, yellow skin, darkened urine, anorexia, nausea, or vomiting to your health care provider.

Miconazole

- If you use the drug (cream or tablet) vaginally, then insert the drug high in the vagina using the applicator provided with the product. Wear a sanitary napkin after insertion of the drug to prevent staining of your clothing and bed linen.
- Continue taking the drug during your menstrual period if you are using the vaginal route.
- Do not have intercourse while taking this drug, or advise your partner to use a condom to avoid reinfection.
- To prevent recurrent infections, avoid nylon and tight-fitting garments. If you have no improvement in 5 to 7 days, then stop using the drug and consult your health care provider because a more serious infection may be present.
- If you experience abdominal pain, pelvic pain, rash, fever, or offensive-smelling vaginal discharge, then do not use the drug but notify your health care provider.

COMPLEMENTARY & ALTERNATIVE MEDICINE

Gentian Violet

Gentian violet is an antibacterial/antifungal that is used for the treatment of superficial fungus infections. It is also used externally for the treatment of abrasions and minor cuts. It is purple in color and will stain anything it touches (skin and clothing) a deep purple. It may be used orally for thrush. It is applied with a cotton-tipped applicator to the specific lesions. It may be used vaginally by soaking a tampon in gentian violet and then inserting it vaginally. It is not used as frequently as the other antifungals.

COMPLEMENTARY & ALTERNATIVE MEDICINE

Antifungal Herbs

Researchers have identified antifungal herbs that are effective against tinea pedis (athlete's foot), such as tea tree oil (*Melaleuca alternifolia*) and garlic (*Allium sativum*).

Tea tree oil comes from an evergreen tree native to Australia. It is used as an antifungal to relieve and control the symptoms of tinea pedis. Topical application is most effective when used in a cream with at least 10% tea tree oil. Several commercially prepared ointments are available. The cream is applied to affected areas twice daily for several weeks.

Garlic is also used as an antifungal. A cream of 0.4% ajoene (the antifungal component of garlic) has been found to relieve symptoms of athlete's foot and, like tea tree oil, is applied twice daily.

Chapter Review

KEY POINTS

- Most antiviral drugs act by inhibiting viral DNA or RNA replication in the virus, causing viral death. Although infections caused by a virus are common, antiviral drugs have limited use because they are effective against only a small number of specific viral infections.
- The most common adverse reactions when these drugs are used systemically are gastrointestinal disturbances, such as nausea, vomiting, diarrhea, and anorexia.
- When administered topically, the antiviral drugs can cause transient burning, stinging, and pruritus.
- Antiviral drugs are contraindicated in patients with congestive heart failure, seizures, and kidney disease and during lactation; are given with caution in patients with kidney impairment; and require dosage adjustments.
- Antiretrovirals are used to decrease the morbidity and mortality associated with HIV infection.
- There are six classes of antiretrovirals. Most patients will be on a combination therapy based on one of the six classes of antiretrovirals.
- Patients who are taking antiretrovirals should take them exactly as prescribed and not skip or discontinue the medication.
- Laboratory tests are performed prior to initiating therapy and continue throughout therapy to determine the patient's viral load and the drug regimen's effectiveness.
- Superficial mycotic (fungal) infections occur on the surface of, or just below, the skin or nails. Deep mycotic infections develop inside the body, such as in the lungs.
- Treatment for deep mycotic infections is often difficult and prolonged.

- When topical antifungal drugs are applied to the skin or mucous membranes, few adverse reactions occur. The vulvovaginal antifungal drugs may cause local irritation, redness, stinging, or abdominal pain. Few adverse reactions occur with the vulvovaginal antifungal drugs.
- The most effective systemic antifungals often cause serious reactions, including fever, shaking, chills, headache, malaise, anorexia, joint and muscle pain, abnormal renal function, nausea, vomiting, and anemia.

CRITICAL THINKING CASE STUDIES

CASE 1

Seasonal Flu

Ms. Jenkins, age 77 years, woke up this morning with flu symptoms. She is aching, fatigued, and has a fever. Her physician has prescribed oseltamivir, but she has some questions.

1. Ms. Jenkins is not sure if she wants to take the medication because her symptoms are not too bad. How soon does oseltamivir need to be started after onset of symptoms?
   a. Within 24 hours
   b. Within 48 hours
   c. Within 72 hours
   d. Within 5 days
2. How should Ms. Jenkins be taking oseltamivir?
   a. Once daily for 5 days
   b. Once daily for 10 days
   c. Twice daily for 5 days
   d. Twice daily for 10 days

3. Ms. Jenkins asks if she should get an annual flu vaccination since she got the vaccination and still got the flu. What should you tell her?

CASE 2
Antifungal Therapy

Ms. Smith has been diagnosed with a vaginal yeast infection. She goes to the pharmacy and purchases Gyne-Lotrimin.

1. How should the vaginal cream be used?
   a. Twice daily
   b. Once daily in the morning
   c. Once daily in the evening
   d. One time as a single dose
2. Ms. Smith decides that she does not want to use a vaginal product. She calls her health care provider and is prescribed Diflucan. She is to take one tablet for a single dose. What adverse effect(s) might she experience?
   a. Nausea
   b. Vomiting
   c. Diarrhea
   d. All of the above
3. Ms. Smith asks you if you know of any things she can do to prevent yeast infections in the future. What can you tell her?

Review Questions

MULTIPLE CHOICE

1. Patients receiving antiretroviral drugs for human immunodeficiency infections should be closely monitored for signs of infection such as
   a. fever
   b. malaise
   c. sore throat
   d. all of the above
2. Zanamivir is taken
   a. via inhalation
   b. by subcutaneous injection
   c. orally with meals
   d. orally mixed with orange juice or apple juice
3. Mr. Carr is receiving amphotericin B for a systemic fungal infection. Which of the following would most likely indicate that Mr. Carr is experiencing an adverse reaction to amphotericin B?
   a. Fever and chills
   b. Back pain
   c. Drowsiness
   d. Flushing of the skin
4. Griseofulvin would not be given to a patient if the patient has
   a. anemia
   b. respiratory disease
   c. a recent myocardial infarction
   d. severe liver disease

5. Patients who are diagnosed as HIV positive, should have which of the following laboratory tests completed?
   a. CDR T-cell count
   b. Plasma HIV RNA
   c. Testing for hepatitis (A, B, and C)
   d. All of the above

MATCHING

Match the antiviral on the left with the correct trade name on the right.

_____ 6. acyclovir   a. Flumadine
_____ 7. cidofovir   b. Tamiflu
_____ 8. ganciclovir   c. Relenza
_____ 9. oseltamivir   d. Vistide
_____ 10. rimantadine   e. Valcyte
_____ 11. valacyclovir   f. Cytovene
_____ 12. valganciclovir   g. Zovirax
_____ 13. zanamivir   h. Valtrex

Match the antiretroviral on the left with the correct trade name on the right.

_____ 14. maraviroc   a. Sustiva
_____ 15. enfuvirtide   b. Epivir
_____ 16. raltegravir   c. Retrovir
_____ 17. efavirenz   d. Crixivan
_____ 18. ritonavir   e. Selzentry
_____ 19. indinavir   f. Fuzeon
_____ 20. zidovudine   g. Norvir
_____ 21. lamivudine   h. Instress

Match the antifungal on the left with the correct trade name on the right.

_____ 22. fluconazole   a. Monistat
_____ 23. griseofulvin   b. Lamisil
_____ 24. ketoconazole   c. Tinactin
_____ 25. miconazole   d. Naftin
_____ 26. terbinafine   e. Diflucan
_____ 27. tolnaftate   f. Grifulvin V
_____ 28. terconazole   g. Nizoral
_____ 29. naftifine   h. Terazol

TRUE OR FALSE

_____ 30. Acyclovir is used to cure herpes simplex.
_____ 31. Patients taking vulvovaginal antifungal drugs may experience local irritation, redness, stinging, or abdominal pain.
_____ 32. The nucleoside/nucleotide analog reverse transcriptase inhibitors may cause redistribution or accumulation of body fat.
_____ 33. Amphotericin B may be given as an oral solution for oral candidiasis.
_____ 34. Current HIV treatment guidelines call for single ingredient therapy upon diagnosis and combination therapy as the disease progresses.

FILL IN THE BLANKS

35. Therapy with the antifungal _____ may cause a _____ in the effects of oral contraceptives, causing breakthrough bleeding, pregnancy, or amenorrhea.

36. Patients taking _____ may experience bone marrow depression, making them susceptible to _____ and easy bruising.

37. Because _____, an antiviral used to treat chronic hepatitis C, is a pregnancy category X drug, it may be teratogenic and embryotoxic and is therefore _____ during pregnancy.

38. The effects of oral hypoglycemic are increased when taken with _____.

39. All of the antiretrovirals are used to decrease morbidity and mortality associated with HIV by preventing viral replication, also referred to as _____ _____.

SHORT ANSWERS

40. What are some common uses of antiviral drugs?

41. What are two types of fungal infections?

42. What are the most common adverse reactions when antiviral drugs are used systemically? Topically?

43. What should you advise patients taking antifungal drugs for ringworm to do to avoid spreading the infection to other family members?

44. For patients who think they may be HIV positive or who are HIV positive, what lifestyle counseling should you offer?

Web Activities

1. Go to the AIDS.gov Web site (www.aids.gov). What is HIV/AIDS? How do you get HIV/AIDS? Where can you get tested for HIV?

2. Go to The American Congress of Obstetricians and Gynecologists Web site (www.acog.org). Conduct a search for "vaginal yeast infections." What can you tell a patient to do to reduce the risk of getting vaginitis? What conditions or diseases increase the risk of a yeast infection?

SUMMARY DRUG TABLE Antifungal Drugs (left, generic; right, trade)

Comprehensive Summary Drug Tables, including uses, adverses effects, dosages, and pregnancy classifications, are provided on the companion website, http://thePoint.lww. com/PharmacologyHP2e

Generic	Trade
amphotericin B *am-foe-ter'-i-sin bee*	Abelcet (lipid), AmBisome (liposome), Amphotec (cholesteryl sulfate complex), *generic*
anidulafungin *ay-nid-yoo-la-fun'-jin*	Eraxis
caspofungin acetate *kass-poe-fun-jin*	Cancidas
fluconazole *floo-kon'-a-zole*	Diflucan, *generic*
flucytosine (5-FC) *floo-sye'-toe-seen*	Ancobon
griseofulvin, microsize *griz-ee-oh-full'-vin*	Grifulvin V, *generic*
griseofulvin, ultramicrosize *griz-ee-oh-full'-vin*	Gris-PEG
itraconazole *eye-tra-kon'-a-zole*	Sporanox, Sporanox PulsePak, *generic*
ketoconazole *kee-toe-koe'-na-zole*	Topical (Rx): Extina, Kuric, Nizoral, Xolegel Topical (OTC): Nizoral A-D Oral: *generic*
micafungin *mi-ka-fun'-gin*	Mycamine
miconazole *mi-kon'-a-zole*	Topical: Cruex, Desenex, Fungoid Tincture, Lotrimin AF, Micatin, Zeasorb, *generic* (OTC) Vaginal: Monistat (OTC) Buccal: Oravig (Rx)
nystatin *nye-stat'-in*	Oral: Bio-Statin, *generic* Topical: Nyamyc, Nystop, *generic* Vaginal: *generic*
posaconazole *poe-sa-kon'-a-zole*	Noxafil
terbinafine *ter'-bin-a-feen*	Lamisil (oral, external Rx), Lamisil Advanced (external OTC), Lamisil AT (external OTC), Terbinex (Rx combination kit), *generic* (Rx and OTC)
voriconazole *vor-i-koe'-na-zole*	Vfend, *generic*

Topical Preparations

Generic	Trade
butenafine *byoo-ten'-a-feen*	Lotrimin Ultra (OTC), Mentax (Rx)
ciclopirox *sye-kloe-peer'-oks*	CNLI Nail, Loprox, Penlac, *generic*
clotrimazole *kloe-trim'-a-zole*	External: Desenex (OTC), FungiCure (Rx), Lotrimin AF (OTC), Mycelex OTC, *generic* Vaginal: Gyne-Lotrimin (OTC), Mycelex-7 (OTC), *generic* Mouth/throat: *generic*
econazole *e-kone'-a-zole*	*generic*
naftifine *naf'-ti-feen*	Naftin
oxiconazole *oks-in-kon'-a-zole*	Oxistat
sertaconazole *ser-ta-koe'-na-zole*	Ertaczo
sulconazole *sul-kon'-a-zole*	Exelderm
tolnaftate *tole-naf'-tate*	Tinactin (OTC), Blis-To-Sol (OTC), Lamisil AF Defense (OTC), Odor Eaters Foot/Sneaker Spray (OTC), Scholls Odor Destroyers Sport (OTC), *generic* (OTC)
undecylenic acid and derivatives *un-de-sil-en'-ik as'-id & dah-riv'-ah-tivs*	Caldesene (OTC), Cruex (OTC), Phicon F (OTC), Blis-To-Sol (OTC), Elon Dual Defense Anti-Fungal Formula (OTC), Gordochom (OTC), Desenex (OTC), Fungi Cure Maximum Strength (OTC)

Vaginal Preparations

Generic	Trade
butoconazole *byoo-toe-koe'-na-zole*	Gynazole-1
terconazole *ter-kone'-a-zole*	Terazol, Zazole, *generic*
tioconazole *tyo-oh-kone'-a-zole*	Monistat-1 (OTC), Vagistat-1 (OTC)

(continued)

SUMMARY DRUG TABLE Antiretroviral Drugs (left, generic; right, trade)

Comprehensive Summary Drug Tables, including uses, adverses effects, dosages, and pregnancy classifications, are provided on the companion website, http://thePoint.lww.com/PharmacologyHP2e

Cellular Chemokine Receptor Antagonist	
maraviroc *mah-rav'-er-rock*	Selzentry

Fusion Inhibitors	
enfuvirtide *en-fyoo'-vir-tide*	Fuzeon

Integrase Inhibitor	
raltegravir *ral-teg'-ra-vir*	Isentress

Nonnucleoside Reverse Transcriptase Inhibitors	
delavirdine mesylate *de-la-vir'-deen*	Rescriptor
efavirenz *e-fav'-e-renz*	Sustiva
efavirenz/emtricitabine/tenofovir disoproxil fumarate *e-fav'-e-renz/em-trye-sye'-ta-been/ te-noe'-fo-veer*	Atripla

Nucleoside Reverse Transcriptase Inhibitors	
etravirine *et-ra-vir'-een*	Intelence
nevirapine *ne-vye'-ra-peen*	Viramune, Viramune XR
abacavir *a-bak'-a-veer*	Ziagen
didanosine *dye-dan'-oh-sin*	Videx, Videx EC, *generic*
emtricitabine *em-trye-sye'-ta-been*	Emtriva
lamivudine *la-mi'-vyoo-deen*	Epivir, Epivir HBV
stavudine *stay-vew'-den*	Zerit, *generic*
telbivudine *tel-bi'-vyoo-deen*	Tyzeka
zidovudine *zye-doe'-vyoo-deen*	Retrovir, *generic*

Nucleoside Analog Reverse Transcriptase Inhibitor Combinations	
abacavir sulfate/lamivudine/zidovudine *a-bak'-a-veer/la-mi'-vyoo-deen/ zye-doe'-vyoo-deen*	Trizivir
abacavir/lamivudine *a-bak'-a-veer/la-mi'-vyoo-deen*	Epzicom
emtricitabine/tenofovir disoproxil fumarate *em-trye-sye'-ta-been/te-noe'-fo-veer*	Truvada
lamivudine/zidovudine *la-mi'-vyoo-deen/zye-doe'-vyoo-deen*	Combivir

Nucleotide Analog Reverse Transcriptase Inhibitors	
tenofovir disoproxil fumarate *te-noe'-fo-veer*	Viread

Protease Inhibitors	
atazanavir *at-a-za-na'-veer*	Reyataz
darunavir *dar-oo'-na-veer*	Prezista
fosamprenavir *fos'-am-pren-a-veer*	Lexiva
indinavir *in-din'-ah-ver*	Crixivan
nelfinavir mesylate *nell-fin'-a-veer*	Viracept
ritonavir *ri-ton'-ah-ver*	Norvir
saquinavir, saquinavir mesylate *sa-kwen'-a-veer*	Invirase
tipranavir *tip-ra'-na-veer*	Aptivus

Protease Inhibitor Combinations	
lopinavir/ritonavir *low-pin'-ah-veer/ rih-ton'-ah-veer*	Kaletra

(continued)

SUMMARY DRUG TABLE Antiviral Drugs (continued)
(left, generic; right, trade)

Comprehensive Summary Drug Tables, including uses, adverses effects, dosages, and pregnancy classifications, are provided on the companion website, http://thePoint.lww.com/PharmacologyHP2e

acyclovir sodium *ay-sye'-kloe-ver*	Zovirax, *generic*
adefovir *a-def'-o-veer*	Hepsera
amantadine *a-man'-ta-deen*	*generic*
boceprevir	Victrelis
cidofovir *si-doh'-foh-vir*	Vistide
entecavir *en-te'-ka-veer*	Baraclude
famciclovir *fam-sye'-kloe-vir*	Famvir, *generic*
foscarnet *foss-kar'-net*	*generic*
ganciclovir *gan-sye'-kloe-vir*	Cytovene and *generic* (IV), sVitrasert (intraocular), Zirgan (ophthalmic), *generic* (oral)
oseltamivir *oh-sell-tam'-ih-veer*	Tamiflu
penciclovir *pen-sye'-kloe-ver*	Denavir
ribavirin *rye-ba-vye'-rin*	Copegus, Rebetol, RibaPak, Ribasphere, RibaTab, Virazole, *generic*
rimantadine HCl *ri-man'-ta-deen*	Flumadine, *generic*
telaprevir	Incivek
valacyclovir *val-ah-sye'-kloe-ver*	Valtrex, *generic*
valganciclovir *val-gan-si'-klo-veer*	Valcyte
zanamivir *zan-am'-ah-ver*	Relenza Diskhaler

38

Antiparasitic Drugs

CHAPTER OBJECTIVES

On completion of this chapter, students will be able to:

1. Define the chapter's key terms.

2. Explain the differences between helminthiasis, malaria, and amebiasis and identify the causative organisms of each infection.

3. Explain the difference between suppression and treatment in the use of antimalarial drugs.

4. Describe the general drug actions, uses, adverse reactions, contraindications, precautions, and interactions of antiparasitic drugs.

5. Discuss important points to keep in mind when educating the patient or family members about the use of antiparasitic drugs.

KEY TERMS

amebiasis—invasion of the body by the ameba *Entamoeba histolytica*
anthelmintic—drugs with actions against helminths
helminthiasis—invasion of the body by helminths (worms)
helminths—worms
parasite—an organism that lives in or on another organism (the host) without contributing to the survival or well-being of the host

CHAPTER OVERVIEW

Drug classes covered in this chapter are:

- Anthelmintic drugs

- Antimalarial drugs

- Amebicides

Drugs by classification are listed on page 420.

thePOINT RESOURCES

- Comprehensive Summary Drug Tables

- Lippincott's Interactive Tutorials: Drugs Used to Treat Infections

- Interactive Practice and Review

- Monographs of Most Commonly Prescribed Drugs

Like viruses and fungi, parasites can also cause infection in humans. This chapter discusses antiparasitic drugs.

A **parasite** is an organism that lives in or on another organism (the host) without contributing to the survival or well-being of the host. **Helminthiasis** (invasion of the body by **helminths** [worms]), malaria (an infectious disease caused by a protozoan and usually transmitted to humans through a bite from an infected mosquito), and **amebiasis** (invasion of the body by the ameba *Entamoeba histolytica*) are worldwide health problems caused by parasites (Key Concepts 38-1).

FACT CHECK

38-1   What is a parasite?

Anthelmintic Drugs

Anthelmintic (against helminths) drugs are used to treat helminthiasis. Roundworms, pinworms, whipworms, hookworms, and tapeworms are examples of helminths (Fig. 38-1). Table 38-1 lists the organisms that cause helminth infections. The anthelmintic drugs are listed in the Summary Drug Table: Anthelmintic Drugs.

Although the actions of anthelmintic drugs vary, their prime purpose is to kill the parasite. Adverse reactions of the anthelmintic drugs, if they do occur, are usually mild when the drug is used in the recommended dosage.

Actions, Uses, and Adverse Reactions of Anthelmintic Drugs

Albendazole

Albendazole (Albenza) interferes with the synthesis of the parasite's microtubules, resulting in death of susceptible larva. This drug is used to treat larval forms of pork tapeworm and to treat liver, lung, and peritoneum disease caused by the dog tapeworm.

Mebendazole

Mebendazole (Vermox) blocks the uptake of glucose by the helminth, resulting in a depletion of the helminth's own gly-

TABLE 38-1   Common Names and Causative Organisms or Parasitic Infections

Common Name	Causative Organism
Roundworm	*Ascaris lumbricoides*
Pinworm	*Enterobius vermicularis*
Whipworm	*Trichuris trichiura*
Threadworm	*Strongyloides stercoralis*
Hookworm	*Ancylostoma duodenale, Necator americanus*
Beef tapeworm	*Taenia saginata*
Pork tapeworm	*Taenia solium*
Fish tape worm	*Diphyllobothrium latum*

cogen. Glycogen depletion results in a decreased formation of adenosine triphosphate, which is required by helminths for reproduction and survival. This drug is used to treat whipworm, pinworm, roundworm, American hookworm, and the common hookworm. Treatment with mebendazole may cause transient abdominal pain and diarrhea.

Ivermectin

Ivermectin binds selectively to glutamate-gated chloride ion channels that occur in invertebrate nerve and muscle cells. This leads to an increase in the permeability of the cell membrane to chloride ions with hyperpolarization of the nerve or muscle cell, resulting in paralysis and death of the parasite.

Ivermectin is active against various life-cycle stages of many but not all roundworms.

Praziquantel

Praziquantel affects the permeability of the cell membrane to cause a rapid contraction of schistosomes (helminths).

KEY CONCEPTS

38-1   Common Parasitic Infections

Pinworm is a helminth infection that is common everywhere, whereas most other helminth infections are predominantly found in countries or areas of the world that lack proper sanitary facilities. Malaria is rare in the United States but sometimes occurs in individuals who have traveled to or lived in areas where this disease is a health problem. The first antimalarial drug, quinine, is derived from the bark of the cinchona tree. Amebiasis is seen throughout the world but is less common in developed countries where sanitary facilities prevent the spread of the causative organism.

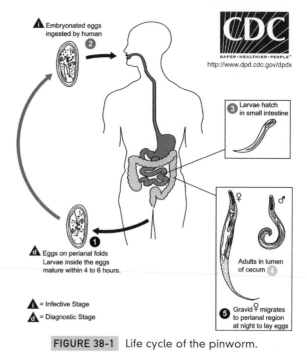

FIGURE 38-1   Life cycle of the pinworm.

Pyrantel

The activity of pyrantel (Antiminth) is probably caused by its ability to paralyze helminths. Paralysis causes the helminth to release its grip on the intestinal wall; it is then excreted in the feces. Pyrantel is used to treat roundworm and pinworm. Some patients receiving pyrantel may experience gastrointestinal side effects, such as nausea, vomiting, abdominal cramps, or diarrhea.

Contraindications, Precautions, and Interactions of Anthelmintic Drugs

Albendazole

- Albendazole is contraindicated in patients with known hypersensitivity.
- The drug has caused embryotoxic and teratogenic effects in experimental animals.
- Albendazole is used cautiously in patients with hepatic impairment and during lactation.
- The effects of albendazole are increased with dexamethasone and cimetidine.

Mebendazole

- Mebendazole is contraindicated in patients with known hypersensitivity.
- Mebendazole, like albendazole, has caused embryotoxic and teratogenic effects in experimental animals.
- Use of mebendazole with the hydantoins and carbamazepine may reduce plasma levels of mebendazole.

Ivermectin

- Ivermectin is contraindicated in patients with known hypersensitivity.
- Ivermectin may cause a Mazzotti reaction, which involves skin, systemic, and ophthalmic reactions likely due to an allergic and inflammatory response.

Praziquantel

- Praziquantel is contraindicated in patients with known hypersensitivity to the drug or any of the product ingredients and in patients with ocular cysticercosis. This drug should not be used in patients with a history of epilepsy or those with signs of potential central nervous system involvement.
- Praziquantel should not be coadministered with drugs that induce cytochrome P450, such as rifampin and phenytoin.
- Praziquantel dose may need to be decreased in patients who are also taking drugs that inhibit cytochrome P450, such as erythromycin and ketoconazole.
- Praziquantel should not be taken with grapefruit juice.

Pyrantel

- Pyrantel is contraindicated in patients with known hypersensitivity.
- Pyrantel is used with caution in individuals with liver dysfunction, malnutrition, or anemia.
- Pyrantel and piperazine are antagonists and should not be given together.

Patient Management Issues with Anthelmintic Drugs

The diagnosis of a helminth infection is made by examination of the stool for ova and all or part of the helminth. Several stool specimens may be necessary before the helminth is seen and identified. The patient history also may lead to a suspicion of a helminth infection, but some patients have no symptoms. When a pinworm infection is suspected, a specimen is taken from the anal area.

Patients with massive helminth infections may or may not be acutely ill. Acutely ill patients require hospitalization, but many individuals with helminth infections can be treated on an outpatient basis.

Gloves are worn when changing bed linens, emptying bedpans, or obtaining or handling stool specimens, and thorough handwashing is required after removing the gloves. Patients should wash their hands thoroughly after personal care and using a bedpan.

Each stool is inspected for passage of the helminth. If stool specimens are to be saved for laboratory examination, then the health care provider should provide procedures to be followed for saving the stool and transporting it to the laboratory. If the patient is acutely ill or has a massive infection, then vital signs are monitored every 4 hours, and fluid intake and output are measured. The patient is observed for adverse drug reactions, as well as severe episodes of diarrhea.

With mebendazole, the patient may chew, swallow whole, or mix the tablets with food. The patient should take this drug with foods high in fat to increase absorption. A complete blood count is obtained before therapy and periodically during therapy because mebendazole can cause leukopenia or thrombocytopenia.

Praziquantel should be taken during meals but not with grapefruit juice. The tablets should not be chewed. Patients should not drive a car or operate machinery on the day that they take praziquantel or the following day.

Patients can take pyrantel anytime without regard to meal or time of day. Patients may take the drug with milk or fruit juices.

Educating the Patient and Family about Anthelmintic Drugs

When an anthelmintic is prescribed on an outpatient basis, the patient or a family member is given complete instructions about household precautions to follow until the helminth is eliminated from the intestine. Following are key points about anthelmintic drugs that the patient and family members should know.

- Report any symptoms of infection (low-grade fever or sore throat) or thrombocytopenia (easy bruising or bleeding).
- Follow the dosage schedule exactly as printed on the prescription container. It is absolutely necessary to follow the directions for taking the drug to eliminate the helminth.
- Follow-up stool specimens will be necessary because this is the only way to determine the success of drug therapy.
- To prevent reinfection and the infection of others in the

household, change and launder your bed linens and undergarments daily, separately from those of other members of your family.

- Daily bathing (showering is best) is recommended. Disinfect toilet facilities daily, and disinfect the bathtub or shower stall immediately after bathing. Use the disinfectant recommended by your health care provider, or use a chlorine bleach solution. Scrub the surfaces thoroughly, and allow the disinfectant to remain in contact with the surfaces for several minutes.
- Wash your hands thoroughly after urinating or defecating and before preparing and eating food.
- Clean under your fingernails daily, and avoid putting your fingers in your mouth or biting your nails.

FACT CHECK

38-2   What are common examples of helminths?
38-3   Which anthelmintic drugs have caused embryotoxic and teratogenic effects in animals?

Antimalarial Drugs

Malaria is transmitted from person to person by a certain species of the *Anopheles* mosquito. The four different protozoans causing malaria are *Plasmodium falciparum*, *P. malariae*, *P. ovale*, and *P. vivax*. Drugs used to treat or prevent malaria are called antimalarial drugs. Three antimalarial drugs are discussed here: chloroquine, artemether/lumefantrine, and quinine sulfate. Other antimalarial drugs in use today are listed in the Summary Drug Table: Antimalarial Drugs.

Actions of Antimalarial Drugs

The plasmodium that causes malaria must enter the mosquito to develop, reproduce, and be transmitted. When the mosquito bites a person infected with malaria, it ingests the male and female forms (gametocytes) of the plasmodium. The gametocytes mate in the mosquito's stomach and ultimately form sporozoites (an animal reproductive cell) that make their way to the salivary glands of the mosquito. When the mosquito bites a noninfected person, the sporozoites enter the person's bloodstream and lodge in the liver and other tissues. The sporozoites

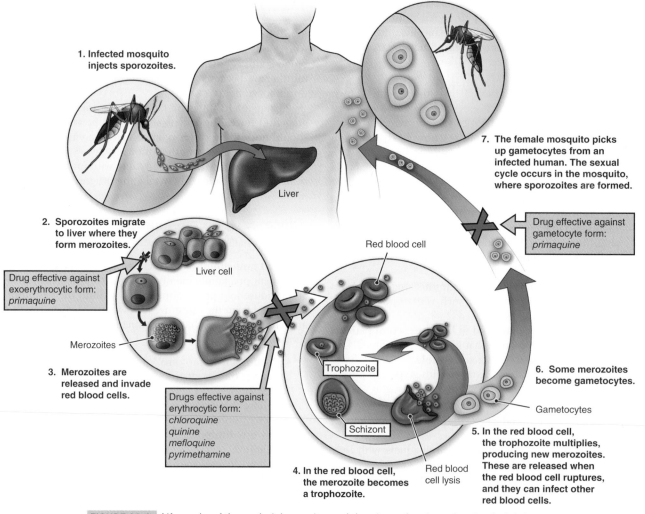

FIGURE 38-2   Life cycle of the malarial parasite and the sites of action of antimalarial drugs.

then undergo asexual cell division and reproduction and form merozoites. The merozoites then divide asexually and enter the red blood cells of the person, where they form the male and female forms of the plasmodium. The symptoms of malaria (shaking, chills, and fever) appear when the merozoites enter the individual's red blood cells.

Antimalarial drugs interfere with the life cycle of the plasmodium, primarily when it is present in red blood cells. Destruction at this stage of the plasmodium life cycle prevents the development of the male and female forms of the plasmodium. This in turn keeps the mosquito (when the mosquito bites an infected individual) from ingesting the male and female forms of the plasmodium, thus effectively ending the plasmodium life cycle (Fig. 38-2).

FACT CHECK

38-4 How do antimalarial drugs act?

Uses of Antimalarial Drugs

Two terms are used when discussing the uses of antimalarial drugs:

1. Suppression: the prevention of malaria
2. Treatment: the management of a malarial attack

Not all antimalarial drugs are effective in suppressing or treating all four of the plasmodium species that cause malaria. In addition, strains have developed that are resistant to some antimalarial drugs. The health care provider must select the antimalarial drug that reportedly is effective, at present, for the type of malaria the individual either has (for treatment) or could be exposed to (for prevention) in a specific area of the world.

Chloroquine (Aralen) is also used in the treatment of extraintestinal amebiasis (see following section on amebicides). Artemether/lumefantrine (Coartem) is used in the treatment of acute, uncomplicated malaria infections in geographic regions where resistance to chloroquine has been reported. Quinine also may be used for the prevention or treatment of nocturnal leg cramps. Quinine may be used in combination with doxycycline, tetracycline, or clindamycin (anti-infectives covered in Chapter 35) as well as alone.

Adverse Reactions of Antimalarial Drugs

Chloroquine

The adverse reactions of chloroquine and hydroxychloroquine include visual disturbances, headache, nausea, vomiting, anorexia, diarrhea, and abdominal cramps.

Artemether/Lumefantrine

The adverse reactions of artemether/lumefantrine in adults include headache, anorexia, dizziness, and asthenia. In children, the most common adverse reactions include pyrexia, cough, vomiting, and anorexia.

Quinine

The use of quinine can cause cinchonism at full therapeutic doses. Cinchonism is a group of symptoms associated with quinine, including tinnitus, dizziness, headache, gastroin-

testinal disturbances, and visual disturbances. These symptoms usually disappear when the dosage is reduced. Other adverse reactions include hematologic changes, vertigo, and skin rash.

Contraindications, Precautions, and Interactions of Antimalarial Drugs

Chloroquine

- Chloroquine is contraindicated in patients with known hypersensitivity.
- Chloroquine is used cautiously in patients with liver disease or bone marrow depression. The drug should be used with extreme caution in children.
- Because the effects of chloroquine during pregnancy are unknown, this drug is given only when clearly needed and the potential benefits outweigh potential hazards to the fetus.
- There is an increased risk of hepatotoxicity when chloroquine is taken with other hepatotoxic drugs.
- Foods that acidify the urine (cranberries, plums, prunes, meats, cheeses, eggs, fish, and grains) may increase excretion and decrease the effectiveness of chloroquine.

Artemether/Lumefantrine

- This drug is contraindicated in patients with known hypersensitivity to either of the ingredients of any of the inactive ingredients in the dosage form.
- Artemether/lumefantrine will prolong the QT interval and should be used with caution in any patients with an existing QT prolongation or those taking other drugs that also cause QT prolongation.
- This drug may decrease the effectiveness of oral contraceptives.
- Artemether/lumefantrine interacts with drugs that are metabolized by CYP2D6 and CYP3A4.
- Patients should not take this drug with grapefruit juice.

Quinine

- Quinine is contraindicated in patients with known hypersensitivity.
- The drug is also contraindicated in patients with myasthenia gravis (may cause respiratory distress and dysphagia).
- Quinine absorption is delayed when taken with antacids containing aluminum.
- Plasma digitalis levels may increase when digitalis preparations and quinine are given concurrently.
- Plasma levels of warfarin are increased when taken with quinine.

Patient Management Issues with Antimalarial Drugs

When an antimalarial drug such as chloroquine is used for prophylaxis (prevention), therapy should begin 2 weeks before exposure and continue for 6 to 8 weeks after the client leaves the area where malaria is prevalent. The patient taking chloroquine may experience a number of visual disturbances, such as disturbed color vision, blurred vision, night blindness, diminished visual fields, or optic atrophy.

Absorption of artemether/lumefantrine is enhanced when taken with food.

ALERT ℞

Chloroquine and Visual Disturbances
Any visual disturbance in patients taking chloroquine should be reported to the health care provider. Irreversible retinal damage has occurred in patients on long-term therapy with these drugs.

Educating the Patient and Family about Antimalarial Drugs

When an antimalarial drug is prescribed for the prevention (suppression) of malaria, the drug regimen is carefully reviewed with the patient. When the drug is to be taken once per week as a prophylactic measure, patients should select a day of the week that will best remind them to take the drug. The importance of taking the drug exactly as prescribed is emphasized because failure to take the drug on an exact schedule will not give protection against malaria.

The program of prevention is usually started 2 weeks before departure to an area where malaria is prevalent.

Following are key points about antimalarial drugs that the patient and family members should know.

Chloroquine

- Take this drug with food or milk. Avoid foods that acidify urine (cranberries, plums, prunes, meats, cheeses, eggs, fish, and grains).
- This drug may cause diarrhea, loss of appetite, nausea, stomach pain, or vomiting. Notify your health care provider if your symptoms become pronounced.
- Chloroquine may cause a yellow or brown discoloration to your urine; this is normal and will go away when the drug therapy is discontinued.
- Notify the health care provider if you experience any of the following:

  - Visual changes
  - Ringing in your ears
  - Difficulty in hearing
  - Fever
  - Sore throat
  - Unusual bleeding or bruising
  - Unusual color (blue–black) of the skin
  - Skin rash
  - Unusual muscle weakness

Artemether/lumefantrine

- Take this drug with food.
- Do not take this drug with grapefruit juice.
- Women who take oral contraceptives should use an alternative form of birth control while on artemether/lumefantrine and until they have had at least one menstrual cycle after the discontinuation of the drug.
- Patients should notify their health care provider if they have any symptoms of QT prolongation, such as heart palpitations or loss of consciousness.

Quinine

- Take this drug with food or immediately after a meal.
- Do not drive or perform other hazardous tasks requiring alertness if you experience blurred vision or dizziness.
- Do not chew the tablet or open the capsule because the drug is irritating to the stomach.
- If you experience itching, rash, fever, difficulty breathing, or vision problems, then stop taking the drug and notify your health care provider.

FACT CHECK

38-5 What is the difference between suppression and treatment of malaria?
38-6 What are the adverse reactions of quinine?

Amebicides

Amebicides (drugs that kill amebas) are used to treat amebiasis caused by the parasite *E. histolytica* (Fig. 38-3). An ameba is a one-celled organism found in soil and water. Examples of amebicides are listed in the Summary Drug Table: Amebicides.

Actions and Uses of Amebicides

The two types of amebiasis are intestinal and extraintestinal. In the intestinal form, the ameba is confined to the intestine. In the extraintestinal form, the ameba is found outside of the intestine, such as in the liver. The extraintestinal form of amebiasis is more difficult to treat.

Iodoquinol (Yodoxin) and metronidazole (Flagyl) are used to treat intestinal amebiasis. Metronidazole is also used to treat infections caused by susceptible microorganisms and is discussed in Chapter 39. Paromomycin is an aminoglycoside with amebicidal activity and is used to treat intestinal amebiasis. Chloroquine hydrochloride (Aralen) is used to treat extraintestinal amebiasis.

Adverse Reactions of Amebicides

Iodoquinol

Various types of skin eruptions, nausea, vomiting, fever, chills, abdominal cramps, vertigo, and diarrhea can occur with iodoquinol use.

Paromomycin

This drug has relatively few adverse reactions. The most common include nausea, vomiting, and diarrhea. More serious adverse reactions, although rare, are nephrotoxicity and ototoxicity.

Contraindications, Precautions, and Interactions of Amebicides

Iodoquinol

- Iodoquinol is contraindicated in patients with known hypersensitivity.

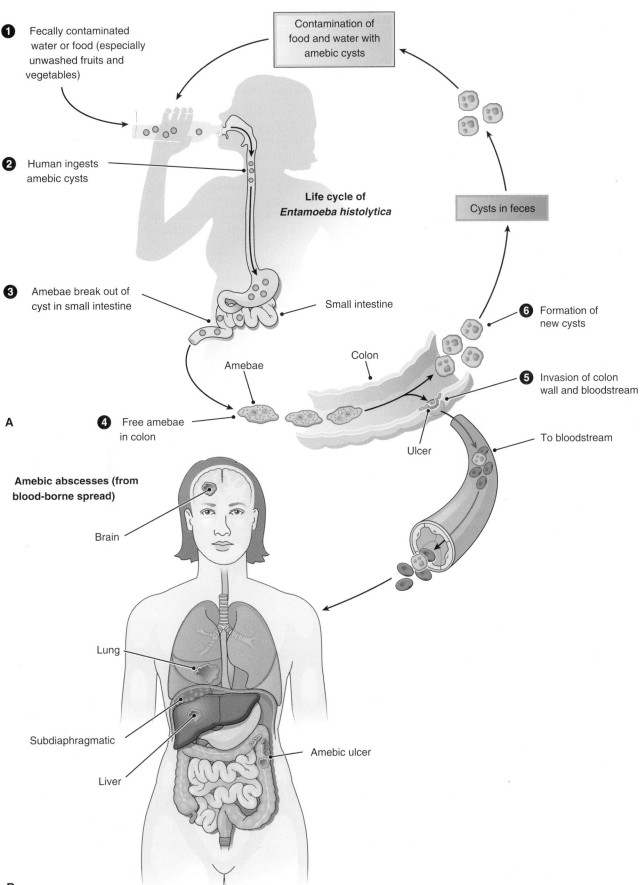

FIGURE 38-3 *Amebiasis.* The protozoan *Entamoeba histolytica* causes *amebiasis*. A. The life cycle of E. *histolytica*. B. Sites of infection.

- Iodoquinol is used with caution in patients with thyroid disease and during lactation.
- Iodoquinol may interfere with the results of thyroid function tests. This interference may last as long as 6 months after iodoquinol therapy is discontinued.

Paromomycin

- Paromomycin is contraindicated in patients with known hypersensitivity.
- Paromomycin is used with caution in patients with bowel disease.
- High doses and prolonged therapy are avoided because the drug may be absorbed in large amounts by patients with bowel disease, causing ototoxicity and kidney impairment.

Patient Management Issues with Amebicides

Diagnosis of amebiasis is made by examining the stool and considering the patient's symptoms. Once the patient has received a diagnosis of amebiasis, local health department regulations often require investigation into the source of infection. A history of foreign travel is necessary. If the patient has not traveled to a foreign country, then further investigation of the patient's lifestyle, such as local travel, use of restaurants, and the local water supply (especially well water) may be necessary to identify the source of the infection. In addition, it is common practice to test immediate family members for amebiasis.

If the patient is acutely ill or has vomiting and diarrhea, then fluid intake and output are measured, and the patient is closely monitored for signs of dehydration. If dehydration is apparent, then the health care provider should be notified.

Patients with amebiasis may or may not be acutely ill. Isolation is usually not necessary, but hospital policy may require isolation procedures. Stool precautions are usually necessary. Thorough handwashing is required after all patient care and handling of stool specimens.

Educating the Patient and Family about Amebicides

The importance of completing the full course of treatment must be stressed. Following are key points about amebicides that the patient and family members should know.

- Follow directions to take the drug exactly as prescribed. Complete the full course of therapy to eradicate the ameba. Failure to complete treatment may result in a return of the infection.
- Follow measures to control the spread of infection. Wash your hands immediately before eating or preparing food and after defecation.
- Food handlers should not resume work until after completing the full course of treatment and stools do not contain the ameba.

Iodoquinol

- Notify your health care provider if you experience nausea, vomiting, or other gastrointestinal distress that becomes severe.

Paromomycin

- Take this drug three times per day with meals.
- Report any ringing in your ears, dizziness, severe gastrointestinal upset, decrease in urinary output, or other urinary difficulties.

FACT CHECK

38-7 Which amebicides are used to treat intestinal amebiasis?

38-8 Which amebicides are used to treat extraintestinal amebiasis?

Chapter Review

KEY POINTS

- Antiparasitic drugs are used to treat parasites, organisms that live in or on another organism (the host) without contributing to the survival or well-being of the host.
- Invasion of the body by helminths, malaria, and amebiasis are problems caused by parasites.
- Anthelmintics are used to kill parasites. Adverse reactions are mild when the drug is used in the recommended dosage. Contraindications, precautions, and interactions are drug specific.
- Antimalarial drugs interfere with the life cycle of the plasmodium and are used for both suppression and treatment.
- Amebicides are used to treat amebiasis.

CRITICAL THINKING CASE STUDY

Malaria Prevention

Mr. Barnes recently traveled to Africa. Upon return, he began exhibiting flu-like symptoms. He is in your clinic today and has been diagnosed with malaria.

The region he visited has a documented resistance to chloroquine.

1. Which of the following would be the drug of choice?
   a. artemether/lumefantrine
   b. mefloquine
   c. primaquine
   d. quinine

2. The health care provider has prescribed Coartem. Mr. Barnes should be warned about all of the following adverse effects EXCEPT
   a. dizziness
   b. asthenia
   c. fatigue
   d. convulsions

3. The health care provider told Mr. Barnes that he will take the medication over 3 days. Mr. Barnes cannot remember the specific information. What should you tell him?

Review Questions

MULTIPLE CHOICE

1. A patient asks how antimalarial drugs prevent or treat malaria. The correct response is that this group of drugs:
   a. kills the mosquito that carries the protozoa
   b. interferes with the life cycle of the protozoa causing malaria
   c. ruptures the red blood cells that contain merozoites
   d. increases the body's natural immune response to the protozoa

2. All of the following drugs are anthelmintic drugs EXCEPT
   a. pyrantel
   b. primaquine
   c. praziquantel
   d. albendazole

3. A patient taking chloroquine for the prevention of malaria should be instructed to
   a. take the drug on an empty stomach
   b. protect the skin from the sun because the drug can cause a severe sunburn
   c. begin therapy 2 weeks before possible exposure
   d. take the drug with a citrus drink to enhance absorption

4. Amebiasis may be intestinal or extraintestinal. Which drug most likely would be prescribed for treatment of a patient experiencing intestinal amebiasis?
   a. quinine
   b. chloroquine phosphate
   c. propranolol
   d. iodoquinol

MATCHING

Match the drug on the left with the correct drug category on the right. Drug categories may be used more than once.

_____ 5. mefloquine   a. anthelmintic
_____ 6. pyrantel   b. antimalarial
_____ 7. paromomycin   c. amebicide
_____ 8. mebendazole
_____ 9. iodoquinol
_____ 10. primaquine

Match the drug on the left with the correct brand name on the right.

_____ 11. albendazole   a. Daraprim
_____ 12. ivermectin   b. Aralen
_____ 13. praziquantel   c. Albenza
_____ 14. iodoquinol   d. Plaquenil
_____ 15. chloroquine phosphate   e. Coartem
_____ 16. hydroxychloroquine   f. Stromectol
_____ 17. artemether/lumefantrine g. Yodoxin
_____ 18. pyrimethamine   h. Biltricide

TRUE OR FALSE

_____ 19. Paromomycin is an aminoglycoside with amebicidal activity that is used to treat intestinal amebiasis.
_____ 20. Long-term therapy for malaria with chloroquine may result in irreversible damage to the retina.
_____ 21. Pinworm is a parasitic infection caused by the ameba E. histolytica.
_____ 22. Chloroquine is a drug that is used to prevent malaria.

FILL IN THE BLANKS

23. Patients taking _____ should be instructed to avoid _____, which may cause a disulfiram-like reaction.
24. Abnormal liver function tests may occur in patients taking the anthelmintic drugs ivermectin, mebendazole, and _____.
25. _____ is used to treat extraintestinal amebiasis as well as malaria.
26. Follow-up stool specimens are necessary for patients taking _____ drugs.

SHORT ANSWERS

27. What are three parasitic infections that are worldwide health problems?
28. Name the two types of amebiasis. How do they differ?
29. When is chloroquine therapy initiated when the drug is used for prevention of malaria?
30. What is the probable action of the anthelmintic drug pyrantel?

Web Activities

1. Go to the Center for Disease Control and Prevention's Web site (http://www.cdc.gov) and conduct a search for "malaria." Find the FAQs for malaria.
   a. How is malaria transmitted?
   b. Who is most at risk of getting very sick and dying from malaria?

2. Return to the CDC Web site home page and conduct a search for "pinworms." Find the FAQs for pinworms.
   a. Who is at risk for pinworm infection?
   b. How is pinworm infection spread?

SUMMARY DRUG TABLE Anthelmintic Drugs
(left, generic; right, trade)

Comprehensive Summary Drug Tables, including uses, adverses effects, dosages, and pregnancy classifications, are provided on the companion website, http://thePoint.lww.com/PharmacologyHP2e

albendazole *al-ben'-dah-zohl*	Albenza
mebendazole *me-ben'-dah-zole*	*generic*
ivermectin *eye-ver-mek'-tin*	Stromectol
praziquantel *pray-zi-kwon'-tel*	Biltricide
pyrantel pamoate *pi-ran'-tel*	Pin-X (OTC), Reese Pinworm Medicine (OTC)

SUMMARY DRUG TABLE Amebicides
(left, generic; right, trade)

Comprehensive Summary Drug Tables, including uses, adverses effects, dosages, and pregnancy classifications, are provided on the companion website, http://thePoint.lww.com/PharmacologyHP2e

chloroquine phosphate *klor'-oh-kwin*	Aralen, *generic*
iodoquinol *eye-oh-doe-kwin'-ole*	Yodoxin
metronidazole *me-troe-ni'-da-zole*	Oral: Flagyl, *generic* IV: Metro, *generic*
paromomycin *par-oh-moe-mye'-sin*	*generic*

SUMMARY DRUG TABLE Antimalarial Drugs
(left, generic; right, trade)

Comprehensive Summary Drug Tables, including uses, adverses effects, dosages, and pregnancy classifications, are provided on the companion website, http://thePoint.lww.com/PharmacologyHP2e

artemether/lumefantrine *ar-tem'-e-ther/loo-me-fan'-treen*	Coartem
atovaquone/proguanil HCl *uh-toe'-vuh-kwone*	Malarone, Malarone Pediatric
chloroquine phosphate *klor'-oh-kwin*	Aralen, *generic*
hydroxychloroquine sulfate *hye-drox-ee-klor'-oh-kwin*	Plaquenil, *generic*
mefloquine HCl *me'-flow-kwin*	*generic*
primaquine phosphate *prim'-a-kween*	*generic*
pyrimethamine *peer-i-meth'-a-mine*	Daraprim
quinine sulfate *kwi'-nine*	Qualaquin

39

Miscellaneous Anti-Infectives

CHAPTER OBJECTIVES

On completion of this chapter, students will be able to:

1. Define the chapter's key terms.

2. Describe the actions and uses of the miscellaneous anti-infectives.

3. Identify common adverse reactions of the miscellaneous anti-infectives.

4. Describe the most common contraindications, precautions, and drug interactions associated with the miscellaneous anti-infectives.

5. Discuss the drug, route of administration, and signs and symptoms associated with "red man syndrome."

6. Discuss important points to keep in mind when educating the patient or family members about the use of miscellaneous anti-infectives.

KEY TERMS

anaerobic—able to live without oxygen
nosocomial pneumonia—hospital-acquired pneumonia
trichomonas—a parasitic protozoan

CHAPTER OVERVIEW

Drug classes covered in this chapter are:

- Miscellaneous anti-infectives

Drugs by classification are listed on page 426.

thePOINT RESOURCES

- Comprehensive Summary Drug Tables

- Lippincott's Interactive Tutorials: Drugs Used to Treat Infections

- Interactive Practice and Review

- Monographs of Most Commonly Prescribed Drugs

The anti-infectives discussed in this chapter are singular drugs; that is, they are not related to each other and do not belong to any one of the drug groups discussed in previous chapters in this unit. Some of these drugs are used only for the treatment of one type of infection, whereas others may be limited to the treatment of serious infections not treatable by other anti-infectives (see Summary Drug Table: Miscellaneous Anti-Infectives).

Miscellaneous Anti-Infectives

The miscellaneous anti-infectives include chloramphenicol, linezolid, meropenem, metronidazole, pentamidine isethionate, and vancomycin.

Actions and Uses of Miscellaneous Anti-Infectives

Chloramphenicol

Chloramphenicol interferes with or inhibits protein synthesis, a process necessary for the growth and multiplication of microorganisms. This is a potentially dangerous drug (see below), and therefore its use is limited to serious infections when less potentially dangerous drugs are ineffective or contraindicated.

Linezolid

Linezolid (Zyvox) is the first of a new classification, an oxazolidinone, that acts by binding to a site on a specific ribosomal RNA and preventing the formation of a component necessary for the bacteria to replicate. It is both bacteriostatic (to enterococci and staphylococci) and bacteriocidal (against streptococci). The drug is used in the treatment of vancomycin-resistant enterococcus, **nosocomial pneumonia** (hospital-acquired) and community-acquired pneumonia, and skin and skin structure infections, including those caused by methicillin-resistant *Staphylococcus aureus*.

Meropenem

Meropenem (Merrem) inhibits synthesis of the bacterial cell wall and causes the death of susceptible cells. This drug is used for intra-abdominal infections caused by *Pseudomonas aeruginosa*, *Escherichia coli*, *Klebsiella pneumoniae*, and other susceptible organisms. Meropenem also is effective against bacterial meningitis caused by *Neisseria meningitidis*, *Streptococcus pneumoniae*, and *Haemophilus influenzae*. It is also used to treat complicated skin and skin structure infections.

Metronidazole

The action of metronidazole (Flagyl) is not well understood, but it is thought to disrupt DNA and protein synthesis in susceptible organisms. This drug may be used in the treatment of serious infections, such as intra-abdominal, bone, soft tissue, lower respiratory, gynecologic, and central nervous system infections caused by susceptible **anaerobic** (able to live without oxygen) microorganisms. It is also used for amebiasis and **trichomonas**. It is available in an extended-release tablet formulation that is used for bacterial vaginosis.

Pentamidine Isethionate

Pentamidine isethionate (Pentam, the parenteral form; Nebu-Pent, the aerosol form) is used in the treatment (parenteral form) or prevention (aerosol form) of *Pneumocystis jiroveci*

(*formerly known as Pneumocystis carinii*) pneumonia, which occurs in those with AIDS. The action of this drug is not fully understood.

Vancomycin

Vancomycin (Vancocin) acts against susceptible gram-positive bacteria by inhibiting bacterial cell wall synthesis and increasing cell wall permeability. This drug is used in the treatment of serious gram-positive infections that do not respond to treatment with other anti-infectives. It also may be used in treating anti-infective–associated pseudomembranous colitis caused by *Clostridium difficile*.

FACT CHECK

39-1   Which drug is used to treat nosocomial and community-acquired pneumonia?

39-2   How does vancomycin act against gram-positive bacteria?

Adverse Reactions of Miscellaneous Anti-Infectives

Chloramphenicol

Serious and sometimes fatal blood dyscrasias (a pathologic disorder of cellular elements of blood) are the chief adverse reaction seen with the use of chloramphenicol. In addition, superinfection, hypersensitivity reactions, nausea, vomiting, and headache may occur. Patients receiving oral chloramphenicol are often hospitalized so that frequent blood studies can be performed during treatment with this drug.

Linezolid

The most common adverse reactions include nausea, vomiting, diarrhea, headache, and insomnia. The drug may also cause fatigue, depression, nervousness, and photosensitivity. Pseudomembranous colitis and thrombocytopenia are the more serious adverse reactions caused by linezolid.

Meropenem

The most common adverse reactions of meropenem include headache, nausea, vomiting, diarrhea, anorexia, abdominal pain, generalized pain, flatulence, anemia, rash, and superinfections. This drug also can cause an abscess or phlebitis at the injection site.

Metronidazole

The most common adverse reactions are related to the gastrointestinal tract and may include nausea, anorexia, and occasionally vomiting and diarrhea. The most serious adverse reactions involve the central nervous system and include seizures and numbness of the extremities. Hypersensitivity reactions also may be seen. Thrombophlebitis may occur with intravenous use of the drug.

Pentamidine Isethionate

More than half of the patients receiving this drug by the parenteral route experience some adverse reaction. Severe and sometimes life-threatening reactions include leukopenia (low white blood cell count), hypoglycemia (low blood sugar), thrombocytopenia (low platelet count), and hypotension (low blood pressure). Moderate or less severe reactions include changes in some laboratory tests, such as the serum creatinine and liver function tests. Other adverse reactions include anxiety, headache, hypotension, nausea, and anorexia. Aerosol use may result in fatigue, a metallic taste in the mouth, shortness of breath, and anorexia.

Vancomycin

Nephrotoxicity (damage to the kidneys) and ototoxicity (damage to the organs of hearing) may occur with this drug. Additional adverse reactions include diarrhea, pseudomembranous colitis, nausea, chills, fever, urticaria, sudden fall in blood pressure with parenteral use (Key Concepts 39-1), and skin rashes.

FACT CHECK

39-3 What is the chief adverse reaction of chloramphenicol?

39-4 Which drug can cause an abscess or phlebitis at the injection site?

Contraindications, Precautions, and Interactions of Miscellaneous Anti-Infectives

Chloramphenicol

- Chloramphenicol is contraindicated in patients with known hypersensitivity.
- This drug is used cautiously in patients with severe liver or kidney disease, in geriatric patients, in individuals with glucose-6-phosphate dehydrogenase deficiency, and during lactation.
- The effects of oral hypoglycemic drugs, oral anticoagulants, and phenytoin may be increased when taken with chloramphenicol.
- Phenobarbital or rifampin may decrease chloramphenicol blood levels.

Linezolid

- The drug is contraindicated in those allergic to it, in lactation, and in those with phenylketonuria (oral form only).
- Linezolid is used cautiously in patients with bone marrow depression, hepatic dysfunction, renal impairment, hypertension, or hyperthyroidism.

KEY CONCEPTS

39-1 Vancomycin and "Red Man Syndrome"

When vancomycin is given intravenously, the infusion rate and the patient's blood pressure are closely monitored. Any decreases in blood pressure or reports of throbbing neck or back pain are reported. These symptoms could indicate a severe adverse reaction referred to as "red man syndrome." Symptoms of this syndrome include a sudden and profound fall in blood pressure, fever, chills, paresthesias, and erythema (redness) of the neck and back.

CONSIDERATIONS | Infants & Children

LIFESPAN

Chloramphenicol

Newborns are at increased risk for experiencing adverse reactions to chloramphenicol because of their inability to metabolize and excrete this drug.

- When linezolid is used with antiplatelet drugs such as aspirin or nonsteroidal anti-inflammatory drugs, there is an increased risk of bleeding and thrombocytopenia.
- When administered with the monoamine oxidase inhibitors (see Chapter 7), the effects of the monoamine oxidase inhibitors are decreased.
- There is a risk of severe hypertension if linezolid is combined with large amounts of food containing tyramine (e.g., aged cheese, caffeinated beverages, yogurt, chocolate, red wine, beer, pepperoni).

Meropenem

- Meropenem is contraindicated in patients who are allergic to cephalosporins and penicillins and in patients with renal failure.
- This drug is not recommended in children younger than 3 months or for women during lactation.
- Meropenem is used cautiously in patients with central nervous system disorders, seizure disorders, or kidney or liver failure.
- When taken with probenecid, the excretion of meropenem is inhibited.

Metronidazole

- This drug is contraindicated in patients with known hypersensitivity and during the first trimester of pregnancy.
- This drug is used cautiously in patients with blood dyscrasias, seizure disorders, or liver dysfunction.
- Safety in children (other than orally for amebiasis) has not been established.
- The metabolism of metronidazole may decrease when used with cimetidine.
- When used with phenobarbital, the effectiveness of metronidazole may decrease.
- When metronidazole is taken with warfarin, the effectiveness of the warfarin is increased.
- Metronidazole should not be combined with alcohol. The combination will result in a disulfiram-like reaction.

Pentamidine Isethionate

- This drug is contraindicated in individuals with hypersensitivity.
- Pentamidine isethionate is used cautiously in patients with hypertension, hypotension, hyperglycemia, renal impairment, diabetes mellitus, liver impairment, bone marrow depression, or lactation.

- An additive nephrotoxicity develops when pentamidine isethionate is used with other nephrotoxic drugs (e.g., aminoglycosides, vancomycin, or amphotericin B).
- An additive bone marrow depression occurs when the drug is used with antineoplastic drugs or when the patient has received radiation therapy recently.

Vancomycin

- This drug is contraindicated in patients with known hypersensitivity.
- Vancomycin is used cautiously in patients with renal or hearing impairment and during lactation.
- When used with other ototoxic and nephrotoxic drugs, additive effects may occur.

FACT CHECK

39-5   Which anti-infective should not be combined with alcohol? Why?

Patient Management Issues with Miscellaneous Anti-Infectives

Before beginning use of these drugs, the patient's vital signs are taken. A thorough allergy history is taken, especially a history of drug allergies. When culture and sensitivity tests are ordered, these procedures must be performed before the first dose of the drug is given. Other laboratory tests such as renal and hepatic function tests, complete blood count, and urinalysis also may be ordered before and during drug therapy for early detection of toxic reactions.

The patient is monitored at frequent intervals, especially during the first 48 hours of therapy. Any adverse reaction should be reported to the health care provider before the next dose of the drug is due.

Chloramphenicol

The oral drug is given when the patient's stomach is empty, 1 hour before or 2 hours after meals. If gastrointestinal distress occurs, then it is acceptable to give the drug with food.

Linezolid

The drug is given orally or intravenously. When the drug is taken orally, it is taken every 12 hours and may be taken with or without food. If nausea develops, then the drug may be taken with food. Foods high in tyramine (see Chapter XX)

are avoided because of the risk of hypertension. The patient's platelet count must be monitored regularly, particularly if the drug is used for longer than 2 weeks.

Meropenem

This drug is used only by the intravenous route.

Metronidazole

The oral form is given with meals to avoid gastrointestinal upset. The patient is informed that an unpleasant metallic taste may be noted. The patient should be advised to avoid alcoholic beverages during and for at least 1 day after treatment. When metronidazole is mixed with alcohol, the patient may experience a disulfiram-like reaction, including flushing, nausea, vomiting, headache, and abdominal cramping.

Patients being treated for gynecologic infections, such as trichomoniasis, should be told that sexual contact with infected partners may lead to reinfection, so sexual partners must be treated concurrently.

Pentamidine Isethionate

This drug may be given by aerosol, and the nebulizer should be explained or demonstrated to the patient. Blood pressure is monitored frequently during use because sudden, severe hypotension may occur. Because hypotension can occur after a single dose, the patient should be lying down when the drug is given. The patient is monitored for signs of hypoglycemia (weakness, diaphoresis, cool skin, shakiness) and hyperglycemia (flushed dry skin, fruity breath odor, increased thirst, and increased urination).

Vancomycin

Vancomycin can be taken orally or by intermittent intravenous infusion.

FACT CHECK

39-6   What information should patients receiving metronidazole for gynecologic infections be given?

Educating the Patient and Family about Miscellaneous Anti-Infectives

When pentamidine is prescribed for aerosol use at home, the use of the special nebulizer is explained, as well as directions for cleaning and maintaining the nebulizer equipment.

ALERT Rx

Chloramphenicol and Blood Dyscrasias
Blood dyscrasias may occur with the use of chloramphenicol during either short- or long-term therapy. Patients are observed closely for signs and symptoms that may indicate a blood dyscrasia: fever, sore throat, sores in the mouth, easy bruising or bleeding (even several weeks after the drug regimen is completed), and extreme fatigue.

ALERT Rx

Intravenous Use of Vancomycin
Patient symptoms of difficulty hearing or tinnitus (ringing in the ears) should be reported to the health care provider before the next dose is due. In addition, fluid intake and output are monitored, and any decrease in urinary output is reported.

When metronidazole is prescribed, the patient is advised to avoid the use of alcoholic beverages because a severe reaction may occur.

Following are key points about miscellaneous anti-infective drugs that the patient and family members should know.

- Take the drug at the prescribed time intervals. These time intervals are important because a certain amount of the drug must be in your body at all times for the infection to be controlled.
- Take the drug with food or on an empty stomach as directed on the prescription container.
- Do not increase or skip a dose unless advised to do so by your health care provider.
- Complete the entire course of treatment. Do not stop the drug, except on the advice of your health care provider, before the course of treatment is complete even if your symptoms have improved or have disappeared. Failure to complete the prescribed course of treatment may result in a return of the infection.
- Notify your health care provider if your symptoms of the infection become worse or do not improve after approximately 5 to 7 days.
- Contact your health care provider as soon as possible if you experience a rash, fever, sore throat, diarrhea, chills, extreme fatigue, easy bruising, ringing in the ears, difficulty hearing, or other problems.
- Do not drink alcoholic beverages unless approved by your health care provider.

Chapter Review

KEY POINTS

- Miscellaneous anti-infectives include chloramphenicol, linezolid, meropenem, metronidazole, pentamidine isethionate, and vancomycin.
- Some of these drugs are used only for the treatment of one type of infection, whereas others may be limited to the treatment of serious infections not treatable by other anti-infectives.
- Headache, nausea, and vomiting are common shared adverse reactions to miscellaneous anti-infectives.
- A severe adverse reaction called "red man syndrome" may occur with intravenous use of vancomycin. Symptoms include a sudden drop in blood pressure, fever, chills, paresthesias, and erythema (redness) of the neck and back.
- All of the miscellaneous anti-infectives are contraindicated in patients with known hypersensitivity.

CRITICAL THINKING CASE STUDY
Serious Unresolved Infection

Mr. Jones has an infection that has not responded to treatment with other anti-infective drugs. His physician has decided to prescribe vancomycin.

1. How is vancomycin administered?
   a. Oral
   b. IM
   c. IV
   d. a and c
2. Which of the following toxicities are associated with vancomycin therapy?
   a. Ototoxicity
   b. Neurotoxicity
   c. Nephrotoxicity
   d. a and c
3. Mr. Jones has started vancomycin therapy. You have been monitoring his blood pressure and notice that it has decreased. He is also complaining of chills and his neck is red. What is Mr. Jones experiencing? Is this a normal adverse reaction with vancomycin?

Review Questions

MULTIPLE CHOICE

1. The oral form of linezolid is contraindicated in patients with
   a. bone marrow depression
   b. hypoglycemia
   c. phenylketonuria
   d. food allergies
2. What must occur before treatment with any of the miscellaneous anti-infectives is started?
   a. Vital signs and an allergy history are taken.
   b. A history of surgical treatments is taken.
   c. Height and weight are measured.
   d. None of the above.
3. Which of the following drugs is used to treat intra-abdominal and dermatologic infections?
   a. pentamidine isethionate
   b. meropenem
   c. linezolid
   d. all of the above
4. Which of the following drugs is available in both parenteral and aerosol forms?
   a. linezolid
   b. vancomycin
   c. pentamidine
   d. metronidazole

MATCHING

_____ 5. linezolid   a. Pentam
_____ 6. meropenem   b. Vancocin
_____ 7. metronidazole   c. Merrem
_____ 8. pentamidine   d. Flagyl
_____ 9. vancomycin   e. Zyvox

TRUE OR FALSE

_____ 10. Vancomycin may be administered orally or intravenously.

_____ 11. All of the miscellaneous anti-infectives are contraindicated in patients with known hypersensitivity.

_____ 12. A patient who has recently received radiation therapy may experience additive bone marrow depression when given chloramphenicol.

_____ 13. An anaerobic microorganism is one that can live without oxygen.

FILL IN THE BLANKS

14. Patients taking _____ may experience thrombophlebitis.

15. Because blood dyscrasias may occur with administration of_____, this drug's use is limited to serious infections that are not treatable by other anti-infectives.

16. Foods that contain high amounts of _____ are avoided with linezolid use because of the increased risk of severe _____.

SHORT ANSWERS

17. Why should patients taking metronidazole avoid alcohol for at least a day after treatment?

18. "Red man" syndrome may occur with IV use of vancomycin. What are the symptoms of this syndrome?

19. Why should patients be lying down when given pentamidine isethionate?

Web Activities

1. Go to the Mayo Clinic Web site (www.mayoclinic.com) and conduct a search for "vancomycin-resistant enterococci" or VRE. What is VRE? What type of infections does VRE cause? How is VRE spread? How can you prevent the spread of VRE?

2. Go to the Centers for Disease Control and Prevention Web site (www.cdc.gov) and conduct a search on "MRSA." What is methicillin-resistant _Staphylococcus aureus_? How can it be prevented? How is it treated?

SUMMARY DRUG TABLE Miscellaneous Anti-Infectives (left, generic; right, trade)

Comprehensive Summary Drug Tables, including uses, adverses effects, dosages, and pregnancy classifications, are provided on the companion website, http://thePoint.lww.com/PharmacologyHP2e

chloramphenicol _klor-am-fen'-i-kole_	Chloramphenicol sodium succinate
linezolid _lah-nez'-oh-lid_	Zyvox
meropenem _meh-row-pen'-em_	Merrem, _generic_
metronidazole _me-troe-nid'-uh- zole_	Oral: Flagyl, _generic_ IV: Metro, _generic_ Topical: MetroCream, Metrogel, MetroLotion, Noritate, Vitazol, _generic_ Vaginal: MetroGel, Vandazole, _generic_
pentamidine isethionate _pen-tam'-ih-deen ice- uh-thigh'-uh-nate_	NebuPent (inhalation), Pentam (injection)
vancomycin HCl _van-koe-mye'-cin_	Vancocin, _generic_

40

Immunologic Agents

CHAPTER OBJECTIVES

On completion of this chapter, students will be able to:

1. Define the chapter's key terms.
2. Compare and contrast cell-mediated and humoral immunity.
3. Discuss active immunity and passive immunity.
4. Explain the difference between a toxin and a toxoid.
5. Describe the general drug actions, uses, adverse reactions, contraindications, precautions, and interactions of immunologic agents.
6. Discuss important points to keep in mind when educating the patient or family members about the use of immunologic agents.

KEY TERMS

active immunity—the reaction of the body when exposed to certain infectious microorganisms (antigens) of forming antibodies to the invading microorganism

antibody—a globulin (protein) produced by the B lymphocytes as a defense against an antigen

antigen—a substance, usually a protein, that stimulates the body to produce antibodies

antigen–antibody response—the reaction of specific circulating antibodies to a specific antigen

antivenin—an antitoxin specific for an animal or insect venom

attenuated—weakened, as in the antigen strain used for vaccine development

booster—the administration of an additional dose of the vaccine to "boost" the production of antibodies to a level that will maintain the desired immunity

CHAPTER OVERVIEW

Drug classes covered in this chapter are:

• Immunologic agents

Drugs by classification are listed on page 436.

thePOINT RESOURCES

• Comprehensive Summary Drug Tables

• Animations: Immune Response; Wound Healing; Acute Inflammation

• Interactive Practice and Review

• Monographs of Most Commonly Prescribed Drugs

cell-mediated immunity—the process of T lymphocytes and macrophages (large cells that surround, engulf, and digest microorganisms and cellular debris) working together to destroy an antigen

globulin—proteins present in blood serum or plasma that contain antibodies

humoral immunity—based on the antigen–antibody response, special lymphocytes (white blood cells) produce circulating antibodies to act against a foreign substance

immune globulin—solutions obtained from human blood containing antibodies that have been formed by the body to specific antigens

immunity—the ability of the body to identify and resist microorganisms that are potentially harmful

immunization—a form of artificial active immunity and an important method of controlling some infectious diseases that can cause serious and sometimes fatal consequences

passive immunity—a type of immunity occurring from the administration of ready-made antibodies from another individual or animal

toxin—a poisonous substance produced by some bacteria

toxoid—a toxin that is weakened but still capable of stimulating the formation of antitoxins

vaccine—artificial active immunity created with killed or weakened antigens for the purpose of creating resistance to disease

mmunity is the ability of the body to identify and resist microorganisms that are potentially harmful. This ability enables the body to fight or prevent infectious disease and inhibit tissue and organ damage. The immune system is not confined to any one part of the body. Immune stem cells, formed in the bone marrow, may remain in the bone marrow until maturation or migrate to different body sites for maturation. After maturation, most immune cells circulate in the body and exert specific effects. The immune system has two distinct, but overlapping, mechanisms with which to fight invading organisms:

- Cell-mediated defenses (cellular immunity)
- Antibody-mediated defenses (humoral immunity)

Cell-Mediated Immunity

Cell-mediated immunity is the result of the activity of many leukocyte actions, reactions, and interactions that range from simple to complex. This type of immunity depends on the actions of the T lymphocytes, which are responsible for a delayed type of immune response (Fig. 40-1). The T lymphocyte becomes sensitized by its first contact with a specific antigen. Subsequent exposure to an antigen stimulates multiple reactions aimed at destroying or inactivating the offending antigen. T lymphocytes and macrophages (large cells that surround, engulf, and digest microorganisms and cellular debris) work together in cell-mediated immunity to destroy the antigen. T lymphocytes attack the antigens directly, rather than produce antibodies (as is performed in humoral immunity). Cellular reactions may also occur without macrophages. Several T lymphocytes (T cells) are involved in cell-mediated immunity:

- Helper T4 cells: function within the bloodstream identifying and destroying antigens
- Helper T1 cells: increase B-lymphocyte antibody production
- Helper T2 cells: increase activity of cytotoxic (killer) T cells, which attack the cell directly by altering the cell membrane and causing cell lysis (destruction)
- Suppressor T cells: suppress the immune response

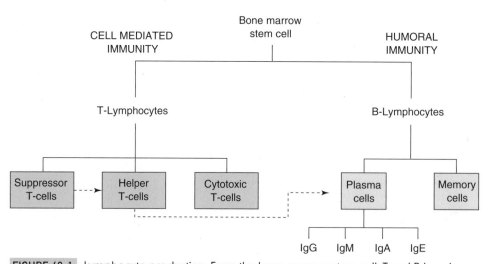

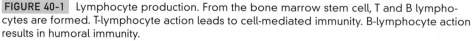

FIGURE 40-1 Lymphocyte production. From the bone marrow stem cell, T and B lymphocytes are formed. T-lymphocyte action leads to cell-mediated immunity. B-lymphocyte action results in humoral immunity.

- Memory T lymphocytes: recognize previous contact with antigens and activate an immune response

T lymphocytes defend against viral infections, fungal infections, and some bacterial infections. If cell-mediated immunity is lost, as in the case of acquired immunodeficiency syndrome, then the body is unable to protect itself against many viral, bacterial, and fungal infections.

Humoral Immunity

In **humoral immunity** special lymphocytes (white blood cells), called B lymphocytes, produce circulating antibodies to act against a foreign substance (see Fig. 40-1). This type of immunity is based on the antigen–antibody response. An **antigen** is a substance, usually a protein, that stimulates the body to produce antibodies. An **antibody** is a globulin (protein) produced by the B lymphocytes as a defense against an antigen. Humoral immunity protects the body against bacterial and viral infections.

Specific antibodies are formed for a specific antigen; for example, chickenpox antibodies are formed when the person is exposed to the chickenpox virus (the antigen). This is called an **antigen–antibody response**. Once manufactured, antibodies circulate in the bloodstream, sometimes for only a short time and at other times for the life of the person. When an antigen enters the body, specific antibodies neutralize the specific invading antigen; this is called immunity (Fig. 40-2). Therefore, the individual with specific circulating antibodies is immune (or has immunity) to a specific antigen. Immunity is the resistance that an individual has against disease.

Cell-mediated immunity and humoral immunity are interdependent. Cell-mediated immunity influences the function of the B lymphocytes, and humoral immunity influences the function of the T lymphocytes.

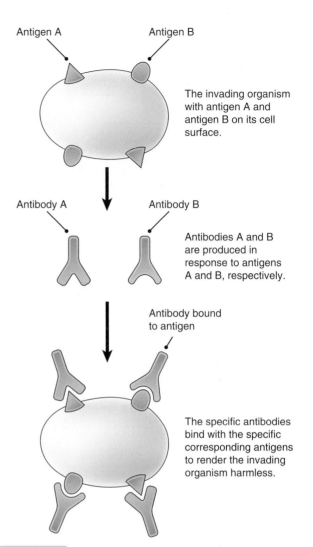

FIGURE 40-2 Antibodies are produced by cells of the immune system to bind with specific antigens.

FACT CHECK

40-1 What is the antigen–antibody response?

Active Immunity and Passive Immunity

Active immunity and passive immunity involve the use of agents that stimulate antibody formation (active immunity) or the injection of ready-made antibodies found in the serum of immune individuals or animals (passive immunity).

Active Immunity

When a person is exposed to certain infectious microorganisms (antigens), the body begins to form antibodies (or build an immunity) to the invading microorganism. This is called **active immunity**. The two types of active immunity are naturally acquired active immunity and artificially acquired active immunity. The Summary Drug Table: Agents for Active Immunization identifies agents that produce active immunity.

Naturally acquired active immunity occurs when a person is exposed to a disease, experiences the disease, and the body manufactures antibodies to provide future immunity to the disease. It is called active immunity because the antibodies were produced by the person who had the disease (Fig. 40-3). Thus, having the disease produces immunity.

Artificially acquired active immunity occurs when an individual is given a killed or weakened antigen, which stimulates the formation of antibodies against the antigen. The antigen does not cause the disease, but the individual will still manufacture specific antibodies against the disease. When a vaccine containing an **attenuated** (weakened) antigen is given, the individual may experience a few minor symptoms of the disease or even a mild form of the disease, but the symptoms are almost always milder and usually last for a short time.

The decision to use an attenuated, rather than a killed, virus as a vaccine to provide immunity is based on research. For example, many antigens, when killed, cause a poor antibody response, whereas when the antigen is merely weakened, a good antibody response occurs. Immunization against a specific disease provides artificially acquired active immunity. As discussed in Key Concepts 40-1, sometimes, a **"booster"** injection is needed to maintain immunity.

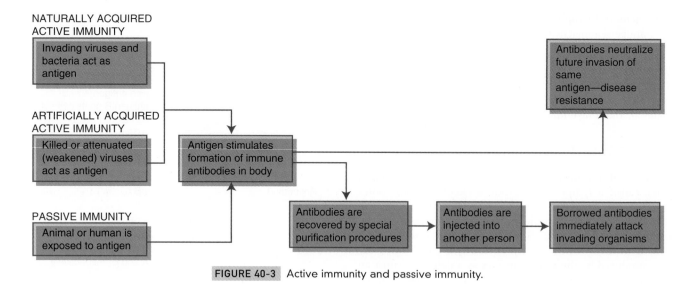

FIGURE 40-3 Active immunity and passive immunity.

The measles vaccine is considered an **immunization.** Immunization is a form of artificial active immunity and an important method of controlling some infectious diseases that can cause serious and sometimes fatal consequences. Currently, many infectious diseases may be prevented by **vaccine** (artificial active immunity), including the following:

- Diphtheria
- H5N1 influenza
- Hepatitis A
- Hepatitis B
- Herpes zoster
- Human papillomavirus
- Influenza (types A and B)
- Japanese encephalitis
- Meningococcal disease
- Mumps
- Measles
- Pertussis
- Pneumococcal disease
- Poliomyelitis
- Rabies
- Rotavirus
- Rubella
- Tetanus
- Typhoid
- Varicella
- Yellow fever

FACT CHECK

40-2 What is an attenuated antigen?
40-3 Why are booster injections sometimes required months or even years aft er the initial immunization?

Passive Immunity

Passive immunity is obtained from the administration of immune globulins or antivenins. This type of immunity provides the individual with ready-made antibodies from another human or an animal. Passive immunity provides immediate immunity to the invading antigen, but lasts for only a short time. The Summary Drug Table: Agents for Passive Immunity identifies agents for passive immunizations. An example of passive immunity is the administration of immune globulins, such as hepatitis B immune globulin. Administration of this vaccine is an attempt to prevent hepatitis B after the individual has been exposed to the virus.

Immunologic Agents

Some immunologic agents capitalize on the body's natural defenses by stimulating the immune response, thereby creating within the body protection to a specific disease. Other immunologic agents supply ready-made antibodies to provide passive immunity. Examples of immunologic agents include vaccines, toxoids, antivenins, and immune globulins.

KEY CONCEPTS

40-1 Booster Injections

Artificially acquired immunity against some diseases may require periodic booster injections to keep an adequate antibody level (or antibody titer) circulating in the blood. A booster injection is the administration of an additional dose of the vaccine to "boost" the production of antibodies to a level that will maintain the desired immunity. The booster is given months or years after the initial vaccine and may be needed because the life of some antibodies is short.

VACCINES AND TOXOIDS

Actions of Vaccines and Toxoids

Antibody-producing tissues cannot distinguish between an antigen that is capable of causing disease (a live antigen), an attenuated antigen, or a killed antigen. Because of this phenomenon, vaccines, which contain either an attenuated or a killed antigen, have been developed to create immunity to certain diseases. The live antigens are either killed or weakened during the manufacturing process. Although the vaccine contains weakened or killed antigens, they do not have sufficient strength to cause disease. Although rare, vaccination with any vaccine may not result in a protective antibody response in all individuals given the vaccine.

A **toxin** is a poisonous substance produced by some bacteria, such as *Clostridium tetani*, the bacteria that cause tetanus. A toxin is capable of stimulating the body to produce antitoxins, which are substances that act in the same manner as antibodies. Toxins are powerful substances, and like other antigens, they can be attenuated. A toxin that is attenuated (or weakened) but still capable of stimulating the formation of antitoxins is called a **toxoid**.

FACT CHECK

40-4 What are toxins and antitoxins?

Uses of Vaccines and Toxoids

An example of passive immunity is the administration of immune globulins (see Summary Drug Table: Agents for Passive Immunity), such as hepatitis B immune globulin. Administration of this vaccine is an attempt to prevent hepatitis B after the individual has been exposed to the virus.

Both vaccines and toxoids are administered to stimulate the immune response within the body to specific antigens or toxins. These agents must be administered before exposure to the pathogenic organism. The initiation of the immune response, in turn, produces resistance to a specific infectious disease. The immunity produced in this manner is active immunity. Uses of vaccines and toxoids include

- Routine immunization of infants and children (Visit the CDC website for current child and adolescent immunization schedules at: http://www.cdc.gov/vaccines/recs/schedules/child-schedule.htm.)
- Immunization of adults against tetanus
- Adults at high risk for certain diseases (e.g., pneumococcal and influenza vaccines for individuals with serious respiratory disorders) (Visit the CDC Web site for the current adult immunization schedule, including the schedule specifically for health care professionals at: http://www.cdc.gov/vaccines/recs/schedules/adult-schedule.htm.)
- Children or adults at risk for exposure to a particular disease (e.g., hepatitis B for health care providers)
- Immunization of prepubertal girls or nonpregnant women of childbearing age against rubella
- Prevention of human papillomavirus in prepubertal girls and nonpregnant young women up to age 25 or 26

Adverse Reactions of Vaccines and Toxoids

Adverse reactions from the administration of vaccines or toxoids are usually mild. Chills, fever, muscular aches and pains, rash, and lethargy may be present. Pain and tenderness at the injection site may also occur. Although rare, a hypersensitivity reaction may occur.

Minor adverse reactions, such as fever, rashes, and aching of the joints, are possible with the administration of a vaccine. In most cases, these reactions subside within 48 hours.

In most cases, the risk of serious adverse reactions from an immunization is much smaller than the risk of contracting the disease for which the immunizing agent is given.

Contraindications, Precautions, and Interactions of Vaccines and Toxoids

- Prior to administering a vaccine, the health care provider is responsible for providing the patient with a Vaccine Information Statement (VIS) specific for that vaccine. These forms are updated regularly and are available from the CDC Web site at http://www.cdc.gov/vaccines/pubs/vis/. The VIS explains which patients should not be vaccinated or should wait as well as the risks of the vaccine and possible severe reactions.
- Immunologic agents are contraindicated in patients with a known hypersensitivity to the agent or any component of it.
- The measles, mumps, rubella, and varicella vaccines are contraindicated in patients who have ever had an allergic reaction to gelatin, neomycin, or a previous dose of one of the vaccines; these vaccines are also contraindicated during pregnancy, especially during the first trimester, because of the danger of birth defects.
- Women are instructed to wait at least 3 months before getting pregnant after receiving these vaccines.
- Vaccines and toxoids are contraindicated during acute febrile illnesses, leukemia, lymphoma, immunosuppressive illness or drug therapy, and nonlocalized cancer.
- The immunologic agents are used with extreme caution in individuals with a history of allergies. Sensitivity testing may be performed in individuals with a history of allergies.
- No adequate studies have been conducted in pregnant women, and it is not known whether these agents are excreted in breast milk. Thus, the immunologic agents are used with caution in pregnant women and during lactation.
- Vaccinations containing live organisms are not administered within 3 months of immune globulin administration because antibodies in the globulin preparation may interfere with the immune response to the vaccination.
- Corticosteroids, antineoplastic drugs, and radiation therapy depress the immune system to such a degree

that insufficient numbers of antibodies are produced to prevent the disease.

- When the salicylates are administered with the varicella vaccination, there is an increased risk of Reye syndrome.

IMMUNE GLOBULINS AND ANTIVENINS

Actions of Globulins and Antivenins

Globulins are proteins present in blood serum or plasma that contain antibodies. **Immune globulins** are solutions obtained from human blood containing antibodies that have been formed by the body to specific antigens. Because they contain ready-made antibodies, they are given for passive immunity against disease. An **antivenin** is an antitoxin specific for an animal or insect venom.

Uses of Globulins and Antivenins

The immune globulins are administered to provide passive immunization to one or more infectious diseases. Those receiving immune globulins receive antibodies only to the diseases to which the donor blood is immune. The onset of protection is rapid but of short duration (1–3 months).

Antivenins are used for passive, transient protection from the toxic effects of bites by spiders (black widow and similar spiders) and snakes (rattlesnakes, copperhead and cottonmouth, and coral). The most effective response is obtained when the drug is administered within 4 hours after exposure.

> ### FACT CHECK
>
> **40-5** What are globulins?

Adverse Reactions of Immune Globulins and Antivenins

Adverse reactions to immune globulins are rare. However, local tenderness and pain at the injection site may occur. The most common adverse reactions include urticaria, angioedema, erythema, malaise, nausea, diarrhea, headache, chills, and fever. Adverse reactions, if they occur, usually last for several hours. Systemic reactions are extremely rare.

The antivenins may cause various reactions, with hypersensitivity being the most severe. Some antivenins are prepared from horse serum, and if a patient is sensitive to horse serum, serious reactions and death may result. The immediate reactions usually occur within 30 minutes after administration of the antivenin. Symptoms include apprehension; flushing; itching; urticaria (hives); edema of the face, tongue, and throat; cough; dyspnea; vomiting; cyanosis (blue coloration of the skin); and collapse.

Contraindications, Precautions, and Interactions of Immune Globulins and Antivenins

- The immune globulins are contraindicated in patients with a history of allergic reactions after administration of human immunoglobulin preparations and individuals with isolated immunoglobulin A deficiency (individuals could have an anaphylactic reaction to subsequent administration of blood products that contain immunoglobulin A).
- The antivenins are contraindicated in patients with hypersensitivity to horse serum or any other component of the serum.
- The immune globulins and antivenins are administered cautiously during pregnancy and lactation and in children.
- Antibodies in the immune globulin preparations may interfere with the immune response to live virus vaccines, particularly measles, but also others, such as mumps and rubella. Live virus vaccines should be administered 14 to 30 days before or 6 to 12 weeks after administration of immune globulins.
- No known interactions have been reported with antivenins.

Patient Management Issues with Immunologic Agents

Before the administration of any vaccine, an allergy history is taken. If a patient is known or thought to have allergies of any kind, then the health care provider must be informed before the vaccine is given. Some vaccines contain antibodies obtained from animals, whereas other vaccines may contain proteins or preservatives to which the individual may be allergic. A highly allergic person may have an allergic reaction that could be serious and even fatal. If the patient has an allergy history, then the health care provider may decide to perform skin tests for allergy to one or more of the components or proteins in the vaccine. It must also be determined whether the patient has any conditions that contraindicate the administration of the agent (e.g., cancer, leukemia, lymphoma, immunosuppressive drug therapy).

A patient is usually not hospitalized after administration of an immunologic agent. However, a patient may be asked to stay in the clinic or office for observation for approximately

> ## ALERT ℞
>
> ### Human Immune Globulin Intravenous Products
> Human immune globulin intravenous products have been associated with renal impairment, acute renal failure, osmotic nephrosis, and death. Individuals with a predisposition to acute renal failure, such as those with preexisting kidney disease, diabetes mellitus, individuals older than 65 years, or patients receiving nephrotoxic drugs should not be given human immune globulin intravenous products.

30 minutes after the injection to observe for any signs of hypersensitivity (e.g., laryngeal edema, hives, pruritus, angioneurotic edema, and severe dyspnea). Emergency resuscitation equipment should be available in the event of a severe hypersensitivity reaction.

It may be beneficial to increase the fluids in the diet, allow for adequate rest, and keep the atmosphere quiet and nonstimulating. The health care provider may prescribe acetaminophen every 4 hours to control these reactions. Local irritation at the injection site may be treated with warm or cool compresses, depending on the patient's preference. A lump may be felt at the injection site after a diphtheria, pertussis, or tetanus injection or other immunization. This is not abnormal and will resolve itself within several days to several months.

Reports of adverse events after immunizations are reported to the Vaccine Adverse Event Reporting System (VAERS), as discussed in Key Concepts 40-2.

Educating the Patient and Family about Immunologic Agents

Because of the effectiveness of various types of vaccines in the prevention of disease, parents are encouraged to have infants and young children receive the immunizations suggested by the health care provider.

Those traveling to a foreign country are urged to contact their health care provider or local health department well in advance of their departure date for information about other immunizations that will be needed. Immunizations should be given well in advance of departure because it may take several weeks to produce adequate immunity.

When an adult or child is receiving a vaccine for immunization, the health care provider explains to the patient or a family member the possible reactions that may occur, such as soreness at the injection site or fever.

Serious viral infections of the central nervous system and fatalities have occurred with the use of some vaccines. Although the number of these incidents is small, a risk factor still remains when some vaccines are given. Parents should understand that a risk is also associated with not receiving immunization against some infectious diseases. That risk may

---

CONSIDERATIONS | Infants & Children

LIFESPAN

Postponing Immunizations

On occasion, it may be necessary to postpone the regular immunization schedule, particularly for children. This is of special concern to parents. The decision to delay immunization because of illness or for other reasons must be discussed with the health care provider. However, the decision to administer or delay vaccination because of febrile illness (illness causing a fever) depends on the severity of the symptoms and the specific disorder. In general, all vaccines can be administered to those with minor illness, such as a cold virus or a low-grade fever. However, moderate or severe febrile illness is a contraindication. In instances of moderate or severe febrile illness, vaccination is performed as soon as the acute phase of the illness is over.

---

be higher and just as serious as the risk associated with the use of vaccines. When a large segment of the population is immunized, the small number of those not immunized are less likely to be exposed to and infected with the disease-producing microorganism. However, when large numbers of the population are not immunized, there is a great increase in the chances of exposure to the infectious disease and a significant increase in the probability that the individual will experience the disease.

Parents or guardians are encouraged to report to their health care provider any adverse reactions or serious adverse events occurring after administration of a vaccine or to report the event to VAERS.

Following are key points about immunologic agents the patient and family members should know when a child is to receive a vaccination:

- If your child is receiving a vaccination:
- The risks of contracting vaccine-preventable diseases are much higher than the adverse reactions associated with immunization.
- Bring all of your child's immunization records to all visits with your health care provider.
- Ask your health care provider to provide you with the date for return for your child's next vaccination.
- Certain adverse reactions (e.g., fever, soreness at the injection site) are common. In general, these reactions are short-lived. Acetaminophen and warm compresses will help to ease these reactions.
- Report any unusual or severe adverse reactions after the administration of a vaccination to your health care provider.

KEY CONCEPTS

40-2 Vaccine Adverse Event Reporting System

The VAERS is a national vaccine safety surveillance program cosponsored by the Centers for Disease Control and Prevention and the Food and Drug Administration. The VAERS collects and analyzes information from reports of adverse reactions after immunization. Anyone can report to the VAERS, and reports are sent in by vaccine manufacturers, health care providers, and vaccine recipients and their parents or guardians. The reporting form can be found at http://vaers.hhs.gov/resources/vaers_form.pdf and in Appendix C.

FACT CHECK

40-6 Why are patients sometimes observed for a short time after receiving immunologic agents?

Chapter Review

KEY POINTS

- The immune system has two distinct but overlapping mechanisms with which to fight invading organisms: cell-mediated defenses (cellular immunity) and antibody-mediated defenses (humoral immunity).
- Cell-mediated immunity and humoral immunity are interdependent: Cell-mediated immunity influences the function of the B lymphocytes, and humoral immunity influences the function of the T lymphocytes.
- Active immunity and passive immunity involve the use of agents that stimulate antibody formation (active immunity) or the injection of ready-made antibodies found in the serum of immune individuals or animals (passive immunity).
- Immunization is a form of artificial active immunity and an important method of controlling some of the infectious diseases that are capable of causing serious and sometimes fatal consequences.
- Passive immunity provides the individual with ready-made antibodies from another human or an animal.
- Some immunologic agents stimulate the immune response, thereby creating within the body protection to a specific disease. Other immunologic agents supply ready-made antibodies to provide passive immunity. Examples of immunologic agents include vaccines, toxoids, and immune globulins.
- A toxin that is attenuated (or weakened) but still capable of stimulating the formation of antitoxins is called a toxoid. Both vaccines and toxoids are administered to stimulate the immune response within the body to specific antigens or toxins. These agents must be administered before exposure to the pathogenic organism. The initiation of the immune response, in turn, produces resistance to a specific infectious disease.
- Adverse reactions from the administration of vaccines or toxoids are usually mild. Chills, fever, muscular aches and pains, rash, and lethargy may occur, along with pain and tenderness at the injection site. The immunologic agents are used with extreme caution in individuals with a history of allergies.
- Immune globulins are solutions obtained from human blood containing antibodies that have been formed by the body to specific antigens. Because they contain ready-made antibodies, they are given for passive immunity against disease. The immune globulins are administered to provide passive immunization to one or more infectious diseases. Those receiving immune globulins receive antibodies only to the diseases to which the donor blood is immune.
- Adverse reactions to immune globulins are rare but may include urticaria, angioedema, erythema, malaise, nausea, diarrhea, headache, chills, and fever.

CRITICAL THINKING CASE STUDY
Childhood Immunizations

Ms. Wilson has brought her 2-month-old daughter, Michelle, to the clinic for the first of her immunizations. Ms. Wilson is nervous about the number of immunizations her child must receive and the effects they will have, and she wonders whether the process is necessary for her daughter's health at such a young age.

1. Ms. Wilson should be told
   a. it is acceptable to postpone the series until her daughter is 1 year old if it will help Ms. Wilson relax
   b. the risk of not having the immunization is greater than the risk of any problem from receiving the vaccine
   c. the vaccines are optional; most of the diseases that these immunizations will prevent are rare
   d. none of the above
2. Ms. Wilson wants to know whether she can expect her daughter to have an adverse reaction to the vaccination. She should be told
   a. there are no adverse reactions associated with vaccines
   b. mild symptoms may occur, but they are rare
   c. possible adverse reactions include local injection-site pain, redness, and swelling
   d. none of the above
3. Ms. Wilson is confused by all of the abbreviations for the immunizations. She notices one is called "DTaP" and asks you what it is for. What would you tell her?
4. At the conclusion of the office visit, Ms. Wilson receives her daughter's immunization record. What should you tell her about this record?

Review Questions

MULTIPLE CHOICE

1. When discussing the possibility of adverse reactions after receiving a vaccine, the parents of a young child are told that
   a. adverse reactions may be severe, and the child should be monitored closely for 24 hours
   b. adverse reactions are usually mild
   c. the child will likely experience a hypersensitivity reaction
   d. the most common adverse reaction is a severe headache
2. Which of the following food allergies would alert the health care provider to a possibility of an allergy to the measles vaccine?
   a. Jell-O gelatin
   b. Peanut butter
   c. Sugar
   d. Corn
3. All of the following are uses of vaccines and toxoids EXCEPT
   a. routine immunization of infants and children
   b. routine immunization of adults
   c. immunization of adults against tetanus
   d. immunization of nonpregnant women of childbearing age against rubella

4. What type of immunity will be produced by the hepatitis B vaccine recombinant?
    a. Artificially acquired active immunity
    b. Naturally acquired active immunity
    c. Passive immunity
    d. Cell-mediated immunity

MATCHING

Match the trade name on the left with the correct category on the right. Categories may be used more than once.

_____	5.	Adacel	a. vaccine, bacterial
_____	6.	RhoGAM	b. vaccine, viral
_____	7.	MMR II	c. toxoid
_____	8.	PEDIARIX	d. immune globulin
_____	9.	Comvax	e. antivenin
_____	10.	CroFab	
_____	11.	Zostavax	
_____	12.	Kinrix	
_____	13.	BabyBIG	
_____	14.	Menactra	
_____	15.	Prevnar	
_____	16.	FluMist	

TRUE OR FALSE

_____ 17. Amphetamines have the potential for abuse and addiction.

_____ 18. Typhoid vaccine may be given orally or parenterally. True

_____ 19. Generally, vaccines can still be administered even if a patient has a low-grade fever. True

_____ 20. A toxoid is a poisonous substance produced by bacteria.

FILL IN THE BLANKS

21. B lymphocytes are involved in _____ immunity.
22. Immune globulin given intramuscularly (IGIM) is used for _____ after exposure to hepatitis ___.
23. Unlike B lymphocytes, T lymphocytes do not produce _____ but directly attack _____.
24. _____ _____ active immunity occurs when a patient experiences a disease for the first time, and the body makes _____ against it.

SHORT ANSWERS

25. Why are the measles, mumps, rubella, and varicella vaccines contraindicated during pregnancy?
26. When should live virus vaccines be administered in relation to administration of immune globulins?
27. Why should a patient traveling to foreign country be advised to get any needed immunizations well in advance of the trip?
28. When providing patient instruction, how would you explain the risk of adverse reactions from an immunization?

Web Activities

1. Go to the VAERS website (http://www.vaers.org) and click on "Frequently Asked Questions." What are the limitations of the VAERS data?
2. Go to the CDC Web site (http://www.cdc.gov) and search for "Vaccine Information Statements." Make note of the VISs available. Have any been recently updated? Choose one and identify who should not get or should wait to get that vaccine, the risks from the vaccine, and what type of reaction to watch for. Also, make note of the date that the VIS was most recently updated (this should be in the lower right-hand corner of the back page).

SUMMARY DRUG TABLE Agents for Active Immunization (left, generic; right, trade)

Comprehensive Summary Drug Tables, including uses, adverses effects, dosages, and pregnancy classifications, are provided on the companion website, http://thePoint.lww. com/PharmacologyHP2e

Vaccines, Bacterial	
anthrax vaccine	BioThrax
bcg vaccine	*generic*
Haemophilus B conjugate vaccine	ActHIB, Hiberix, Liquid PedvaxHIB
Haemophilus influenzae type b conjugate and hepatitis B vaccine	Comvax
meningococcal vaccine	Menactra, Menomune
pneumococcal vaccine, polyvalent	Pneumova× 23
pneumococcal 7-valent conjugate vaccine (diphtheria CRM197 protein)	Prevnar
pneumococcal 13-valent conjugate vaccine	Prevnar 13
typhoid vaccine	Typhim VI, Vivotif Berna
Vaccines, Viral	
H5N1 influenza vaccine	H5N1 influenza vaccine
hepatitis A (inactivated)/hepatitis B (recombinant) vaccine	Twinrix
hepatitis A vaccine, inactivated	Havrix, Vaqta
hepatitis B vaccine recombinant	Engerix-B, Recombivax HB
human papillomavirus (type S 16, 18) bivalent vaccine, recombinant	Cervarix
human papillomavirus quadrivalent vaccine, recombinant	Gardasil
influenza type A and B vaccine	Injection: Afluria, Agriflu, Fluarix, FluLaval, Fluvirin, Fluzone Intranasal: FluMist

japanese encephalitis virus vaccine	JE-Vax
measles, mumps, and rubella virus vaccine, live	MMR II
measles, mumps, rubella, and varicella virus vaccine, live, attenuated	ProQuad
poliovirus vaccine, inactivated (IPV)	Ipol
rabies vaccine	Imovax Rabies, RabAvert
rotavirus vaccine, live	Rotarix, Rota Teq
varicella virus vaccine	Varivax
yellow fever vaccine	YF-VAX
zoster vaccine, live, attenuated	Zostavax
Toxoids	
diphtheria and tetanus toxoids adsorbed	Decavac, *generic* (adult and pediatric)
diphtheria and tetanus toxoids and acellular pertussis adsorbed, hepatitis B (recombinant) and inactivated poliovirus vaccine combined	PEDIARIX
diphtheria and tetanus toxoid/acellular pertussis adsorbed/inactivated poliovirus/*Haemophilus influenzae* type B conjugate vaccine combined	Pentacel
diphtheria toxoid/tetanus toxoid/acellular pertussis vaccine, adsorbed (DTaP/Tdap)	Adacel, Boostrix, Daptacel, Infanrix, Tripedia
diphtheria toxoid/tetanus toxoid/acellular pertussis, adsorbed/inactivated poliovirus combination vaccine (DTaP, IPV)	Kinrix

SUMMARY DRUG TABLE Agents for Passive Immunity (left, generic; right, trade)

Comprehensive Summary Drug Tables, including uses, adverses effects, dosages, and pregnancy classifications, are provided on the companion website, http://thePoint.lww. com/PharmacologyHP2e

Immune Globulins	
antithymocyte globulin (rabbit) (ATG rabbit)	Thymoglobulin
botulism immune globulin IV (human) (BIG-IV)	BabyBIG
cytomegalovirus immune globulin IV, human (CMV-IGIV)	CytoGam
hepatitis B immune globulin (human) (HBIG)	HepaGam B, HyperHEP B S/D, Nabi-HB
immune globulin (human) IM (IG, IGIM, IMIG, gamma globulin, IgG)	GamaSTAN S/D
immune globulin IV (human)	Carimune, Flebogamma, Flebogamma DIF, GamaSTAN S/D, Gammagard, Gammagard S/D, Gammagard S/D less IgA, Gammaplex, Gamunex, octagam, Privigen
immune globulin (human) subcutaneous (IGSC, SCIG)	Hizentra, Vivaglobin

lymphocyte immune globulin, antithymocyte globulin (equine) (LIG, ATG, ATG equine)	Atgam
rabies immune globulin, human (RIGH)	HyperRAB S/D, Imogam Rabies-HT
Rh₀ (D) immune globulin IM (human)	HyperRHO S/D, MICRhoGAM Ultra-Filtered Plus, RhoGAM Ultra-Filtered Plus
Rh₀ (D) immune globulin IV (human) (Rh [D] IGIV)	Rhophylac, WinRho SDF
vaccinia immune globulin IV (VIGIV) (human)	*generic*
Antivenins	
antivenin (*Latrodectus mactans*) (black widow spider antivenin) (equine origin)	Antivenin (*Latrodectus mactans*)
antivenin (*Micrurus fulvius*) (North American coral snake antivenin) (equine origin)	Antivenin (*Micrurus fulvius*)
crotalidae polyvalent immune FAB (ovine origin)	CroFab

41

Antineoplastic Drugs

CHAPTER OBJECTIVES

On completion of this chapter, students will be able to:

1. Define the chapter's key terms.
2. Explain why chemotherapy is administered in a series of cycles.
3. Compare and contrast the actions of various antineoplastic drugs.
4. Describe the general drug actions, uses, adverse reactions, contraindications, precautions, and interactions of antineoplastic drugs.
5. Discuss important points to keep in mind when educating the patient and family members about the use of antineoplastic drugs.

KEY TERMS

alopecia—the loss of hair
anemia—decrease in red blood cells
anorexia—loss of appetite
antineoplastic drugs—drugs used for cure, control, or palliative (relief of symptoms) treatment of malignancies
bone marrow suppression—a potentially dangerous adverse reaction to antineoplastic drugs resulting in decreased production of blood cells
chemotherapy—drug therapy with antineoplastic drugs
extravasation—escape of fluid from a blood vessel into surrounding tissues
leukopenia—a decrease in the white blood cells or leukocytes; a symptom of bone marrow suppression
oral mucositis—inflammation of the oral mucous membranes
stomatitis—inflammation of the mouth
thrombocytopenia—a decrease in the thrombocytes; a symptom of bone marrow suppression
vesicant—an adverse drug reaction resulting in tissue necrosis, which is caused by the infiltration or extravasation of the drug out of a blood vessel and into soft tissue

CHAPTER OVERVIEW

Drug classes covered in this chapter are:

• Antineoplastic drugs

Drugs by classification are listed on pages 446-448.

thePOINT RESOURCES

• Comprehensive Summary Drug Tables

• Interactive Practice and Review

• Monographs of Most Commonly Prescribed Drugs

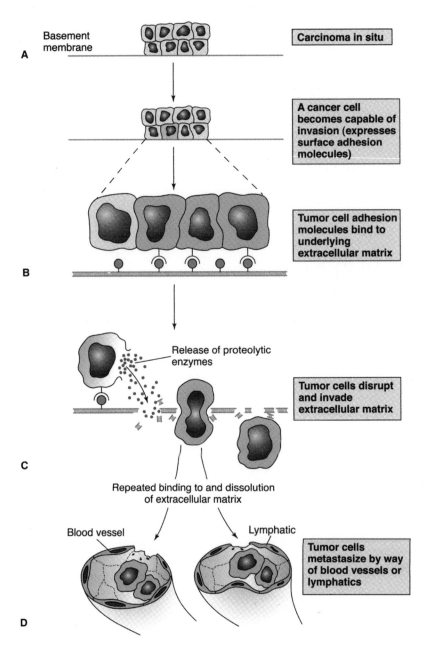

Basement
membrane

A

Carcinoma in situ

**A cancer cell
becomes capable of
invasion (expresses
surface adhesion
molecules)**

**Tumor cell adhesion
molecules bind to
underlying
extracellular matrix**

B

Release of proteolytic
enzymes

**Tumor cells disrupt
and invade
extracellular matrix**

C

Repeated binding to and dissolution
of extracellular matrix

Blood vessel   Lymphatic

**Tumor cells
metastasize by way
of blood vessels or
lymphatics**

D

FIGURE 41-1   Metastasis of cancer cells. A. Growth of primary tumor and invasion of surrounding tissues. B. Movement of tumor cells into the endothelium and basement membrane of the surrounding capillary. C. Shed tumor cells in lungs, brain, and liver become trapped and penetrate the capillary wall to establish themselves in this new environment. D. Proliferation at the new site, which requires a conducive environment with blood supply and nutrition.

Antineoplastic drugs are used in the treatment of malignant diseases (cancer). These drugs can be used for cure, control, or palliative (relief of symptoms) therapy. Although these drugs may not always lead to a complete cure of the malignancy, they often slow the rate of tumor growth and delay metastasis (spreading of the cancer to other sites) (Fig. 41-1). Use of these drugs is one of the tools in the treatment of cancer. The term **chemotherapy** is often used to refer to therapy with antineoplastic drugs.

Antineoplastic Drugs

Many antineoplastic drugs are available to treat malignancies. The antineoplastic drugs covered in this chapter include the alkylating drugs, antibiotics, antimetabolites, hormones, mitotic inhibitors, and selected miscellaneous drugs. Antineoplastic drugs not specifically discussed in this chapter are listed in the Summary Drug Table: Antineoplatic Drugs.

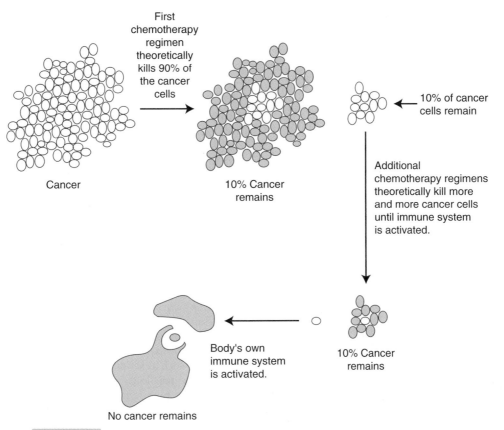

FIGURE 41-2 Cell kill theory describing activity of repeated chemotherapy regimens.

Actions of Antineoplastic Drugs

Generally, most antineoplastic drugs affect cells that rapidly proliferate (divide and reproduce). Malignant neoplasms or cancerous tumors usually consist of rapidly proliferating aberrant (abnormal) cells. Cancer cells have no biological feedback controls that stop their aberrant growth or proliferation. Cancer cells are more sensitive to antineoplastic drugs when the cells are in the process of growing and dividing. Chemotherapy (Key Concepts 41-1) is administered at the time the cell population is dividing as part of a strategy to optimize cell death.

However, the normal cells that line the mouth and gastrointestinal tract and cells of the gonads, bone marrow, hair follicles, and lymph tissue are also rapidly dividing cells and are usually affected by these drugs. Thus, antineoplastic drugs may affect normal as well as malignant (cancerous) cells.

FACT CHECK

41-1 Antineoplastic drugs generally affect which type of cells?

Alkylating Drugs

Alkylating drugs interfere with the process of cell division of malignant and normal cells. The drug binds with DNA, causing breaks and preventing DNA replication. Malignant cells appear to be more susceptible to the effects of alkylating drugs. Examples of alkylating drugs include busulfan (Myleran, Busulfex) and chlorambucil (Leukeran).

KEY CONCEPTS

4-1 Chemotherapy

Chemotherapy is administered in a series of cycles to allow for recovery of the normal cells and to destroy more of the malignant cells (Fig. 41-2). According to cell kill theory, a drug regimen is intended to kill 90% of the cancer cells during the first course of treatment. The second course, according to this theory, targets the remaining cancer cells and reduces those cells by 90%. Further courses of chemotherapy continue to reduce the number of cancer cells, until all cells are killed. This theory is the rationale for using repeated doses of chemotherapy with several antineoplastic drugs. Every malignant cell must be destroyed for the cancer to be cured. Each cycle of treatment with the antineoplastic drugs kills some, but by no means all, of the malignant cells. Therefore, repeated courses of chemotherapy are used to kill more and more of the malignant cells, until theoretically none is left.

Antineoplastic Antibiotics

The antineoplastic antibiotics, unlike their anti-infection antibiotic relatives, do not have anti-infective (against infection) ability. Their action is similar to the alkylating drugs. Antineoplastic antibiotics appear to interfere with DNA and RNA synthesis and therefore delay or inhibit cell division, including the reproducing ability of malignant cells. Examples of antineoplastic antibiotics include bleomycin and doxorubicin (Adriamycin).

Antimetabolites

The antimetabolites interfere with various metabolic functions of cells, thereby disrupting normal cell functions. They inactivate enzymes or alter the structure of DNA, changing the ability of DNA to replicate. These drugs are most effective in the treatment of rapidly dividing neoplastic cells. Examples of the antimetabolites include methotrexate and fluorouracil.

Hormones

The exact method of antineoplastic action of hormones is unclear. These drugs also appear to counteract the effect of male or female hormones in hormone-dependent tumors (see Chapter 33). They appear to alter the hormonal environment of the cell. Examples of hormones used as antineoplastic drugs include the antiandrogens (abiraterone acetate), progestins (megestrol acetate), estrogens (estramustine), and antiestrogens (tamoxifen).

Gonadotropin-releasing hormone analogs, for example, goserelin (Zoladex), appear to act by inhibiting the anterior pituitary secretion of gonadotropins, thus suppressing the release of pituitary gonadotropins. These drugs primarily decrease serum testosterone levels and therefore are used in the treatment of advanced prostatic carcinomas.

Mitotic Inhibitors

Mitotic inhibitors (antimitotics) interfere with or stop cell division. Examples of mitotic inhibitors include paclitaxel (Abraxane), vincristine (Vincasar PFS), and vinblastine.

Miscellaneous Antineoplastic Drugs

In addition to the types of antineoplastics already covered, there are a number of miscellaneous antineoplastics. While some have multiple drugs that appear to work similarly, many are the only one in a particular category. The miscellaneous antineoplastic drugs are covered in the Summary Drug Table: Antineoplastic Drugs. The mechanisms of action of some of these drugs are not entirely clear.

FACT CHECK

41-2 What are five commonly used types of antineoplastic drugs?

Uses of Antineoplastic Drugs

Antineoplastic drugs may be given alone or in combination with other antineoplastic drugs. In many instances, a combination of these drugs produces better results than the use of a single antineoplastic drug.

Although many antineoplastic drugs share a similar activity (i.e., they interfere in some way with cell division), their uses are not necessarily similar.

Adverse Reactions of Antineoplastic Drugs

Antineoplastic drugs often produce a wide variety of adverse reactions (Key Concepts 41-2). Some of these reactions are dose dependent; that is, their occurrence is more common or their intensity is more severe with higher doses. Other adverse reactions occur primarily because of the effect the drug has on many cells of the body. Because the antineoplastic drugs affect cancer cells and rapidly proliferating normal cells (e.g., cells in the bone marrow, gastrointestinal tract, reproductive tract, and the hair follicles), adverse reactions occur as the result of the action on these cells. Adverse reactions common to many of the antineoplastic drugs include bone marrow suppression, nausea, vomiting, stomatitis, diarrhea, and hair loss.

Some adverse reactions are desirable, for example, the depressing effect of certain antineoplastic drugs on the bone marrow, because this adverse drug reaction is essential in the treatment of the leukemias. Other adverse reactions are not desirable, such as severe vomiting or diarrhea.

Adverse reactions occurring with the administration of these drugs may range from very mild to life threatening. Some of these reactions, such as the loss of hair (**alopecia**), may have little effect on the physical status of the patient but may affect the patient's mental health.

Because a hemorrhagic syndrome may occur with plicamycin, assessments for hemorrhage are planned. Hyperuricemia (elevated blood uric acid levels) may occur with some drugs, such as melphalan (Alkeran) or mercaptopurine (Purinethol), so fluid intake and output measurements are planned. Because other antineoplastic drugs are nephrotoxic, blood urea nitrogen levels and serum creatinine are monitored closely during therapy.

Alopecia

Alopecia (loss of hair) is a common adverse reaction of some antineoplastic drugs. Some drugs cause severe hair loss, whereas others cause gradual thinning. Drugs causing severe

KEY CONCEPTS

41-2 Handling Adverse Effects of Antineoplastic Drugs

Antineoplastic drugs are potentially toxic and often cause many serious adverse reactions. Some of these adverse effects must be accepted because the only alternative is to stop treatment of the malignancy. A treatment plan is developed that will prevent, lessen, or treat most or all of the symptoms of a specific adverse reaction. An example of prevention is giving an antiemetic before administering an antineoplastic drug known to cause severe nausea and vomiting.

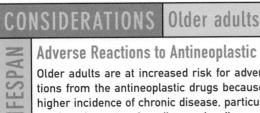

CONSIDERATIONS | Older adults

Adverse Reactions to Antineoplastic Drugs

Older adults are at increased risk for adverse reactions from the antineoplastic drugs because of their higher incidence of chronic disease, particularly kidney impairment and cardiovascular disease. A lower dosage of an antineoplastic may be used for patients with renal impairment. Creatinine clearance is used to monitor renal function in older adults.

hair loss include doxorubicin and vinblastine. Methotrexate, bleomycin, vincristine, and etoposide cause gradual hair loss.

A patient given these drugs should be informed that hair loss may occur. This problem occurs 10 to 21 days after the treatment cycle is completed. Hair loss is temporary, and hair will grow again when the drug therapy is completed.

Anorexia

Anorexia (loss of appetite resulting in an inability to eat) is common with antineoplastic drugs. Patients often report alterations in their sense of taste during the course of chemotherapy. Small, frequent meals (five to six meals daily) are usually better tolerated than three large meals. Breakfast is often the best-tolerated meal of the day. The patient is taught the importance of eating meals high in nutritive value, particularly protein (e.g., eggs, milk products, tuna, beans, peas, and lentils). Some patients can eat high-protein finger foods such as cheese or peanut butter and crackers. Nutritional supplements may also be prescribed. The patient's body weight is monitored at least weekly, and any weight loss is reported. If the patient continues to lose weight, then a feeding tube may be used to administer a nutritionally complete liquid. Although this is not ideal, a hospitalized patient who is malnourished and weak may benefit from this intervention.

Bone Marrow Suppression

Bone marrow suppression is a potentially dangerous adverse reaction of decreased production of blood cells. Bone marrow suppression is manifested by abnormal laboratory test results and clinical evidence of leukopenia, thrombocytopenia, or anemia. For example, there is a decrease in the white blood cells or leukocytes **(leukopenia),** a decrease in the thrombocytes **(thrombocytopenia),** and a decrease in the red blood cells, resulting in anemia. Patients with leukopenia have a lower resistance to infection and must be monitored closely for any signs of infection.

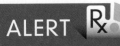

ALERT

Signs of Infection

Any of the following signs of infection should be reported to the health care provider immediately: a temperature of 100.4°F or higher, cough, sore throat, chills, frequent urination, or a low white blood cell count.

ALERT

Symptoms of Thrombocytopenia

Thrombocytopenia is characterized by a decrease in the platelet count. Patients with thrombocytopenia are monitored for bleeding tendencies, and precautions are taken to prevent bleeding. The patient should not use razors, nail trimmers, dental floss, firm toothbrushes, or any sharp objects. The patient is monitored closely for easy bruising, skin lesions, and bleeding from any orifice (opening) of the body. Any of the following should be reported to the health care provider immediately: bleeding gums, easy bruising, petechiae (pinpoint hemorrhages), increased menstrual bleeding, tarry stools, bloody urine, or coffee-ground emesis.

Anemia occurs as the result of a decreased production of red blood cells in the bone marrow and is characterized by fatigue, dizziness, shortness of breath, and palpitations. Blood transfusions may sometimes be necessary to correct the anemia.

Nausea and Vomiting

Nausea and vomiting are common adverse reactions of antineoplastic drugs. The health care provider may order an antiemetic approximately 30 minutes before treatment begins and continue the antiemetic for several days after administration of the chemotherapy. Small, frequent meals are provided as the patient can tolerate food. Greasy or fatty foods and unpleasant sights, smells, and tastes should be avoided. Cold foods, dry foods, and salty foods may be better tolerated.

Stomatitis

Because the cells in the mouth grow rapidly, they are particularly sensitive to the effects of antineoplastic drugs. **Stomatitis** (inflammation of the mouth) or **oral mucositis** (inflammation of the oral mucous membranes) may occur 5 to 7 days after chemotherapy and continue up to 10 days after therapy. This adverse reaction can also affect the patient's nutrition. The patient must avoid any foods or products that are irritating to the mouth, such as alcoholic beverages, spices, strong mouthwashes, or toothpaste. Soft or liquid foods high in nutritive value should be given. Any white patches on the tongue, throat, or gums; any burning sensation; and bleeding from the mouth or gums should be reported to the health care provider. The health care provider may order a topical viscous anesthetic, such as lidocaine viscous, before meals to decrease discomfort when eating.

Diarrhea

Measures to manage diarrhea include a low-residue diet while the bowel rests. Electrolytes are monitored and supplemented as needed. Adequate hydration must be maintained; intravenous fluids may be necessary. If diarrhea is severe, then therapy may be delayed or stopped, or the dose decreased.

Tissue Integrity

Some antineoplastic drugs are **vesicants** (i.e., they cause tissue necrosis if they infiltrate or extravasate out of the blood vessel and into the soft tissue). If **extravasation** occurs, then underlying tissue is damaged. The damage can be severe, causing physical deformity or loss of vascularity or tendon function. Examples of vesicant drugs are daunorubicin, doxorubicin, and vinblastine.

When the patient is receiving a vesicant, the intravenous site should be monitored continuously. Extravasation may occur without warning, or signs may be detected. The earlier the extravasation is detected, the less likely soft tissue damage will occur. If an extravasation is suspected, then the infusion is stopped immediately and the extravasation reported to the health care provider.

FACT CHECK

41-3 What are common adverse reactions to many of the antineoplastic drugs?

Contraindications, Precautions, and Interactions of Antineoplastic Drugs

The information provided here is general, and the contraindications, precautions, and interactions for each antineoplastic drug vary.

- Antineoplastic drugs are contraindicated in patients with leukopenia, thrombocytopenia, anemia, serious infections, serious renal disease, or known hypersensitivity to the drug and during pregnancy.
- Antineoplastic drugs are used cautiously in patients with renal or hepatic impairment, active infection, or other debilitating illnesses, or in those who have recently completed treatment with other antineoplastic drugs or radiation therapy.
- Prior to initiating antineoplastic therapy, a complete medication history should be performed to ensure that the antineoplastic does not interact with any current medication and vice versa.

Alkylating Drugs

- The alkylating drugs may antagonize the effects of antigout drugs by increasing serum uric acid levels. Dosage adjustment of the antigout drug may be needed.
- If cisplatin is used concurrently with aminoglycosides, then there may be an increase in nephrotoxicity and ototoxicity.

- When cisplatin is used concurrently with loop diuretics, there is an increased risk of ototoxicity.
- Administering live viral vaccines with cyclophosphamide may decrease the antibody response of the vaccine.

Antineoplastic Antibiotics

- Plasma digoxin levels may decrease when the drug is administered with bleomycin.
- When bleomycin is used with cisplatin, there is an increased risk of bleomycin toxicity.
- Pulmonary toxicity may occur when bleomycin is administered with other antineoplastic drugs.
- Mitomycin and dactinomycin have an additive bone marrow depressant effect when administered with other antineoplastic drugs.
- Mitomycin, mitoxantrone, and dactinomycin decrease antibody response to live virus vaccines.
- Dactinomycin potentiates or reactivates skin or gastrointestinal reactions of radiation therapy.
- There is an increased risk of bleeding when plicamycin is administered with aspirin, warfarin, heparin, or a nonsteroidal anti-inflammatory drug.

Antimetabolite Drugs

- Antimetabolite drugs may antagonize the effects of antigout drugs by increasing serum uric acid concentration.
- Toxicity from methotrexate may be increased by other nephrotoxic drugs.
- When the antimetabolites are administered with other antineoplastic drugs, bone marrow suppression is additive.
- Vitamin preparations containing folic acid may decrease the effects of methotrexate.
- Alcohol ingestion while taking methotrexate may increase the risk of hepatotoxicity.
- Concurrent use of methotrexate and a nonsteroidal anti-inflammatory drug may cause severe methotrexate toxicity.
- Fluorouracil is not compatible with diazepam, doxorubicin, and methotrexate.
- Food decreases the absorption of fluorouracil.
- Live viral vaccines should not be administered if a patient is receiving fluorouracil, because a decrease in antibody production may occur, causing the vaccine to be ineffective.
- Severe cardiomyopathy with left ventricular failure has occurred when fluorouracil and cisplatin are given together.

Hormones

- Bicalutamide may increase the effect of oral anticoagulants.
- Flutamide enhances the action of leuprolide.
- Additive antineoplastic effects may occur when leuprolide is administered with megestrol or flutamide.
- Estrogens decrease the effectiveness of tamoxifen.

Mitotic Inhibitors

- Additive bone marrow depressive effects occur when a mitotic inhibitor drug is administered with another antineoplastic drug or radiation therapy.
- Administration of vincristine with digoxin results in a decreased therapeutic effect of the digoxin and decreased plasma digoxin levels.

- There is a decrease in serum concentrations of phenytoin when administered with vinblastine.

FACT CHECK

41-4 In which patients are antineoplastic drugs used cautiously?

Patient Management Issues with Antineoplastic Drugs

After the administration of an antineoplastic drug, the patient assessment is based on the following:

- General condition
- The individual response to the drug
- Adverse reactions that may occur
- Guidelines established by the primary health care provider or hospital
- Results of periodic laboratory tests

A complete blood count may be used to determine the response of the bone marrow to an antineoplastic drug. Liver function tests may be used to detect liver toxicity, which may be an adverse reaction that can be seen with the administration of some of these drugs.

If laboratory tests indicate a severe depressant effect on the bone marrow or other test abnormalities, then the health care provider may reduce the next drug dose or temporarily stop chemotherapy to allow the affected body systems to recover.

Administration of Antineoplastic Drugs

Antineoplastic drugs such as melphalan, busulfan, and chlorambucil are usually given orally. (Melphalan and busulfan are also available as injectable products for specific indications.) Most oral drugs are taken by the patient at home. The section on Educating the Patient and Family provides information to include in helping the patient and family members understand the treatment.

Although some of these drugs are given orally, others are given by the parenteral route. Goserelin (Zoladex), a hormonal antineoplastic drug used to treat breast cancer, is administered subcutaneously in an unusual way. The drug is contained in a dry pellet that is implanted in the soft tissue of the abdomen, where it is gradually absorbed over 1 to 3 months. After a local anesthetic, such as lidocaine, is administered, a large needle (usually 16 gauges) is used to insert the pellet.

The intravenous route of drug delivery is the most common and most reliable method of drug delivery.

Educating the Patient and Family about Antineoplastic Drugs

When the patient is hospitalized, all treatments and possible adverse effects are explained to the patient before the initiation of therapy.

Some of these drugs are taken orally at home. Some hospitals or health care providers give printed instructions to the patient. The patient has a right to know the dangers associated with these drugs and what adverse reactions may occur.

Some patients are given antineoplastic drugs in the medical office or outpatient clinic. Again, the treatment regimen is explained thoroughly to the patient and family members. In some instances, a drug to prevent nausea may be taken before administration of the drugs in the medical office or clinic. Most patients are compliant with therapy, although some patients might decide to skip a dose to feel better temporarily. The importance of maintaining the dosing schedule exactly as prescribed must be emphasized. A calendar marked with the doses to take, the dates the drug is to be taken, and space to record each dose may help the patient. One course of therapy is generally prescribed at a time to avoid inadvertent overdosing that could be life threatening.

Following are key points about antineoplastic drugs the patient and family members should know.

- Take the drug only as directed on the prescription container. Unless otherwise indicated, take the drug on an empty stomach with water to enhance absorption. However, you should follow any specific directions, such as "take on an empty stomach" or "take at the same time each day"; they are extremely important.
- Never increase, decrease, or skip a dose unless advised to do so by your health care provider.
- If you experience any problems (adverse reactions), no matter how minor, contact your health care provider immediately.
- Follow all recommendations from your health care provider, such as increasing your fluid intake, eating, or avoiding certain foods.
- The effectiveness or action of the drug could be altered if you do not follow these directions. Additional recommendations, such as checking the mouth for sores, rinsing the mouth thoroughly after eating or drinking, or drinking extra fluids, help identify or minimize some of the effects these drugs have on the body.
- Keep all your appointments for chemotherapy. These drugs must be given at certain intervals to be effective.
- Do not take any nonprescription drug unless approved by your health care provider.

COMPLEMENTARY & ALTERNATIVE MEDICINE

Green Tea

The beneficial effects of green tea lie in the polyphenols, or flavonoids, that have antioxidant properties. Antioxidants are thought to play a major role in preventing disease (e.g., colon cancer) and reducing the effects of aging. Green tea polyphenols are powerful antioxidants. The polyphenols are thought to act by inhibiting the reactions of free radicals within the body thought to play a role in aging. The benefits of green tea include an overall sense of well-being, cancer prevention, dental health, and maintenance of heart and liver health. Green tea used as directed is safe and well tolerated. It contains as much as 50 mg of caffeine per cup. Decaffeinated green tea retains all of the polyphenol content. The recommended dosage is two to five cups per day. Standardized green tea extracts vary in strength, so dosages may need to be adjusted.

- Do not drink alcoholic beverages unless your health care provider approves.
- Always inform other physicians, dentists, and medical personnel of your therapy with this drug.
- Keep all appointments for the laboratory tests ordered by your health care provider. If unable to keep a laboratory appointment, notify your health care provider immediately.

> **FACT CHECK**
>
> **41-5** After receiving therapy with an antineoplastic drug, why would a patient also likely have a complete blood count and liver function tests?

Chapter Review

KEY POINTS

- Antineoplastic drugs may be given alone or in combination with other antineoplastic drugs. Although many antineoplastic drugs share a similar activity (i.e., they interfere in some way with cell division), their uses are not necessarily similar.
- Alkylating drugs interfere with the process of cell division of malignant and normal cells. The alkylating drugs may antagonize the effects of antigout drugs by increasing serum uric acid levels.
- The antineoplastic antibiotics include bleomycin and doxorubicin (Adriamycin). Contraindications of the antineoplastic antibiotics include a decrease in plasma digoxin levels, pulmonary toxicity, an additive bone marrow depressant effect, a decreased antibody response to live virus vaccines, and an increased risk of bleeding. Adverse reactions and contraindication are drug specific.
- The antimetabolites interfere with various metabolic functions of cells, thereby disrupting normal cell functions. These drugs are most effective in the treatment of rapidly dividing neoplastic cells. Antimetabolite drugs may antagonize the effects of antigout drugs by increasing the serum uric acid concentration. When the antimetabolites are administered with other antineoplastic drugs, bone marrow suppression is additive.
- The exact method of antineoplastic action of hormones is unclear. These drugs also appear to counteract the effect of male or female hormones in hormone-dependent tumors. Examples of hormones used as antineoplastic drugs include the antiandrogens (abiraterone acetate), progestins (megestrol acetate), estrogens (estramustine), and antiestrogens (tamoxifen).
- Mitotic inhibitors (antimitotics) interfere with or stop cell division. Examples of mitotic inhibitors include paclitaxel (Abaxane), vincristine (Vincasar PFS), and vinblastine. Additive bone marrow depressive effects occur when the mitotic inhibitor drugs are administered with other antineoplastic drugs or radiation therapy.
- Because the antineoplastic drugs affect cancer cells and rapidly proliferating normal cells (i.e., cells in the bone marrow, gastrointestinal tract, reproductive tract, and the hair follicles), adverse reactions occur as the result of the action on these cells. Adverse reactions common to many of the antineoplastic drugs include bone marrow suppression, nausea, vomiting, stomatitis, diarrhea, and hair loss.

CRITICAL THINKING CASE STUDY

Leukemia Treatment

Dennis, age 10 years, has leukemia and is to begin chemotherapy with chlorambucil (Leukeran). His parents are anxious about the treatment and have many questions.

1. One question they have involves potential adverse reactions to Leukeran. They should be told
   a. bone marrow depression, nausea, diarrhea, and alopecia are possible
   b. bone marrow depression, muscular twitching, and tremors are possible
   c. bone marrow depression, nausea, diarrhea, and cystitis are possible
   d. none of the above
2. Dennis's parents wonder if Dennis will lose his appetite. They should be told
   a. it is not uncommon for patients to experience alterations in their sense of taste
   b. small, frequent meals are usually better tolerated than two or three big meals
   c. it is important that Dennis eat foods with high nutritional quality
   d. all of the above
3. Dennis's parents are curious as to why antineoplastics are given in cycles. What should you tell them?

Review Questions

MULTIPLE CHOICE

1. Which of the following findings would be most indicative that the patient has thrombocytopenia?
   a. Nausea
   b. Blurred vision
   c. Headaches
   d. Easy bruising
2. Which of the following adverse reactions to the antineoplastic drugs is most likely to affect the patient's mental health and self-esteem?
   a. Hematuria
   b. Alopecia
   c. Nausea
   d. Diarrhea

3. When assessing a patient for leukopenia, the health care provider
   a. checks the patient every 8 hours for hematuria
   b. monitors the patient for fever, sore throat, and chills
   c. checks female patients for increased menstrual bleeding
   d. asks about frequency of skin rashes
4. Which of the following interventions would be most helpful for a patient with stomatitis?
   a. Avoiding foods that irritate the mouth
   b. Eating soft or liquid foods
   c. Avoiding alcohol and strong mouthwashes
   d. All of the above

MATCHING

_____ 5. busulfan   a. Leukeran
_____ 6. doxorubicin   b. Arimidex
_____ 7. methotrexate   c. Abraxane
_____ 8. mercaptopurine   d. Alkeran
_____ 9. vincristine   e. Lupron
_____ 10. chlorambucil   f. Purinethol
_____ 11. leuprolide   g. Rheumatrex
_____ 12. paclitaxel   h. Myleran
_____ 13. anastrazole   i. Adriamycin
_____ 14. melphalan   j. Vincasar PFS

TRUE OR FALSE

_____ 15. Antineoplastic antibiotics have anti-infective ability.
_____ 16. Swelling around the injection site is the most common symptom of extravasation.
_____ 17. Certain adverse reactions of antineoplastic drugs are more common or severe with higher doses.
_____ 18. To temporarily prevent nausea or vomiting, patients taking antineoplastic drugs at home may decrease or skip a dose.

FILL IN THE BLANKS

19. Antineoplastic drugs are _____ in patients with leukopenia, thrombocytopenia, or serious renal disease.
20. _____ _____ bind with DNA, thus preventing DNA replication.
21. In a patient receiving antineoplastic drugs for leukemia, _____ _____ _____ is a desirable adverse reaction.
22. The risk of ototoxicity increases when _____ is used concurrently with loop diuretics.

SHORT ANSWERS

23. Why is chemotherapy administered in repeated doses or cycles?
24. Why is chemotherapy administered when cells are dividing?
25. Goserelin is a hormone used to treat breast cancer. How is it administered?
26. How can nausea and vomiting be prevented in a patient receiving antineoplastic drug therapy?

Web Activities

1. Go to the National Comprehensive Cancer Network Web site (http://www.nccn.org) and click on "About NCCN." Read about the mission of NCCN, when it was established, and the types of organizations that comprise its membership.
2. Return to the starting page and click on "Network Hospitals." Select the member hospital nearest your area and read the opening section in its profile. Write a brief statement about the focus of that cancer center.

SUMMARY DRUG TABLE Antineoplastic Drugs (left, generic; right, trade)

Comprehensive Summary Drug Tables, including uses, adverses effects, dosages, and pregnancy classifications, are provided on the companion website, http://thePoint.lww.com/PharmacologyHP2e

Alkylating Agents	
altretamine (hexamethylmelamine) *al-tret'-a-meen*	Hexalen
bendamustine *ben-da-mus'-teen*	Treanda
busulfan *byoo-sul'-fan*	Busulfex, Myleran
carmustine (BCNU) *kar-mus'-teen*	IV: BiCNU Implant: Gliadel Wafer
chlorambucil *klor-am'-byoo-sill*	Leukeran
cyclophosphamide *sye-klo-foss'-fam- ide*	*generic*
dacarbazine (DTIC; imidazole carboxamide) *da-kar'-ba-zeen*	generic

Estrogens	
estramustine phosphate sodium *ess-tra-muss'-teen*	Emcyt
ifosfamide *eye-fos'-fam-ide*	Ifex, *generic*
lomustine (CCNU) *loe-mus'-teen*	CeeNU
mechlorethamine hydrochloride (nitrogen mustard; HN$_2$) *me-klor-eth'-a-meen*	Mustargen
melphalan (L-PAM; L-Phenylalanine Mustard; L-Sarcolysin) *mel'-fa-lan*	Alkeran, *generic*
streptozocin *strep-toe-zoe'-sin*	Zanosar
thiotepa (triethylenethiophosphoramide; TSPA: TESPA) *thye-oh-tep'-a*	*generic*

Anthracenedione	
mitoxantrone HCl *mye-toe-zan'-trone*	Novantrone, *generic*

Antimetabolites	
capecitabine *kap-ah-seat'-ah-bean*	Xeloda
cladribine *kla'-dri-bean*	Leustatin, *generic*
clofarabine *klo-fare'-a-been*	Clolar
cytarabine *sye-tare'-a-bean*	DepoCyt (liposome injection), *generic (injection)*
floxuridine *floks-yoor'-i-deen*	FUDR, generic
fludarabine *floo-dar'-a-bean*	Fludara, Oforta, *generic*
fluorouracil (5-FU) *flure-oh-yoor'-a-sill*	Topical: Carac, Efudex, Fluoroplex, *generic* Injection: Adrucil, *generic*

gemcitabine HCl *jem-site'-ah-ben*	Gemzar
mercaptopurine (6-mercaptopurine, 6-MP) *mer-kap-toe- pyoor'-een*	Purinethol, *generic*
methotrexate *meth-o-trex'-ate*	Rheumatrex, Trexall, *generic*
pemetrexed *pem-e-treks'-ed*	Alimta
pentostatin *pen'-toe-stat-in*	Nipent, *generic*
pralatrexate *pral-a-trex'-ate*	Folotyn
thioguanine (TG) *thye-oh-gwon'-een*	Tabloid

Mitotic Inhibitors (Antimitotic Agents)	
cabazitaxel *ca-baz-i-taks'-el*	Jevtana
docetaxel *dohs-eh-tax'-el*	Taxotere, *generic*
eribulin mesylate	Halaven
ixabepilone *ix-ab-ep'-i-lone*	Ixempra Kit
paclitaxel *pass-leh-tax'-ell*	Abraxane, *generic*
vinblastine sulfate (VLB) *vin-blas'-teen*	*generic*
vincristine sulfate (VCR; LCR) *vin-kris'-teen*	Vincasar PFS, *generic*
vinorelbine tartrate *vi-nor'-el-been*	Navelbine, *generic*

Antineoplastic Antibiotics	
bleomycin sulfate *blee-oh-my'-sin*	*generic*
dactinomycin *dak-ti-no-my'-sin*	Cosmegen, *generic*
daunorubicin citrate liposome *daw-noe-roo'-bi-sin*	DaunoXome
daunorubicin HCl *daw-noe-roo'-bi-sin*	Ceruibidine, *generic*
doxorubicin HCl *dox-oh-roo'-by-sin*	Adriamycin, *generic*
doxorubicin HCl liposomal (pegylated liposomal doxorubicin) *dox-oh-roo'-by-sin HCl lip-pah-sow'-mal*	Doxil
epirubicin HCl *ep-ee-roo'-by-sin*	Ellence, *generic*
idarubicin HCl *eye-da-roo'-by-sin*	Idamycin PFS, *generic*

SUMMARY DRUG TABLE Antineoplastic Drugs (continued)

mitomycin *mye-toe-my'-sin*	*generic*
valrubicin *val-roo'-by-sin*	Valstar
Biological Response Modifiers	
aldesleukin *al-dess-loo'-kin* (interleukin-2; IL-2)	Proleukin
BCG, intravesical	TheraCys, Tice BCG
denileukin diftitox *deh-nih-loo'- kin diff'-tih-tox*	Ontak
Cytoprotective Agents	
amifostine *am-ih-foss'-teen*	Ethyol, *generic*
dexrazoxane *dex-ray-zox'-ane*	Totect, Zinecard, *generic*
levoleucovorin calcium *lee-voe-loo-koe-vor'-in*	*Fusilev*
mesna *mes'-na*	Mesnex, *generic*
DNA Demethylation Agents	
azacitidine *ay-za-sye'-ti-deen*	Vidaza
decitabine *de-sye'-ta-been*	Dacogen
nelarabine *nel-ay'-re-been*	Arranon
DNA Topoisomerase Inhibitors	
irinotecan HCl *eh-rin-oh'-te-kan*	Camptosar, *generic*
topotecan HCl *toe-poh'-te-kan*	Hycamtin, *generic*
Enzymes	
asparaginase *a-spare'-a-gi-nase*	Elspar
pegaspargase (PEG-asparaginase) *peg-ass-par'-jase*	Oncaspar
Epipodophyllotoxins	
etoposide *e-toe-poe'-side*	Etopophos, Toposar, *generic*
teniposide (VM-26) *teh-nip-oh-side*	Vumon
Histone Deacetylase Inhibitors	
romidepsin *roe-mi-dep'-sin*	Istodax
vorinostat *vor-in'-oh-stat*	Zolinza
HORMONES	
Antiandrogens	
abiraterone acetate	Zytiga
bicalutamide *bye-cal-loo'-ta- mide*	Casodex, *generic*
flutamide *flu'-ta-mide*	*generic*

nilutamide *nah-loo'-ta-mide*	Nilandron
Progestins	
medroxyprogesterone acetate *me-drox'-ee-proe- jess'-te-rone*	Depo-Provera
megestrol acetate *me-jess'-trole*	*generic*
Antiestrogens	
fulvestrant *fool-ves'-trant*	Faslodex
tamoxifen citrate *|ta-mox'-i-fen*	*generic*
toremifene citrate *tore-em'-ah-feen*	Fareston
Gonadotropin-Releasing Hormone Analogues	
goserelin acetate *goe'-se-rel-in*	Zoladex
histrelin acetate	Supprelin LA, Vantas
leuprolide acetate *loo-proe'-lide*	Eligard, Lupron, Lupron Depot, Lupron Depot-Ped, *generic*
triptorelin pamoate *trip-toe-rell'-in*	Trelstar Depot, Trelstar Depot Mixject, Trelstar LA, Trelstar LA Mixject, Trelstar Mixject
Aromatase Inhibitors	
anastrazole *|an-ahs'-troh-zol*	Arimidex, *generic*
exemestane *ex-ah'-mess-tane*	Aromasin, *generic*
letrozole *le'-tro-zol*	Femara, *generic*
Imidazotetrazine Derivatives	
temozolomide *te-moe-zoe'-loe-mide*	Temodar
Kinase Inhibitors	
dasatinib *da-sa'-ti-nib*	Sprycel
erlotinib *er-loe'-tye-nib*	Tarceva
everolimus *e-ver-oh'-li-mus*	Afinitor, Zortress
gefitinib *ge-fi'-tye-nib*	Iressa
imatinib mesylate *eh-mat'-eh-nib*	Gleevec
lapatinib *la-pa-ti'-nib*	Tykerb
nilotinib *nye-loe'-ti-nib*	Tasigna
pazopanib *paz-oh'-pa-nib*	Votrient
sorafenib *sor-af'-e-nib*	NexAVAR
sunitinib *su-nit'-e-nib*	Sutent

(continued)

SUMMARY DRUG TABLE　Antineoplastic Drugs (continued)

HORMONES	
Kinase Inhibitors *(continued)*	
temsirolimus *tem-sir-oh'-li-mus*	Torisel
vandetanib	*generic*
Methylhydrazine Derivatives	
procarbazine HCl *proe-kar'-ba-zeen*	Matulane
Monoclonal Antibodies	
alemtuzumab *ay-lem-tuh'-zoo-mab*	Campath
bevacizumab *be-vuh-siz'-un-mab*	Avastin
cetuximab *se-tuk'-see-mab*	Erbitux
ibritumomab tiuxetan *ib-ri-tu'-moe-mab tie-ux-eh'-tan*	Zevalin
ipilimumab ofatumumab *oh-fa-toom'-yoo-mab*	Yervoy Arzerra
panitumumab *pan-i-toom'-yoo-mab*	Vectibix
rituximab *ri-tuk'-si-mab*	Rituxan
tositumomab and iodine ¹³¹I-tositumomab *toe-si-tyoo'-mo-mab*	Bexxar, *generic*
trastuzumab *trass-to-zoo'-mab*	Herceptin
Platinum Coordination Complex	
carboplatin *kar'-boe-pla-tin*	*generic*
cisplatin (CDDP) *sis'-pla-tin*	*generic*
oxaloplatin *ox-al'-i-pla-tin*	Eloxatin, *generic*

Proteasome Inhibitors	
bortezomib *bore-tez'-oh-mib*	Velcade
Radiopharmaceuticals	
samarium SM 153 lexidronam	Quadramet
sodium iodide I 131	Hicon, *generic*
strontium-89 chloride	Metastron
Retinoids	
tretinoin *tret'-i- noyn*	Vesanoid, *generic*
Rexinoids	
bexarotene *bex-air'-oh-teen*	Targretin
Substituted Ureas	
hydroxyurea *hye-drox-ee- yoor-ee'-ah*	Droxia, Hydrea, *generic*
Unclassified Antineoplastics	
arsenic trioxide *ar'-se-nik tri-oks'-id*	Trisenox
porfimer sodium *poor-fi'-mer*	Photofrin
mitotane *mye'-toe-tane*	Lysodren
sipuleucel-T *si-pu-loo'-sel*	Provenge
sterile talc powder	Sclerosol Intrapleural, *generic*

DRUGS THAT AFFECT OTHER BODY SYSTEMS

XI

42

Musculoskeletal System Drugs

CHAPTER OBJECTIVES

On completion of this chapter, students will be able to:

1 Define the chapter's key terms.

2 Identify and describe common musculoskeletal disorders.

3 Describe the general drug actions, uses, adverse reactions, contraindications, precautions, and interactions of drugs that affect the musculoskeletal system.

4 Discuss important points to keep in mind when educating the patient or family members about the use of drugs that affect the musculoskeletal system.

KEY TERMS

chrysiasis—gray to blue pigmentation of the skin that may occur from gold deposits in tissues

corticosteroids—hormones secreted from the adrenal cortex that contain potent anti-inflammatory action

gout—a form of arthritis in which uric acid accumulates in increased amounts in the blood and often is deposited in the joints

musculoskeletal—the bone and muscular structure of the body

osteoarthritis—a noninflammatory joint disease resulting in degeneration of the articular cartilage and changes in the synovial membrane

rheumatoid arthritis—a chronic disease characterized by inflammatory changes within the body's connective tissue

CHAPTER OVERVIEW

Drug classes covered in this chapter are:

- Bisphosphonates
- Skeletal muscle relaxants
- Corticosteroids
- Drugs used for gout
- Gold compounds
- Miscellaneous drugs

Drugs by classification are listed on page 460.

thePOINT RESOURCES

- Comprehensive Summary Drug Tables
- Animations: Muscle Contraction
- Interactive Practice and Review
- Monographs of Most Commonly Prescribed Drugs

A variety of drugs are used in the treatment of **muscu-loskeletal** (bone and muscle) disorders. Examples of the musculoskeletal disorders discussed in this chapter include osteoarthritis (Fig. 42-1), **rheumatoid arthritis,** gout, and Paget disease. These and other musculoskeletal disorders are described in Table 42-1. The drug selected is based on the musculoskeletal disorder being treated, the severity of the disorder, and the patient's positive or negative response to past therapy. For example, early cases of rheumatoid arthritis (a chronic disease characterized by inflammatory changes within the body's connective tissue) may respond well to the salicylates, whereas advanced rheumatoid arthritis not responding to other drug therapies may require the use of one of the gold compounds.

The salicylates and nonsteroidal anti-inflammatory drugs are important in the treatment of arthritic conditions. For example, the salicylates and nonsteroidal anti-inflammatory drugs are used in the treatment of rheumatoid arthritis and **osteoarthritis** (a noninflammatory joint disease resulting in degeneration of the articular cartilage and changes in the synovial membrane), as well as relief of pain or discomfort resulting from musculoskeletal injuries such as sprains. Chapter 8 discusses these drugs in detail.

Bisphosphonates

The bisphosphonates are used to treat musculoskeletal disorders such as osteoporosis and Paget disease. This chapter discusses the use of these drugs in the treatment of osteoporosis.

Actions of Bisphosphonates

The bisphosphonates act primarily on the bone by inhibiting normal and abnormal bone resorption. This results in increased bone mineral density, reversing the progression of osteoporosis.

Uses of Bisphosphonates

The bisphosphonates are used to treat osteoporosis in postmenopausal women, Paget disease of the bone, and postoperative treatment after total hip replacement (etidronate).

Adverse Reactions of Bisphosphonates

Adverse reactions with the bisphosphonates include nausea, diarrhea, increased or recurrent bone pain, headache, dyspepsia, acid regurgitation, dysphagia, and abdominal pain. An analgesic may be used for headache. The health care provider must be notified of adverse reactions such as the return of bone pain or severe diarrhea.

Contraindications, Precautions, and Interactions of Bisphosphonates

- All of the bisphosphonates are contraindicated in patients with known hypersensitivity.
- Alendronate and risedronate are contraindicated in patients with hypocalcemia.
- These drugs are contraindicated in patients with significant renal impairment.
- Concurrent use of these drugs with hormone replacement therapy is not recommended.
- These drugs are used cautiously in patients with gastrointestinal disorders or renal function impairment and during pregnancy and lactation.
- When administered with ranitidine, alendronate bioavailability is increased.
- When calcium supplements or antacids are administered with risedronate or alendronate, absorption of the bisphosphonates is decreased.
- In addition, risedronate absorption is inhibited when the drug is administered with magnesium and aluminum.
- There is an increased risk of gastrointestinal effects when a bisphosphonate is administered with aspirin.

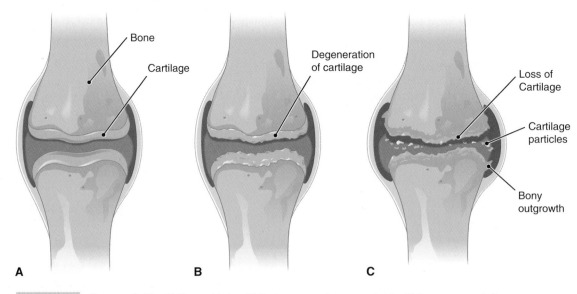

FIGURE 42-1   Osteoarthritis. (A) Normal joint. (B) Early stage of osteoarthritis. (C) Late stage of disease.

TABLE 42-1 Selected Musculoskeletal Disorders

Disorder	Description
Synovitis	Synovitis is an inflammation of the synovial membrane of a joint resulting in pain, swelling, and inflammation. It occurs in disorders such as rheumatic fever, rheumatoid arthritis, and gout.
Arthritis	Arthritis is the inflammation of a joint. The term is frequently used to refer to any disease involving pain or stiffness of the musculoskeletal system.
Osteoarthritis or degenerative joint disease (DJD)	Osteoarthritis is a noninflammatory degenerative joint disease marked by degeneration of the articular cartilage, changes in the synovial membrane, and hypertrophy of the bone at the margins.
Rheumatoid arthritis (RA)	RA is a chronic systemic disease that produces inflammatory changes throughout the connective tissue in the body. It affects joints and other organ systems of the body. Destruction of articular cartilage occurs, affecting joint structure and mobility. RA primarily affects individuals between 20 and 40 y/o.
Gout	Gout is a form of arthritis in which uric acid accumulates in increased amounts in the blood and often is deposited in the joints. The deposit or collection of urate crystals in the joints causes the symptoms (pain, redness, swelling, joint deformity).
Osteoporosis	Osteoporosis is a loss of bone density occurring when the loss of bone substance exceeds the rate of bone formation. Bones become porous, brittle, and fragile. Compression fractures of the vertebrae are common. This disorder occurs most often in postmenopausal women but can occur in men as well.
Paget disease (osteitis deformans)	Paget disease is a chronic bone disorder characterized by abnormal bone remodeling. The disease disrupts the growth of new bone tissue causing the bone to thicken and become soft. This weakens the bone, which increases susceptibility of fracture even with slight trauma or collapse of the bone (e.g., the vertebrae).
Multiple sclerosis	Multiple sclerosis is a common demyelinating disorder of the CNS, causing patches of sclerosis (plaques), in the brain and spinal cord; typical symptoms include visual loss, diplopia, nystagmus, dysarthria, weakness, paresthesias, bladder abnormalities, and mood alterations.

Patient Management Issues with Bisphosphonates

The health care provider should be notified if the patient experiences chest pain, heartburn, or trouble or pain when swallowing. Lifestyle modifications that will help prevent or treat osteoporosis include stopping smoking, reducing the use of alcohol, exercising regularly, and eating a balanced diet.

Box 42-1 outlines additional general management considerations for patients receiving musculoskeletal system drugs.

Educating the Patient and Family about Bisphosphonates

Following are key points about bisphosphonates that the patient and family members should know.

Alendronate and risedronate:

- These drugs are taken with 6 to 8 oz of water first thing in the morning.
- Do not lie down for at least 30 minutes after taking the drug and wait at least 30 minutes before taking any other food or drink.
- Do not take with mineral water, coffee, tea, or juice.
- Take the drugs exactly as prescribed.
- Your health care provider may prescribe alendronate as a once-weekly dose or to be taken daily. Risedronate is taken daily.
- Take supplemental calcium and vitamin D if dietary intake is inadequate. Take all medications, including vita-

min and mineral supplements, at a different time of the day to prevent interference with absorption of the drug.

FACT CHECK

42-1 How do bisphosphonates act?

Skeletal Muscle Relaxants

Actions of Skeletal Muscle Relaxants

The mode of action of many skeletal muscle relaxants, such as carisoprodol (Soma), baclofen (Lioresal), and chlorzoxazone (Parafon Forte DSC), is not clearly understood. Many of these drugs do not directly relax skeletal muscles, but their ability to relieve acute painful musculoskeletal conditions may be attributable to their sedative action. Cyclobenzaprine (Flexeril) appears to have an effect on muscle tone, thus reducing muscle spasm.

The exact mode of action of diazepam (Valium), an antianxiety drug (see Chapter 7), in the relief of painful musculoskeletal conditions is unknown. The drug does have a sedative action, which may account for some of its ability to relieve muscle spasm and pain.

Uses of Skeletal Muscle Relaxants

Skeletal muscle relaxants are used in various acute, painful musculoskeletal conditions, such as muscle strains and back pain.

BOX 42-1

Drug Therapy for Musculoskeletal Disorders: General Considerations

- Periodic evaluation is an important part of therapy for musculoskeletal disorders. With some disorders such as acute gout, the patient can be expected to respond to therapy in hours, and the joints are inspected every 1 to 2 hours to identify a response or nonresponse to therapy. At this time, the patient is questioned regarding the relief of pain, as well as adverse drug reactions. In other disorders, response is gradual and may take days, weeks, and even months of treatment. Depending on the drug and the disorder, the evaluation of therapy may be daily or weekly.
- Some of these drugs are toxic. The patient is closely observed for adverse reactions. Should any one or more adverse reactions occur, the health care provider is notified before the next dose is due.
- A patient with a musculoskeletal disorder may be in acute pain or have long-standing mild to moderate pain, which can be just as difficult to tolerate as severe pain. Along with pain, there may be skeletal deformities, such as the joint deformities seen with advanced rheumatoid arthritis (Fig. 42-2). For many musculoskeletal conditions, drug therapy is a major treatment modality. Therapy with these drugs may keep the disorder under control (e.g., therapy for gout), improve the patient's ability to perform the activities of daily living, or make the pain and discomfort tolerable.
- Patients with an arthritis disorder may experience much pain or discomfort and may require assistance with activities, such as walking, eating, and grooming. Patients with osteoporosis may require a brace or corset when out of bed.
- Patients with a musculoskeletal disorder often have anxiety related to the symptoms and the chronicity of their disorder. In addition to physical care, these patients often require emotional support, especially when a disorder is disabling and chronic. It is explained to the patient that therapy may take weeks or longer before any benefit is noted.

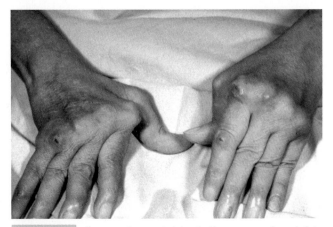

FIGURE 42-2 Severe rheumatoid arthritis may produce joint deformities.

Adverse Reactions of Skeletal Muscle Relaxants

Drowsiness is the most common reaction occurring with the use of skeletal muscle relaxants. Some of the adverse reactions that may occur with the administration of diazepam include drowsiness, sedation, sleepiness, lethargy, constipation or diarrhea, bradycardia or tachycardia, and rash.

Because of the risk of injury caused by drowsiness, the patient is carefully monitored before being allowed to walk or perform self-care activities alone. If drowsiness does occur, then assistance with activities is necessary. If drowsiness is severe, then the health care provider should be notified before the next dose is due.

Contraindications, Precautions, and Interactions of Skeletal Muscle Relaxants

All of the skeletal muscle relaxants are contraindicated in patients with known hypersensitivity. See Chapter 7 for information on contraindications, precautions, and interactions of diazepam.

- Baclofen is contraindicated in skeletal muscle spasms caused by rheumatic disorders.
- Carisoprodol is contraindicated in patients with a known hypersensitivity to meprobamate.
- Cyclobenzaprine is contraindicated in patients with a recent myocardial infarction, cardiac conduction disorders, and hyperthyroidism. In addition, cyclobenzaprine is contraindicated within 14 days of the administration of a monoamine oxidase inhibitor.
- Oral dantrolene is contraindicated in patients with active hepatic disease and muscle spasm caused by rheumatic disorders and during lactation.
- The skeletal muscle relaxants are used with caution in patients with a history of cerebrovascular accident, cerebral palsy, Parkinsonism, or seizure disorders and lactation.
- Carisoprodol is used with caution in patients with severe liver or kidney disease and during lactation.
- Cyclobenzaprine is used cautiously in patients with cardiovascular disease and during and lactation.
- An increased central nervous system depressant effect occurs when a skeletal muscle relaxant is administered with another central nervous system depressant, such as alcohol, antihistamines, opiates, and sedatives.
- There is an additive anticholinergic effect when cyclobenzaprine is administered with another drug with anticholinergic effects (e.g., antihistamines, antidepressants, atropine, haloperidol).

Patient Management Issues with Skeletal Muscle Relaxants

Because these medications cause drowsiness, the patient should not drive or operate heavy machinery. Patients should not combine skeletal muscle relaxants with alcohol or other CNS depressants.

Educating the Patient and Family about Skeletal Muscle Relaxants

Following are key points about skeletal muscle relaxants that the patient and family members should know.

- This drug may cause drowsiness. Do not drive or perform other hazardous tasks if you feel drowsy.
- This drug is for short-term use. Do not use the drug for longer than 2 to 3 weeks.
- Avoid alcohol or other depressants while taking this drug.

FACT CHECK

42-2   Skeletal muscle relaxants are used with caution in which patients?

Corticosteroids

Actions of Corticosteroids

Corticosteroids are hormones secreted from the adrenal cortex. These hormones arise from the cortex of the adrenal gland and are made from the crystalline steroid alcohol cholesterol. Synthetic forms of the natural adrenal cortical hormones are available. The potent anti-inflammatory action of the corticosteroids makes these drugs useful in the treatment of many types of musculoskeletal disorders. The corticosteroids are discussed in Chapter 31.

Uses of Corticosteroids

The corticosteroids may be used to treat rheumatic disorders such as ankylosing spondylitis, rheumatoid arthritis, gout, bursitis (inflammation of the bursa, usually the bursa of the shoulder), and osteoarthritis.

Adverse Reactions of Corticosteroids

Corticosteroids may be given in high doses for some arthritic disorders. Many adverse reactions are associated with high-dose and long-term corticosteroid therapy. A comprehensive list of adverse reactions is provided along with contraindications, precautions, and interactions of the corticosteroids in Chapter 31.

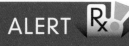

ALERT

Corticosteroids
When corticosteroid use is discontinued, the dosage must be tapered gradually over several days. If high dosages have been given, then it may take a week or more to taper the dosage.

Patient Management Issues with Corticosteroids

Details about patient management issues with corticosteroids are addressed in Chapter 31.

Educating the Patient and Family about Corticosteroids

Key points about corticosteroid use that the patient and family members should know are covered in Chapter 31.

FACT CHECK

42-3   What are corticosteroids used to treat?

Drugs Used for Gout

Gout is a form of arthritis in which uric acid accumulates in increased amounts in the blood and often is deposited in the joints. The deposit or collection of urate crystals in the joints causes the symptoms (pain, redness, swelling, joint deformity) of gout (Fig. 42-3).

Actions of Drugs Used for Gout

Allopurinol (Zyloprim) reduces the production of uric acid crystals in the joints. This probably accounts for its ability to relieve the severe pain of acute gout. Colchicine has no effect on uric acid metabolism.

In those with gout, the serum uric acid level is usually elevated. Probenecid works in the same manner and may be given alone or with colchicine as combination therapy when the patient has frequent, recurrent attacks of gout. Probenecid also has been used to prolong the plasma levels of the penicillins and cephalosporins. Febuxostat is a xanthine derivative, like allopurinol, which decreases serum uric acid concentrations. Pegloticase is a recombinant uricase and decreases serum uric acid concentrations by catalyzing the oxidation of uric acid to

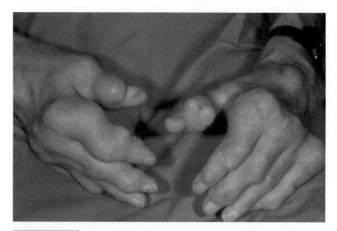

FIGURE 42-3   Gout often produces swollen joints.

allantoin. Allantoin is a metabolite of uric acid that is readily eliminated by the kidneys and has no activity.

Uses of Drugs for Gout

Drugs indicated for treatment of gout may be used to manage acute attacks of gout or in preventing acute attacks of gout (prophylaxis).

Adverse Reactions of Drugs for Gout

One adverse reaction associated with allopurinol is skin rash, which in some cases has been followed by serious hypersensitivity reactions such as exfoliative dermatitis and Stevens-Johnson syndrome (see Chapter 35 for a description of this syndrome). Other adverse reactions include nausea, vomiting, diarrhea, abdominal pain, and hematologic changes.

Colchicine administration may result in nausea, vomiting, diarrhea, abdominal pain, and bone marrow depression. When this drug is given to patients with an acute attack of gout, the health care provider may order the drug given at frequent intervals until gastrointestinal symptoms occur. Probenecid administration may cause headache, gastrointestinal symptoms, urinary frequency, and hypersensitivity reactions.

Contraindications, Precautions, and Interactions of Drugs for Gout

All of the drugs used for gout are contraindicated in patients with known hypersensitivity.

- Probenecid is contraindicated in patients with blood dyscrasias or uric acid kidney stones and in children younger than 2 years.
- Colchicine is contraindicated in patients with serious gastrointestinal, renal, hepatic, or cardiac disorders and those with blood dyscrasias.
- Allopurinol is used cautiously in patients with liver and renal impairment and during lactation.
- Probenecid is used cautiously in patients with renal impairment, previous hypersensitivity to sulfa drugs, and peptic ulcer disease.
- Colchicine is used with caution in older adults and during lactation.
- There is an increased incidence of skin rash when allopurinol and ampicillin are administered concurrently.
- Concurrent administration of allopurinol and theophylline increases the risk of theophylline toxicity.
- When angiotensin-converting enzyme inhibitors or the thiazide diuretics are administered with allopurinol, there is an increased risk of hypersensitivity reactions.
- Administration of allopurinol with aluminum salts may decrease the effectiveness of allopurinol.
- Salicylates antagonize probenecid's uricosuric action.
- Concurrent administration of probenecid increases the effects of acyclovir, barbiturates, benzodiazepines, dapsone, methotrexate, nonsteroidal anti-inflammatory drugs, rifampin, and the sulfonamides.

Patient Management Issues with Drugs for Gout

A liberal fluid intake is encouraged, and the patient's intake and output should be measured. The daily urine output should be at least 2 L. An increased urinary output is necessary to excrete the urates (uric acid) and prevent uric acid stone formation in the genitourinary tract. Allopurinol should be taken with food or milk.

Educating the Patient and Family about Drugs for Gout

Following are key points about drugs for gout that the patient and family members should know.

- Drink at least 10 glasses of water per day until the acute attack has subsided.
- Take this drug with food to minimize gastrointestinal upset.
- If you feel drowsy, do not drive or perform other hazardous tasks.
- Acute gout: Notify your health care provider if your pain is not relieved in a few days.
- Colchicine for acute gout: Take this drug at the intervals prescribed by your health care provider, and stop taking the drug when the pain is relieved or if diarrhea or vomiting occurs. If the pain is not relieved in approximately 12 hours, notify your health care provider.
- Allopurinol: Notify your health care provider if a skin rash occurs, if urination is painful or contains blood, the eyes become irritated, or there is swelling of the lips or mouth.
- Colchicine: Notify your health care provider if skin rash, sore throat, fever, unusual bleeding or bruising, unusual fatigue, or weakness occurs.

> ## FACT CHECK
> 42-4 How do drugs used for gout act?

Gold Compounds

Gold suppresses or prevents, but does not cure, arthritis and synovitis (inflammation of the joints). The therapeutic effects from gold compounds occur slowly. Early improvement is often limited to reduction in morning stiffness. The full effects of gold therapy do not occur for 6 to 8 weeks or in some cases after 6 months of therapy.

Actions of Gold Compounds

The exact mechanism of action of the gold compounds (e.g., gold sodium thiomalate, aurothioglucose, and auranofin) in the suppression or prevention of inflammation is unknown. Gold compounds decrease synovial inflammation and retard cartilage and bone destruction. Gold decreases the concentration of rheumatoid factor and immunoglobulins.

Uses of Gold Compounds

Gold compounds are used to treat active juvenile and adult rheumatoid arthritis not controlled by other anti-inflammatory drugs. When cartilage and bone damage has already occurred, however, gold cannot reverse structural changes to the joints. The greatest benefit appears to occur in patients in the early stages of disease.

Adverse Reactions of Gold Compounds

Adverse reactions to the gold compounds may occur any time during therapy, as well as many months after therapy has been discontinued. Dermatitis (inflammation of the skin) and stomatitis (inflammation of mucosa of the mouth, gums, and possibly the tongue) are the most common adverse reactions. Pruritus (itching) often occurs before the skin eruption becomes apparent. Photosensitivity reactions (exaggerated sunburn reaction when the skin is exposed to sunlight or ultraviolet light) may also occur. **Chrysiasis** (gray to blue pigmentation of the skin) may occur and is caused by gold deposits in tissues. Gold dermatitis is exacerbated by exposure to sunlight.

Contraindications, Precautions, and Interactions of Gold Compounds

- The gold compounds are contraindicated in patients with a known hypersensitivity.
- Parenteral administration is contraindicated in patients with uncontrolled diabetes, hepatic disease, uncontrolled hypertension, uncontrolled congestive heart failure, systemic lupus erythematosus, or blood dyscrasias and in those having recent radiotherapy.
- Oral administration is contraindicated in patients with necrotizing enterocolitis, pulmonary fibrosis, or hematologic disorders and during lactation.
- The gold compounds are used cautiously in patients with a history of hypersensitivity to other drugs, previous kidney or liver disease, diabetes, or hypertension.
- Concurrent administration of auranofin with phenytoin may increase phenytoin blood levels.

Patient Management Issues with Gold Compounds

The patient is closely observed for evidence of dermatitis. Itching may occur before a skin reaction and should be

CONSIDERATIONS | Older adults

LIFESPAN

Gold Compounds
Gold compounds are given cautiously to older adults. Tolerance for gold therapy decreases with advancing age.

ALERT Rx

Symptoms of Thrombocytopenia
If the patient experiences signs and symptoms of thrombocytopenia (e.g., easy bruising, bleeding gums, epistaxis, melena) when taking gold compounds, then the health care provider should be notified immediately.

reported to the health care provider immediately. If itching occurs, then a soothing lotion or an antiseptic cream may be used. The environment should be kept free of irritants that aggravate itching, such as rough fabrics, excessive warmth, or excessive dryness.

The patient's mouth should be inspected daily for ulceration of mucous membranes. A metallic taste may occur before stomatitis becomes evident. The patient should inform the health care provider if a metallic taste occurs. Good oral care is necessary. Teeth should be brushed after each meal and the mouth rinsed with plain water to remove food particles. Mouthwash may also be used, but excessive use may result in oral infections caused by the destruction of the normal bacteria present in the mouth.

Educating the Patient and Family about Gold Compounds

Following are key points about gold compounds that the patient and family members should know.

- Toxic reactions are possible when taking gold compounds. Report adverse reactions to your health care provider as soon as possible.
- Contact your health care provider if you note a metallic taste.
- Arthralgia (pain in the joints) may occur for 1 to 2 days after the parenteral form is given.
- Chrysiasis (gray to blue pigmentation of the skin) may occur, especially on areas exposed to sunlight. Avoid exposure to sunlight or ultraviolet light.

FACT CHECK
42-5 What are gold compounds used to treat?

Miscellaneous Drugs

The miscellaneous drugs are used to treat a variety of musculoskeletal disorders. Penicillamine, methotrexate, and hydroxychloroquine are used to treat rheumatoid arthritis in patients who have had an insufficient therapeutic response to or are intolerant of other antirheumatic drugs such as the salicylates and nonsteroidal anti-inflammatory drugs. Immunomodulators are used to treat rheumatoid arthritis and multiple sclerosis.

Actions of Miscellaneous Drugs

The mechanisms of action of penicillamine, methotrexate, and hydroxychloroquine in the treatment of rheumatoid arthritis are unknown.

Uses of Miscellaneous Drugs

Penicillamine, methotrexate, and hydroxychloroquine are used in the treatment of rheumatoid arthritis. Methotrexate is reserved for severe, disabling disease that is not responsive to other treatment.

Adverse Reactions of Miscellaneous Drugs

Hydroxychloroquine may result in irritability, nervousness, anorexia, nausea, vomiting, and diarrhea. This drug also may have adverse effects on the eye, including blurred vision, corneal edema, halos around lights, and retinal damage. Hematologic effects, such as aplastic anemia and leukopenia, may also occur.

The adverse reactions seen with penicillamine include pruritus, rash, anorexia, nausea, vomiting, epigastric pain, bone marrow depression, proteinuria, hematuria, increased skin friability, and tinnitus. Penicillamine may cause a severe toxic reaction.

Methotrexate is a potentially toxic drug that is also used in the treatment of malignancies and psoriasis. Nausea, vomiting, a decreased platelet count, leukopenia (decreased white blood cell count), stomatitis (inflammation of the oral cavity), rash, pruritus, dermatitis, diarrhea, alopecia (loss of hair), and diarrhea may occur with the administration of this drug.

Contraindications, Precautions, and Interactions of Miscellaneous Drugs

- These drugs are contraindicated in patients with known hypersensitivity.
- Hydroxychloroquine is contraindicated in patients with porphyria (a group of serious inherited disorders affecting the bone marrow or the liver), psoriasis (chronic skin disorder), and retinal disease (may cause irreversible retinal damage).
- Methotrexate is contraindicated during pregnancy because it is a pregnancy category X drug and may cause birth defects in the developing fetus.
- Penicillamine is contraindicated in patients with a history of allergy to penicillin.
- Hydroxychloroquine is used cautiously in patients with hepatic disease or alcoholism and during lactation.
- Methotrexate is used cautiously in patients with renal impairment, women of childbearing age, and older adults or individuals who are chronically ill or debilitated.
- Penicillamine is used with extreme caution during lactation.
- There is an increased risk of toxicity of methotrexate when administered with a nonsteroidal anti-inflammatory drug, salicylate, oral antidiabetic drug, phenytoin, tetracycline, or probenecid.
- There is an additive bone marrow depressant effect when administered with other drugs known to depress the bone marrow or with radiation therapy.
- There is an increased risk for nephrotoxicity when methotrexate is administered with another drug that causes nephrotoxicity.
- When penicillamine is administered with digoxin, decreased blood levels of digoxin may occur.
- There is a decreased absorption of penicillamine when the drug is administered with food, iron preparations, and antacids.

Patient Management Issues with Miscellaneous Drugs

Patients taking hydroxychloroquine are closely observed for adverse reactions such as skin rash, fever, cough, easy bruising or unusual bleeding, or symptoms of sore throat, visual changes, mood changes, loss of hair, tinnitus, or hearing loss. Any adverse reactions should be reported immediately. Particularly important are visual changes because irreversible retinal damage may occur. The patient is observed for signs of easy bruising and infection, which may indicate bone marrow depression, an adverse reaction related to the platelets and white blood cells. A decreased platelet count may cause the patient to bleed easily. The mouth is inspected daily for signs of inflammation or ulceration. Stools are also inspected for diarrhea or signs of gastrointestinal bleeding.

Methotrexate is potentially toxic. Therefore, development of adverse reactions, such as thrombocytopenia and leukopenia, are closely monitored. Hematology, liver, and renal function studies are monitored every 1 to 3 months with methotrexate therapy. The health care provider is notified of abnormal hematology, liver function, or kidney function findings. All adverse reactions or suspected adverse reactions should immediately be reported to the health care provider.

Educating the Patient and Family about Miscellaneous Drugs

Following are key points about miscellaneous drugs that the patient and family members should know.

Hydroxychloroquine

- Take hydroxychloroquine with food or milk.
- Contact your health care provider immediately if you experience any of the following: hearing or visual changes, skin rash or severe itching, hair loss, change in the color of the hair (bleaching), changes in the color of the skin, easy bruising or bleeding, fever, sore throat, muscle weakness, or mood changes. It may be several weeks before symptoms are relieved.

Methotrexate

- Take methotrexate exactly as directed. If a weekly dose is prescribed, then use a calendar or some other method to take the drug on the same day each week. Never increase the prescribed dose of this drug. Mistaken daily use has led to fatal toxicity.
- Notify your health care provider immediately if you experience any of the following: sore mouth, sores in the mouth, diarrhea, fever, sore throat, easy bruising, rash, itching, or nausea and vomiting.

- Women of childbearing age should use an effective contraceptive during therapy with methotrexate and for 8 weeks after therapy.

Penicillamine

- Your health care provider will explain the treatment regimen and adverse reactions before therapy is started.
- You must know which toxic reactions require contacting your health care provider immediately.
- Take penicillamine on an empty stomach, 1 hour before or 2 hours after a meal. If other drugs are prescribed, then penicillamine is taken 1 hour apart from any other drug.
- Observe skin areas over the elbows, shoulders, and buttocks for evidence of bruising, bleeding, or break in the skin (delayed wound healing may occur). If these occur, then do not self-treat the problem, but notify your health care provider immediately.
- An alteration in taste perception may occur. Taste perception should return to normal within 2 to 3 months.

KEY CONCEPTS

42-1   Providing Patient Information

The information given a patient and family members depends on the type and severity of the musculoskeletal disorder. It must be carefully explained to the patient that treatment for the disorder includes drug therapy, as well as other medical management, such as diet, exercise, limitations or nonlimitations of activity, and periodic physical therapy treatments. Patients need to understand the importance of not taking any nonprescription drugs unless the health care provider has approved their use.

FACT CHECK

42-6   Why should women of childbearing age use an effective contraceptive during therapy with methotrexate and for 8 weeks afterward?

COMPLEMENTARY & ALTERNATIVE MEDICINE

Glucosamine and Chondroitin

Both glucosamine and chondroitin are used, in combination or alone, to treat arthritis, particularly osteoarthritis. Chondroitin acts as the flexible connecting matrix between the protein filaments in cartilage. Chondroitin can be produced in the laboratory or be derived from natural sources (e.g., shark cartilage). Some studies suggest that if chondroitin sulfate is available to the cell matrix, synthesis of the matrix can occur. For this reason, it is used to treat arthritis. Although there is not much information on chondroitin's long-term effects, it is generally not considered to be harmful.

Glucosamine is found in mucopolysaccharides, mucoproteins, and chitin. Chitin is found in various marine invertebrates and other lower animals and members of the plant family. In osteoarthritis, there is a progressive degeneration of cartilage glycosaminoglycans. Oral glucosamine theoretically provides a building block for regeneration of damaged cartilage. The absorption of oral glucosamine is 90% to 98%, making it widely accepted for use. However, chondroitin molecules are very large (50–300 times larger than glucosamine), and only 0% to 13% of chondroitin is absorbed. These larger molecules may not be undelivered to cartilage cells. Glucosamine is generally well tolerated, and no adverse reactions have been reported with its use.

Chapter Review

KEY POINTS

- The bisphosphonates are used to treat musculoskeletal disorders, such as osteoporosis and Paget disease, and act primarily on the bone by inhibiting normal and abnormal bone resorption, thereby increasing bone density. These drugs are used to treat osteoporosis in postmenopausal women, Paget disease of the bone, and postoperative treatment after total hip replacement (etidronate). Adverse reactions include nausea, diarrhea, increased or recurrent bone pain, headache, dyspepsia, acid regurgitation, dysphagia, and abdominal pain.
- Skeletal muscle relaxants are used in various acute, painful musculoskeletal conditions, such as muscle strains and back pain. Drowsiness is the most common reaction seen with the use of skeletal muscle relaxants. There is an increased central nervous system depressant effect when the skeletal muscle relaxants are administered with another central nervous system depressant such as alcohol, antihistamines, opiates, and sedatives.
- Corticosteroids are hormones secreted from the adrenal cortex. The potent anti-inflammatory action of corticosteroids makes these drugs useful in the treatment of many types of musculoskeletal disorders. Corticosteroids may be given in high doses for some arthritic disorders, and many adverse reactions are associated with high-dose and long-term corticosteroid therapy.
- Drugs may be used to manage acute attacks of gout or prevent acute attacks (prophylaxis). Allopurinol is used to reduce the production of uric acid, and colchicine is used to reduce inflammation. Probenecid increases the

excretion of uric acid by the kidneys. Probenecid may be given alone or with colchicine as combination therapy for frequent, recurrent attacks of gout. Adverse reactions to these drugs include skin rash, nausea, vomiting, diarrhea, and abdominal pain.

- Gold suppresses or prevents, but does not cure, arthritis and synovitis (inflammation of the joints). The exact mechanism of action of the gold compounds (e.g., gold sodium thiomalate, aurothioglucose, and auranofin) in the suppression or prevention of inflammation is unknown. Adverse reactions to the gold compounds may occur any time during therapy, as well as many months after therapy has been discontinued, and include dermatitis, stomatitis, pruritus, and chrysiasis.
- Miscellaneous drugs are used to treat a variety of musculoskeletal disorders, such as rheumatoid arthritis in patients who have had an insufficient therapeutic response to or are intolerant of other antirheumatic drugs such as salicylates and nonsteroidal anti-inflammatory drugs.
- Penicillamine, methotrexate, and hydroxychloroquine are used in the treatment of rheumatoid arthritis. Hydroxychloroquine may result in irritability, nervousness, anorexia, nausea, vomiting, and diarrhea. Adverse reactions to penicillamine include pruritus, rash, anorexia, nausea, vomiting, epigastric pain, bone marrow depression, proteinuria, hematuria, increased skin friability, and tinnitus. Methotrexate is a potentially toxic drug that is also used in the treatment of malignancies and psoriasis. Adverse reactions include nausea, vomiting, a decreased platelet count, leukopenia, stomatitis, rash, pruritus, dermatitis, diarrhea, alopecia, and diarrhea.

CRITICAL THINKING CASE STUDY
Rheumatoid Arthritis

Ms. Leeds is prescribed methotrexate for rheumatoid arthritis that has not responded to other therapies. She is nervous about starting the drug after she was told that the drug can cause many serious adverse reactions.

1. Ms. Leeds wonders what the adverse effects of methotrexate may include. She should be told
   a. ulcerative stomatitis, leukopenia, nausea and abdominal distress
   b. rash, anorexia, hematuria
   c. emesis and Stevens-Johnson syndrome
   d. none of the above
2. Ms. Leeds asks why she is being asked to take methotrexate. She is told
   a. methotrexate is used to treat rheumatoid arthritis when other treatments are not working
   b. methotrexate is used for patients intolerant of the salicylates and nonsteroidal anti-inflammatory drugs
   c. methotrexate is used primarily in older patients; it is most effective in patients older than 60
   d. a and b

3. Ms. Leeds asks if methotrexate is used to treat anything other than rheumatoid arthritis. You tell her
   a. methotrexate is also used for dialysis patients
   b. methotrexate is used solely for rheumatoid arthritis treatment
   c. methotrexate is also used to treat malignancies and psoriasis
   d. all of the above
4. Ms. Leeds cannot remember how many times a day she should take the methotrexate that she was prescribed. What should you tell her?

Review Questions

MULTIPLE CHOICE

1. When taking a skeletal muscle relaxant, the most common adverse reaction is
   a. drowsiness
   b. gastrointestinal bleeding
   c. vomiting
   d. constipation
2. A corticosteroid may be prescribed for what condition?
   a. Rheumatoid arthritis
   b. Gout
   c. Osteoarthritis
   d. All of the above
3. When allopurinol (Zyloprim) is used for the treatment of gout, what adverse effect may occur?
   a. Rash
   b. Nausea and vomiting
   c. Hematologic changes
   d. All of the above
4. What should a patient prescribed risedronate be educated about?
   a. The drug is taken once weekly.
   b. Take a daily laxative because the drug will likely cause constipation.
   c. Take the drug in the morning before breakfast and immediately lie down for 30 minutes to facilitate absorption.
   d. After taking the drug, remain upright for at least 30 minutes.

MATCHING

_____ 5.	carisoprodol	a.	Zyloprim
_____ 6.	alendronate	b.	Flexeril
_____ 7.	adalimumab	c.	Enbrel
_____ 8.	infliximab	d.	Boniva
_____ 9.	allopurinol	e.	Soma
_____ 10.	etanercept	f.	Humira
_____ 11.	ibandronate	g.	Imuran
_____ 12.	hydroxychloroquine	h.	Fosamax
_____ 13.	cyclobenzaprine	i.	Plaquenil
_____ 14.	azathioprine	j.	Remicade

TRUE OR FALSE

_____ 15. Many skeletal muscle relaxants do not directly relax skeletal muscles; however, their sedative action may relieve acute painful musculoskeletal conditions.

_____ 16. It may take weeks before patients with acute gout can be expected to respond to therapy.

_____ 17. In addition to experiencing pain, patients with musculoskeletal disorders may also have skeletal deformities.

_____ 18. Rheumatoid arthritis is a noninflammatory joint disease.

FILL IN THE BLANKS

19. A patient who is taking _____ _____ on an outpatient basis for arthritis should be told to contact the health care provider if a _____ in the mouth occurs.

20. The gout drug _____ may cause a skin rash, which may precede a serious adverse reaction called Stevens-Johnson syndrome.

21. Penicillamine is contraindicated in patients with a history of allergy to _____.

22. _____ _____ is characterized by inflammatory changes within the body's connective tissue.

SHORT ANSWERS

23. What should you instruct a patient taking drugs for gout about fluid intake?

24. Should therapy with corticosteroids be stopped abruptly?

25. What is chrysiasis and what causes it?

26. Which miscellaneous drug may affect the eye, and what are the possible adverse effects?

Web Activities

1. Go to the National Library of Medicine NIH Senior Health website (http://nihseniorhealth.gov/). Explore the information on arthritis. What information does this Web site offer about the causes and risk factors for osteoarthritis?

2. At the same Web site, what information is available about the risk factors and prevention of osteoporosis?

SUMMARY DRUG TABLE: Drugs Used to Treat Musculoskeletal Disorders (left, generic; right, trade)

Comprehensive Summary Drug Tables, including uses, adverse effects, dosages, and pregnancy classifications, are provided on the companion website, http://thePoint.lww.com/PharmacologyHP2e

DRUGS USED TO TREAT OSTEOPOROSIS

Bisphosphonates

alendronate sodium *ah-len'-drew-nate*	Fosamax, *generic*
etidronate disodium *e-tid'-ro-nate*	Didronel *generic*
ibandronate *eye-ban'-droh-nate*	Boniva
pamidronate disodium *pa-mi-droe'-nate*	Aredia
risedronate sodium *rah-sed'-dro-nate*	Actonel, Atelvia
tiludronate *tye-loo'-droe-nate*	Skelid
zoledronic acid *zoe-le-dron'-ik*	Reclast, Zometa

Skeletal Muscle Relaxants

baclofen *bak'-loe-fen*	Gablofen, Lioresal, *generic*
carisoprodol *ker-eye-soe-proe'-dol*	Soma, *generic*
chlorzoxazone *klor-zox'-a-zone*	Parafon Forte DSC, *generic*
cyclobenzaprine HCl *sye-kloe-ben'-za-preen*	Amrix, Fexmid, Flexeril, *generic*
dantrolene sodium *dan'-troe-leen*	Dantrium, Revonto, generic
diazepam *dye-az'-e-pam*	Diazepam Intensol, Valium, *generic (C-IV)*
metaxalone *me-taks'-a-lone*	Skelaxin, generic
methocarbamol *meth-oh-kar'-ba-mol*	Robaxin, *generic*
orphenadrine citrate *or-fen'-a-dreen*	Norflex, *generic*
tizanadine *tye-zan'-i-deen*	Zanaflex

Corticosteroids

Glucocorticoids

betamethasone *bay-ta-meth'-a-zone*	Oral: Celestone Topical: Beta-Val, Luxiq, and generic
betamethasone sodium phosphage/ betamethasone acetate	Celestone Soluspan
budesonide *bue-des'-oh-nide*	Oral: Entocort EC; Inhalation Pulmicort; Nasal: Rhinocort Aqua

cortisone *kor'-ti-sone*	*generic*
dexamethasone *dex-a-meth'-a-sone*	Oral: Baycadron, Dexamethasone Intensol, DexPak, *generic* Injection: *generic* Ophthalmic: Maxidex, *generic* Intraocular: Ozurdex
Hydrocortisone (cortisol) *hye-droe-kor-ti-zone*	Oral: *generic* Topical: many trade names, *generic* (Rx and OTC) Rectal: many trade names, *generic* Injection: Solu-Cortef Enema: Cortenema, Colocort, *generic*
methylprednisolone *meth-ill-pred-niss'-oh-lone*	Oral: Medrol, *generic* Injection: A-Methapred, Depo-Medrol, Solu-Medrol, *generic*
prednisolone *pred-niss'-oh-lone*	Oral: AsmaPred Plus, Millipred, Orapred, Pediapred,Prelone, Veripred, *generic* Ophthalmic, Pred Forte, Pred Mild, Prelone, *generic*
prednisone *pred'-ni-sone*	Prednisone Intensol, Sterapred,, Sterapred DS, *generic*
triamcinolone *trye-am-sin'-oh-lone*	Injection: Aristospan, Kenalog, *generic* Topical: Kenalog, Triderm, *generic* Nasal: Nasacort AQ; Oral Paste: Oralone Intraocular: Triesence

Mineralocorticoid

fludrocortisone acetate *floo-droe-kor9-te-sone*	*generic*

Immunomodulators

abatacept *ab-a-ta'-sept*	Orencia
adalimumab *a-da-lim'-yoo-mab*	Humira
anakinra *an-a-kin'-ra*	Kineret
certolizumab pegol *cer-to-liz'-u-mab peg'-ol*	Cimzia

etanercept *ee-tah-ner'-sept*	Enbrel,
fingolimod	Gilenya
golimumab *goe-lim'-ue-mab*	Simponi
infliximab *in-fliks'-e-mab*	Remicade
interferon beta-1A	Avonex, Rebif
interferon beta-1b	Betaseron, Extavia
mitoxantrone *mye-toe-zan'-trone*	Novantrone, *generic*
natalizumab *na-ta-liz'-u-mab*	Tysabri
Tocilizumab *toe-si-liz'-soo-mab*	Actemra

Drugs Used to Treat Gout

Allopurinol *al-oh-pure'-i-nole*	Zyloprim, *generic*
colchicine *kol'-chi-seen*	Colcrys, generic
febuxostat *feb-ux'-oh-stat*	Uloric
pegloticase	Krystexxa
probenecid *proe-ben'-e-sid*	*generic*

Gold Compounds

auranofin *au-rane'-oh-fin*	Ridaura
gold sodium thiomalate *thi-oh-ma'-late*	Myochrysine, *generic*

Miscellaneous Drugs

Azathioprine *ay-za-thye'-oh-preen*	Azasan, Imuran, *generic*
Cyclosporine *sye'-kloe-spor-een*	Gengraf, Neoral, Sandimmune, *generic*
Dalfampridine *dal-fam'-pri-deen*	Ampyra
glatiramer acetate *gla-tir'-a-mer as'-e-tate*	Copaxone
hyaluronic acid derivatives *hye-al-yoor-on'-ic*	Euflexxa, Hyalgan, Supartz, Orthovisc, Synvisc
hydroxychloroquine *hye-droks-ee-klor'-oh-kwin*	Plaquenil, *generic*
Leflunomide *le-floo'-noh-mide*	Arava, *generic*
Methotrexate *meth-oh-treks'-ate*	Rheumatrex, Trexall, *generic*
penicillamine *pen-i-sil'-a-meen*	Cuprimine, Depen Titratabs
Sulfasalazine *sul-fa-sal'-a-zeen*	Azulfidine, *generic*

43

Integumentary System Topical Drugs

CHAPTER OBJECTIVES

On completion of this chapter, students will be able to:

1. Define the chapter's key terms.
2. Identify the classes of topical dermatological drugs.
3. Describe the general drug actions, uses, adverse reactions, contraindications, precautions, and interactions of topical drugs used in the treatment of skin disorders.
4. Discuss important points to keep in mind when educating the patient or family members about the use of topical drugs used in the treatment of skin disorders.

KEY TERMS

antipsoriatics—drugs used to treat psoriasis

antiseptic—a drug that stops, slows, or prevents the growth of microorganisms

dermis—the layer of skin below the epidermis that contains small capillaries, which supply nourishment to the dermis and epidermis

epidermis—the outermost layer of the skin

germicide—a drug that kills bacteria

immunocompromised—patients with an immune system not fully capable of fighting infection

keratolytic—a drug that removes excess growth of the epidermis (top layer of skin) in disorders such as warts

necrotic—dead, as in dead tissue

proteolysis—the process of hastening the reduction of proteins into simpler substances

purulent exudates—pus-containing fluid

CHAPTER OVERVIEW

Drug classes covered in this chapter are:

- Topical anti-infectives
- Topical antiseptics and germicides
- Topical corticosteroids
- Topical antipsoriatics
- Topical enzymes
- Keratolytics
- Topical local anesthetics

Drugs by classification are listed on pages 469-470.

thePOINT RESOURCES

- Comprehensive Summary Drug Tables
- Interactive Practice and Review
- Monographs of Most Commonly Prescribed Drugs

The skin forms a barrier between the outside environment and the structures located beneath the skin (Fig. 43-1). The **epidermis** is the outermost layer of the skin. Immediately below the epidermis is the dermis. The **dermis** contains small capillaries, which supply nourishment to the dermis and epidermis, sebaceous (oil-secreting) glands, sweat glands, nerve fibers, and hair follicles. Because the skin interacts with the outside environment, it is subject to various types of injury and trauma, as well as changes in the skin itself. Each of the following sections discusses only select topical drugs for various skin conditions. See the Summary Drug Table: Dermatologic Drugs for a more complete listing of the drugs.

Topical Anti-Infectives

Localized skin infections may require the use of a topical anti-infective. The topical anti-infectives include antibiotic, antifungal, and antiviral drugs.

Actions and Uses of Topical Anti-Infectives

Topical Antibiotic Drugs

Topical antibiotics exert a direct local effect on specific microorganisms and may be bactericidal (a substance that destroys bacteria) or bacteriostatic (the slowing or retarding of the multiplication of bacteria). Bacitracin inhibits the cell wall synthesis. Bacitracin, gentamicin, erythromycin (Erymax), and metronidazole are examples of topical antibiotics.

These drugs are used to prevent superficial infections in minor cuts, wounds, skin abrasions, and minor burns. Erythromycin is also used to treat acne vulgaris.

Topical Antifungal Drugs

Antifungal drugs exert a local effect by inhibiting growth of the fungi. Examples of antifungal drugs are miconazole, ciclopirox

(Loprox), and econazole. They are used for treatment of tinea pedis (athlete's foot), tinea cruris (jock itch), tinea corporis (ringworm) (Fig. 43-2), and superficial candidiasis.

Topical Antiviral Drugs

Acyclovir (Zovirax) and penciclovir (Denavir) are the only topical antiviral drugs currently available by prescription. Docosanol (Abreva) is the only topical antiviral that is available over-the-counter. These drugs inhibit viral replication.

Acyclovir is used in the treatment of initial episodes of genital herpes, as well as herpes simplex virus infections in **immunocompromised** patients (patients with an immune system not fully capable of fighting infection). Penciclovir and docosanol are used for the treatment of recurrent herpes labialis (cold sores) in adults.

Adverse Reactions of Topical Anti-Infectives

Adverse reactions to topical anti-infectives are usually mild. Occasionally, the patient may experience a skin rash, itching, urticaria (hives), dermatitis, irritation, or redness, which may indicate a hypersensitivity (allergic) reaction to the drug. Prolonged use of topical antibiotic preparations may result in a superficial superinfection (an overgrowth of bacterial or fungal microorganisms not affected by the antibiotic being administered).

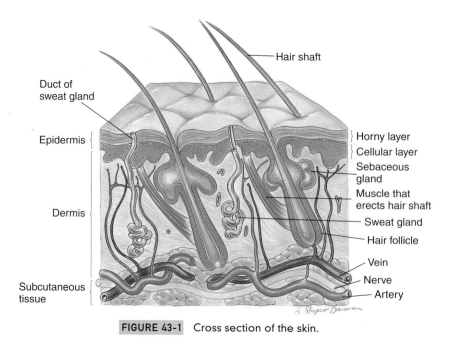

Duct of sweat gland

Epidermis

Dermis

Subcutaneous tissue

Hair shaft

Horny layer
Cellular layer
Sebaceous gland
Muscle that erects hair shaft
Sweat gland
Hair follicle
Vein
Nerve
Artery

FIGURE 43-1   Cross section of the skin.

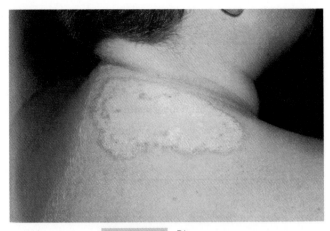

FIGURE 43-2   Ringworm.

Contraindications, Precautions, and Interactions of Topical Anti-Infectives

- These drugs are contraindicated in patients with known hypersensitivity.
- Because neomycin toxicity can cause nephrotoxicity and ototoxicity, it is used cautiously in patients with extensive burns or trophic ulceration when extensive absorption can occur.
- There are no significant interactions with the topical anti-infectives.

FACT CHECK

43-1   What are the three types of topical anti-infective drugs?

Topical Antiseptics and Germicides

An **antiseptic** is a drug that stops, slows, or prevents the growth of microorganisms. A **germicide** is a drug that kills bacteria.

Actions of Topical Antiseptics and Germicides

The exact mechanism of action of topical antiseptics and germicides is not well understood. These drugs affect a variety of microorganisms. Some of these drugs have a short duration of action, whereas others have a long duration of action. The action of these drugs may depend on the strength used and the time the drug is in contact with the skin or mucous membrane.

Benzalkonium is a rapid-acting preparation with a moderately long duration of action. It is active against bacteria and some viruses, fungi, and protozoa. Benzalkonium solutions are bacteriostatic or bactericidal, depending on their concentration.

Chlorhexidine gluconate affects a wide range of microorganisms, including gram-positive and gram-negative bacteria. Iodine has anti-infective action against many bacteria, fungi, viruses, yeasts, and protozoa. Povidone–iodine (Betadine) is a combination of iodine and povidone, which liberates free iodine. Povidone–iodine is often preferred over iodine solution or tincture because it is less irritating to the skin. Unlike the use of iodine alone, treated areas may be bandaged or taped.

Uses of Topical Antiseptics and Germicides

Topical antiseptics and germicides are primarily used to reduce the number of bacteria on skin surfaces. Some of these drugs, such as chlorhexidine gluconate, may be used as a surgical scrub, as a preoperative skin cleanser, for washing the hands before and after caring for patients, and in the home to cleanse the skin. Others may be applied to minor cuts and abrasions to prevent infection. Some of these drugs may also be used on mucous membranes. Chlorhexidine gluconate is used both topically and orally as a rinse.

Adverse Reactions of Topical Antiseptics and Germicides

Topical antiseptics and germicides have few adverse reactions. Occasionally, an individual may be allergic to the drug, and a skin rash or itching may occur. If an allergic reaction is noted, then the topical drug is discontinued.

Contraindications, Precautions, and Interactions of Topical Antiseptics and Germicides

- These drugs are contraindicated in patients with known hypersensitivity.
- There are no significant precautions or interactions when used as directed.

FACT CHECK

43-2   Why is povidone–iodine often preferred over iodine solution or tincture?

Topical Corticosteroids

Topical corticosteroids vary in potency, depending on the concentration of the drug (percentage), the vehicle in which the drug is suspended (lotion, cream, aerosol spray), and the area to which the drug is applied (open or denuded skin, unbroken skin, thickness of the skin over the treated area).

Examples of topical corticosteroids include amcinonide, betamethasone dipropionate, fluocinolone acetonide, hydrocortisone, and triamcinolone acetate.

Actions and Uses of Topical Corticosteroids

Topical corticosteroids exert localized anti-inflammatory activity. When applied to inflamed skin, they reduce itching, redness, and swelling.

These drugs are useful in treating skin disorders, such as psoriasis, dermatitis, rashes, eczema, insect bite reactions, and superficial and partial-thickness burns, including sunburns.

Adverse Reactions of Corticosteroids

Localized reactions may include burning, itching, irritation, redness, dryness of the skin, and secondary infection.

Contraindications, Precautions, and Interactions of Corticosteroids

- Topical corticosteroids are contraindicated in patients with known hypersensitivity; as monotherapy for bacterial skin infections; for use on the face, groin, or axilla (only the high-potency corticosteroids); and for ophthalmic use (may cause steroid-induced glaucoma or cataracts).
- Avoid contact with eyes or mucous membranes.
- There are no significant interactions when administered as directed.

FACT CHECK

43-3   What are topical corticosteroids used to treat?

Topical Antipsoriatics

Actions and Uses of Antipsoriatics

Topical **antipsoriatics** are drugs used in the treatment of psoriasis (Fig. 43-3). Topical antipsoriatics help remove the plaques associated with psoriasis (a chronic skin disease manifested by bright red patches covered with silver scales or plaques). Examples of antipsoriatics include anthralin (Anthra-Derm) and calcipotriene (Dovonex).

Adverse Reactions of Antipsoriatics

These drugs may cause burning, itching, and skin irritation. Anthralin may cause skin irritation, as well as temporary discoloration of the hair and fingernails.

Contraindications, Precautions, and Interactions of Antipsoriatics

- These drugs are contraindicated in patients with known hypersensitivity to the drugs.

CONSIDERATIONS | Older adults

LIFESPAN

Calcipotriene

Adults older than 65 years have more skin-related adverse reactions to calcipotriene. Calcipotriene should be used cautiously in older adults.

FACT CHECK

43-4   What are common adverse reactions of antipsoriatics?

Topical Enzymes

Actions and Uses of Topical Enzymes

A topical enzyme aids in the removal of dead soft tissues by hastening the reduction of proteins into simpler substances. This is called **proteolysis** or a proteolytic action.

The components of certain types of wounds, namely **necrotic** (dead) tissues and **purulent exudates** (pus-containing fluid), prevent effective wound healing. Removal of this type of debris by application of a topical enzyme aids in healing. Examples of conditions that may respond to application of a topical enzyme include partial-thickness and full-thickness burns, pressure ulcers (Fig. 43-4), and ulcers caused by peripheral vascular disease. An example of a topical enzyme is collagenase (Santyl).

Adverse Reactions of Topical Enzymes

The application of collagenase may cause mild, transient pain. Numbness and dermatitis also may occur. Collagenase has a low incidence of adverse reactions.

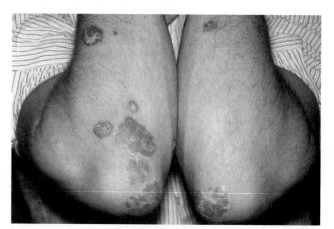

FIGURE 43-3 Psoriasis.

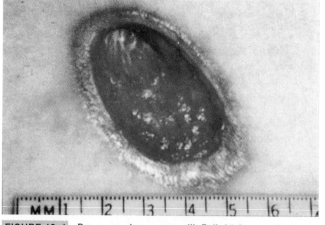

FIGURE 43-4 Pressure ulcers stage III. Full-thickness skin loss, with damage to or necrosis of subcutaneous tissue that may extend to, but not through, underlying muscle.

Contraindications, Precautions, and Interactions of Topical Enzymes

- Topical enzyme preparations are contraindicated in patients with known hypersensitivity, in wounds in contact with major body cavities or where nerves are exposed, and in fungating neoplastic ulcers.
- Enzymatic activity may be impaired when these agents are administered with several detergents and antiseptics (benzalkonium chloride, hexachlorophene, iodine, and nitrofurazone).

FACT CHECK

43-5 How do topical enzymes affect proteolysis?

Keratolytics

Actions and Uses of Keratolytics

A **keratolytic** is a drug that removes excess growth of the epidermis (top layer of skin) in disorders such as warts.

These drugs are used to remove warts, calluses, corns, and seborrheic keratoses (benign variously colored skin growths arising from oil glands of the skin) (Fig. 43-5). Examples of keratolytics include salicylic acid, masoprocol (Actinex), and diclofenac (Solaraze). Some strengths of salicylic acid are available as nonprescription products for the removal of warts on the hands and feet.

Adverse Reactions of Keratolytics

These drugs are usually well tolerated. Occasionally, a transient burning sensation, rash, dry skin, scaling, or flu-like syndrome may occur. Dry skin increases the risk of skin breakdown caused by scratching. The patient can be advised to keep nails short, to use warm water with mild soap for cleaning the skin, and to rinse and dry the skin thoroughly. Bath oils, creams, and lotions may be applied if necessary as long as the health care provider is consulted first. Dry, flaky skin is subject to breakdown and infection. The skin is observed for signs of infection (e.g., redness, heat, pus, and elevated temperature and pulse), and any sign of infection is immediately reported.

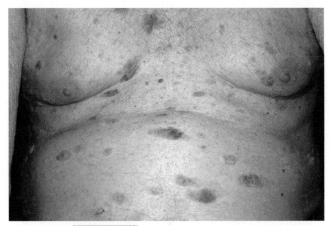

FIGURE 43-5 Seborrheic keratoses.

ALERT Rx

Salicylic Acid
Salicylic acid may cause salicylate toxicity (see Chapter 8) with prolonged use.

Contraindications, Precautions, and Interactions of Keratolytics

- Keratolytics are contraindicated in patients with known hypersensitivity and for use on moles, birthmarks, or warts with hair growing from them; on genital or facial warts; on warts on mucous membranes; or on infected skin.
- Prolonged use of the keratolytics in infants or patients with diabetes or impaired circulation is contraindicated.
- Do not apply to open skin wounds, areas that are infected, or exfoliative dermatitis.
- Do not apply external heat or an occlusive dressing.
- Avoid contact with eyes or mucous membranes.
- There are no significant interactions when applied as directed.

FACT CHECK

43-6 How do keratolytics act?

Topical Local Anesthetics

A topical anesthetic may be applied to the skin or mucous membranes.

Actions and Uses of Topical Local Anesthetics

Topical anesthetics temporarily inhibit the conduction of impulses from sensory nerve fibers. Examples of local anesthetics include benzocaine, dibucaine (Nupercainal), and lidocaine. These drugs may be used to relieve itching and pain caused by skin conditions, such as minor burns, fungus infections, insect bites, rashes, sunburn, and plant poisoning such as poison ivy. Some are applied to mucous membranes as local anesthetics.

Adverse Reactions of Topical Local Anesthetics

Occasionally, local irritation, dermatitis, rash, burning, stinging, and tenderness may occur.

Contraindications, Precautions, and Interactions of Topical Local Anesthetics

- These drugs are contraindicated in those with a known hypersensitivity.
- The topical anesthetics are used cautiously in patients receiving class I antiarrhythmic drugs, such as tocainide

and mexiletine, because the toxic effects are additive and potentially synergistic.

- There are no significant interactions when applied as directed.

Patient Management Issues with Topical Drugs

These solutions are not kept at the bedside of any patient who is confused or disoriented because the solution may be mistaken and used inappropriately.

The health care provider usually orders the patient to apply topical corticosteroids sparingly. The health care provider also may order the area of application to be covered or left exposed to the air. Some corticosteroids are applied as an occlusive dressing. In such a situation, the drug is applied while the skin is still moist after washing with soap and water. The area is covered with a plastic wrap, sealed with tape or bandage, and the drug left in place for the prescribed period of time.

Certain types of wounds may require special preparations before applying the topical enzyme. The area is cleaned or prepared and the topical enzyme applied as directed by the health care provider. If bleeding occurs with the use of sutilains, then the ointment is discontinued and the health care provider is contacted.

When applying antipsoriatics, care is exercised so that the product is applied only to the psoriatic lesions and not to surrounding skin. Signs of excessive irritation should be reported to the health care provider.

When a topical gel, such as lidocaine viscous, is used for oral anesthesia for the control of pain, the patient is instructed not to eat food for 1 hour after use because local anesthesia of the mouth or throat may impair swallowing and increase the possibility of aspiration.

Educating the Patient and Family about Topical Drugs

Following are key points about topical drugs used in the treatment of skin disorders that the patient and family members should know.

- Wash your hands thoroughly before and after applying the product.
- If the enclosed directions state that the product will stain clothing, then be sure clothing is moved away from the treated area. If the product stains your skin, then wear disposable gloves when applying the drug.
- Follow the directions on the label or use as directed by your health care provider. Read any enclosed directions for use of the product carefully.
- Prepare the area to be treated as recommended by your health care provider or as described in the directions supplied with the product.
- Do not apply to areas other than those specified by your health care provider. Apply the drug as directed (e.g., thin layer, apply liberally, and so on).
- Follow the directions of your health care provider regarding covering the treated area or leaving it exposed to air. The effectiveness of certain drugs depends on keeping the area covered or leaving it open.
- Keep this product away from your eyes (unless use in or around your eye has been recommended or prescribed). Do not rub or put your fingers near your eyes unless your hands have been thoroughly washed and all remnants of the drug removed from the fingers. If the product is accidentally spilled, sprayed, or splashed in your eye, then wash your eye immediately with copious amounts

of running water. Contact your health care provider immediately if burning, pain, redness, discomfort, or blurred vision persists for more than a few minutes.

- The drug may cause momentary stinging or burning when applied.
- Discontinue use of the drug and contact your health care

provider if rash, burning, itching, redness, pain, or other skin problems occur.

- Gentamicin, and other topical drugs, may cause photosensitivity. Take measures to protect your skin from ultraviolet rays (e.g., wear protective clothing and use a sunscreen when out in the sun).

Chapter Review

KEY POINTS

- Topical anti-infectives include antibiotic, antifungal, and antiviral drugs. Topical antibiotic drugs may be either bactericidal or bacteriostatic and are used to prevent superficial infections in minor cuts, wounds, skin abrasions, and minor burns and for treatment of acne vulgaris. Antifungal drugs exert a local effect by inhibiting growth of the fungi. Antiviral drugs inhibit viral replication.
- Topical antiseptics and germicides affect a variety of microorganisms, although the exact mechanism is not clearly understood. The action of these drugs may depend on the strength used and the time the drug is in contact with the skin or mucous membrane. Topical antiseptics and germicides are primarily used to reduce the number of bacteria on skin surfaces.
- Topical corticosteroids exert localized anti-inflammatory activity, and when applied to inflamed skin, they reduce itching, redness, and swelling. These drugs are useful in treating skin disorders, such as psoriasis, dermatitis, rashes, eczema, insect bite reactions, and first- and second-degree burns, including sunburns.
- Topical antipsoriatics help remove the plaques associated with psoriasis and may cause burning, itching, and skin irritation.
- A topical enzyme aids in the removal of dead soft tissues by hastening the reduction of proteins into simpler substances. Removal of this type of dead skin debris by application of a topical enzyme aids in healing for certain types of wounds. Collagenase may cause mild, transient pain, numbness, and dermatitis.
- Keratolytics are drugs that remove excess growth of the epidermis (top layer of skin) in disorders such as warts.
- Topical anesthetics temporarily inhibit the conduction of impulses from sensory nerve fibers. These drugs may be used to relieve itching and pain due to skin conditions, such as minor burns, fungus infections, insect bites, rashes, sunburn, and plant poisoning such as poison ivy.

CRITICAL THINKING CASE STUDY

Ringworm

Mr. Davies, age 42 years, has a rash on his arm that has been diagnosed as ringworm.

1. Which of the following drug classifications would be used to treat ringworm?
   a. Antibiotic
   b. Antifungal
   c. Antiviral
   d. Antiseptic

2. Mr. Davies's health care provider has recommended that he get Lotrimin Ultra, which is available over the counter. How should Mr. Davies use it?
   a. Once a day until clear, which may take up to 4 weeks
   b. Twice a day until clear, which may take up to 4 weeks
   c. Three times a day until clear, which may take up to 4 weeks
   d. Four times a day until clear, which may take up to 4 weeks

3. What should you tell Mr. Davies about using the Lotrimin Ultra?

Review Questions

MULTIPLE CHOICE

1. What reaction could occur with prolonged use of the topical antibiotics?
   a. Water intoxication
   b. Superficial superinfection
   c. An outbreak of eczema
   d. Cellulitis

2. Which of the following drugs has a proteolytic action?
   a. amcinonide
   b. collagenase
   c. bacitracin
   d. ciclopirox

3. What type of action do the corticosteroids have when used topically?
   a. Bactericidal activity
   b. Anti-inflammatory activity
   c. Antifungal activity
   d. Antiviral activity

4. Which of the following drugs is best suited to be used as a topical antiseptic?
   a. amphotericin B
   b. belnzocaine
   c. clindamycin
   d. povidone–iodine

MATCHING

Match the drug on the left with the classification on the right.

_____ 5. chlorhexidine
              gluconate   a. antibiotic
_____ 6. lidocaine   b. antifungal
_____ 7. hydrocortisone   c. antiviral
_____ 8. anthralin   d. antiseptic
_____ 9. bacitracin   e. corticosteroid
_____ 10. collagenase   f. antipsoriatic
_____ 11. acyclovir   g. enzyme preparation
_____ 12. salicylic acid   h. keratolytic
_____ 13. econazole   i. local anesthetic

Match the generic name on the left with the trade name on the right.

_____ 14. dibucaine   a. Dovonex
_____ 15. docosanol   b. Santyl
_____ 16. diclofenac   c. Halog
_____ 17. sulconazole   d. Betadine
_____ 18. mupirocin   e. Exelderm
_____ 19. halcinonide   f. Solaraze
_____ 20. calcipotriene   g. Bactroban
_____ 21. povidone–iodine   h. Abreva
_____ 22. collagenase   i. Nupercainal

TRUE OR FALSE

_____ 23. A keratolytic agent is safe to use on moles and birthmarks.
_____ 24. The epidermis is the innermost layer of the skin.
_____ 25. Chlorhexidine is used as a surgical scrub or as a preoperative skin cleanser.
_____ 26. Topical corticosteroids exert anti-infective activity.

FILL IN THE BLANKS

27. The _____ contains small capillaries, sebaceous and sweat glands, nerve fibers, and hair follicles.
28. _____ _____ are contraindicated for ophthalmic use because they may cause glaucoma or cataracts.
29. _____ are drugs that kill bacteria, while _____ are drugs that stop or slow the growth of microorganisms.
30. Benzocaine is used for topical _____ in local skin disorders.

SHORT ANSWERS

31. What conditions are topical enzymes used for, and why?
32. A patient using a topical drug accidentally splashes some of the drug in his eyes. What should the patient be instructed to do?
33. What factors affect the potency of topical corticosteroids?
34. How do topical antipsoriatics work?

Web Activities

1. Go to the National Psoriasis Foundation Web site (www.psoriasis.org), click on the "Research" tab, and then choose "Clinical Trials." This section describes drugs currently being tested. Choose any one clinical trial and read about it. Write a brief statement about what the trial is testing.
2. At the same Web site, return to the home page and click on "News and Events," and then "News Stories." Choose any news story about a drug, and write a brief summary about the use of that drug for psoriasis.

SUMMARY DRUG TABLE: Dermatologic Drugs (left, generic; right, trade)

Comprehensive Summary Drug Tables, including uses, adverses effects, dosages, and pregnancy classifications, are provided on the companion website, http://thePoint.lww.com/PharmacologyHP2e

Antibiotic Drugs

azelaic acid *az-e-lak'*	Azelex, Finacea, Finacea Plus
bacitracin *ba-ci-tra'-sin*	*generic* (OTC)
benzoyl peroxide *been'-zoyl per-ox'-ide*	Many trade names (Rx and OTC), *generic*
clindamycin, topical *clin'-da-my-sin*	Cleocin T, Clinda-Derm, Clindagel, Clindets, C/T/S, Evoclin, *generic*
erythromycin *ee-rith-ro-my'-sin*	Akne-Mycin, Emcin, Ery 2% Pad, Erymax, *generic*
gentamicin *jen-ta-my'-sin*	*generic*
metronidazole *meh-trow-nye'-dah-zoll*	MetroLotion, Nydamax, Noritate, Metrocream, Vitazol, *generic*
mupirocin *mew'-pie-ro-sin*	Bactroban, Centany, Centany AT, *generic*
sulfacetamide sodium *sul-fah-see'-ta-mide*	Mexar, Ovace Plus, Seb-Prev, Klaron, *generic*

Antifungal Drugs

butenafine HCl *beu-ten'-ah-feen*	Lotrimin Ultra (OTC), Mentax (Rx)
ciclopirox *sic-lo-peer'-ox*	Ciclodan, Loprox, Penlac Nail, *generic*
clotrimazole *kloe-trim'-a-zole*	*Cruex, Lotrimin AF, generic* (OTC)
econazole nitrate *ee-kon'-a-zole*	*generic*
ketoconazole *kee-toe-koe'-na-zole*	Extina (Rx), Kuric (Rx), Nizoral A-D (OTC), Xolegel (Rx), *generic* (Rx and OTC)
miconazole nitrate *mi-kon'-a-zole*	*Numerous trade names, generic* (OTC)
naftifine HCl *naf'-ti-feen*	Naftin
nystatin *nye-stat'-in*	Pediaderm AF, Nyamyc, Nystop, Pedi-Dri, *generic*
oxiconazole *ox-ee-kon'-ah-zole*	Oxistat
sertaconazole *ser-ta-koe'-na-zole*	Ertaczo
sulconazole *sue-kon'-ah-zole*	Exelderm
terbinafine HCl *ter-ben'-a-feen*	Lamisil AT, *generic* (OTC)
tolnaftate *tole-naf'-tate*	Numerous trade names, *generic* (OTC)

undecylenic acid and derivatives *un-de-sil-en'-ik*	Variety of trade names (OTC)

Antiviral Drugs

acyclovir *ay-sye'-kloe-veer*	Zovirax
docosanol *doe-koe'-san-ole*	Abreva (OTC)
penciclovir *pen-sye'-kloe-veer*	Denavir

Antiseptic and Germicides

benzalkonium chloride (BAC) *benz-al-cone'-e-um*	Variety of trade names, *generic*
chlorhexidine gluconate *klor-hex'-e-deen*	Betasept (OTC)
hexachlorophene *heks-a-klor'-o-feen*	pHisoHex
povidone–iodine *pov-e-don*	Betadine, *generic*
silver nitrate	*generic*
sodium hypochlorite	Dakin solution, Di-Dak-Sol
triclosan *trye'-klo-san*	Variety of trade names (OTC)
zinc acetate	Ivy-Dry (OTC)

Corticosteroids, Topical

alclometasone dipropionate *al-kloe-met-a-sone die-pro'-pee-oh-nate*	Aclovate, *generic*
amcinonide *am-sin'-oh-nide*	*generic*
augmented betamethasone dipropionate	Diprolene, AF, Diprolene, *generic*
betamethasone dipropionate *bay-ta-meth'-a-sone*	Betanate, Del-Beta, *generic*
betamethasone valerate *bay-ta-meth'-a-sone- val'-eh-rate*	BETADERM, Luxiq, *generic*
clobetasol propionate *kloe-bay'-ta-sol*	Clobex, Cormax, Olux, Olux-E, Temovate, Temovate E, *generic*
clocortolone pivalate *klor-kor'-toe-lone*	Cloderm
desonide *des'-oh-nide*	Desonate, DesOwen, Desonil, LoKara, Verdeso, *generic*

desoximetasone *dess-ox-i-met'-a-sone*	Topicort, Topicort LP, *generic*
diflorasone diacetate *dye-flor'-a-sone*	ApexiCon, ApexiCon E, *generic*
fluocinolone acetonide *floo-oh-sin'-oh-lone*	Capex, Derma-Smoothe/FS, *generic*
fluocinonide *floo-oh-sin'-oh-nide*	Vanos, *generic*
flurandrenolide *floor-an-dren'-oh-lide*	Cordran, Cordran SP
fluticasone propionate *floo-tik'-a-sone*	Cutivate, *generic*
halcinonide *hal-sin'-oh-nide*	Halog
halobetasol propionate *hal-oh-bay'-ta-sol*	Ultravate, *generic*
hydrocortisone *hye-droe-kor'-ti-sone*	Various trade names (Rx and OTC)
hydrocortisone acetate *hye-droe-kor'-ti-sone*	Caldecort, CortAlo, NuCort, NuZon, *generic*
hydrocortisone buteprate	Pandel
hydrocortisone butyrate	Locoid, *generic*
hydrocortisone probutate	Pandel
hydrocortisone valerate	Westcort, *generic*
mometasone furoate *moe-met'-a-sone*	Elocon, *generic*
prednicarbate *pred-ni-kar'-bate*	Dermatop
triamcinolone acetonide *trye-am-sin'-oh-lone*	Pediaderm, SP Rx 228, Triderm, Kenalog, *generic*
triamcinolone acetonide, augmented *trye-am-sin'-oh-lone*	Trianex

Antipsoriatic Drugs

anthralin *an-thra'-lin*	Dritho-Creme, Dritho-Scalp, Psoriatec
calcipotriene *cal-cip-o-tri-een*	Dovonex, Calcitrene, *generic*

(continued)

SUMMARY DRUG TABLE: Dermatologic Drugs (continued)

Antipsoriatic Drugs *(continued)*	
calcipotriene/ betamethasone dipropionate *kal-si-poe'-try-een/ bay-ta-meth'-a-sone*	Taclonex, Taclonex Scalp
coal tar	Variety of trade names, *generic* (OTC)
selenium sulfide *se-le'-ne-um*	Dandrex, Tersi, *generic* (Rx and OTC)

Enzyme Preparations	
collagenase *koll-ah-gen'-ase*	Santyl
enzyme combinations, topical	Granulex, Optase, Xenaderm, AllanDerm-T, Revina, Granul-Derm, TBC Topical Spray

Keratolytic Drugs	
diclofenac sodium *dye-kloe'-fen-ak*	Solaraze, Flector, Voltaren, Pennsaid
salicylic acid *sal-i-sill'-ik*	Various trade names, *generic* (OTC)

Local Anesthetics	
benzocaine *benz-o-kaine*	Various trade names, *generic* (OTC)
dibucaine *di-bu-kaine*	Nupercainal, *generic*
lidocaine *lie'-doe-kaine*	Various trade names, *generic* (Rx and OTC)
pramoxine *pra-moks'-een*	Variety of trade names, *generic* (Rx and OTC)
pramoxine, calamine	Caladryl (OTC)

44

Otic and Ophthalmic Preparations

CHAPTER OBJECTIVES

On completion of this chapter, students will be able to:

1. Define the chapter's key terms.
2. Describe the general drug actions, uses, adverse reactions, contraindications, precautions, and interactions of otic and ophthalmic preparations.
3. Describe how to properly use ophthlamic solutions, suspensions, and ointments.
4. Discuss important points to keep in mind when educating the patient or family members about the use of otic and ophthalmic preparations.

KEY TERMS

cycloplegia—paralysis of the ciliary muscle, resulting in an inability to focus the eye
intraocular pressure—the pressure within the eye
miosis—the contraction of the pupil of the eye
miotics—drugs used to help contract the pupil of the eye
mydriasis—dilation of the pupil
mydriatics—drugs that dilate the pupil, constrict superficial blood vessels of the sclera, and decrease the formation of aqueous humor
ophthalmic—eye
otic—ear

CHAPTER OVERVIEW

Drug classes covered in this chapter are:

- Otic Preparations
- Ophthalmic Preparations

Drugs by classification are listed on pages 481–482.

thePOINT RESOURCES

- Comprehensive Summary Drug Tables
- Interactive Practice and Review
- Monographs of Most Commonly Prescribed Drugs

The eyes and ears are subject to various disorders, which range from mild to serious. Because the eyes and ears provide an interpretation of our outside environment, any disease or injury that has the potential for partial or total loss of function of these organs must be treated.

Otic Preparations

Actions of Otic Preparations

Various types of preparations are used for the treatment of **otic** (ear) disorders. There are three categories of otic preparations: (1) antibiotics, (2) antibiotic and steroid combinations, and (3) miscellaneous preparations. The miscellaneous preparations usually contain one or more of the following ingredients:

- Benzocaine: a local anesthetic
- Phenylephrine: a vasoconstrictor decongestant
- Hydrocortisone, desonide: corticosteroids for anti-inflammatory and antipruritic effects
- Glycerin: an emollient and a solvent
- Antipyrine: an analgesic
- Acetic acid, boric acid, benzalkonium chloride, aluminum acetate, benzethonium chloride: provide antifungal or antibacterial action
- Carbamide peroxide: aids in removing earwax by softening and breaking up the wax
- Isopropyl alcohol and glycerin: aids in removal of water after swimming and other water-based activities

Examples of otic preparations are listed in the Summary Drug Table: Otic Preparations.

Uses of Otic Preparations

Otic preparations are instilled in the external auditory canal and may be used to relieve pain, treat infection and inflammation, and aid in the removal of earwax and water (Fig. 44-1). When a patient has an inner ear infection, systemic antibiotic therapy is indicated.

Adverse Reactions of Otic Preparations

When otic drugs are applied topically, the amount of drug that enters the systemic circulation is not sufficient to produce adverse reactions. Prolonged use of otic preparations containing an antibiotic may result in a superinfection (an overgrowth of bacterial or fungal microorganisms not affected by the antibiotic being administered).

Contraindications, Precautions, and Interactions of Otic Preparations

- These drugs are contraindicated in patients with a known hypersensitivity.
- Drugs to remove cerumen are not used if ear drainage, discharge, pain, or irritation is present; if the eardrum is perforated; or if after ear surgery.
- No significant interactions have been reported with use of the otic preparations.

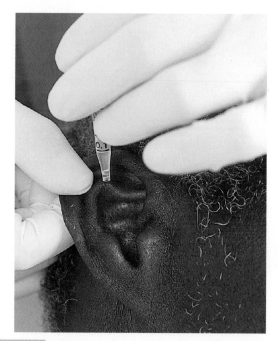

FIGURE 44-1 Instilling ear drops. With the patient's head turned toward the unaffected side, the cartilaginous portion of the outer ear (pinna) is pulled up and back in an adult, and the prescribed number of drops is instilled on the side of the auditory canal.

Patient Management Issues with Otic Preparations

Ear disorders may result in symptoms such as pain, a feeling of fullness in the ear, tinnitus, dizziness, or a change in hearing. Before an otic solution is instilled, the patient should be informed that a feeling of fullness may be felt in the ear and that hearing in the treated ear may be impaired while the solution remains in the ear canal.

Educating the Patient and Family about Otic Preparations

The patient and family members are given instructions or a demonstration of the installation technique of an otic preparation. Following are key points about otic preparations that the patient and family members should know.

- Cold and warm (above body temperature) preparations may cause dizziness or other sensations after being instilled into your ear. Warm preparations before use by holding the container in your hand or gently rubbing it between both hands.

ALERT ℞

Drugs for Otic Use

Only preparations labeled as otic are instilled in the ear. The label of the preparation must be checked carefully for the name of the drug and a statement indicating that the preparation is for otic use.

ALERT Rx

Otic Drugs and Child Safety

Otic drugs available in dropper bottles may be dangerous if ingested by young children; therefore, the drugs must be stored safely out of the reach of children.

- Wash your hands thoroughly before cleansing the area around your ear (when necessary) and instilling ear drops or ointment.
- Instill the prescribed number of drops or amount of ointment in your ear. Do not put the applicator or dropper tip in your ear.
- Immediately after use, replace the cap or dropper and store the solution according to the directions on the label.
- If the drops are in a suspvension form, shake well for 10 seconds before using.
- Keep your head tilted or lie on the untreated side for 2 to 3 minutes to allow the solution to remain in contact with your ear. Excess solution and solution running out of your ear can be wiped off with a tissue.
- Do not insert anything into the ear canal before or after applying the prescribed drug unless advised to do so by your health care provider. At times, a soft cotton plug may be inserted into the affected ear to prevent the solution from draining from the ear.
- Complete a full course of treatment with the prescribed drug to achieve satisfactory results.
- Do not use nonprescription ear products during or after treatment unless such use has been approved by your health care provider.
- Temporary changes in hearing or a feeling of fullness in the ear may occur for a short time after the drug has been instilled.
- Notify your health care provider if your symptoms do not improve or become worse.

Drugs Used to Remove Cerumen

- Do not use if ear drainage, discharge, pain, or irritation occurs.
- Do not use for more than 4 days. If excessive cerumen remains, consult your health care provider.
- Any wax remaining after the treatment may be removed by gently flushing the ear with warm water using a soft rubber bulb ear syringe.
- Drugs that loosen cerumen work by softening the dried earwax inside the ear canal. Cerumenex is available by prescription and is not allowed to stay in the ear canal more than 30 minutes before irrigation. When Cerumenex is administered, your ear canal is filled with the solution and a cotton plug is inserted. The drug is allowed to remain in your ear for 15 to 30 minutes, and then your ear is flushed with warm water using a soft rubber bulb ear syringe.
- If you become dizzy, consult a physician.

FACT CHECK

44-1 What are the three categories of drugs used to treat otic disorders?

44-2 What are the common uses of otic preparations?

Ophthalmic Preparations

Various types of preparations are used for the treatment of ophthalmic disorders such as glaucoma to lower the **intraocular pressure** (IOP) (the pressure within the eye), bacteria or viral infections of the eye, inflammatory conditions, and symptoms of allergy related to the eye.

Glaucoma is a condition of the eye in which there is an increase in the intraocular pressure, causing progressive atrophy of the optic nerve with deterioration of vision and, if untreated, blindness. The higher the intraocular pressure, the greater the risk of optic nerve damage, visual loss, and blindness. There are two types of glaucoma: angle-closure glaucoma and open-angle, or chronic, glaucoma. Box 44-1 describes the two types of glaucoma.

BOX 44.1

Glaucoma

The eye's lens, iris, and cornea are continuously bathed and nourished by a fluid called aqueous humor. As aqueous humor is produced, excess fluid normally flows out through a complex network of tissue called trabecular meshwork. An angle is formed where the trabeculum and iris meet. This forms a filtration angle that maintains the normal pressure within the eye by allowing excess aqueous humor to leave the anterior chamber of the eye (Fig. 44-2). In chronic or open-angle glaucoma, the angle that permits the drainage of aqueous humor appears to be normal but does not function properly. In angle-closure glaucoma, the iris blocks the trabecular meshwork and limits the flow of aqueous humor from the anterior chamber of the eye. This limitation of outflow causes an accumulation of intraocular fluid, followed by increased intraocular pressure. Some individuals have an anatomical defect that causes the angle to be more narrow than normal but do not have any symptoms and glaucoma does not develop under normal circumstances. However, certain situations, such as medication that causes dilation of the eye, fear, or pain, that cause the eye to dilate may precipitate an attack. The aim of treatment in glaucoma is to lower the intraocular pressure. For more information on glaucoma, see Chapter 13.

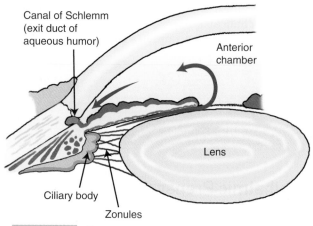

Canal of Schlemm
(exit duct of
aqueous humor)

Anterior
chamber

Lens

Ciliary body

Zonules

FIGURE 44-2 Flow of aqueous humor in the normal eye.

Most of the drug classifications used to treat **ophthalmic** (eye) conditions have already been discussed in previous chapters. The following sections provide a short summary of these drugs in ophthalmic use. The Summary Drug Table: Select Ophthalmic Preparations provides examples of the drugs used to treat ophthalmic problems.

The incidence of adverse reactions associated with ophthalmic drugs is usually small (Key Concepts 44-1). Some ophthalmic preparations produce momentary stinging or burning on instillation. The stinging and burning should resolve soon after use. If not, the health care provider should be contacted.

FACT CHECK

44-3 What is intraocular pressure, and which ophthalmic disorder increases it?

ANTIGLAUCOMA AGENTS

α$_2$-Adrenergic Drugs

Brimonidine tartrate is an α$_2$-adrenergic receptor agonist that acts to reduce aqueous humor production and increase the outflow of aqueous humor. It is used to lower intraocular pressure in patients with open-angle glaucoma or ocular hypertension.

Although adverse reactions are usually mild, treatment with brimonidine tartrate includes oral dryness, ocular hyperemia, burning and stinging, headache, visual blurring, foreign

KEY CONCEPTS

44-1 Ophthalmic Drugs and Systemic Effects

Because small amounts of the ophthalmic preparation may be absorbed systemically, some of the adverse effects associated with systemic administration of the particular drug may be observed.

body sensation, fatigue, drowsiness, ovular allergic reactions, and ocular pruritus.

This drug is contraindicated in patients with hypersensitivity and in patients taking the monoamine oxidase inhibitors. Patients should wait at least 15 minutes after instilling brimonidine before inserting soft contact lenses because the preservative in the drug may be absorbed by soft contact lenses. It is used cautiously during lactation and in patients with cardiovascular disease, depression, cerebral or coronary insufficiency, orthostatic hypotension, or Raynaud phenomenon. When brimonidine is used with central nervous system depressants such as alcohol, barbiturates, opiates, sedatives, or anesthetics, there is a risk for an additive central nervous system depressant effect. The drug is used cautiously in combination with the β-blockers, antihypertensive drugs, and cardiac glycosides because a synergistic effect may occur.

FACT CHECK

44-4 Why should patients wait at least 15 minutes after instilling brimonidine before inserting soft contact lenses?

Sympathomimetic Drugs

Sympathomimetics have α-adrenergic and β-adrenergic activity (see Chapter 11 for a detailed discussion of adrenergic drugs). These drugs lower intraocular pressure by increasing the outflow of aqueous humor in the eye and are used to treat glaucoma. Apraclonidine is used to control or prevent postoperative elevations in intraocular pressure.

These drugs may cause transient local reactions such as hyperemia, pruritus, increased tear production, foreign body sensation, ocular pain, and edema. With prolonged use, adrenochrome (a red pigment contained in epinephrine) deposits may occur in the conjunctiva and cornea. Although rare, systemic reactions may occur such as headache, palpitations, tachycardia, extrasystoles, cardiac arrhythmia, hypertension, and faintness.

These drugs are contraindicated in patients with hypersensitivity to the drug.

Sympathomimetic drugs are used cautiously during lactation and in patients with hypertension, diabetes, hyperthyroidism, heart disease, cerebral arteriosclerosis, or bronchial asthma. Some of these drugs contain sulfites that may cause allergic-like reactions (hives, wheezing, anaphylaxis) in patients with sulfite sensitivity. See Chapter 11 for information on interactions.

β-Adrenergic Blocking Drugs

The β-adrenergic blocking drugs decrease the rate of production of aqueous humor and thereby lower the intraocular pressure. These drugs are used in the treatment of glaucoma.

Adverse reactions associated with the β-adrenergic blocking drugs include eye irritation, burning, tearing, conjunctivitis, decreased night vision, ptosis, abnormal corneal staining, and corneal sensitivity. Systemic reactions, although rare, include arrhythmias, palpitation, headache, nausea, and dizziness. See Chapter 12 for additional systemic adverse reactions.

β-adrenergic blocking drugs are contraindicated in patients with bronchial asthma, obstructive pulmonary disease, sinus bradycardia, heart block, cardiac failure, or cardiogenic shock, and in patients with hypersensitivity to the drug or any components of the drug. These drugs are used cautiously during lactation and in patients with cardiovascular disease, diabetes (may mask the symptoms of hypoglycemia), and hyperthyroidism (may mask symptoms of hyperthyroidism). A patient taking β-adrenergic blocking drugs for ophthalmic reasons may experience increased or additive effects when the drugs are administered with the oral β-blockers. Coadministration of timolol maleate and calcium antagonists may cause hypotension, left ventricular failure, and conduction disturbances within the heart. There is a potential additive hypotensive effect when the β-blocking ophthalmic drugs are administered with the phenothiazines.

FACT CHECK

44-5 How do sympathomimetics lower IOP?
44-6 How do β-adrenergic blocking drugs lower IOP?

Direct-Acting Miotics

Miotics contract the pupil of the eye, a condition called **miosis**, resulting in an increase in the space through which the aqueous humor flows. This increased space and improved flow results in a decrease in the intraocular pressure. Miotics may be used in the treatment of glaucoma (see Chapter 13). The miotics were, for a number of years, the drug of choice for glaucoma. These drugs have lost that first-choice treatment status to the β-adrenergic blocking drugs.

Direct-acting miotics may cause stinging on instillation, transient burning, tearing, headache, brow ache, and decreased night vision. Systemic adverse reactions include hypotension, flushing, breathing difficulties, nausea, vomiting, diarrhea, cardiac arrhythmias, and frequent urge to urinate.

These drugs are contraindicated in patients with hypersensitivity to the drug and in conditions in which constriction is undesirable (e.g., iritis, uveitis, and acute inflammatory disease of the anterior chamber). The drugs are used cautiously in patients with corneal abrasion, lactation, cardiac failure, bronchial asthma, peptic ulcer, hyperthyroidism, gastrointestinal spasm, urinary tract infection, Parkinson disease, recent myocardial infarction, hypotension, or hypertension. These drugs are also used cautiously in patients with angle-closure glaucoma because miotics can occasionally precipitate angle-closure glaucoma by increasing the resistance to aqueous flow from posterior to anterior chamber. See Chapter 13 for information on interactions.

FACT CHECK

44-7 What are common adverse reactions of direct-acting miotics?

Cholinesterase Inhibitor Miotics

The cholinesterase inhibitors are more potent and longer acting than the direct-acting miotics and are used to treat open-angle glaucoma. When administered into the eye, these drugs produce intense miosis (constriction of the pupil) and muscle contractions, causing a decreased resistance to aqueous outflow.

Adverse reactions and systemic toxicity are more common in the cholinesterase inhibitor ophthalmic preparations than in the direct-acting miotics. Ophthalmic adverse reactions include blurred vision, myopia, painful accommodative or ciliary body spasm, and night blindness. Systemic adverse reactions include nausea, vomiting, abdominal cramps, diarrhea, urinary incontinence, fainting, salivation, difficulty breathing, and cardiac irregularities. Iris cysts may form, enlarge, and obstruct vision. The iris cyst usually shrinks on discontinuation of use of the drug or after a reduction in strength of the drops or frequency of instillation.

Cholinesterase inhibitors are contraindicated in patients with hypersensitivity to the drug or any components of the drug. Some of these products contain sulfites, and patients with sulfite sensitivity may experience allergic-type reactions. The drugs are also contraindicated in patients with any active inflammatory disease of the eye and during lactation. The cholinesterase inhibitors are used cautiously in patients with myasthenia gravis (may cause additive adverse effects), before and after surgery, and in patients with chronic angle-closure (narrow angle) glaucoma or those with narrow angles (may cause papillary block and increase the angle blockage). When the cholinesterase inhibitors are administered with systemic anticholinesterase drugs, there is a risk for additive effects. Individuals, such as farmers, warehouse workers, or gardeners, working with carbamate or organophosphate insecticides or pesticides are at risk for systemic effects of the cholinesterase inhibitors from absorption of the pesticide or insecticide through the respiratory tract or the skin. Individuals working with pesticides or insecticides containing carbamate or organophosphate and taking a cholinesterase inhibitor should be advised to wear respiratory masks, change clothes frequently, and wash exposed clothes thoroughly.

FACT CHECK

44-8 Cholinesterase inhibitor miotics are used to treat which type of glaucoma?

Carbonic Anhydrase Inhibitors

Except for dorzolamide and brinzolamide, carbonic anhydrase inhibitors are administered systemically. Carbonic anhydrase is an enzyme found in many tissues of the body, including the eye. Inhibition of carbonic anhydrase in the eye decreases aqueous humor secretion, resulting in a decrease of intraocular pressure.

These drugs are used in the treatment of elevated intraocular pressure seen in open-angle glaucoma.

Adverse reactions associated with use of the carbonic anyhydrase inhibitors include ocular burning, stinging, or discomfort immediately after administration, bitter taste, ocular allergic reaction, blurred vision, tearing, dryness, dermatitis, foreign body sensation, ocular discomfort, photophobia, and headache.

Use of the carbonic anhydrase inhibitors is contraindicated in patients with known hypersensitivity and during lactation. The drugs are used cautiously in patients with renal and hepatic impairment. When high doses of the salicylates are administered concurrently, toxic levels of the carbonic anhydrase inhibitors have been reported. See Chapter 25 for more information on interactions of carbonic anhydrase inhibitors.

FACT CHECK
44-9   How do carbonic anhydrase inhibitors work?

Prostaglandin Agonists

Prostaglandin agonists act to lower intraocular pressure by increasing the outflow of aqueous humor through the trabecular meshwork. Prostaglandin agonists are used to lower intraocular pressure in patients with open-angle glaucoma and ocular hypertension in patients who do not tolerate other intraocular pressure–lowering medications or have an insufficient response to these medications.

Adverse reactions associated with the prostaglandin agonists include blurred vision, burning and stinging, foreign body sensation, itching, increased pigmentation of the iris, dry eye, excessive tearing, lid discomfort and pain, and photophobia.

MYDRIATICS

Vasoconstrictors/Mydriatics

Vasoconstrictors and **mydriatics** dilate the pupil **mydriasis,** constrict superficial blood vessels of the sclera, and decrease the formation of aqueous humor. Depending on the specific drug and strength, these drugs may be used before eye surgery in the treatment of glaucoma, for relief of minor eye irritation, redness, and to dilate the pupil for examination of the eye.

Adverse reactions include transitory stinging on initial instillation, blurring of vision, mydriasis, increased redness, irritation, discomfort, and increased intraocular pressure. Systemic adverse reactions include headache, brow ache, palpitations, tachycardia, arrhythmias, hypertension, myocardial infarction, and stroke.

These drugs are contraindicated in individuals with hypersensitivity, in patients with narrow-angle glaucoma or anatomically narrow-angle and no glaucoma, and in patients with sulfite sensitivity (some of these products contain sulfite). The drugs are used cautiously in patients with hypertension, diabetes, hyperthyroidism, cardiovascular disease, and arteriosclerosis.

Local anesthetics can increase absorption of topical drugs. Systemic adverse reactions may occur more frequently when these drugs are administered with the β-adrenergic blocking drugs. When mydriatics (drugs that dilate the pupil) are administered with monoamine oxidase inhibitors or as long as 21 days after monoamine oxidase inhibitors administration, exaggerated adrenergic effects may occur.

Antimuscarinics/Cycloplegic Mydriatics

Cycloplegic mydriatics cause mydriasis and **cycloplegia** (paralysis of the ciliary muscle, resulting in an inability to focus the eye). These drugs (see Chapter 14) are used in the treatment of inflammatory conditions of the iris and uveal tract of the eye and for examination of the eye.

Local adverse reactions associated with administration of the cycloplegic mydriatics include increased intraocular pressure, transient stinging or burning, and irritation with prolonged use (e.g., conjunctivitis, edema, exudates). Systemic adverse reactions include dryness of the mouth and skin, blurred vision, photophobia, corneal staining, tachycardia, headache, parasympathetic stimulation, and somnolence.

These drugs are contraindicated in patients with hypersensitivity and in patients with glaucoma. Some of these preparations contain sulfite, and individuals who are allergic to sulfites may have allergic-like symptoms. The cycloplegic mydriatics are used cautiously in elderly patients and during pregnancy and lactation. No significant interactions have been reported when the drugs are given topically.

FACT CHECK
44-10   What is cycloplegia?

ANTIHISTAMINES AND MAST CELL STABILIZERS

Antihistamines and mast cell stabilizers are used to treat the signs and symptoms of allergic conjuctivits (excessive watering or tearing and itching) as well as ocular pruritus. Mast cell stabilizers act by inhibiting the antigen-induced release of inflammatory mediators (e.g., histamine) from human mast cells.

Antihistamines used ophthalmically work the same as those taken orally; they compete with histamine at the receptor site. The antihistamines block the receptor and prevent histamine from causing its action, which results in watery, itchy eyes. Although mild, the adverse reactions associated with the mast cell inhibitors include headache, rhinitis, unpleasant taste, asthma, and cold/flu symptoms. These drugs may also cause ocular burning or irritation, dry eye, eye redness, foreign body sensation, and ocular discomfort.

In addition to single-ingredient products, the antihistamines are also used in combination with vasoconstrictors (decongestants) to relieve the symptoms of allergic conjunctivitis.

These drugs are contraindicated in patients with hypersensitivity. Mast cell stabilizers are used cautiously in patients who wear contact lenses (preservative may be absorbed by the soft contact lenses). They are all used with caution during lactation. There have been no significant drug–drug interactions associated with these drugs.

FACT CHECK

44-11 What are antihistamines and mast cell stabilizers used to treat?

ANTI-INFECTIVES

Antibiotics

Antibiotics have antibacterial activity and are used in the treatment of eye infections. See the Summary Drug Table: Select Ophthalmic Preparations.

Antibiotic ophthalmics are usually well tolerated, and few adverse reactions occur. Occasional transient irritation, burning, itching, stinging, inflammation, or blurring of vision may occur. With prolonged or repeated use, a superinfection may occur.

Antibiotic ophthalmics are contraindicated in patients with hypersensitivity. These drugs are also contraindicated in patients with epithelial herpes simplex keratitis, varicella, mycobacterial infection of the eye, and fungal diseases of the eye. There are no significant precautions or interactions when the drugs are administered as directed by the health care provider.

Antifungal Drugs

Antifungal drugs act against a variety of yeast and fungi. Natamycin is the only ophthalmic antifungal in use.

Adverse reactions are rare. Occasional local irritation to the eye may occur. Natamycin is contraindicated in patients with hypersensitivity. It is used cautiously during pregnancy and lactation.

Antiviral Drugs

Antiviral drugs interfere with viral reproduction by altering DNA synthesis. These drugs are used for the treatment of herpes simplex infections of the eye, treatment of immunocompromised patients with cytomegalovirus retinitis, and prevention of cytomegalovirus retinitis in patients undergoing transplantation.

The use of the antiviral ophthalmics may cause occasional irritation, pain, pruritus, inflammation, or edema of the eyes or lids; allergic reactions; foreign body sensation; photophobia; and corneal clouding.

These drugs are contraindicated in patients with hypersensitivity to the drug and are used cautiously in immunocompromised patients and during lactation. Some of these solutions contain boric acid and may result in a precipitate that causes irritation.

FACT CHECK

44-12 What are antibiotics used to treat?

ANTI-INFLAMMATORY AGENTS

Corticosteroids

Corticosteroids possess anti-inflammatory activity. They are used for inflammatory conditions, such as allergic conjunctivitis, keratitis, herpes zoster keratitis, and inflammation of the iris. Corticosteroids also may be used after injury to the cornea or after corneal transplants to prevent rejection.

Adverse reactions associated with administration of the corticosteroid ophthalmic preparations include elevated intraocular pressure with optic nerve damage, loss of visual acuity, cataract formation, delayed wound healing, secondary ocular infection, exacerbation of corneal infections, dry eyes, ptosis, blurred vision, discharge, ocular pain, foreign body sensation, and pruritus.

Corticosteroid ophthalmic preparations are contraindicated in patients with acute superficial herpes simplex keratitis, fungal disease of the eye, or viral diseases of the eye, and after removal of a superficial corneal foreign body. Corticosteroid ophthalmic preparations are used cautiously in patients with infectious conditions of the eye. These drugs are used cautiously during lactation. Prolonged use of the corticosteroids may result in elevated intraocular pressure and optic nerve damage.

Nonsteroidal Anti-Inflammatory Drugs

Nonsteroidal anti-inflammatory drugs inhibit prostaglandin synthesis (see Chapter 8 for a discussion), thereby exerting anti-inflammatory action. These drugs are used to treat postoperative inflammation after cataract surgery (diclofenac), for the relief of itching of the eyes caused by seasonal allergies (ketorolac), and during eye surgery to prevent miosis (flurbiprofen).

The most common adverse reactions associated with nonsteroidal anti-inflammatory drugs include transient burning and stinging on instillation and other minor ocular irritation.

These drugs are contraindicated in individuals with known hypersensitivity. Nonsteroidal anti-inflammatory drug flurbiprofen is contraindicated in patients with herpes simplex keratitis. Diclofenac and ketorolac are contraindicated in patients who wear soft contact lenses (may cause ocular irritation). Nonsteroidal anti-inflammatory drugs are used cautiously during pregnancy and lactation. Nonsteroidal anti-inflammatory drugs are used cautiously in patients with bleeding tendencies. When used topically, there is less risk of interactions with drugs or other substances. There is a possibility of a cross-sensitivity reaction when nonsteroidal anti-inflammatory drugs are administered to patients allergic to the salicylates. Corticosteroids and antibiotics are used cautiously in patients with sulfite sensitivity because an allergic-type reaction may result. Coadministration of idoxuridine with solutions containing boric acid may cause irritation.

LUBRICANTS

These products lubricate the eyes. Inactive ingredients may be found in some preparations. Examples of these drugs include preservatives, antioxidants, which prevent deterioration of the product, and drugs that slow drainage of the drug from the eye into the tear duct. Examples of the types of eye preparations are found in the Summary Drug Table: Select Ophthalmic Preparations. Artificial tear solutions are used for conditions such as dry eyes and eye irritation caused by inadequate tear production.

Adverse reactions are rare, but on occasion, redness or irritation may occur. Artificial tears are contraindicated in patients with hypersensitivity. No precautions or interactions have been reported.

Patient Management Issues with Ophthalmic Preparations

Before being placed in the eye, ophthalmic solutions and ointments can be warmed by hand for a few minutes. Ophthalmic ointments are applied to the eyelids or dropped into the lower conjunctival sac; ophthalmic solutions are dropped into the middle of the lower conjunctival sac (Fig. 44-3). Wash hands prior to inserting the drops or ointment and repeat afterward. Do not touch the tip of the dropper bottle or tube to the eye or anything else because it is sterile and touching could cause contamination. When two eye drops are prescribed for use at the same time, it is important to wait at least 5 minutes before instilling the second drug. This help

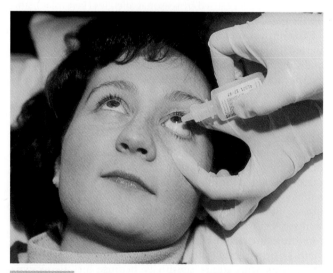

FIGURE 44-3 Instilling eye medication. While the patient looks upward, the lower lid is gently pulled down and the correct number of drops is instilled into the lower conjunctival sac.

prevents dilution of the drug and loss of some therapeutic effect from tearing.

Some ophthalmic drugs produce blurring of vision, which can result in falls and other injuries. Patients should be warned to be careful getting out of bed when their vision is impaired by these drugs.

Educating the Patient and Family about Ophthalmic Preparations

The patient or a family member requires instruction in the technique of instilling an ophthalmic preparation. In addition, following are key points about ophthalmic preparations the patient and family members should know:

- Eye preparations may cause a momentary stinging or burning sensation; this is normal.
- Temporary blurring of vision may occur. Avoid activities requiring clear vision until vision returns to normal.
- If more than one topical ophthalmic drug is being used, administer the drugs at least 5 to 10 minutes apart or as directed by the health care provider.
- Complete a full course of treatment with the prescribed drug to achieve satisfactory results.
- Do not rub your eyes, and keep your hands away from your eyes.
- Do not use nonprescription eye products during or after treatment unless your health care provider approves.
- Some of these preparations cause sensitivity (photophobia) to light; to minimize this, wear sunglasses.
- Notify your health care provider if your symptoms do not improve or if they worsen.
- Brimonidine patients should wait at least 15 minutes after instilling brimonidine before inserting soft contact lenses.

ALERT Rx

Ophthalmic Drops Used Otically
While otic drops should *never* be used ophthalmically, occasionally an ophthalmic drop may be used otically. Since the variety of drugs that are available in otic drops are limited, an ophthalmic drop may be used to deliver a medication to the ear that would otherwise not be possible given commercially available products. It is very important to read the label and ensure that the drops are being instilled correctly.

Prostaglandin Agonists

- Remove contact lenses before administration and leave them out at least 15 minutes before reinserting them.
- The color of your iris may change because of an increase of the brown pigment and cause different eye coloration. This may be more noticeable in patients with blue, green, gray-brown or other light-colored eyes.

Chapter Review

KEY POINTS

- Various preparations are used for the treatment of otic disorders. Three categories are antibiotics, antibiotic and steroid combinations, and miscellaneous preparations.
- Otic preparations are instilled in the external auditory canal and may be used to relieve pain, treat infection and inflammation, and aid in the removal of earwax.
- Various types of preparations are used for the treatment of ophthalmic disorders such as glaucoma (to lower the intraocular pressure), bacterial or viral infections of the eye, inflammatory conditions, and symptoms of allergy related to the eye.
- The incidence of adverse reactions associated with ophthalmic drugs is usually small. Because small amounts of the ophthalmic preparation may be absorbed systemically, some of the adverse effects associated with systemic administration of the particular drug may occur. Some ophthalmic preparations produce momentary stinging or burning on instillation.
- When administering an ophthalmic drop or ointment, the tip of the dropper or tube must not be touched. If it is touched, then it should be discarded and a new product purchased. Contamination of the dropper or tube could lead to an eye infection.

CRITICAL THINKING CASE STUDY
CASE 1

Otic Infection

Ms. Kassidy swims three times a week for exercise. Today she is in your clinic complaining of a feeling of fullness in her right ear. She is afraid that she might have water in her ear.
1. Which of the following would be appropriate for removing water from the ear?
   a. Antipyrine/benzocaine
   b. Isopropyl alcohol/glycerin
   c. Ciprofloxacin
   d. Hydrocortisone, neomycin, polymyxin

2. A couple of days later, Ms. Kassidy sees her physician because she now has ear pain in the same ear that she thought had water in it. Which of the following would NOT be appropriate for a bacterial ear infection?
   a. Antipyrine/benzocaine
   b. Isopropyl alcohol/glycerin
   c. Ciprofloxacin
   d. Hydrocortisone, neomycin, polymyxin
3. What would be appropriate counseling for otic drops used to treat an otic infection?

CASE 2

Glaucoma

Ms. Stone, age 76 years, has glaucoma and is prescribed timolol (Timoptic) eye drops. The initial assessment of Ms. Stone reveals that she also has severe arthritis and appears to have difficulty following instructions.
1. What other information should be obtained from Ms. Stone before beginning treatment?
   a. Whether she feels comfortable administering the eye drops
   b. Whether there is a family member who may be able to assist her should her arthritis make inserting the drops into her eye difficult
   c. Whether Ms. Stone lives alone
   d. All of the above
2. Ms. Stone looks perplexed about proper use of timolol. She wonders whether the number of drops she inserts into her eye matters. She should be told
   a. it is important to try to insert the prescribed amount in each eye
   b. there is no precise measure; she should attempt to insert enough that her eye feels moist from the medication
   c. she should insert a drop, rub her eye, and insert another drop
   d. none of the above

3. Ms. Stone wonders whether there are any potential adverse reactions to timolol. You tell her
   a. eye pain or dryness are common adverse reactions
   b. there are no known adverse reactions
   c. adverse reactions exist only when timolol is combined with antidiabetic drugs
   d. a and c
4. How would you instruct Ms. Stone to put the drops in her eye?

Review Questions

MULTIPLE CHOICE

1. What is the rationale for warming an otic solution that has been refrigerated before instilling the drops into a patient's ear?
   a. The drug becomes thick when refrigerated, and warming liquefies the solution.
   b. It helps to prevent dizziness on instillation.
   c. A cold solution can significantly increase the patient's blood pressure.
   d. A cold solution could damage the tympanic membrane.
2. An otic preparation is instilled into the
   a. inner ear
   b. middle ear
   c. external auditory canal
   d. pinna
3. An ophthalmic solution is instilled into the
   a. inner canthus
   b. upper conjunctival sac
   c. lower conjunctival sac
   d. upper canthus
4. Which of the following instructions would be included for a patient prescribed an ophthalmic solution?
   a. Squeeze your eyes tightly after the solution is instilled.
   b. Immediately wipe your eye using pressure to squeeze out excess medication.
   c. After the drug is instilled, remain upright with your head bent slightly forward for approximately 2 minutes.
   d. Temporary stinging or burning may be felt at the time the drug is inserted in your eye.

MATCHING

Match the otic preparation on the left with the correct trade name on the right.

_____ 5. hydrocortisone/neomycin/
　　　　 polymyxinB　　　　　　a. Swim-Ear
_____ 6. hydrocortisone/　　　　b. Ciprodex
　　　　 acetic acid　　　　　　c. DermOtic
_____ 7. ciprofloxacin　　　　　d. Cetraxal
_____ 8. ciprofloxacin/　　　　　e. Cortisporin Otic
　　　　 dexamethasone　　　　f. Otoalgan
_____ 9. acetic acid
_____ 10. isoporpyl alcohol/
　　　　　glycerin

_____ 11. antipyrine/benzocaine　g. Acetasol HC
_____ 12. fluocinolone　　　　　h. VoSol

Match the ophthalmic preparation on the left with the correct trade name on the right.

_____ 13. betaxolol　　　　　　a. Alomide
_____ 14. bimatoprost　　　　　b. Betagan
_____ 15. azelastine　　　　　　c. Ciloxan
_____ 16. brinzolamide　　　　　d. Natacyn
_____ 17. levobunolol　　　　　e. Betoptic-S
_____ 18. lodoxamide　　　　　f. Vitrasert
_____ 19. natamycin　　　　　　g. Lumigan
_____ 20. ciprofloxacin　　　　　h. Optivar
_____ 21. diclofenac　　　　　　i. Azopt
_____ 22. ganciclovir　　　　　　j. Voltaren

TRUE OR FALSE

_____ 23. Otic preparations have no significant interactions with other drugs.
_____ 24. A patient with allergic conjunctivitis would likely be prescribed mast cell stabilizers to prevent eye itching.
_____ 25. A patient with an inner ear infection would likely be treated with a topical otic preparation.
_____ 26. Mydriatics contract the pupil of the eye.

FILL IN THE BLANKS

27. Treatment for a patient with herpes simplex infection of the eye would likely include _____ _____.
28. _____, which is used to soften earwax, should not remain in the ear canal for more than _____ minutes.
29. A patient receiving prolonged treatment with an antibiotic otic drug might experience _____ as an adverse reaction.
30. Miotics are drugs used for glaucoma that _____ the pupil, thus allowing increased space for _____ _____ to flow through.

SHORT ANSWERS

31. After an otic medication is instilled, how should the patient be positioned?
32. A patient has been prescribed two eye drops for use at the same time. How would you advise the patient to instill the drugs? Why?

Web Activities

1. Go to the American Optometric Association Web site (http://www.aoa.org). Under "Eye & Vision Problems," go to the information on conjunctivitis. What are the causes of conjunctivitis? How is conjunctivitis diagnosed? Are there any special precautions for contact lens wearers? What can a person do to reduce the spread of conjunctivitis?
2. At the same website, return to the "Eye & Vision Problems" tab and go to the information on dry eye. What are the causes of dry eye? How is dry eye treated? What can a person do to reduce the symptoms?

SUMMARY DRUG TABLE Otic Preparations (left, generic; right, trade)

Comprehensive Summary Drug Tables, including uses, adverses effects, dosages, and pregnancy classifications, are provided on the companion website, http://thePoint.lww.com/PharmacologyHP2e

Steroid and Antibiotic Combinations, Solutions	
hydrocortisone 1%, acetic acid 2% solution *hye-droe-kor'-ti-sone*	Acetasol HC, Otomycet-HC, VSol HC
hydrocortisone, neomycin sulfate, polymyxin B	Cortisporin Otic, Oticin HC, Otimar, Otocidin, *generic*

Steroid and Antibiotic Combinations, Suspensions	
ciprofloxacin, hydrocortisone suspension *sip-roe-floks'-a-sin*	Cipro HC
ciprofloxacin, dexamethasone suspension	Ciprodex
hydrocortisone, neomycin sulfate, polymyxin B	Aural, Cortomycin, Oticin HC, Otimar, *generic*

Otic Antibiotics	
ciprofloxacin solution	Cetraxal
ofloxacin solution *oh-floks'-a-sin*	*generic*

Miscellaneous Otic Preparations	
acetic acid 2% solution *a-see'-tik*	VoSol, *generic*

antipyrine, benzocaine *an-tee-pye'-reen/ben'-zoe-kane*	Aurodex, Auroguard, Dolotic, Oto Care, Otoalgan, Pro-Otic, *generic*
antipyrine, benzocaine, u-polycosanol 410 solution	Auralgan, Otic Care, Treagan
antipyrine, benzocaine, phenylephrine solution	Otogesic
carbamide peroxide, anhydrous glycerin *kar'-ba-mide*	E-R-O Ear, Mollifene Ear Wax Removing Formula, Murine Ear, Debrox
chloroxylenol, glycerin, pramoxine, zinc solution	Zinotic, Zinotic ES
fluocinolone acetonide iol *floo-oh-sin'-oh-lone*	DermOtic
hydrocortisone, pramoxine, chloroxylenol solution	Aero Otic HC, Cortane B, Exotic-HC, Mediotic-HC, Oto-End, Otomar
isopropyl alcohol 95%, glycerin 5%	Swim-Ear, Auro-Dri, Ear Dry, Dri/Ear

SUMMARY DRUG TABLE Select Ophthalmic Preparations (left, generic; right, trade)

Comprehensive Summary Drug Tables, including uses, adverses effects, dosages, and pregnancy classifications, are provided on the companion website, http://thePoint.lww.com/PharmacologyHP2e

ANTIGLAUCOMA AGENTS	
α₂ Adrenergic Receptor Agonists	
brimonidine *bri-moe'-ni-deen*	Alphagan P, *generic*
Carbonic Anhydrase Inhibitors	
brinzolamide *brin-zoh'-la-mide*	Azopt
Dorzolamide *dor-zole'-a-mide*	Trusopt, *generic*
Miotics, Direct-Acting	
carbachol *kar'-ba-kole*	Isopto Carbachol (ophthalmic solution), Miostat (injection)
pilocarpine *pye-loe-kar'-peen*	Isopto Carpine, Pilopine-HS, *generic*
acetylcholine chloride *a-se-teel-koe'-leen*	Miochol-E
Sympathomimetic	
apraclonidine *a-pra-kloe'-ni-deen*	Iopidine, *generic*
Miotics, Cholinesterase Inhibitors	
echothiophate *ek-oh-thye'-oh-fate*	Phospholine Iodide
α-Agonist/β-Blocker Combinations	
brimonidine, timolol *bri-moe'-ni-deen/ tim'-oh-lol*	Combigan

β-Blocker/Carbonic Anhydrous Inhibitor Combinations	
dorzolamide/timolol *dor-zole'-a-mide/ tim'-oh-lol*	Cosopt, *generic*
β-Blockers	
betaxolol *be-taks'-oh-lol*	Betoptic S, *generic*
carteolol *kar'-tee-oh-lole*	*generic*
levobunolol *lee-voe-byoo'-noe-lole*	Betagan, *generic*
metipranolol *met-i-pran'-oh-lol*	Optipranolol, *generic*
timolol *tim'-oh-lol*	Betimol, Istalol, *generic*
Prostaglandins	
bimatoprost *bi-mat'-oh-prost*	Lumigan, Latisse
latanoprost *la-ta'-noe-prost*	Xalatan, *generic*
travoprost *tra'-voe-prost*	Travatan Z
Mydriatics Adrenergic Agonists	
Mydriatic combination hydroxyamphetamine, tropicamide *hye-droks-ee-am-fet'-a-meen / troe-pik'-a-mide*	Paremyd

phenylephrine *fen-il-ef'-rin*	AK-Dilate, Mydfrin, Neo-Synephrine, Neofrin, *generic*
Mydriatic combination phenylephrine, cyclopentolate *fen-il-ef'-rin* *sye-kloe-pen'-toe-late*	Cyclomydril
phenylephrine, scopolamine *fen-il-ef'-rin/ skoe-pol'-a-meen*	Murocoll-2
Antimuscarinics/Cycloplegic Mydriatics	
atropine *a'-troe-peen*	Isopto Atropine, *generic*
cyclopentolate *sye-kloe-pen'-toe-late*	AK-Pentolate, Cyclogyl, Cylate, *generic*
homatropine hydrobromide *hoe-ma'-troe-peen*	Isopto Homatropine
scopolamine *skoe-pol'-a-meen*	Isopto Hyoscine
tropicamide *troe-pik'-a-mide*	Mydral, Mydriacil, Tropicacyl, *generic*
Ophthalmic Anesthetics	
lidocaine *lye'-doe-kane*	Akten
proparacaine *proe-par'-a-kane*	Alcaine, Parcaine, *generic*

(contiued)

SUMMARY DRUG TABLE: Select Ophthalmic Preparations (continued)

ANTIGLAUCOMA AGENTS

Ophthalmic Anesthetics (continued)

Drug	Trade Name
proparacaine/ fluorescein *proe-par'-a-kane/* *flure'-e-seen*	Flucaine, Fluoracaine
tetracaine *tet'-ra-kane*	Tetcaine, TetraVisc, *generic*

Antihistamines and Mast Cell Stabilizers

Drug	Trade Name
azelastine *a-zel'-as-teen*	Optivar, *generic*
bepotastine *be-poe-tas'-teen*	Bepreve
cromolyn sodium *kroe'-moe-line*	Crolom, *generic*
emedastine *em-e-das'-teen*	Emadine
epinastine *ep-i-nas'-teen*	Elestat, *generic*
ketotifen *kee-toe-tye'-fen*	Alaway, Clairitin Eye, Itchy Eye, Zaditor, Zyrtec Itchy Eye, *generic*
lodoxamide *loe-doks'-a-mide*	Alomide
nedocromil *ne-doe-kroe'-mil*	Alocril
olopatadine *oh-la-pat'-a-deen*	Pataday, Patanol
pemirolast *pe-mir'-oh-last*	Alamast

Vasoconstrictors (Decongestants)

Drug	Trade Name
naphazoline *naf-az'-oh-leen*	AK-Con, All Clear, All Clear AR, Napha Forte, *generic* (OTC)
oxymetazoline *oks-i-met-az'-oh-leen*	Visine L.R. (OTC)
phenylephrine *fen-in-ef'-rin*	Ak-Dilate, Mydfrin, Neofrin, *generic*
tetrahydrozoline *tet-ra-hye-droz'-a-leen*	Opti-Clear, Visine Original, *generic* (OTC)

Antihistamine/Vasoconstrictor (Decongestant) Combination

Drug	Trade Name
naphazoline/ pheniramine *naf-az'-oh-leen/* *fen-nir'-a-meen*	Naphcon A, Opcon-A, Visine-A

ANTINFECTIVES

Antibiotics

Drug	Trade Name
bacitracin *bas-i-tray'-sin*	*generic*
besifloxacin *be-si-flox'-a-sin*	Besivance
ciprofloxacin *sip-roe-floks'-a-sin*	Ciloxan, *generic*
erythromycin *er-ith-roe-mye'-sin*	Ilotycin, Romycin, *generic*
gatifloxacin *gat-i-floks'-a-sin*	Zymaxid
gentamicin *jen-ta-mye'-sin*	Garamycin, Gentak, *generic*
levofloxacin *lee-voe-floks'-a-sin*	Iquix, Quixin, *generic*
moxifloxacin *moks-i-floks'-a-sin*	Moxeza, Vigamox
ofloxacin *oh-floks'-a-sin*	Ocuflox, *generic*
tobramycin *toe-bra-mye'-sin*	AK-Tob, Tobrasol, Tobrex, *generic*

Antifungals

Drug	Trade Name
natamycin *na-ta-mye'-sin*	Natacyn

Antivirals

Drug	Trade Name
ganciclovir *gan-sye'-kloe-veer*	Vitrasert, Zirgan
trifluridine *trye-flure'-i-deen*	Viroptic, *generic*

ANTIINFLAMMATORY AGENTS

Corticosteroids

Drug	Trade Name
dexamethasone *deks-a-meth'-a-sone*	Maxidex, Ozurdex, *generic*
difluprednate *dye-floo-pred'-nate*	Durezol
fluocinolone *floo-oh-sin'-oh-lone*	Retisert
fluorometholone *flure-oh-meth'-oh-lone*	Flarex, FML Forte, *generic*
loteprednol *loe-te-pred'-nol*	Alrex, Lotemax
prednisolone *pred-niss'-oh-lone*	Econopred Plus, Omnipred, Pred Mild, Pred-Forte, Pred-Phosphate, *generic*
rimexolone *ri-meks'-oh-lone*	Vexol

NSAIDS

Drug	Trade Name
bromfenac *brome'-fen-ak*	Bromday, *generic*
diclofenac *dye-kloe'-fen-ak*	Voltaren, *generic*
flurbiprofen *flure-bi'-proe-fen*	Ocufen, *generic*
ketorolac *kee'-toe-role-ak*	Acular, Acular LS, Acuvail, *generic*
nepafenac *ne-pa-fen'-ak*	Nevanac

Antiinfective/Antiinflammatory Combinations

Drug	Trade Name
loteprednol/ tobramycin *Loe-te-pred'-nol/* *toe-bra-mye'-sin*	Zylet
neomycin/polymyxin B/hydrocortisone *nee-oh-mye'-sin/* *pol-i-miks'-in bee/* *hye-droe-kor'-ti-sone*	*generic*
neomycin/polymyxin B/dexamethasone *nee-oh-mye'-sin/* *pol-i-miks'-in bee/* *deks-a-meth'-a-sone*	Maxitrol, Poly-Dex, *generic*
neomycin/polymyxin B/bacitracin/ hydrocortisone *nee-oh-mye'-sin/* *pol-i-miks'-in bee/* *bas-i-tray'-sin/* *hye-droe-kor'-ti-sone*	*Generic*
prednisolone/ sulfacetamide *pred-niss'-oh-lone*	Blephamide, *generic*
tobramycin/ dexamethasone *toe-bra-mye'-sin/* *deks-a-meth'-a-sone*	Tobradex, *generic*
fluorometholone, sulfacetamide *flure-oh-meth'-oh-lone*	FML S
neomycin, polymyxin B, prednisolone *nee-oh-mye'-sin/* *pol-i-miks'-in bee/* *pred-nis'-oh-lone*	Poly-Pred
gentamicin, prednisolone *jen-ta-mye'-sin/* *pred-nis'-oh-lone*	Pred-G

Lubricants

Drug	Trade Name
Artificial Tears	Variety of trade names (OTC)
cyclosporine *cye-kloe-spor'-een*	Restasis

45

Fluids, Electrolytes, and Total Parenteral Nutrition

CHAPTER OBJECTIVES

On completion of this chapter, students will be able to:

1. Define the chapter's key terms.
2. Describe the general drug actions, uses, adverse reactions, contraindications, precautions, and interactions of fluids and electrolytes.
3. Discuss important points to keep in mind when educating the patient or family members about the use of fluids and electrolytes.

KEY TERMS

electrolyte—an electrically charged particle (ion) that is essential for normal cell function and is involved in various metabolic activities

fluid overload—a condition when the body's fluid requirements are met and the administration of fluid occurs at a rate that is greater than the rate at which the body can use or eliminate the fluid

half-normal saline—solution containing 0.45% NaCl

hypocalcemia—low blood calcium

hypokalemia—low blood potassium

hyponatremia—low blood sodium

normal saline—solution containing 0.9% NaCl

protein substrates—amino acid preparations that act to promote the production of proteins and are essential to life

substrate—a substance that is the basic component of an organism

CHAPTER OVERVIEW

Drug classes covered in this chapter are:

- Solutions Used in the Management of Body Fluids
- Electrolytes
- Total Parenteral Nutrition

Drugs by classification are listed on page 494.

thePOINT RESOURCES

- Comprehensive Summary Drug Tables
- Interactive Practice and Review
- Monographs of Most Commonly Prescribed Drugs

483

The composition of body fluids remains relatively constant despite the many demands placed on the body each day. On occasion, these demands cannot be met, and electrolytes and fluids must be given in an attempt to restore equilibrium.

Electrolytes are electrically charged particles (ions) that are essential for normal cell function and are involved in various metabolic activities. This chapter discusses the use of electrolytes to replace one or more electrolytes that may be lost by the body.

Solutions Used in the Management of Body Fluids

When body fluids are depleted, they can be replaced using a number of solutions that increase the volume of fluid in circulation at any given time. The solutions used in the management of body fluids discussed in this chapter include blood plasma, plasma protein fractions, protein substrates, energy substrates, plasma proteins, electrolytes, and miscellaneous replacement fluids.

Actions and Uses of Solutions Used in the Management of Body Fluids

Blood Plasma

Blood plasma is the liquid part of blood, containing water, sugar, electrolytes, fats, gases, proteins, bile pigment, and clotting factors. Human plasma, also called human pooled plasma, is obtained from donated blood. Although whole blood must be typed and cross-matched because it contains red blood cells carrying blood type and Rh factors, human plasma does not require this procedure. Therefore, plasma can be given quickly in acute emergencies.

Plasma administered intravenously is used to increase blood volume when severe hemorrhage has occurred, and it is necessary to partially restore blood volume while waiting for whole blood to be typed and cross-matched. Another use of plasma is in treating conditions when plasma alone has been lost, as may occur with severe burns.

Plasma Protein Fractions

Plasma protein fractions include human plasma protein fraction 5% and normal serum albumin 5% (Albuminar-5, Buminate 5%) and 25% (Albuminar-25, Buminate 25%). Plasma protein fraction 5% is an intravenous solution containing 5% human plasma proteins. Serum albumin is obtained from donated whole blood and is a protein found in plasma. The albumin fraction of human blood acts to maintain plasma colloid osmotic pressure and as a carrier of intermediate metabolites in the transport and exchange of tissue products. It is critical in regulating the volume of circulating blood. When blood is lost from shock, such as in hemorrhage, the person has a reduced plasma volume. When blood volume is reduced, albumin quickly restores the volume in most situations.

Plasma protein fractions are used to treat hypovolemic (low blood volume) shock that occurs as the result of burns, trauma, surgery, and infections, or in conditions in which shock is not currently present but likely to occur. Plasma protein fractions are also used to treat hypoproteinemia (a deficiency of protein in the blood), as might occur in patients with nephrotic syndrome and hepatic cirrhosis, as well as other diseases or disorders. A blood type and cross-match is not needed when plasma protein fractions are given.

Protein Substrates

A **substrate** is a substance that is the basic component of an organism. **Protein substrates** are amino acid preparations that act to promote the production of proteins (anabolism). Amino acids are necessary to promote synthesis of structural components, reduce the rate of protein breakdown (catabolism), promote wound healing, and act as buffers in extracellular and intracellular fluids. Crystalline amino acid preparations are hypertonic solutions of balanced essential and nonessential amino acid concentrations that provide substrates for protein synthesis or act to conserve existing body protein.

Amino acids promote the production of proteins, enhance tissue repair and wound healing, and reduce the rate of protein breakdown. Amino acids are used in certain disease states, such as severe kidney and liver disease, as well as in total parenteral nutrition solutions (see the last section of this chapter). Total parenteral nutrition may be used in patients with conditions such as impairment of gastrointestinal absorption of protein; in patients with an increased requirement for protein, as seen in those with extensive burns or infections; and in patients with no available oral route for nutritional intake.

Energy Substrates

Energy substrates include dextrose solutions and fat emulsion. Solutions used to supply energy and fluid include dextrose (glucose) in water or sodium chloride, alcohol in dextrose, and intravenous fat emulsion. Dextrose is available in various strengths in a fluid, which may be water or saline. Dextrose and dextrose in alcohol are available in various strengths in water. Dextrose solutions also are available with electrolytes, for example, Plasma-Lyte 56 and 5% Dextrose.

An intravenous fat emulsion contains soybean or safflower oil and a mixture of natural triglycerides, predominately unsaturated fatty acids. No more than 60% of the patient's total caloric intake should come from fat emulsion, with carbohydrates and amino acids comprising the remaining 40% or more of caloric intake.

Dextrose is a carbohydrate used to provide a source of calories and fluid. Alcohol (in dextrose) also provides calories.

Intravenous fat emulsion is used in the prevention and treatment of essential fatty acid deficiency. It also provides nonprotein calories for those receiving total parenteral nutrition when calorie requirements cannot be met by glucose. Fat emulsion is used as a source of calories and essential fatty acids for patients requiring parenteral nutrition for extended periods (usually more than 5 days).

Plasma Expanders

The intravenous solutions of plasma expanders include hetastarch (Hespan), low-molecular-weight dextran (Dextran 40), and high-molecular-weight dextran (Dextran 70, Dextran 75).

Plasma expanders are used to expand plasma volume when shock is caused by burns, hemorrhage, surgery, and other trauma and for prophylaxis of venous thrombosis and thromboembolism. When used in the treatment of shock, plasma expanders are not a substitute for whole blood or plasma, but they are of value as emergency measures until those substances can be used.

Intravenous Replacement Solutions

Intravenous replacement solutions are a source of electrolytes and water for hydration and used to facilitate amino acid utilization and maintain electrolyte balance.

Dextrose and electrolyte solutions such as Plasma-Lyte R and 5% dextrose are used as a parenteral source of electrolytes, calories, or water for hydration. Invert sugar–electrolyte solutions, such as Multiple Electrolytes and Travert 5% and 10%, contain equal parts of dextrose and fructose and are used as a source of calories and hydration.

Adverse Reactions of Solutions Used in the Management of Body Fluids

Blood Plasma

When a patient receives a transfusion of blood plasma, he or she can experience a hemolytic transfusion reaction. This reaction is caused by the antibodies in the patient's blood reacting to antigens in the plasma. Patients with an immunoglobulin A (IgA) deficiency may have an anaphylactic reaction to donor plasma as well.

Plasma Protein Fractions

Adverse reactions are rare when plasma protein fractions are administered, but nausea, chills, fever, urticaria, and hypotensive episodes may occur occasionally.

Protein Substrates

Use of protein substrates (amino acids) may result in nausea, fever, flushing of the skin, metabolic acidosis or alkalosis, and decreased phosphorus and calcium blood levels.

Energy Substrates

The most common adverse reaction associated with the administration of fat emulsion is sepsis caused by administration equipment and thrombophlebitis caused by vein irri-

tations. Less frequently occurring adverse reactions include dyspnea, cyanosis, hyperlipidemia, hypercoagulability, nausea, vomiting, headache, flushing, increase in temperature, sweating, sleepiness, chest and back pain, slight pressure over the eyes, and dizziness.

Plasma Expanders

Use of hetastarch, a plasma expander, may cause vomiting, a mild temperature elevation, itching, and allergic reactions. Allergic reactions are evidenced by wheezing, edema around the eyes (periorbital edema), and urticaria. Other plasma expanders may result in mild cutaneous eruptions, generalized urticaria, hypotension, nausea, vomiting, headache, dyspnea, fever, tightness of the chest, bronchospasm, wheezing, and, rarely, anaphylactic shock.

Intravenous Replacement Solutions

Intravenous replacement solutions are generally well tolerated.

Contraindications, Precautions, and Interactions of Solutions Used in the Management of Body Fluids

All of the solutions used in the management of body fluids are contraindicated in patients with hypersensitivity to any component of the solution.

Blood Plasma

- Blood plasma is used cautiously during pregnancy and lactation.
- No interactions have been reported in the use of blood plasma.

Plasma Protein Fractions

- Plasma proteins are contraindicated in those with a history of allergic reactions to albumin, severe anemia, or cardiac failure; in the presence of normal or increased intravascular volume; and in patients on cardiopulmonary bypass.
- Plasma protein fractions are used cautiously in patients who are in shock or dehydrated, and in those with congestive cardiac failure or liver or kidney failure.
- These solutions are used cautiously during pregnancy and lactation.

Protein Substrates

- These solutions are used cautiously during pregnancy and lactation.

Energy Substrates

- Dextrose solutions are contraindicated in patients with diabetic coma with excessively high blood sugar.
- Concentrated dextrose solutions are contraindicated in patients with increased intracranial pressure, delirium tremens (if patient is dehydrated), hepatic coma, or glucose–galactose malabsorption syndrome.
- Alcohol dextrose solutions are contraindicated in patients with epilepsy, urinary tract infections, alcoholism, and diabetic coma.

- Alcohol dextrose solutions are used cautiously in patients with hepatic and renal impairment, vitamin deficiency (may cause or potentiate vitamin deficiency), diabetes, or shock; during postpartum hemorrhage; and after cranial surgery.
- Dextrose solutions are used cautiously in patients receiving a corticosteroid or corticotropin.
- Dextrose and alcohol dextrose solutions are incompatible with blood (may cause hemolysis).
- Intravenous fat emulsions are contraindicated in conditions that interfere with normal fat metabolism (e.g., acute pancreatitis) and in patients allergic to eggs.
- Intravenous fat emulsions are used with caution in those with severe liver impairment, pulmonary disease, anemia, and blood coagulation disorders. They also are used cautiously during pregnancy and lactation.

Plasma Expanders

- Plasma expanders are contraindicated in patients with severe bleeding disorders, severe cardiac failure, renal failure with oliguria, or anuria.
- Plasma expanders are used cautiously in patients with renal disease, congestive heart failure, pulmonary edema, and severe bleeding disorders.
- Plasma expanders are used cautiously during pregnancy and lactation.

Intravenous Replacement Solutions

If too much solution is given, it is possible for the patient to experience fluid overload or circulatory overload.

Patient Management Issues with Solutions Used in the Management of Body Fluids

Before intravenous use of fluids and electrolytes, the patient's blood pressure, pulse, and respiratory rate are taken to provide a baseline, which is especially important when the patient is receiving blood plasma, plasma expanders, or plasma protein fractions for shock or other serious disorders. Ongoing measurements are important also. A patient in shock and receiving a plasma expander may require monitoring of the blood pressure and pulse rate every 5 to 15 minutes, whereas the patient receiving dextrose 3 days after surgery may require monitoring every 30 to 60 minutes.

One adverse reaction common to all solutions administered by the parenteral route is **fluid overload**, that is, the administration of more fluid than the body is able to handle. Patients

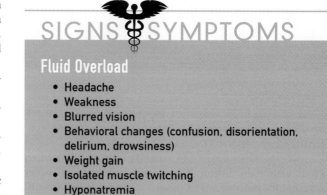

SIGNS & SYMPTOMS

Fluid Overload

- Headache
- Weakness
- Blurred vision
- Behavioral changes (confusion, disorientation, delirium, drowsiness)
- Weight gain
- Isolated muscle twitching
- Hyponatremia
- Rapid breathing
- Wheezing
- Coughing
- Rise in blood pressure
- Distended neck veins
- Elevated central venous pressure
- Convulsions

receiving intravenous solutions are observed at frequent intervals for signs of fluid overload. If signs of fluid overload (Signs and Symptoms box) are observed, the intravenous infusion rate is slowed and the health care provider is notified immediately.

Educating the Patient and Family about Solutions Used in the Management of Body Fluids

The patient and family members are given a brief explanation of the reason for and the method of administration of an intravenous solution. Sometimes, patients or family members tamper with or adjust the rate of flow of intravenous administration sets. They need to understand the importance of not touching the intravenous administration set or the equipment used to administer intravenous fluids.

Electrolytes

Along with a disturbance in fluid volume (e.g., loss of plasma, blood, or water) or a need for parenteral nutrition, an electrolyte imbalance may exist (Key Concepts 45-1). An electrolyte is an electrically charged substance essential to the normal

---

ALERT ℞

Infusion with a Fat Solution

During the first 30 minutes of infusion of a fat solution, the patient is carefully observed for difficulty in breathing, headache, flushing, nausea, vomiting, or signs of a hypersensitivity reaction. If any of these reactions occur, the infusion is discontinued and the health care provider is notified immediately.

CONSIDERATIONS | Older adults

LIFESPAN

Increased Risk of Fluid Overload

Older adults are at increased risk for fluid overload because of the increased incidence of cardiac disease and decreased renal function that may accompany old age. Careful monitoring for signs and symptoms of fluid overload is extremely important when administering fluids to older adults.

KEY CONCEPTS

45-1   Electrolyte Imbalance

In some instances, an electrolyte imbalance may be present without an appreciable disturbance in fluid balance. For example, a patient taking a diuretic is able to maintain fluid balance by an adequate oral intake of water, which replaces the water lost through diuresis. However, the patient is likely to be unable to replace the potassium that is also lost during diuresis. When the potassium concentration in the blood is too low, as may occur with the use of a diuretic, an imbalance may occur that requires the addition of potassium.

functioning of all cells. Electrolytes circulate in the blood at specific levels where they are available for use when needed by the cells. An electrolyte imbalance occurs when the concentration of an electrolyte in the blood is either too high or too low. Commonly used electrolytes are listed in the Summary Drug Table: Electrolytes. Combined electrolyte solutions are also available (Box 45-1).

Actions and Uses of Electrolytes

Bicarbonate (HCO$_3^-$)

This electrolyte plays a vital role in the acid–base balance of the body. Bicarbonate may be given intravenously as sodium bicarbonate (NaHCO$_3$) in the treatment of metabolic acidosis, a state of imbalance that may be seen in

BOX 45.1

Combined Electrolyte Solutions

- Combined electrolyte solutions are available for oral and intravenous use. The intravenous solutions contain various electrolytes and dextrose.
- Intravenous solutions are used to replace fluid and electrolytes that have been lost and to provide calories by means of their carbohydrate content. Examples of intravenous electrolyte solutions are dextrose 5% with 0.9% sodium chloride, lactated Ringer injection, Plasma-Lyte, and 10% Travert (invert sugar—a combination of equal parts of fructose and dextrose), and Electrolyte No. 2. The health care provider selects the type of combined electrolyte solution to meet the patient's needs.
- Oral electrolyte solutions contain a carbohydrate and various electrolytes. Examples of combined oral electrolyte solutions are Pedialyte and Rehydralyte. Oral electrolyte solutions are most often used to replace lost electrolytes, carbohydrates, and fluid in conditions such as severe vomiting or diarrhea.

diseases or situations such as severe shock, diabetic acidosis, severe diarrhea, extracorporeal circulation of blood, severe renal disease, and cardiac arrest. Oral sodium bicarbonate is used as a gastric and urinary alkalinizer. It may be used as a single drug or may be found as one of the ingredients in some antacid preparations. It is also useful in treating severe diarrhea accompanied by bicarbonate loss.

Bicarbonate is no longer used as the first-line treatment during cardiopulmonary resuscitation after cardiac arrest. According to the American Heart Association, bicarbonate is used when all other treatment options have failed.

Calcium (Ca^{++})

Calcium is necessary for the functioning of nerves and muscles, the clotting of blood (see Chapter 23), the building of bones and teeth, and other physiologic processes. Examples of calcium salts are calcium gluconate and calcium carbonate.

Calcium may be given for the treatment of **hypocalcemia** (low blood calcium), which may be seen in patients with parathyroid disease or after accidental removal of the parathyroid glands during surgery of the thyroid gland. Calcium may also be given during cardiopulmonary resuscitation, particularly after open heart surgery, when epinephrine fails to improve weak or ineffective myocardial contractions. Calcium may be used as adjunct therapy of insect bites or stings to reduce muscle cramping, such as occurs with black widow spider bites. Calcium may also be recommended for those eating a diet low in calcium or as a dietary supplement when there is an increased need for calcium, such as during pregnancy.

FACT CHECK

45-6 Sodium bicarbonate is given intravenously to treat what disorder?

45-7 What is low blood calcium called?

Magnesium (Mg^{++})

Magnesium plays an important role in the transmission of nerve impulses. It is also important in the activity of many enzyme reactions, such as carbohydrate metabolism.

Magnesium sulfate is used as replacement therapy in hypomagnesemia. Magnesium sulfate is used in the prevention and control of seizures in obstetric patients with pregnancy-induced hypertension, also referred to as eclampsia and preeclampsia. It may also be added to total parenteral nutrition mixtures.

Potassium (K$^+$)

Potassium is necessary for the transmission of impulses; the contraction of smooth, cardiac, and skeletal muscles; and other important physiologic processes. Potassium as a drug is available as potassium chloride (KCl) and potassium gluconate.

Potassium may be given for **hypokalemia** (low blood potassium). Examples of causes of hypokalemia are a marked loss of gastrointestinal fluids (severe vomiting, diarrhea, nasogastric suction, draining intestinal fistulas), diabetic acidosis, marked diuresis, and severe malnutrition.

Sodium (Na⁺)

Sodium is essential for the maintenance of normal heart action and in the regulation of osmotic pressure in body cells. Sodium, as sodium chloride, may be given intravenously. A solution containing 0.9% sodium chloride is called **normal saline**, and a solution containing 0.45% NaCl is called **half-normal saline**. Sodium also is available combined with dextrose, such as dextrose 5% and sodium chloride 0.9%.

Sodium is used to treat **hyponatremia** (low blood sodium). Examples of causes of hyponatremia are excessive diaphoresis, severe vomiting or diarrhea, excessive diuresis, and draining intestinal fistulas.

Adverse Reactions of Electrolytes

Bicarbonate (HCO₃⁻)

In some instances, excessive oral use may produce nausea and vomiting. Some individuals may use sodium bicarbonate (baking soda) for the relief of gastric disturbances, such as pain, discomfort, symptoms of indigestion, and gas. Prolonged use of oral sodium bicarbonate or excessive doses of intravenous sodium bicarbonate may result in systemic alkalosis.

Calcium (Ca⁺⁺)

Irritation of the vein, tingling, a metallic or chalky taste, and "heat waves" may occur when calcium is given intravenously.

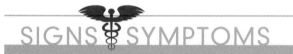

SIGNS & SYMPTOMS

Electrolyte Imbalances

Calcium

Normal laboratory values: 4.5 to 5.3 mEq/L or 9 to 11 mg/dL*

Hypocalcemia

Hyperactive reflexes, carpopedal spasm, perioral paresthesias, positive Trousseau sign, positive Chvostek sign, muscle twitching, muscle cramps, tetany (numbness, tingling, and muscular twitching usually of the extremities), laryngospasm, cardiac arrhythmias, nausea, vomiting, anxiety, confusion, emotional lability, convulsions

Hypercalcemia

Anorexia, nausea, vomiting, lethargy, bone tenderness or pain, polyuria, polydipsia, constipation, dehydration, muscle weakness and atrophy, stupor, coma, cardiac arrest

Magnesium

Normal laboratory values: 1.5 to 2.5 mEq/L or 1.8 to 3 mg/dL*

Hypomagnesemia

Leg and foot cramps, hypertension, tachycardia, neuromuscular irritability, tremor, hyperactive deep tendon reflexes, confusion, disorientation, visual or auditory hallucinations, painful paresthesias, positive Trousseau sign, positive Chvostek sign, convulsions

Hypermagnesemia

Lethargy, drowsiness, impaired respiration, flushing, sweating, hypotension, weak to absent deep tendon reflexes

Potassium

Normal laboratory values: 3.5 to 5 mEq/L*

Hypokalemia

Anorexia, nausea, vomiting, mental depression, confusion, delayed or impaired thought processes, drowsiness, abdominal distention, decreased bowel sounds, paralytic ileus, muscle weakness or fatigue, flaccid paralysis, absent or diminished deep tendon reflexes, weak irregular pulse, paresthesias, leg cramps, electrocardiograph (ECG) changes

Hyperkalemia

Irritability, anxiety, listlessness, mental confusion, nausea, diarrhea, abdominal distress, gastrointestinal hyperactivity, paresthesias, weakness and heaviness of the legs, flaccid paralysis, hypotension, cardiac arrhythmias, ECG changes

Sodium

Normal laboratory values: 132 to 145 mEq/L*

Hyponatremia

Cold clammy skin, decreased skin turgor, apprehension, confusion, irritability, anxiety, hypotension, postural hypotension, tachycardia, headache, tremors, convulsions, abdominal cramps, nausea, vomiting, diarrhea

Hypernatremia

Fever, hot dry skin, dry sticky mucous membranes, rough dry tongue, edema, weight gain, intense thirst, excitement, restlessness, agitation, oliguria or anuria

*These laboratory values may not concur with the normal range of values in all hospitals and laboratories. The hospital policy manual or laboratory values sheet should be consulted for the normal ranges of all laboratory tests.

Rapid intravenous administration (calcium gluconate) may result in bradycardia, vasodilation, decreased blood pressure, cardiac arrhythmias, and cardiac arrest. Oral administration may result in gastrointestinal disturbances. Use of calcium chloride may cause peripheral vasodilation, temporary decline in blood pressure, and a local burning. See the Signs and Symptoms Box for adverse reactions associated with hypercalcemia and hypocalcemia.

Magnesium (Mg++)

Adverse reactions seen with magnesium administration are rare. If they do occur, they are most likely related to overdose and may include flushing, sweating, hypotension, depressed reflexes, muscle weakness, and circulatory collapse (see Signs and Symptoms Box: Electrolyte Imbalances).

Potassium (K+)

Nausea, vomiting, diarrhea, abdominal pain, and phlebitis have been seen with oral and intravenous use of potassium. Adverse reactions related to hypokalemia or hyperkalemia are listed in Signs and Symptoms Box: Electrolyte Imbalances.

If extravasation (escape of fluid from a vessel into surrounding tissues) of the intravenous solution should occur, local tissue necrosis (death of tissue) may occur. If extravasation occurs, the health care provider should be contacted immediately and the infusion slowed to a rate that keeps the vein open.

Sodium (Na+)

Sodium as the salt (e.g., NaCl) has no adverse reactions except those related to overdose (see Signs and Symptoms Box: Electrolyte Imbalances). In some instances, excessive oral use may cause nausea and vomiting.

Contraindications, Precautions, and Interactions of Electrolytes

Bicarbonate (HCO$_3^-$)

- Bicarbonate is contraindicated in patients losing chloride by continuous gastrointestinal suction or through vomiting; in patients with metabolic or respiratory alkalosis, hypocalcemia, renal failure, or severe abdominal pain of unknown cause; and in those on sodium-restricted diets.
- Bicarbonate is used cautiously in patients with congestive heart failure or renal impairment and with glucocorticoid therapy.
- Bicarbonate is used cautiously during pregnancy.
- Oral administration of bicarbonate may decrease the absorption of ketoconazole.
- Increased blood levels of quinidine, flecainide, or sympathomimetics may occur when these agents are taken with bicarbonate
- There is an increased risk of crystalluria when bicarbonate is taken with the fluoroquinolones.
- Possible decreased effects of lithium, methotrexate, chlorpropamide, salicylates, and tetracyclines may occur when these drugs are taken with sodium bicarbonate.
- Sodium bicarbonate is not used within 2 hours of enteric-coated drugs; the protective enteric coating may disintegrate before the drug reaches the intestine.

Calcium (Ca++)

- Calcium is contraindicated in patients with hypercalcemia or ventricular fibrillation and in patients taking digitalis.
- Calcium is used cautiously in patients with cardiac disease.
- Hypercalcemia may occur when calcium is taken with the thiazide diuretics.
- When calcium is used with atenolol, there is a decrease in the effect of atenolol, possibly resulting in decreased beta blockade.
- There is an increased risk of digitalis toxicity when digitalis preparations are administered with calcium.
- The clinical effect of verapamil may be decreased when the drug is used with calcium.
- Concurrent ingestion of spinach or cereal may decrease the absorption of calcium supplements.

Magnesium (Mg++)

- Magnesium sulfate is contraindicated in patients with heart block or myocardial damage and in women with pregnancy-induced hypertension during the 2 hours before delivery.
- In addition, magnesium chloride is contraindicated in patients with renal impairment or marked myocardial disease and those in a coma.
- Magnesium (sulfate) is used with caution in patients with renal function impairment.
- Prolonged respiratory depression and apnea may occur when magnesium is administered with the neuromuscular blocking agents.

Potassium (K+)

- Potassium is contraindicated in patients who are at risk for experiencing hyperkalemia, such as those with renal failure, oliguria, or azotemia (the presence of nitrogen-containing compounds in the blood), anuria, severe hemolytic reactions, untreated Addison disease, acute dehydration, heat cramps, and any form of hyperkalemia.
- Potassium is used cautiously in patients with renal impairment or adrenal insufficiency, heart disease, metabolic acidosis, or prolonged or severe diarrhea.
- Concurrent use of potassium with angiotensin-converting enzyme inhibitors may result in elevated serum potassium.
- Potassium-sparing diuretics and salt substitutes used with potassium can produce severe hyperkalemia.
- The use of digitalis with potassium increases the risk of digoxin toxicity.

Sodium (Na+)

- Sodium is contraindicated in patients with hypernatremia or fluid retention and when the administration of sodium or chloride could be detrimental.
- Sodium is used cautiously in surgical patients and those with circulatory insufficiency, hypoproteinemia, urinary tract obstruction, congestive heart failure, edema, or renal impairment.
- Sodium is used cautiously during pregnancy.

Patient Management Issues with Electrolytes

When bicarbonate is given in the treatment of metabolic acidosis, the drug may be added to the intravenous fluid or given as a prepared intravenous sodium bicarbonate solution. The patient is observed for signs of clinical improvement, and the blood pressure, pulse, and respiratory rate are monitored every 15 to 30 minutes or as ordered by the health care provider. Extravasation of the drug requires selection of another needle site because the drug is irritating to the tissues.

Before, during, and after the use of calcium, blood pressure, pulse, and respiratory rate are monitored every 30 minutes until the patient's condition has stabilized. After administration of calcium, the patient is observed for signs of hypercalcemia. Patients receiving oral potassium are observed for signs of hyperkalemia, which would indicate that the dose of potassium is too high. Signs of hypokalemia may also occur during therapy and may indicate that the dose of potassium is too low and must be increased. In some instances, frequent laboratory monitoring of the serum potassium may be ordered.

When magnesium sulfate is ordered to treat convulsions or severe hypomagnesemia, the patient requires constant observation. The patient's blood pressure, pulse, and respiratory rate are obtained immediately before the drug is administered, as well as every 5 to 10 minutes during the time of intravenous infusion or after the drug is given directly intravenously.

The patient is observed for early signs of hypermagnesemia, and the health care provider is contacted immediately if this imbalance is suspected.

When sodium is administered by intravenous infusion, the patient is observed during and after administration for signs of hypernatremia. Patients receiving a 3% or 5% sodium chloride solution by intravenous infusion are observed closely for signs of pulmonary edema (dyspnea, cough, restlessness, bradycardia). If any one or more of these symptoms should occur, the intravenous infusion is slowed to keep the vein open, and the health care provider is contacted immediately.

Oral sodium bicarbonate tablets are taken with a full glass of water. If the urine remains acidic, the health care provider is notified because an increase in the dose of the drug may be necessary. Intravenous sodium bicarbonate is given in emergency situations, such as metabolic acidosis or certain types of drug overdose, when alkalization of the urine is necessary to hasten drug elimination.

When given orally, potassium may cause gastrointestinal distress. Therefore, it is given immediately after meals or with food and a full glass of water. Oral potassium must not be crushed or chewed.

Magnesium sulfate may be ordered intramuscularly, intravenously, or by intravenous infusion diluted in a specified type and amount of intravenous solution. When ordered to be given intramuscularly, this drug is given undiluted as a 50% solution for adults and a 20% solution for children. Magnesium sulfate is given deep intramuscularly in a large muscle mass, such as the gluteus muscle.

Educating the Patient and Family about Electrolytes

Because overdose (which can be serious) may occur if the patient does not adhere to the prescribed dosage and schedule, it is most important that the patient completely understands how much and when to take the drug.

The health care provider may order periodic laboratory and diagnostic tests for some patients receiving oral electrolytes (Key Concepts 45-2). The patient is encouraged to keep all appointments for these tests, as well as health care provider or clinic visits. Patients with a history of using sodium bicarbonate (baking soda) as an antacid are warned that overuse can result in alkalosis and could disguise a more serious problem. Those with a history of using salt tablets (sodium chloride) are advised not to do so during hot weather unless the health care provider recommends it. Excessive use of salt tablets can result in a serious electrolyte imbalance.

Following are key points about electrolytes the patient and family members should know:

Calcium

- Contact your health care provider if you experience any of the following: nausea, vomiting, anorexia, constipation, abdominal pain, dry mouth, thirst, or polyuria (symptoms of hypercalcemia).
- Do not exceed the dosage recommendations.

Potassium

- Take the drug exactly as directed on the prescription container. Do not increase, decrease, or omit doses of the drug unless advised to do so by your health care provider. Take the drug immediately after meals or with food and a full glass of water. Avoid the use of nonprescription drugs and salt substitutes (many contain potassium) unless use of a specific drug or product is approved by your health care provider.
- Contact your health care provider if you experience tingling of your hands or feet, a feeling of heaviness in your legs, vomiting, nausea, abdominal pain, or black stools.
- If the tablet has a coating (enteric-coated tablets), swallow it whole. Do not chew or crush the tablet.
- If you are to use effervescent tablets, place the tablet in 4 to 8 oz of cold water or juice. Wait until the fizzing stops before drinking. Sip the liquid during a period of 5 to 10 minutes.
- If you are to use an oral liquid or a powder, add the dose to 4 to 8 oz of cold water or juice and sip slowly during a period of 5 to 10 minutes. Measure the dose accurately.

Magnesium

- Do not take oral magnesium sulfate if you are experiencing abdominal pain, nausea, or vomiting. If you experience diarrhea and abdominal cramping, discontinue the drug.

Total Parenteral Nutrition

When normal eating is not possible or is inadequate to meet an individual's nutritional needs, intravenous nutritional therapy or total parenteral nutrition is required. Products used to meet the intravenous nutritional requirements of a patient include protein substrates (amino acids), energy substrates (dextrose and fat emulsions), fluids, electrolytes, and trace minerals (see the Summary Drug Table: Electrolytes).

Total parenteral nutrition is used to prevent nitrogen and weight loss or to treat negative nitrogen (mineral

---

LIFESPAN CONSIDERATIONS | **Infants & Children**

TPN for Neonates

The TPN formula for neonates must be very precise. The infant must be weighed daily, and the daily weight is used in TPN calculations.

---

component in protein and amino acids) balance (a situation in which more nitrogen is used by the body than is taken in) when

- The oral, gastrostomy, or jejunostomy route cannot or should not be used
- Gastrointestinal absorption of protein is impaired by obstruction
- Inflammatory disease or antineoplastic therapy prevents normal gastrointestinal functioning.
- Bowel rest is needed (e.g., after bowel surgery)
- Metabolic requirements for protein are significantly increased (e.g., in hypermetabolic states such as serious burns, infections, or trauma)
- Morbidity and mortality may be reduced by replacing amino acids lost from tissue breakdown (e.g., renal failure)
- Tube feeding alone cannot provide adequate nutrition

Total parenteral nutrition may be administered through a peripheral vein or through a central venous catheter. Peripheral total parenteral nutrition is used for patients requiring parenteral nutrition for relatively short periods of time (no more than 5–14 days) and when the central venous route is not possible or necessary. Peripheral total parenteral nutrition is used when the patient's caloric needs are minimal and can be partially met by normal means (through the alimentary tract); it prevents protein catabolism (breakdown of cells) in patients who have adequate body fat and no clinically significant protein malnutrition. These solutions may be used alone or combined with dextrose (5% or 10%) solutions.

ALERT Rx

Hyperglycemia

Hyperglycemia is the most common metabolic complication of total parenteral nutrition. A too-rapid infusion of amino acid–carbohydrate mixtures may result in hyperglycemia, glycosuria, mental confusion, and loss of consciousness. Blood glucose levels may be obtained every 4 to 6 hours to monitor for hyperglycemia and guide the dosage of dextrose and insulin (if required). To minimize these complications, the health care provider may decrease the rate of administration, reduce the dextrose concentration, or administer insulin.

Total parenteral nutrition through a central vein is indicated in patients to promote protein synthesis in those who are severely hypercatabolic, severely depleted of nutrients, or require long-term nutritional parenteral nutrition. For example, amino acids combined with hypertonic dextrose and intravenous fat emulsions are infused through a central venous catheter to promote protein synthesis. Vitamins, trace minerals, and electrolytes may be added to the total parenteral nutrition mixture to meet the patient's individual needs. The daily dose depends on a patient's daily protein requirement, metabolic state, and clinical responses. Various laboratory studies and assessments are required before and during administration of total parenteral nutrition.

To prevent a rebound hypoglycemic reaction from the sudden withdrawal of total parenteral nutrition containing a concentrated dose of dextrose, the rate of administration is slowly reduced or the concentration of dextrose gradually decreased.

FACT CHECK

45-11 How may total parenteral nutrition be administered?

Chapter Review

KEY POINTS

- Blood plasma is the liquid part of blood. Human plasma is obtained from donated blood and can be given in acute emergencies because it does not require a donor match.
- Plasma protein fractions are critical in regulating the volume of circulating blood. Plasma protein fractions are used to treat hypovolemic (low blood volume) shock that occurs as the result of burns, trauma, surgery, and infections. Plasma protein fractions do not require a donor match.
- Protein substrates are amino acid preparations that promote the production of proteins (anabolism). Amino acids promote the production of proteins, enhance tissue repair and wound healing, and reduce the rate of protein breakdown. Amino acids are used in certain disease states, such as severe kidney and liver disease, as well as in total parenteral nutrition solutions.
- Energy substrates include dextrose solutions and fat emulsion. Intravenous fat emulsion is used in the prevention and treatment of essential fatty acid deficiency.
- Plasma expanders are used to expand plasma volume when shock is caused by burns, hemorrhage, surgery, and other trauma and for prophylaxis of venous thrombosis and thromboembolism.
- Intravenous replacement solutions are a source of electrolytes and water for hydration and used to facilitate amino acid utilization and maintain electrolyte balance. Dextrose and electrolyte solutions are used as a parenteral source of electrolytes, calories, or water for hydration.
- Bicarbonate plays a vital role in the acid–base balance of the body. Bicarbonate may be given intravenously as sodium bicarbonate, which may be given intravenously in the treatment of metabolic acidosis, a state of imbalance that may occur in severe shock, diabetic acidosis, severe diarrhea, extracorporeal circulation of blood, severe renal disease, and cardiac arrest.
- Calcium may be given for the treatment of hypocalcemia, which may occur in patients with parathyroid disease or after removal of the parathyroid glands, and during cardiopulmonary resuscitation when epinephrine fails to improve weak or ineffective myocardial contractions.
- Magnesium is used as replacement therapy in hypomagnesemia. Magnesium sulfate is used in the prevention and control of seizures in obstetric patients with pregnancy-induced hypertension.

- Potassium is necessary for the transmission of impulses; the contraction of smooth, cardiac, and skeletal muscles; and other important physiologic processes. It is also given for hypokalemia.
- Sodium is essential for the maintenance of normal heart action and in the regulation of osmotic pressure in body cells. Sodium is used to treat hyponatremia.
- Combined electrolyte solutions are available for oral and intravenous use. Intravenous solutions are used to replace fluid and electrolytes that have been lost and to provide calories by means of their carbohydrate content.
- Total parenteral nutrition is used to prevent nitrogen and weight loss or to treat negative nitrogen balance. Peripheral total parenteral nutrition is used for patients requiring parenteral nutrition for relatively short periods of time and when the central venous route is not possible or necessary. Peripheral total parenteral nutrition is used when the patient's caloric needs are minimal and can be partially met by normal means.

CRITICAL THINKING CASE STUDY

Potassium Chloride Therapy

Mr. Kendall is prescribed an oral potassium chloride liquid. He has questions about the drug and why it was prescribed.

1. Mr. Kendall asks why his health care provider chose potassium chloride liquid. He should be told
   a. potassium is important in physiologic processes, such as helping the cardiac muscle contract
   b. potassium is necessary for the transmission of impulses
   c. potassium helps relieve hyperkalemia
   d. a and b
2. Mr. Kendall wonders if adverse reactions may occur with this drug. He should be told
   a. there are no known adverse reactions
   b. nausea and vomiting sometimes occur with potassium chloride
   c. headache, fatigue, and confusion are common adverse reactions
   d. none of the above

3. Mr. Kendall is taking an extended-release potassium chloride tablet. What should he be told about taking his daily potassium dose?

Review Questions

MULTIPLE CHOICE

1. Which of the following is a symptom of fluid overload?
   a. Tinnitus
   b. Hypotension
   c. Decreased body temperature
   d. Behavioral changes
2. Which of the following symptoms may result from hypocalcemia?
   a. Tetany
   b. Constipation
   c. Muscle weakness
   d. Hypertension
3. Sodium is used
   a. to treat hyponatremia
   b. to treat hypokalemia
   c. to treat hypocalcemia
   d. none of the above
4. Which of the following symptoms are most likely related to hypernatremia?
   a. Fever, increased thirst
   b. Cold, clammy skin
   c. Decreased skin turgor
   d. Hypotension
5. Which of the following is the most common metabolic complication of total parenteral nutrition?
   a. Hypomagnesemia
   b. Hypermagnesemia
   c. Hypoglycemia
   d. Hyperglycemia

MATCHING

Match the electrolyte on the left with the adverse reaction(s) on the right.

_____	6.	calcium carbonate
_____	7.	sodium chloride
_____	8.	potassium chloride
_____	9.	magnesium oxide
_____	10.	sodium bicarbonate

a. nausea, vomiting, diarrhea
b. diarrhea, abdominal cramping
c. fluid overload
d. sodium and fluid retention
e. constipation

TRUE OR FALSE

_____ 11. A patient receiving total parenteral nutrition is likely to experience hypoglycemia as a common complication.

_____ 12. Pedialyte is an example of a combined electrolyte solution.

_____ 13. Hypokalemia is low blood calcium.

_____ 14. Potassium that is given intravenously must always be diluted before administration.

FILL IN THE BLANKS

15. After undergoing bowel surgery, a patient may require _____ _____ _____ in order to allow the bowel to rest.
16. Soybean or safflower oil and natural triglycerides are contained in an intravenous _____ _____.
17. A patient receiving calcium who has elevated plasma calcium, weakness, and severe nausea and vomiting may be experiencing _____ _____, which requires immediate notification of the health care provider.
18. When severe hemorrhage occurs, intravenous administration of _____ _____ is used to help increase the patient's blood volume.

SHORT ANSWERS

19. What are six solutions that are used in the management of body fluids?
20. Why are older adults at greater risk for fluid overload?
21. Compare and contrast the administration instructions on the various dosage forms of potassium.
22. When is total parenteral nutrition indicated?

Web Activities

1. Go to the Kids Health Web site (http://www.kidshealth.org) and enter as "Parents." Conduct a search on "blood tests," and read the information about a "Comprehensive Metabolic Panel." What does the CMP help the doctors look at? How long does it take to get the results?
2. Go to the American Society for Parenteral and Enteral Nutrition Web site (www.nutritioncare.org). Click on the tab "About A.S.P.E.N." Discuss the core values, vision, mission, and history of A.S.P.E.N.

SUMMARY DRUG TABLE Electrolytes (left, generic; right, trade)

Comprehensive Summary Drug Tables, including uses, adverses effects, dosages, and pregnancy classifications, are provided on the companion website, http://thePoint.lww.com/PharmacologyHP2e

calcium acetate	Eliphos, PhosLo, Phoslyra, Calphron, *generic*	magnesium	*generic*
calcium carbonate	Many trade names, *generic* (OTC)	magnesium chloride	Mag-64, Mag-SR, *generic*
calcium chloride	*generic*	magnesium gluconate	Mag-G, *generic*
calcium citrate	*generic*	magnesium lactate	Mag-Tab SR
calcium glubionate	Calcionate	magnesium oxide	Uro-Mag, MagOx, Phillips' Cramp-Free, *generic*
calcium gluconate	Cal-Glu (OTC), *generic* (Rx and OTC)	magnesium sulfate	Epsom salt (OTC), *generic* (Rx)
calcium glycerophosphate	Prelief (OTC)	potassium acetate	*generic*
calcium lactate	Cal-Lac, *generic* (OTC)	potassium bicarbonate	Klor-Con, Effer-K, *generic*
calcium microcrystalline hydroxyapatite	Calcium Microcrystalline Hydroxyapatite	potassium chloride	Micro-K, Klor-Con, K-Tab, Epiklor, *generic*
oral electrolyte mixtures	Infalyte Oral Solution, Naturalyte Solution, Pedialyte, Pedialyte Solution, Pedialyte Freezer, Pops, Rehydralyte, Resol Solution	potassium gluconate	*generic*
		sodium chloride	Slo-Salt, Slo-Salt-K, Sustain, *generic*
		sodium bicarbonate	Alka-Seltzer Heartburn Relief (OTC), Baros (Rx), *generic* (Rx)

XII

46

Complementary and Alternative Medicine

CHAPTER OBJECTIVES

On the completion of this chapter, students will be able to:

1. Define the chapter's key terms.
2. Discuss federal regulation and research related to CAM.
3. Discuss the Dietary Supplement Health and Education Act.
4. Identify nutritional supplements and discuss the importance of nutritional and herbal supplement usage.
5. Describe why and how consumers should be more vigilant in the use of herbal products.
6. Categorize vitamins as water soluble or fat soluble.
7. List vitamins and their sources and function, and recognize signs and symptoms of deficiencies and overdose.
8. Identify and distinguish between the various minerals important for good health.
9. Discuss the uses, contraindications, precautions, interactions, and adverse reactions associated with herbal remedies.
10. Discuss the Food and Drug Administration (FDA) ban of various herbal remedies.

KEY TERMS

alternative therapies—therapies used instead of conventional or Western medical therapies

complementary and alternative medicine (CAM)—a group of nontraditional therapies

complementary therapies—therapies such as relaxation techniques, massage, dietary supplements, healing touch, and herbal therapy used together or to "complement" traditional health care

CHAPTER OVERVIEW

Drug classes covered in this chapter are:

- Nutritional supplements
- Herbal remedies

thePOINT RESOURCES

- Interactive Practice and Review

dietary supplement—substances such as herbs, vitamins, minerals, amino acids, and other natural substances; also referred to as nutritional supplements

efficacy—effectiveness

fat-soluble vitamins—vitamins that are generally metabolized slowly and are stored in the liver

herb—plant used in medicine or as seasoning

herbal remedies—plants or herbs used to treat various disorders

herbal therapy—a type of complementary or alternative therapy that uses plants or herbs to treat various disorders; also called botanical medicine

minerals—in terms of nutrition, are inorganic nutrients necessary to maintain health in the human body

nutritional supplements—substances such as herbs, vitamins, minerals, amino acids, and other natural substances; also referred to as dietary supplements

vitamin—organic substance needed by the body in small amounts for normal growth and nutrition

water-soluble vitamins—vitamins that are rapidly metabolized and are readily excreted in the urine

Complementary and alternative medicine (CAM) is broadly defined as a group of nontraditional therapies. **Complementary therapies** are used with traditional health care and include therapies such as relaxation techniques, massage, dietary supplements, healing touch, and herbal therapy, while **alternative therapies** are used instead of conventional or Western medical therapies. The term "complementary/alternative therapy" often is used as an umbrella term for many therapies from all over the world.

The use of CAM by American adults has increased in recent years. According to the National Center for Complementary and Alternative Medicine (NCCAM), an agency of the National Institutes of Health, adults in the United States spent about $33.9 billion on CAM therapies and products in 2009. Americans use CAM therapies to treat conditions such as back, neck, and joint pain, as well as anxiety, stress, insomnia, and high cholesterol levels. According to the 2007 National Health Statistics Report prepared by the U.S. Department of Health and Human Services and the Centers for Disease Control, about 38% of adults and about 12% of children in the United States used CAM therapy in some form in the preceding year. Natural products, deep breathing exercises, meditation, chiropractic therapy, and massage were among the most populart CAM therapies in the United States. Fish oil, glucosamine, echinacea, flaxseed, and ginseng were among the most common natural products used by Americans.

Federal Regulation and Research Related to CAM

As more Americans turn to CAM therapies, confusion has arisen as to which products and practices are and are not regulated by the Food and Drug Administration (FDA). Depending upon their use, CAM products may be regulated by either the Federal Food, Drug, and Cosmetic Act or the Public Health Service Act, or they may not be subject to FDA regulation at all. The Federal Food, Drug, and Cosmetic Act was passed in 1938 and has been amended several times. The most recent amendments were made in 2009. With regard to CAM, the Federal Food, Drug, and Cosmetic Act defines the following terms: cosmetics, devices, dietary supplements, drugs, foods, and food additives. Complementary and alternative medicine

products that fall into these categories may be regulated under this act. Acupuncture needles, for example, are classified as devices by the FDA because they "are intended for use in the cure, mitigation, treatment, or prevention of disease." Certain CAM products that are sold as food are also regulated under this act. The Public Health Service Act, passed in 1999, defines biological products, which can include "botanicals, animal-derived extracts, vitamins, minerals, fatty acids, amino acids, proteins, prebiotics and probiotics, whole diets, and functional foods."

Dietary supplements, such as herbal remedies, are often not regulated by the FDA because these products are not considered drugs. It is also important to realize that neither of these acts exempts a CAM product from regulation. For example, raw vegetable juice sold as a CAM therapy is still subject as a food product and therefore subject to the requirements set aside for foods in the Act.

FDA and Dietary Supplement Health and Education Act

The FDA has the responsibility of approving new drugs and monitoring drugs for adverse or toxic reactions. In 1994, the US government passed the Dietary Supplement Health and Education Act (DSHEA), which defines substances such as herbs, vitamins, minerals, amino acids, and other natural substances as **dietary supplements.** Under DSHEA, the initial responsibility for the safety of a dietary supplement rests with the manufacturer. After a dietary supplement has been marketed to the public, the FDA is responsible for monitoring its safety. Dietary Supplement Health and Education Act outlines the types of claims that manufacturers can make about a supplement.

In order to insure the safety of their products, manufacturers of dietary supplements are required to follow current good manufacturing practices (cGMP). As of June 2008, the FDA requires all dietary supplements to be evaluated based on their identity, purity, quality, strength, and composition. Since December 2007, the FDA requires manufacturers to report all notifications that they receive of adverse reactions to dietary supplements. Before marketing any dietary supplement containing new dietary ingredients (NDIs), manufacturers are also required to provide the FDA with information pertaining to the safety of the ingredient. New dietary ingredients include most ingredients introduced into the food supply after DSHEA was passed in 1994, although some ingredients introduced after 1994 are excluded if they were used in conventional foods.

The act permits general health claims such as "improves memory" or "promotes regularity" as long as the label also has a disclaimer stating that the supplements are not approved by the FDA and are not intended to diagnose, treat, cure, or prevent disease. The claims must be truthful and not misleading and must be supported by scientific evidence.

National Center for Complementary and Alternative Medicine

In 1992, the National Institutes of Health (NIH) established an Office of Alternative Medicine (OAM) to facilitate the study of alternative medical treatments and to disseminate information to the public. In 1998, the name was changed to NCCAM. The mission of NCCAM is to scientifically explore CAM practices, to train CAM researchers, and to share information with the public and with professionals. This office was established partly because of the increased interest and use of CAM in the United States.

One of the purposes of NCCAM is to evaluate the safety and **efficacy,** or effectiveness, of widely used natural products, such as herbal remedies and nutritional and food supplements, and to share this information with the public and with health professionals. The Center is also dedicated to developing programs and encouraging scientists to investigate CAM treatments that show promise. National Center for Complementary and Alternative Medicine has funded more than 2500 scientific research projects. Research conducted by NCCAM's Laboratory of Clinical Investigation includes the endocrine section and the diabetes unit. Both groups conduct research to determine the effects of CAM practices on their respective conditions. National Center for Complementary and Alternative Medicine also conducts clinical trials for conditions including asthma, arthritis, memory disorders, a variety of cancers, and pain, among others.

FACT CHECK

46-1 How does the Federal Food, Drug, and Cosmetic Act affect the regulation of CAM products?

46-2 The Public Health Service Act defines biological products. What are some products defined under this act?

46-3 After a dietary supplement has been marketed to the public, which federal agency is responsible for monitoring its safety?

Nutritional Supplements

Nutritional supplements are substances such as herbs, vitamins, minerals, amino acids, and other natural substances (Box 46-1).

Herbs are used for various effects, such as to boost the immune system, treat depression, or promote relaxation.

BOX 46.1

Recommended Dietary Allowances (RDAs)

- Tables listing the latest information on recommended dietary allowances (RDAs) of vitamins and minerals for infants, children, males, females, and pregnant and lactating females can be found at the U.S. Department of Agriculture Web site: http://fnic.nal.usda.gov.

Growing awareness about the benefits of **herbal therapies** and nutritional supplements has led to increased use of these products to treat various disorders. However, while much information is available about herbs and supplements, some of it may be misleading, so it is important to verify its accuracy.

Medicinal herbs and nutritional substances are available at supermarkets, pharmacies, health food stores, specialty herb stores, and through the Internet. Dietary supplements are not preapproved by the government for safety or effectiveness before marketing, and unlike drugs, supplements are not intended to treat, diagnose, prevent, or cure diseases. Because these substances are "natural products," many individuals may incorrectly assume that they are without adverse effects (Key Concepts 46-1).

Considerations for Supplement Use

The decision to use a nutritional supplement should be based on several factors. First, people should consider their diet as a whole. As the name implies, supplements are intended to enhance, not replace, a well-balanced diet. People should also understand the supplement's purpose as well as its potential for side effects (Box 46-2). Chamomile, for example, is a

KEY CONCEPTS

46-1 Ask Patients about Herbal Products When Obtaining a Drug History

Many botanicals have strong pharmacological activity, and some may interact with prescription drugs or be toxic in the body. For example, comfrey, an herb that was once widely used to promote digestion, can cause liver damage. Although it may still be available in some areas, it is a dangerous herb and is not recommended for use as a supplement. Patients should always be questioned about the use of herbs, teas, vitamins, or other nutritional or dietary supplements as part of a drug history. Many patients consider herbs as natural and therefore safe. Some also have trouble thinking about their use of an herbal tea as a part of their health care regimen. Any patient use of herbal remedies or dietary supplements should be reported to the health care provider.

BOX 46.2

Supplement Use: When to Involve a Health Care Professional

- Certain people, including children, women who are pregnant or breastfeeding, and people who have chronic medical conditions, should always include a health care professional in the decision-making process for supplement use. For example, black cohosh should not be taken by women who are pregnant, and echinacea should not be taken by individuals with autoimmune diseases such as multiple sclerosis, SLE, RA, AIDS, and HIV infection. Individuals who are considering substituting a dietary supplement for their regular medication should also talk with their health care provider.

KEY CONCEPTS

46-2 Water-Soluble Vitamins

Because water-soluble vitamins are excreted in the urine when in excess, patients may notice that their urine appears more concentrated when taking a multivitamin supplement.

member of the ragweed family and should not be taken by those allergic to ragweed.

Individuals who take over-the-counter or prescription medications must consider carefully when choosing a dietary supplement because negative interactions can occur. Gingko, for example, should not be taken with antidepressant drugs, such as MAOIs, or antiplatelet drugs, such as coumadin, unless advised to do so by the primary care provider. In fact, a number of dietary supplements interact with antiplatelet drugs, including St. John's wort, motherwort, ginseng, garlic, hawthorn, and saw palmetto. Individuals who expect to have surgery should be aware that some dietary supplements, including gingko, garlic, and ginger, may increase the risk of bleeding. Other dietary supplements, including valerian, can unpredictably alter the effects of common anesthetics. Due to their effects on enzymes that regulate metabolism of medications, grapefruit juice, black cohosh, and St. John's wort have a number of drug interactions to be cautious about.

After deciding to use a particular dietary supplement, individuals should be sure to read the label and follow the directions. Overdosing on a dietary supplement is possible—and the reaction can be just as serious as a drug overdose. For example, high doses of omega-3 fatty acids may lead to an increased risk of bleeding. High doses of caffeine in black tea may cause anxiety. High doses of turmeric, used to treat upset stomach and arthritis pain, may actually cause stomach upset and ulcers.

Vitamins

Vitamins are a group of unrelated organic substances that are essential in small amounts for the regulation of normal metabolism, growth, and function of the human body. Vitamins are usually classified as either fat soluble (vitamins A, D, E, and K) or water soluble (vitamins B and C). The **fat-soluble vitamins** are generally metabolized slowly and are stored in the liver, whereas the **water-soluble vitamins** are rapidly metabolized and are readily excreted in the urine.

Toxic effects have been observed when large dosages of some vitamins are ingested. Generally, the water-soluble vitamins

are less toxic since excess quantities are usually excreted in the urine (Key Concepts 46-2). Excessive amounts of fat-soluble vitamins, however, are stored in the body, which makes toxic levels of these vitamins easier to achieve. Also, fat-soluble vitamins interact with drugs that prevent their absorption from the gut, such as orlistat and bile acid sequestrants.

Fat-Soluble Vitamins

Vitamin A

Vitamin A, or retinol, is essential for maintaining the functional and structural integrity of epithelial cells; it also plays a major role in epithelial differentiation. Bone development and growth in children have also been linked to adequate vitamin A intake. Vitamin A, when reduced to the aldehyde 11-*cis*-retinal, combines with opsin to produce the visual pigment rhodopsin. This pigment is present in the rods of the retina and is partly responsible for the process of dark adaptation.

Principal dietary sources of vitamin A are milk fat (cheese and butter) and eggs. Since it is stored in the liver, inclusion of liver in the diet also provides vitamin A. A plant pigment, carotene, is a precursor for vitamin A and is present in highly pigmented vegetables, such as carrots, rutabaga, and red cabbage.

Acute hypervitaminosis A results in drowsiness, headache, vomiting, papilledema, and a bulging fontanel in infants. The symptoms of chronic toxicity include scaly skin, hair loss, brittle nails, and hepatosplenomegaly. Anorexia, irritability, and swelling of the bones have been seen in children. Retardation of growth also may occur. Liver toxicity has been associated with excessive vitamin A intake. Vitamin A is teratogenic in large amounts.

Vitamin D

Vitamin D is the collective term for a group of compounds formed by the action of ultraviolet irradiation on sterols. Cholecalciferol (vitamin D_3) and calciferol (vitamin D_2) are formed by irradiation of the provitamins 7-dehydrocholesterol and ergosterol, respectively. Food sources of vitamin D include fish, eggs, and milk. Another source of vitamin D is sunlight. The conversion to vitamin D_3 occurs in the skin. The liver is the principal storage site for vitamin D, and it is here that the vitamin is hydroxylated to form 25-hydroxyvitamin D. Additional hydroxylation to form 1,25-dihydroxyvitamin D occurs in the kidney in response to the need for calcium and phosphate. Vitamin D also aids bone growth and helps prevent rickets in children and osteomalacia and osteoporosis in adults.

The hypercalcemia resulting from hypervitaminosis D is responsible for toxic symptoms such as muscle weakness, bone pain, anorexia, ectopic calcification, hypertension, and cardiac arrhythmias. Toxicity in infants can result in mental and physical retardation, renal failure, and death.

Vitamin E

Vitamin E is a potent antioxidant that is capable of protecting polyunsaturated fatty acids from oxidative breakdown. This vitamin also functions to enhance vitamin A use. Vitamin E is believed to be useful in preventing and treating some diseases, such as coronary heart disease; however, the physiological actions that might provide these benefits are not fully known. Vitamin E is found in a variety of foodstuffs, the richest sources being plant oils, including wheat germ and rice, and the lipids of green leaves.

Prolonged administration of large dosages of vitamin E may result in muscle weakness, fatigue, headache, and nausea. This toxicity can be reversed by discontinuing the large-dose supplementation.

Vitamin K

Vitamin K activity is associated with several quinones, including phylloquinone (vitamin K_1), menadione (vitamin K_3), and a variety of menaquinones (vitamin K_2). These quinones promote the synthesis of proteins that are involved in the coagulation of blood. These proteins include prothrombin, factor VII (proconvertin), factor IX (plasma thromboplastin), and factor X (Stuart factor). The vitamin K quinones are obtained from three major sources. Vitamin K is present in various plants, especially green vegetables. The menaquinones that possess vitamin K_2 activity are synthesized by bacteria, particularly gram-positive organisms; the bacteria in the gut of animals produce useful quantities of this vitamin. Vitamin K_3 is a chemically synthesized quinone that possesses the same activity as vitamin K_1.

Vitamin K is available by prescription and over-the-counter as phytonadione in oral tablets and injection dosage forms. Toxicity of vitamin K has not been well defined. It is not known if vitamin K will cause harm to the fetus if used during pregnancy and therefore should be used only when absolutely needed. Caution should be used in lactating females because it is unknown whether vitamin K is excreted in breast milk or not.

ALERT ℞

Vitamin K

Studies indicate that diet can influence a patient's prothrombin time (PT). In patients receiving warfarin, a diet high in vitamin K may increase the risk of clot formation. A diet low in vitamin K may increase the risk of hemorrhage. Significant changes in vitamin K intake may necessitate warfarin dose adjustment. For patients receiving warfarin, maintaining a consistent daily intake of vitamin K and avoiding large fluctuations is key. To ensure this, patients need to know the vitamin K content of food. For example, green leafy vegetables and some vegetable oils (soybean and canola oil) are high in vitamin K. Root vegetables, fruits, cereals, dairy products, and meats are generally low in vitamin K.

FACT CHECK

46-4 What are the fat-soluble vitamins?
46-5 How are fat-soluble vitamins metabolized and stored?

Water-Soluble Vitamins

The B Vitamins

The B-vitamin group is made up of substances that tend to occur together in foods and are given the collective name vitamin B complex. The vitamins of the B group usually have to be converted to an active form, and most of them play a vital role in intracellular metabolism. The B vitamins are obtained from both meat and vegetable products, except for vitamin B_{12}, which occurs only in animal products. The richest source of the B-vitamin group is seeds, including the germ of wheat or of rice.

- Thiamine (B_1)

Vitamin B_1, also known as thiamine, is found in brewer's yeast, some meats (pork, ham, liver), whole grains, peas, beans, and milk. It is necessary for glucose metabolism. Thiamine deficiency is known as "beriberi," which can result in nerve damage, dementia, and heart failure if left untreated.

- Riboflavin (B_2)

Vitamin B_2 is also known as riboflavin. Dietary sources include beef, liver, almonds, milk, dairy products, egg, fish, and spinach. Although rare, riboflavin deficiency may cause swelling of lining of mouth and nose, mouth and lip sores, inflammation of tongue, dermatitis, and anemia.

- Niacin (B_3)

Vitamin B_3, more commonly known as niacin, is found in some meats (beef, liver, chicken breast), eggs, legumes, some cereals, and peanuts. Among its many functions in the body, niacin decreases hepatic LDL (low-density lipoprotein) and VLDL (very-low-density lipoprotein) production, which is why many patients use it to reduce their cholesterol.

Niacin deficiency, though rare, results in pellagra, which is characterized by diarrhea, dementia, and dermatitis. Left untreated, pellagra can ultimately result in death. Other symptoms of niacin deficiency include inflammation of mouth, tongue, and vagina and nerve pain. Niacin is available in both prescription and over-the-counter formulations. A common adverse reaction of niacin is flushing, which is discussed in Key Concepts 46-3.

- Pantothenic Acid (B_5)

Vitamin B_5, also called pantothenic acid, is found in milk, lean beef, eggs, cabbage, broccoli, and legumes. It helps with metabolism of carbohydrates, proteins, and lipids and is a precursor of an essential coenzyme required for life-sustaining reactions. It also is required for normal epithelial function. Pantothenic acid deficiency is rare but can result in abdominal pain, vomiting, and insomnia.

- Pyridoxine (B_6)

Vitamin B_6 is also called pyridoxine. Food sources include beef liver, pork, baked potato, spinach, banana, cereals, milk, fish, and avocado. Pyridoxine is involved in some of the body's enzymatic reactions. Inflammation of the mouth, lips, and tongue; psychological disorders (anxiety, depression, confusion); anemia; and, rarely, seizures may occur with

KEY CONCEPTS

46-3   Niacin and Flushing

A common adverse reaction associated with niacin therapy is flushing. The flushing is a sensation of warmth, especially of the face and upper body, which may also be accompanied by itching, tingling, or headache. It begins approximately 20 minutes after administration and can last between 30 and 60 minutes. The effect will usually subside after 3 to 6 weeks of therapy. It can be minimized by slowly increasing the dose, taking with food or milk, taking 325 mg of aspirin about an hour prior to administration, or using a sustained-release dosage formulation.

pyridoxine deficiency. Pyridoxine levels in the body can be reduced by some medications including isoniazid, alcohol, penicillamine, and theophylline.

• Cyanocobalamin (B_{12})

Vitamin B_{12}, also called cyanocobalamin, is found in meat, liver, kidney, fish, poultry, and dairy products. It is also available both over the counter and by prescription.

Vitamin B_{12} deficiency may result from impaired absorption of the vitamin due to diseases including pernicious anemia or inadequate pancreatic function. Vitamin B_{12} deficiency causes macrocytic anemia, nerve damage, and dementia.

Overdoses of B Vitamins

The effects of most vitamin B overdoses have not been documented, although large dosages of pyridoxine have been reported to cause peripheral neuropathies. Ataxia and numbness of the hands and feet and impairment of the senses of pain, touch, and temperature may result. Excessive niacin intake may result in flushing, pruritus, and gastrointestinal disturbances. These symptoms are due to niacin's ability to cause the release of histamine. Large dosages of niacin can result in hepatic toxicity.

Vitamin C

Vitamin C (ascorbic acid) is essential for the maintenance of the ground substance, or extracellular matrix, that binds cells together and for the formation and maintenance of collagen. The exact biochemical role it plays in these functions is not known, but it may be related to its ability to act as an oxidation–reduction system.

Vitamin C is found in fresh fruit and vegetables. It is very water soluble, is readily destroyed by heat, especially in an alkaline medium, and is rapidly oxidized in air. Fruit and vegetables that have been stored in air, cut or bruised, washed, or cooked may have lost much of their vitamin C content.

Megavitamin intake of vitamin C may result in diarrhea due to intestinal irritation. Since ascorbic acid is partially metabolized and excreted as oxalate, renal oxalate stones may form in some patients.

FACT CHECK

46-6   What are the water-soluble vitamins?
46-7   How are water-soluble vitamins metabolized and excreted?
46-8   Which B vitamin has been shown to lower LDL cholesterol?

Minerals

Minerals, in terms of nutrition, are inorganic nutrients necessary to maintain health in the human body. Minerals perform functions that include building bones and regulating the heartbeat.

Minerals are divided into two categories: macrominerals and trace minerals. The human body requires larger amounts of macrominerals, which include calcium, magnesium, phosphorus, potassium, and sodium. The human body only requires small amounts of trace minerals, which include iodine, iron, and zinc, among others.

Macrominerals

Calcium

The human body contains more calcium than any other mineral. It is stored mostly in bones and teeth and is required for muscle contraction, secretion of hormones and enzymes, transmission of pulses through the nervous system, and the expansion and contraction of blood vessels. Calcium is found in dairy products, including cheese, yogurt, and milk, and in green, leafy vegetables.

Potassium

Potassium, classified as an electrolyte in the body, is important for regulating the acid–base balance, for synthesizing amino acids, for metabolizing carbohydrates, and for building muscle. Potassium is found in meats, fish, vegetables, fruits, milk, yogurt, and nuts.

Other Macrominerals

The body requires magnesium to contract and relax muscles, to produce and transport energy, to produce protein, and

ALERT ℞

Potassium

Potassium may sometimes be given intravenously for severe potassium deficiency. Potassium chloride vials have an outer cap that has "Must Be Diluted" printed on it. This cap must be removed before reaching the vial stopper to withdraw the drug via syringe and needle. It is important to dilute potassium for injection because potassium is important for the heart to function properly, and too much potassium will cause the heart to stop.

for the function of enzymes. Fruits and vegetables, legumes, soy products, whole grains, and nuts are good sources of magnesium.

One percent of an individual's body weight consists of phosphorus. It is mostly found in bones and teeth; however, it exists in every cell of the body. Phosphorus is important for forming teeth and bones, and it helps the body synthesize proteins. The main sources of phosphorus are milk and meat.

Sodium regulates blood pressure and blood volume in the body and is also important for the functioning of nerves and muscles. Sodium is found naturally in most foods, as well as in sodium chloride, commonly known as table salt.

Trace Minerals

The body uses iodine to metabolize food into energy. It is also important to thyroid function. Iodine is most commonly found in iodized salt, or table salt with iodine added.

Iron

Iron is found in each cell in the human body and is essential for making hemoglobin and myoglobin. Iron can be found in many foods including dried beans and fruit, egg yolks, liver, lean red meat, whole grains, and fish, including salmon and tuna.

Zinc

Zinc helps the body's immune system work correctly. It is involved in cell division and growth, it helps wounds heal, it breaks down carbohydrates, and it is important for the senses of smell and taste. Zinc is found in meat, nuts, and legumes.

FACT CHECK

46-9 Why is it so important to dilute potassium for injection?

46-10 What is the function of iron?

Herbal Remedies

Herbal remedies use plants or herbs to treat various disorders. People around the world use herbal remedies extensively. Herbs have been used by virtually every culture in the world throughout known history. For example, Hippocrates prescribed St. John's wort, an herbal remedy for depression that is still popular. Native Americans used plants such as coneflower, ginseng, and ginger for therapeutic purposes.

Although herbs have been used for thousands of years, most of what we know has come from observation rather than clinical study. Most herbs have not been scientifically studied for safety and efficacy. In the United States, the following herbal remedies are classified by the FDA as dietary supplements rather than drugs.

Herbal remedies affect various body systems. Many commonly used herbs are discussed below and are listed in Table 46-1. For certain herbs, additional information regarding uses may also be found in the table.

Herbs That Affect the Neurologic System

The brain, spinal cord, and nerves form the neurologic system. Its two anatomic divisions are the central nervous system (which includes the brain and spinal cord) and the peripheral nervous system (which includes the body's nerves). The central function of the peripheral nervous system is to carry impulses to and from the central nervous system. Several herbal remedies that can affect the neurologic system are described below (also see Table 46-1).

Gingko Biloba

Gingko biloba, one of the oldest known herbs in the world, is used to improve symptoms associated with reduced blood flow to the brain, including short-term memory loss and dizziness. It is also a frequent treatment for headache, depression, erectile dysfunction, and anxiety. It is also sometimes used for tinnitus. It is commercially available over-the-counter in liquid, capsule, or tablet form.

The leaves of the gingko plant contain insufficient quantities of active ingredients for effective use as medical treatment. Gingko extract is most commonly used. Clinical studies of the extract suggest that it is effective in treating established dementia. However, a recent study in the *Journal of the American Medical Association* indicated that for elderly patients with normal memory, gingko did not improve learning, memory, attention, or concentration.

The health improvements associated with gingko are not immediate but may begin after 4 to 24 weeks. The potential adverse effects of regular use of gingko include mild gastrointestinal upset, headache, rash, muscle spasms, cramps, dizziness, palpitations, constipation, and bleeding. Large doses reportedly cause diarrhea, nausea, vomiting, weakness, lack of muscle tone, and restlessness.

Patients taking anticlotting medication, including over-the-counter treatments such as aspirin and ibuprofen, should avoid taking gingko. Taking gingko with a thiazide diuretic will increase blood pressure. Patients taking monoamine oxidase inhibitors (MAOIs) should not take gingko because of increased risk of toxic reaction. Moderate interactions may occur with alprazolam, anticonvulsants, antidiabetic meds, buspirone, efavirenz, fluoxetine, and drugs metabolized by cytochrome P450 (various substrates).

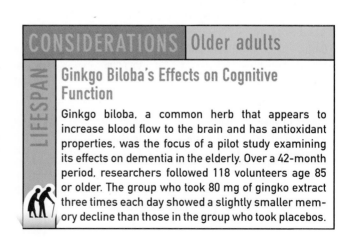

CONSIDERATIONS | **Older adults**

LIFESPAN

Ginkgo Biloba's Effects on Cognitive Function

Ginkgo biloba, a common herb that appears to increase blood flow to the brain and has antioxidant properties, was the focus of a pilot study examining its effects on dementia in the elderly. Over a 42-month period, researchers followed 118 volunteers age 85 or older. The group who took 80 mg of gingko extract three times each day showed a slightly smaller memory decline than those in the group who took placebos.

TABLE 46-1   Common Herbal Remedies

Common Name	Scientific Name	Body Systems Affected	Uses	Adverse Reactions	Significant Considerations
Aloe vera	*Aloe vera*	Skin	Inhibits infection and promotes healing of minor burns and wounds	None significant if used as directed; may cause burning sensation in wound	Rare reports of delayed healing when used in the gel form on a wound; taken internally, aloe gel may have laxative effect
Bilberry	*Vaccinium myrtillus*	Various	Vision enhancement and eye health, microcirculation, spider veins and varicose veins, capillary strengthening before surgery	No adverse effects have been reported in clinical studies	None
Black cohosh, (black snakeroot, squawroot)	*Cimicifuga racemosa*	Endocrine Reproductive	Management of some symptoms of menopause	Overdose causes nausea, dizziness, nervous system and visual disturbances, decreased pulse rate, and increased perspiration	Should not be used during pregnancy; possible interactions with hormone therapy
Chamomile	*Matricaria chamomilla*	Gastrointestinal Various	Colic, dyspepsia, oral mucositis	Possible contact dermatitis and, in rare instances, anaphylaxis	Chamomile is a member of the ragweed family, and those allergic to ragweed should not take the herb
Cranberry	*Vaccinium macrocarpon*	Urinary	Urinary tract infection (UTI)	Large doses can produce gastrointestinal symptoms (e.g., diarrhea)	None
Echinacea (American coneflower, black susans)	*Echinacea angustifolia*	Immune	Prevents and shortens symptoms and duration of upper respiratory infections (URIs) including colds	Rare; nausea and mild gastrointestinal (GI) upsets	Should not be used by individuals with autoimmune diseases such as multiple sclerosis, SLE, and RA, AIDS, and HIV infection
Elderberry	*Sambucus canadensis, Sambucus nigra, Sambucus racemosa*	Immune	Reduce flu-like symptoms	Nausea, vomiting, diarrhea when raw	May interfere with immunosuppressant therapy
Garlic	*Allium sativum*	Cardiovascular Immune	Oral: lowers blood sugar, cholesterol, and lipids. Topical: antifungal	Oral form: may cause abnormal blood glucose levels	Oral form: increased risk of bleeding in patients taking the coumarins, salicylates, or antiplatelet drugs
Ginger (ginger root, black ginger)	*Zingiber officinale*	Neurologic Immune Gastrointestinal	Antiemetic, cardiotonic, antithrombotic, antibacterial, antioxidant, antitussive, anti-inflammatory, GI disturbances, lower cholesterol, prophylaxis for nausea and vomiting, colic, bronchitis	Excessive doses may cause CNS depression and interfere with cardiac functioning or anticoagulant activity	Theoretically, ginger could enhance the effects of the antiplatelet drugs, such as coumarin

TABLE 46-1 Common Herbal Remedies *(continued)*

Common Name	Scientific Name	Body Systems Affected	Uses	Adverse Reactions	Significant Considerations
Ginkgo (maiden hair tree, kew tree)	*Ginkgo biloba*	Neurologic	Age-related memory impairment, cognitive function, dementia, diabetic retinopathy, glaucoma, PVD, PMS, Raynaud syndrome, vertigo	Rare if used as directed; possible effects include headache, dizziness, heart palpitations, GI effects, rash, allergic dermatitis	Do not take with antidepressant drugs, such as the MAOIs, or the antiplatelet drugs, such as coumarin, unless advised by the primary care provider
Ginseng	*Panax quinquefolius, Panax ginseng*	Neurologic Cardiovascular	Diabetes, respiratory tract infections, athletic performance, ADHD	Most common: nervousness, excitation, hypoglycemia	Taking ginseng in combination with stimulants such as caffeine is not advised; do not use for longer than 3 mo (some herbalists recommend use for 1 mo followed by no use for 2 mo)
Goldenseal	*Hydrastis canadensis*	Immune Skin Various	Uses: common cold, upper respiratory tract infections, swine flu, nasal congestion, allergic rhinitis, gastritis, peptic ulcers, colitis, diarrhea, constipation, flatulence, inflammation of vaginal and urethral mucous membranes, UTIs, menorrhagia, dysmenorrhea Topical: mouthwash for sore gums and mouth Topical: skin rashes, ulcers, wound infections, itching, eczema, acne, dandruff, ringworm, herpes blisters, herpes labialis Ophthalmic: eyewash for eye inflammation, conjunctivitis Otological: ringing of the ears, earache	Large doses may cause dry or irritated mucous membranes and injury to the gastrointestinal system; may reduce the beneficial bacteria in the intestines	Should not be taken for more than 3–7 d; do not use during pregnancy or if lactating
Grape seed extract	*Vitis vinifera*	Cardiovascular	Atherosclerosis, high blood pressure, high cholesterol	Headache; dry, itchy scalp; dizziness; nausea	Interactions between grape seed extract and medicines or other supplements have not been studied
Green tea	*Camellia sinensis*	Immune	May reduce the risk of some cancers, lowers lipid levels, helps prevent dental carries, antimicrobial and antioxidative effects	Contains caffeine (may cause mild stimulant effects such as anxiety, nervousness, heart irregularities, restlessness, insomnia, and digestive irritation)	Interactions: anemia, anxiety disorders, bleeding disorders, cardiac conditions, diabetes glaucoma, hypertension, liver disease, osteoporosis

(continues)

TABLE 46-1   Common Herbal Remedies *(continued)*

Common Name	Scientific Name	Body Systems Affected	Uses	Adverse Reactions	Significant Considerations
Kava (kawa, kava-kava, awa yanggona)	*Piper methysticum*	Neurologic	Mild to moderate anxiety and as a sedative	GI upset, headache, dizziness, drowsiness, enlarged pupils and disturbances of oculomotor equilibrium and accommodation, dry mouth, allergic skin reactions	Limit use to no more than 3 mo
Lemon balm (balm, melissa, sweet balm)	*Melissa officinalis*	Immune	Graves disease, sedative, antispasmodic, cold sores (topical)	Topical: none Oral: GI effects, dizziness	None
Milk thistle	*Silybum marianum*	Gastrointestinal	Used to treat liver disease; milk thistle seed extract has been used in the treatment of alcoholic and other cirrhoses	Loose stools due to increased bile solubility	Appears to be safe but has not been studied in pregnant women or children
Saw palmetto (cabbage palm, fan palm, scrub palm)	*Serenoa repens*	Endocrine Reproductive	Symptoms of benign prostatic hyperplasia	Generally well tolerated; occasional gastrointestinal effects	May interact with hormones such as oral contraceptive drugs and hormone replacement therapy, and anticoagulant and antiplatelet drugs
St. John's wort (Klamath weed, goat weed, rosin rose)	*Hypericum perforatum*	Neurologic	Antidepressant	Insomnia, vivid dreams, restlessness, anxiety, agitation, irritability, GI discomfort, diarrhea, fatigue, dry mouth, dizziness, headache, skin rash, paresthesia, hypoglycemia	May decrease efficacy of theophylline, warfarin, and digoxin; use with other prescriptions is not recommended
Tea tree oil	*Melaleuca alternifolia*	Immune Skin	Topical antimicrobial	Contact dermatitis	For topical use only; do not take orally
Valerian	*Valeriana officinalis*	Neurologic	Restlessness, sleep disorders	Rare if used as directed	May interact with the barbiturates (e.g., phenobarbital), the benzodiazepines (e.g., diazepam), and the opiates (e.g., morphine)
Willow bark (weidenrinde, white willow, purple osier willow, crack willow)	*Salix alba, S. purpurea, S. fragilis*	Neurologic	Analgesic	Adverse reactions are those associated with the salicylates	Do not use with aspirin or other NSAIDs; do not use in patients with peptic ulcers and other medical conditions in which the salicylates are contraindicated

ALERT Rx

Ginseng

Ginseng is contraindicated in individuals with high blood pressure and during pregnancy.

Ginseng

Ginseng has been called the "king of herbs" because of its wide use and benefits attributed to the herb. In early times in China, ginseng was valued as much as gold. Hundreds of ginseng products (e.g., gum, teas, chewing gum, juices) are sold throughout the United States. Two species of ginseng are American and Panax, with Panax believed to be the better species of the two. The primary use of ginseng is to improve energy and mental performance. The benefits of ginseng are said to include improving endurance during exercise, reducing fatigue, boosting stamina and reaction times, and increasing feelings of well-being. Recent studies indicate that ginseng is effective in lowering the levels of postprandial glucose in type 2 diabetics.

Additional research is needed before definitive statements can be made about the value of ginseng for improving cognitive performance in Alzheimer patients or others. Some studies have shown improved memory, for example, whereas others have not.

The herb should not be taken in combination with stimulants, including substances containing caffeine. Because ginseng can lower blood sugar levels in people with type 2 diabetes, it should not be used by those taking insulin or oral antidiabetic medications without careful glucose monitoring. Ginseng may also interfere with the heart medication digoxin. Warfarin therapy effectiveness is decreased with concurrent ginseng therapy.

Kava

Kava has been used by many Pacific Island cultures for thousands of years as a psychoactive beverage. It is currently available over-the-counter in pill, tincture, tea, and topical forms. Kava is a popular treatment for reducing stress, anxiety, and depression; for promoting sleep; and for relieving menstrual symptoms. Kava is promoted as a natural alternative to anxiety drugs, including Xanax (alprazolam) and Valium (diazepam), and also has a reputation as an aid to feeling "high" and for being an aphrodisiac.

The FDA has issued an alert that the use of kava may cause liver damage. Because kava-containing products have been associated with liver-related injuries such as hepatitis, cirrhosis, and liver failure, the safest use of kava seems to be using the herb occasionally for episodes of anxiety rather than on a regular basis.

St. John's Wort

St. John's wort has been used for centuries for medicinal purposes, including the treatment of depression, as a sedative, and as a balm for burns, wounds, and insect bites. In Europe, it is prescribed widely as a treatment for depression. In the United States, it is one of the top-selling herbal products. People also use St. John's wort for many other uses, including anxiety and sleep disorders. It is commercially available over-the-counter in capsules, in a dried form used to make teas, and in concentrated extracts.

ALERT Rx

Kava and Liver Disease

Individuals using a kava-containing dietary supplement who experience symptoms of liver disease should immediately consult their health care provider. Symptoms of liver disease include jaundice, urine with a brown discoloration, nausea, vomiting, light-colored stools, weakness, and loss of appetite.

Kava may increase one's drowsiness when taken with other substances that cause drowsiness, such as antidepressants, sedatives, pain relievers, antianxiety drugs, seizure medications, muscle relaxants, and others. Because of both increased drowsiness and liver effects, kava should not be combined with alcohol.

Identifying kava-containing products can be difficult. Careful reading of the "Supplement Facts" information on the label may identify kava by any of the following names: ava, ava pepper, awa, kava root, kava-kava, kew, piper methysticum, sakau, tonga, or yanggona. Using multiple forms of kava simultaneously increases the risk of adverse effects and overdose.

Kava should not be used for longer than 3 months without supervision by a health care provider. Long-term use of kava has reportedly led to "kawaism." The symptoms of "kawaism" include dry, flaking, discolored skin; a scaly skin rash; red eyes; puffy face; muscle weakness; blood abnormalities; and general feelings of poor health.

BOX 46.3

St. John's Wort and Drug Interactions

- Major Drug Interactions
  - alprazolam, aminolevulinic acid, amitriptyline, antidepressants, barbiturates, oral contraceptive drugs, cyclosporine, amitriptyline, carisoprodol, citalopram, diazepam, lansoprazole, omeprazole, phenytoin, warfarin, some calcium channel blockers, chemotherapeutic agents, antifungals, glucocorticoids, cisapride, alfentanil, fentanyl, losartan, fluoxetine, midazolam, ondansetron, propranolol, fexofenadine, digoxin, fenfluramine, imatinib, irinotecan, meperidine, mephenytoin, narcotics, nefazodone, NNRTIs, nortriptyline, paroxetine, pentazocine, p-glycoprotein substrates, phenobarbital, phenprocoumon, phenytoin, photosensitizing drugs, protease inhibitors, reserpine, sertraline, tacrolimus, tramadol

- Moderate Drug Interactions
  - "triptans" (5-HT1 agonists), clopidogrel, celecoxib, diclofenac, fluvastatin, glipizide, ibuprofen, irbesartan, losartan, phenytoin, piroxicam, tamoxifen, tolbutamide, torsemide, warfarin, DXM, MAOIs, procainamide, simvastatin

Scientific studies have shown that St. John's wort is useful for treating mild to moderate depression but is ineffective for more severe depression. Its mechanism of action is not precisely known but is thought that the compounds in this plant may prevent nerve cells in the brain from reabsorbing serotonin.

This herb has become popular for a number of reasons. Some people do not experience relief from prescribed antidepressants and turn to St. John's wort instead. Others who experience adverse effects from prescribed antidepressants prefer to use St. John's wort because it has fewer and less severe adverse effects. It is also less expensive than prescribed drugs. In 2001, the National Institute of Mental Health issued a public alert that warned about serious adverse interactions that have been reported between St. John's wort and a number of drugs (Box 46-3). Potentially dangerous effects can occur in patients taking indinavir (a protease inhibitor used to treat HIV), cyclosporine (used to reduce the risk of organ transplant rejection), digoxin, and warfarin.

Valerian

Valerian first arrived in America with the landing of the Mayflower. In Europe, it is widely used for its sedative effects, including the treatment of insomnia, nervousness, and anxiety and is growing in popularity in the United States as a sleep aid. Valerian works by relaxing muscles and improves the quality of sleep by shortening the length of time it takes to fall asleep and reducing the number of awakenings through the night. Unlike sedative drugs, valerian does not cause sluggishness on awakening and does not lead to dependence. It is commercially available over the counter in tea, capsule, or tincture form.

When treating anxiety, it is safe and potentially more effective to combine valerian with other calming herbs such as chamomile or lemon balm. It may take 2 to 4 weeks before an improvement in symptoms is noticeable.

Valerian interacts with a number of other medications, specifically CNS depressants. Valerian should not be taken concurrently with drugs that have sedative or anesthetic properties, including alcohol, alprazolam, and benzodiazepines.

Willow Bark

Willow bark has a long history of use as an analgesic, dating back to the time of Hippocrates, when it was common for patients to chew on the bark to reduce fever or inflammation. Its other important medicinal quality is to relieve pain. When

ALERT ℞

St. John's Wort Contraindications and Precautions
None of the antidepressants should be administered with herbal preparations containing St. John's wort because of the potential for adverse reactions. In fact, this herb interacts with many commonly prescribed drugs and should be used with caution (see Box 46-1). Any patient who wants to initiate St. John's wort therapy should discuss it with a health care provider first.

ALERT ℞

Willow Bark
Although adverse reactions are rare with willow bark, it should be used with caution in patients with peptic ulcers and medical conditions in which aspirin is contraindicated, including patients taking blood-thinning medications such as warfarin. Patients taking anticoagulant or antiplatelet medications should avoid the use of willow bark altogether. Willow bark should not be combined with aspirin, choline magnesium trisalicylate, salsalate, or any other salicylate-containing drugs.

Willow bark is also purported to help with sexual dysfunction, diarrhea, tendonitis, bursitis, and some forms of arthritis. Scientific study has been insufficient to verify the accuracy of these claims. It is available as an over the counter and is commonly consumed in tea and tincture form.

used as a medicinal herb, willow bark is collected in early spring from young willow branches, when the bark is most tender. White willow in particular is used medicinally.

Salicylate was originally isolated from willow bark and identified as the most likely source of the bark's anti-inflammatory effects. Its chemical structure was replicated in the laboratory and mass-produced as synthetic salicylic acid. Years later, a modified version (acetylsalicylic acid) was first sold as aspirin. Aspirin became the most widely used pain reliever, fever reducer, and anti-inflammatory agent, and willow bark lost popularity. Synthetic anti-inflammatory drugs work quickly and have a higher potency than willow bark. Willow bark takes longer to work and may have to be taken in fairly high doses to achieve a noticeable effect. However, willow bark has fewer adverse reactions than salicylates.

Herbs That Affect the Cardiovascular System

The cardiovascular system pumps blood through the lungs and the rest of the body, providing it with oxygen and nutrients and disposing of waste products such as carbon dioxide. It includes the heart, arteries, capillaries, and veins. Several herbal remedies that can affect the cardiovascular system are described below (also see Table 46-1).

Garlic

Garlic is commonly used as a food product and an herbal supplement. It has been used for many years throughout the world. Although garlic has many medicinal purposes, its positive effect on cardiovascular health is the most well-known and has been extensively researched. Other benefits of garlic are that it helps to lower serum cholesterol and triglyceride levels, improves the ratio of HDL (high-density lipoprotein) to LDL (low-density lipoprotein) cholesterol, lowers blood pressure, and helps to prevent atherosclerosis. It is often used as an antioxidant, to protect the liver, as an effective antifungal, antiviral, and antibiotic, to reduce blood sugar levels, to strengthen the immune system, and to reduce menstrual pain. Garlic has also been used topically to treat warts, corns, calluses, ear infections, muscle pain, nerve pain, arthritis, and sciatica.

Generally, garlic taken orally is in the form of enteric-coated odorless garlic or fresh pressed garlic. Although no serious reactions have occurred in pregnant women taking garlic, its use is not recommended. Major drug interactions occur with isoniazid, NNRTIs, and saquinavir. Moderate drug interactions occur with anticoagulant/antiplatelet drugs, warfarin, contraceptive drugs, cyclosporine, and drugs metabolized by cytochrome P450. Garlic is excreted in breast milk and may cause colic in some infants.

Grape Seed Extract

Grape leaves and fruit have been used as medicine since ancient Greece. As the name implies, grape seed extract comes from the seeds of grapes. It is still not clear exactly how grape seed extract affects health, but studies have shown that antioxidants contained in grape seed can prevent cell damage caused by free radicals. Most studies have not yet explored the relationship between antioxidants and specific diseases or conditions. Grape seed extract is available commercially in capsule and tablet form. It has been used safely for up to 8 weeks in clinical trials and has been generally well tolerated when taken orally. It does interact with warfarin and drugs metabolized by cytochrome P450, including some antidepressants.

Herbal Remedies for Hypertension

Various herbs and supplements, such as hawthorn extracts, garlic, onion, and gingko biloba, may be used by herbalists for hypertension. Although these substances may lower blood pressure in some individuals, their use is not recommended because the effect is slight and usually too gentle to affect moderate to severe hypertension.

Herbs That Affect the Gastrointestinal and Urinary Systems

The gastrointestinal system consists of the digestive tract, which breaks down food so that it can be absorbed into the bloodstream. The urinary system eliminates waste from the human body and consists of the kidneys, the ureters, the bladder, and the urethra. Several herbal remedies can affect the gastrointestinal and urinary systems and are discussed below (also see Table 46-1).

Chamomile

Chamomile is an herb extract from two varieties of chamomile plant. When taken orally, it reduces flatulence and diarrhea caused by a nervous stomach, reduces stomach upset, helps to control travel sickness, reduces restlessness and irritability, treats the common cold and fever, reduces cough, liver, and gallbladder symptoms, increases appetite, and acts as a mild sedative. It has also been used for menstrual cramps and, when applied topically, soothes skin irritation and inflammation.

Chamomile is on the FDA's list of herbs generally regarded as safe. It is available in pill, liquid, and tea formulations. When used as a tea, chamomile appears to produce an anti-spasmodic effect on the smooth muscle of the gastrointestinal tract and to protect against the development of stomach ulcers. It is one of the most popular teas in Europe.

ALERT Rx

Chamomile and Allergic Reactions
Although chamomile is generally safe and nontoxic, the tea is prepared from the pollen-filled flower heads and has resulted in mild symptoms of contact dermatitis to severe anaphylactic reactions in individuals hypersensitive to ragweed, asters, and chrysanthemums. Although uncommon, allergic reaction to any form of chamomile is possible. Symptoms include difficulty breathing; closing of the throat; swelling lips, tongue, or face; and hives or vomiting. A physician should be consulted before consuming chamomile if a patient is being treated with warfarin (Coumadin), ardeparin (Normiflo), dalteparin (Fragmin), danaparoid (Orgarin), enoxaparin (Lovenox), heparin, or any other blood thinner, or if a patient is hypersensitive to ragweed, asters, and chrysanthemums. Moderate drug interactions may occur with benzodiazepines, CNS depressants, contraceptive drugs metabolized by cytochrome P450, estrogens, and tamoxifen.

Cranberry

Cranberry juice has long been recommended for preventing and treating urinary tract infections. In fact, clinical studies have confirmed that it is beneficial to individuals with frequent urinary tract infections. Cranberries inhibit bacteria from attaching to the walls of the urinary tract and prevent certain bacteria from forming dental plaque in the mouth. Cranberry juice and capsules have no contraindications, no known adverse reactions, and no drug interactions.

Although cranberry juice may help to prevent the occurrence and relieve the symptoms of a urinary tract infection, no evidence suggests it works as a cure. If a urinary tract infection is thought to be present, then it is necessary to seek medical treatment.

Ginger

Ginger, a medicinal herb, is derived from the root of the ginger plant. It has been used safely as a food by millions of individuals for hundreds of years. When dried for consumption, it resembles an ash-colored powder, smells like pepper, and has a spicy taste. Ginger is usually taken to reduce nausea, vomiting, and indigestion. Clinical studies suggest that ginger can be effective in preventing the nausea associated with motion sickness, seasickness, and anesthesia, although results are unclear whether ginger helps people already experiencing the symptoms of seasickness. Ginger is commercially available over the counter in dried form (chopped, powdered, powdered extract), candied ginger, and tea.

Although conclusive studies have not yet shown that ginger is also effective as a treatment for arthritis pain and inflammation, anecdotal evidence points to that conclusion.

Ginger may be used for morning sickness associated with pregnancy. Small amounts present in food preparation are generally regarded as safe. The medicinal use of ginger should cease 2 to 3 weeks before surgery to reduce the risk of bleeding.

The only known adverse effects of ginger are heartburn, diarrhea, and heightened taste sensitivity. Ginger may affect platelet aggregations and should not be used with anticoagulants including warfarin. In addition, ginger may cause hypoglycemia and interact with antidiabetic drugs.

Milk Thistle

Milk thistle, a flowering herb commonly found in the Mediterranean, has been used for centuries to treat a variety of conditions, including liver problems. There is no conclusive evidence to show that milk thistle improves liver function, but promising data has shown a positive effect on liver disease in humans. At this time, however, few studies have been conducted, and the results are mixed. National Center for Complementary and Alternative Medicine and the National Institute of Diabetes and Digestive and Kidney Diseases are currently cofunding research on the effects of milk thistle on hepatitis C and nonalcoholic liver disease, while the National Cancer Institute and the National Institute of Nursing Research are investigating its uses for cancer prevention and for the treatment of HIV complications. Milk thistle has been shown as useful in type 2 diabetic patients in combination with their current medications in lowering fasting blood glucose, hemoglobin A1c, and cholesterol levels. It is also useful in improving symptoms of dyspepsia in combination with other natural medications in a product known as Iberogast. Milk thistle is available commercially in capsule, extract, and tea form.

Herbal Remedies as Diuretics

Numerous herbal diuretics, substances that help rid the body of excess water, are available as over-the-counter products, and most are nontoxic. However, most are either ineffective or no more effective than caffeine. The following are some of the herbals reported to have diuretic activity: celery, chicory, sassafras, juniper berries, St. John's wort, foxglove, horsetail, licorice, dandelion, digitalis purpurea, ephedra, hibiscus, parsley, and elderberry.

There is very little and in many instances no scientific evidence to justify the use of these plants as diuretics. For example, dandelion root is a popular preparation once thought to be a strong diuretic, but scientific research has found dandelion root, although safe, to be ineffective as a diuretic. No herbal diuretic should be taken unless approved by the health care provider.

Diuretic teas such as juniper berries and shave grass or horsetail should be avoided. Juniper berries have been associated with renal damage, and horsetail contains severely toxic compounds. In 1994, the FDA banned dietary supplements containing ephedra, or ma huang, due to dangerous and sometimes fatal side effects, which include raising blood pressure and stressing the circulatory system.

Herbs That Affect the Endocrine and Reproductive Systems

The endocrine system is responsible for secreting hormones. The pituitary gland, the adrenal gland, the pancreas, the thyroid gland, and the ovaries and testes are included in the endocrine system. The reproductive system is responsible for human reproduction. Herbal remedies that can affect the endocrine and reproductive systems are described below (also see Table 46-1).

Black Cohosh

Black cohosh grows in North America and has been used for centuries for a variety of medicinal purposes. Black cohosh is generally regarded as safe when used as directed. Today, it is used primarily for hot flashes and other menopausal symptoms, muscular and arthritic pain, headache, and eyestrain. It is available over-the-counter in the form of tablets, capsules, tinctures, and tea. Black cohosh tea is not considered as effective as other forms.

This herb is popular as an alternative to hormone replacement therapy, which may increase a woman's risk of serious illness, including cancer, depression, and high blood pressure.

Black cohosh is thought to increase diminished estrogen levels in menopausal women. When taken orally, it may reduce physical menopausal symptoms, including night sweats, hot flashes, headaches, heart palpitations, dizziness, vaginal atrophy, and tinnitus (ringing in the ears). It may improve the regularity of menstrual cycles by balancing hormones and reducing uterine spasms. Black cohosh may also reduce the psychological symptoms associated with menopause, including insomnia, nervousness, irritability, and depression.

Black cohosh interacts with atorvastatin, cisplatin, hepatotoxic drugs, and drugs metabolized by cytochrome P450. Women taking hormone alternative replacement therapy should consult with their health care provider before taking black cohosh.

Saw Palmetto

Saw palmetto is derived from the berries of the saw palm tree and is used to treat benign prostatic hypertrophy, commonly known as enlargement of the prostate. Half of all men older than 60 have some symptoms of benign prostatic hypertrophy and must cope with a more urgent and more frequent needt to urinate, often interrupting sleep, creating urinary leaking, a feeling of not having completely emptied the bladder, and a stop-and-start flow of urine. Although commercially available over-the-counter in tea form, saw palmetto should be taken as a tincture, capsule, or tablet because the active agents in the herb are not water soluble.

Although scientific study is far from complete, encouraging evidence reported in the *Journal of the American Medical Association* suggests that saw palmetto is effective in the treatment of benign prostatic hypertrophy, increases the flow of urine, and reduces urinary frequency and the sleep interruption associated with it. It often takes 1 to 3 months of treatment before an improvement in symptoms occurs. After 6 months of treatment with saw palmetto, a health care provider should assess the person's condition.

Saw palmetto when used in combination with anticoagulant or antiplatelet drugs may increase the risk of bleeding.

Herbs That Affect the Immune System

The immune system helps the body to defend itself against foreign substances or organisms. Several herbal remedies that can affect the immune system are described below (see also Table 46-1).

Echinacea

Echinacea, a frequently used herb, is taken to stimulate the immune system function by increasing the number and activity of immune cells and to stimulate phagocytosis (ingestion and destruction of bacteria and other harmful substances). It may shorten the duration of colds and influenza.

Echinacea is available in pill, tincture, and tea form. Most herbalists recommend that echinacea should be taken at the initial signs of infection, when symptoms first become apparent. Small repeated doses throughout the day may be better than taking larger doses less frequently. The herb should not be taken for more than eight consecutive weeks. The standard recommendation is 7 to 14 days of treatment.

Individuals with allergies to daisy-type plants are more susceptible to reactions, and if a patient has lupus, rheumatoid arthritis, multiple sclerosis, tuberculosis, or HIV, then echinacea intake should be limited. Drugs that interact with echinacea include caffeine, drugs metabolized by cytochrome P450, and immunosuppressants.

Elderberry

Elderberry is an immunostimulant that is used to reduce flu-like symptoms. It must be given within 24 to 48 hours of the onset of symptoms. Elderberry comes in liquid and lozenge dosage forms that are taken four times daily. Significant symptom relief can be expected after 2 to 4 days of use. Use during pregnancy and lactation is not recommended due to insufficient information.

Goldenseal

Goldenseal, also called *Hydrastis canadensis*, is an herb found growing in certain areas of the northeastern United States. Goldenseal has long been used alone or in combination with Echinacea for colds and influenza. However, there is no scientific evidence to support the use of goldenseal for cold and influenza or as a stimulant, as there is for the use of echinacea. Similarly, goldenseal is touted as an "herbal antibiotic," although there is no scientific evidence to support this use. Another myth surrounding goldenseal use is that taking the herb masks the presence of illicit drugs in the urine.

There are many traditional uses of the herb, such as an antiseptic for the skin, mouthwash for canker sores, wash for inflamed or infected eyes, and the treatment of sinus infections and digestive problems, such as peptic ulcers and gastritis. Some evidence supports the use of goldenseal to treat diarrhea caused by bacteria or intestinal parasites, such as Giardia. The herb is contraindicated during pregnancy and in patients with hypertension. It should not be used during pregnancy, lactation, or in newborn infants because it can cause kernicterus in newborn babies. Moderate drug interactions may occur with cyclosporine and drugs metabolized by cytochrome P450. Because of widespread use, destruction of its natural habitats, and renewed interest in its use as a herbal remedy, goldenseal was classified as an "endangered" plant in 1997 by the US government.

Green Tea

Green tea and black tea come from the same plant. The difference is in the processing. Green tea is simply dried tea leaves, whereas black tea is fermented, giving it the dark color, the stronger flavor, and the lowest amount of tannins and polyphenols. The beneficial effects of green tea lie in the polyphenols, or flavonoids, that have antioxidant properties. Antioxidants are thought to play a major role in preventing disease (e.g., colon cancer) and reducing the effects of aging. Green tea polyphenols are thought to act by inhibiting the reactions of free radicals within the body thought to play a role in aging. The benefits of green tea include an overall sense of well-being, cancer prevention, dental health, and maintenance of heart and liver health. Green tea used as directed is safe and well tolerated. It contains as much as 50 mg of caffeine per cup. Decaffeinated green tea retains all of the polyphenol content. Standardized green tea extracts vary in strength, so dosages may need to be adjusted. Patients with hypertension, cardiac conditions, anxiety, insomnia, diabetes, and ulcers should use green tea with caution. Major drug interactions occur with amphetamines, cocaine, and ephedrine. Moderate interactions occur with adenosine, cimetidine, clozapine, contraceptives, dipyridamole, disulfiram, estrogens, fluvoxamine, hepatotoxic drugs, lithium, MAOIs, nicotine, pentobarbital, quinolones, theophylline, verapamil, and warfarin.

Lemon Balm

Lemon balm is a perennial herb with heart-shaped leaves that has been used for hundreds of years. Traditionally, the herb has been used for Graves disease and as a sedative, antispasmodic, and an antiviral agent. Lemon balm is possibly effective for Alzheimer disease, colic, dyspepsia, and sleep. When used topically, lemon balm has antiviral activity against herpes simplex virus. Lemon balm when taken with CNS depressants will cause an additive effect.

Herbs That Affect Other Body Systems

Several herbal remedies that can affect other body systems are described below (also see Table 46-1).

Aloe Vera

Aloe is used to prevent infection and promote healing of minor burns (e.g., sunburn) and wounds. When used externally, the herb helps repair skin tissue and reduce inflammation. It aids in the healing of dermal ulcers, wounds, and frostbite. A regular ingredient in face and hand creams, lotions, and skin moisturizers, it is also used in diapers, wipes, and bandages to soothe, reduce inflammation, and protect the skin. Aloe gel is naturally thick when taken from the leaf but quickly becomes watery because of the action of enzymes in the plant. Commercially available preparations have additive thickeners to make the aloe appear like the fresh gel. The herb can be applied directly from the fresh leaf by cutting the leaf in half lengthwise and gently rubbing the inner gel directly onto the skin. Commercially prepared products are applied externally as needed.

Although available as an oral juice, its benefits have not been confirmed. Some individuals have reported the oral juice effective in healing and preventing stomach ulcers. The FDA regulates aloe in drink form. Historically, it was used in the United States as a powerful laxative and is currently approved as a natural flavoring substance in foods. Although available as a juice that is promoted to help heal and prevent stomach ulcers, no research exists to support this claim. When aloe vera is taken orally, major drug interactions occur with digoxin;

moderate drug interactions occur with antidiabetic drugs, diuretics, stimulant laxatives, and warfarin.

Bilberry

Bilberry, also known as whortleberry, blueberry, trackleberry, and huckleberry, is a shrub with blue flowers that appear in early spring and ripen in July and August. Although bilberry is given to improve capillary strength and flexibility and as an antioxidant, the most beneficial use appears to be in promoting healthy eyes. Bilberry is thought to increase production of the enzymes responsible for energy production in the eye and promote capillary blood flow in the eyes, hands, and feet. Bilberry extract has been shown to increase the flexibility of the cell walls of both red blood cells and endothelial cells, making the cells better able to stretch and squeeze through tighter spaces. With increased flexibility in the red blood cells, more oxygen reaches the tissues, including the retina of the eye. A component of bilberry also speeds the regeneration of rhodopsin (visual purple), which is a critical protein found in the rods of the eye. Bilberry interacts with anticoagulant/antiplatelet drugs and antidiabetic drugs.

Natural Remedies as Antifungal Treatments

Researchers have identified several antifungal herbs that are effective against pedis (athlete's foot), such as tea tree oil

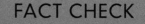

FACT CHECK

46-11   What conditions has the herb gingko biloba been used to treat? What are its adverse effects?

46-12   What is the herb ginseng used for? What are its contraindications?

and garlic. Tea tree oil comes from an evergreen tree native to Australia. The herb has been used as a nonirritating antimicrobial for cuts, stings, wounds, burns, and acne. It can be found in shampoos, soaps, and lotions. Tea tree oil should not be ingested orally, but it is effective when used topically for minor cuts and stings. Tea tree oil is used as an antifungal to relieve and control the symptoms of tinea pedis. Topical application is most effective when used in a cream with at least 10% tea tree oil. Several commercially prepared ointments are available. The cream is applied to affected areas twice daily for several weeks.

Garlic is used as an antifungal. A cream of 0.04% ajoene (the antifungal component of garlic) has been found to relieve symptoms of athlete's foot and, like tea tree oil, is applied twice daily.

Chapter Review

KEY POINTS

- The DSHEA of 1994 makes the distinction between dietary supplements, food additives, and drugs.
- It is important to differentiate between water-soluble and fat-soluble vitamins in order to avoid excessive buildup in the body and overdose.
- Herbal therapy may be an important complementary or alternative to drug therapy, but herbs can have many effects and interactions and should be used as carefully as drugs, based on available information and safety warnings. Patients frequently view herbs as harmless and may need to be taught cautions to take with any herbal product.

CRITICAL THINKING CASE STUDY
CASE 1
Taking Herbal Supplements for Depression

Mrs. Lawrence, age 56, visits the doctor for an annual checkup. When asked if she takes any drugs, she answers no. However, toward the end of the conversation, she mentions that she takes an herbal supplement to treat mild depression.

1. Why should patients always be questioned specifically about the use of herbs, teas, vitamins, or other nutritional or dietary supplements as part of a drug history?
2. How should the physician address the use of herbal supplements with this patient?

CASE 2
Immune System Remedies

During his clinic visit, Mr. Davidson complains of a sore throat and says he thinks he is coming down with a cold.

1. What natural remedies could Mr. Davidson take to help boost his immune system and decrease the severity and length of a cold?
   a. Vitamin C
   b. Zinc
   c. Echinacea
   d. All of the above
2. If Mr. Davidson was allergic to daisy-type plants, he should be instructed to limit his intake of which of the following natural remedies?
   a. Vitamin C
   b. Zinc
   c. Echinacea
   d. All of the above
3. Mr. Davidson asks about drugs that interact with Echinacea. What should you tell him?

Review Questions

MULTIPLE CHOICE

1. Which herb is said to help lower blood cholesterol and reduce high blood pressure?
   a. Black cohosh
   b. Valerian
   c. Garlic
   d. Ginkgo biloba
2. Which natural remedy contains polyphenols, or flavonoids, that have antioxidant properties?
   a. Green tea
   b. Niacin
   c. Vitamins A and D
   d. Zinc
3. Together with calcium, this is an essential constituent of bones and teeth. It is present in all living cells where it is involved in the release of energy.
   a. Iron
   b. Zinc
   c. Phosphorus
   d. Sodium
4. A lack of which fat-soluble vitamin can cause impaired vision in reduced light?
   a. Vitamin B_2 (riboflavin)
   b. Vitamin D (cholecalciferol)
   c. Vitamin C (ascorbic acid)
   d. Vitamin A (retinol)

MATCHING

Match the vitamin on the left with the correct category on the right. Categories may be used more than once.

_____ 5. vitamin A	a.	water soluble
_____ 6. vitamin B	b.	fat soluble
_____ 7. vitamin C		
_____ 8. vitamin D		
_____ 9. vitamin E		
_____ 10. vitamin K		

Match the vitamin on the left with the correct name on the right

_____ 11. vitamin A	a.	ascorbic acid
_____ 12. vitamin B1	b.	riboflavin
_____ 13. vitamin B2	c.	phylloquinone
_____ 14. vitamin B3	d.	cholecalciferol
_____ 15. vitamin B5	e.	retinol
_____ 16. vitamin B6	f.	pyridoxine
_____ 17. vitamin B12	g.	cyanocobolamin
_____ 18. vitamin C	h.	menaquinones
_____ 19. vitamin D2	i.	niacin
_____ 20. vitamin D3	j.	calciferol
_____ 21. vitamin K1	k.	thiamine
_____ 22. vitamin K2	l.	pantothenic acid
_____ 23. vitamin K3	m.	menadione

Match the mineral on the left with the correct category on the right. Categories may be used more than once.

_____ 24. calcium	a.	macromineral
_____ 25. iron	b.	trace mineral
_____ 26. magnesium		
_____ 27. phosphorous		
_____ 28. potassium		
_____ 29. sodium		
_____ 30. zinc		

TRUE OR FALSE

_____ 31. Dietary supplements are regulated by the government.

_____ 32. As part of a drug history, patients should always be questioned about the use of herbs, teas, vitamins, or other nutritional or dietary supplements.

_____ 33. The water-soluble vitamins are generally metabolized slowly and are stored in the liver.

_____ 34. Cranberry juice and capsules have no contraindications, no known adverse reactions, and no drug interactions.

FILL IN THE BLANKS

35. In patients receiving warfarin, a diet high in vitamin _____ may increase the risk of clot formation.
36. _____ is used to treat benign prostatic hypertrophy, commonly known as enlargement of the prostate.
37. To manage the symptoms of menopause, female patients may use the herb _____ _____.
38. The macromineral_____ is important for regulating the acid–base balance, for synthesizing amino acids, for metabolizing carbohydrates, and for building muscle.

SHORT ANSWERS

39. What are the risks of overdosing on fat-soluble vitamin A?
40. What are the two categories of minerals?
41. What is a common adverse reaction associated with niacin therapy? How can it be minimized?
42. Why should the herb St. John's wort be used with caution?

Web Activities

1. Go to the Web site of the National Center for Complementary and Alternative Medicine (http:// nccam.nih.gov). Go to "Herbs at a Glance." Choose any herb and look for information on what it is used to treat. Briefly answer these questions based on what you learn from this site:
   a. Name the herb.
   b. What are other common names of the herb?

  c. What are the Latin names, if any?
  d. What is the herb used for?
  e. How is the herb used?
  f. What does science say about the herb?
  g. Does the herb have any side effects or cautions?
2. Go to the United States Department of Agriculture National Agricultural Library homepage (fnic.nal. usda.gov). Browse for "Dietary Guidance." Find the Dietary Reference Intake (DRI) information.
  a. How do the DRIs compare with RDAs for both vitamins and minerals?

Find the DRI table.
  b. What are your DRIs?
  c. How are they different from someone who is older?
  d. How are they different from someone who is pregnant?
  e. How are they different from when you were 9 years old?
  f. How are they different from what they will be when you are older than 70?

A

Glossary

A

absence seizures—previously referred to as petit mal seizures; are characterized by a brief loss of consciousness, during which physical activity ceases, and may last a few seconds and happen multiple times a day

acetylcholine—a natural chemical in the brain that is required for memory and thinking; a neurotransmitter in the parasympathetic nervous system

acetylcholinesterase—a neurotransmitter that inactivates acetylcholine

acquired immunodeficiency syndrome (AIDS)—syndrome of the immune system caused by an infection of HIV that is characterized by opportunistic infections

action potential—an electrical impulse that passes from cell to cell in the myocardium, stimulating fibers to shorten and causing muscular contraction (systole)

active immunity—the reaction of the body when exposed to certain infectious microorganisms (antigens) of forming antibodies to the invading microorganism

acute pain—pain that is of short duration and lasts less than 3 to 6 months and can be from mild to severe

addiction—physical drug dependence

additive drug reaction—a reaction that occurs when the combined effect of two drugs is equal to the sum of each drug given alone

adrenal insufficiency—a critical deficiency of the mineralocorticoids and the glucocorticoids that requires immediate treatment

adrenergic blocking drugs—drugs that impede certain sympathetic nervous system functions

adrenergic drugs—drugs with effects similar to those that occur in the body when the adrenergic nerves are stimulated

adverse reaction—undesirable drug effects

agonist—a drug that binds with a receptor to produce a therapeutic response

agonist–antagonist—a narcotic analgesic that has properties of both the agonist and antagonist

akathisia—extreme restlessness and increased motor activity

alanine aminotransferase (ALT)—an enzyme found predominantly in the liver; high levels may indicate liver damage

aldosterone—a hormone that promotes the retention of sodium and water, which may contribute to a rise in blood pressure

allergic reaction—a drug reaction that occurs because the individual's immune system views the drug as a foreign substance; also called adverse effect

alopecia—the loss of hair

alternative therapies—therapies used instead of conventional or Western medical therapies

Alzheimer disease—a disease of the elderly causing progressive deterioration of mental and physical abilities

amebiasis—invasion of the body by the ameba *Entamoeba histolytica*

anaerobic—able to live without oxygen

analeptics—drugs that stimulate the respiratory center

analgesia—absence of pain

analgesic—a drug that alleviates pain

anaphylactic shock—a severe form of hypersensitivity reaction; an extremely serious allergic drug reaction

anaphylactoid reaction—unusual or exaggerated allergic reaction

androgens—hormones that stimulate activity of the accessory male sex organs

anemia—a decrease in the number of red blood cells (RBCs), a decrease in the amount of hemoglobin in RBCs, or both a decrease in the number of RBCs and hemoglobin

anesthesia—a loss of feeling or sensation

anesthesiologist—a physician with special training in administering anesthetics

anesthetist—a nurse with special training who is qualified to administer anesthetics

angina—a disorder often caused by atherosclerotic plaque formation in the coronary arteries, which causes decreased oxygen supply to the heart muscle and results in chest pain or pressure

angiotensin-converting enzyme—a naturally occurring enzyme that converts angiotensin I to angiotensin II, which is a powerful vasoconstrictor

anorexia—a diminished appetite or loss of appetite

anorexiants—drugs used to suppress the appetite

antacids—drugs that neutralize or reduce the acidity of stomach and duodenal contents

antagonist—a drug that joins with a receptor to prevent the action of an agonist at that receptor; a substance that counteracts the action of something else

anthelmintic—drugs with actions against helminths

antianxiety drugs—drugs used to treat anxiety

antibacterial—active against bacteria

antibodies—immune system molecules produced in reaction to an antigen

antibody—a globulin (protein) produced by the B lymphocytes as a defense against an antigen

anticonvulsants—drugs used for the management of convulsive disorders

antidepressants—drugs used to treat depression

antiemetic—a drug used to treat or prevent nausea or vomiting

antiflatulents—drugs that remove flatus or gas in the stomach and small intestine

antigen—a substance, usually a protein, that the immune system perceives as foreign and that causes the body to produce antibodies

antigen–antibody response—the reaction of specific circulating antibodies to a specific antigen

antihistamine—a drug used to counteract the effects of histamine on body organs and structures

anti-infective—a drug used to treat infections and bacteria; another word for antibacterial

antineoplastic drugs—drugs used for cure, control, or palliative (relief of symptoms) treatment of malignancies

antipsoriatics—drugs used to treat psoriasis

antipsychotic drugs—drugs used to treat psychotic disorders

antipyretic—a drug that reduces elevated body temperature

antiseptic—a drug that stops, slows, or prevents the growth of microorganisms

antitubercular drugs—drugs used to treat active cases of tuberculosis

antitussive—a drug used to relieve coughing

antivenin—an antitoxin specific for an animal or insect venom

antivertigo—a drug used to treat or prevent vertigo

anxiety—a feeling of apprehension, worry, or uneasiness that may or may not be based on reality

anxiolytics—another term that refers to antianxiety drugs

arrhythmia—a disturbance or irregularity in the heart rate or rhythm, or both

asthma—a reversible obstructive disease of the lower airway

ataxia—a loss of control of voluntary movements, especially producing an unsteady gait

atelectasis—reduction of air in the lung

atherosclerosis—a disorder in which lipid deposits accumulate on the lining of the blood vessels, eventually producing degenerative changes and obstruction of blood flow; a disease characterized by deposits of fatty plaques on the inner wall of arteries

atrial fibrillation—a cardiac arrhythmia characterized by rapid contractions of the atrial myocardium, resulting in an irregular and often rapid ventricular rate

attention deficit hyperactivity disorder (ADHD)—a disorder manifested by a short attention span, hyperactivity, impulsiveness, and emotional lability

attenuated—weakened, as in the antigen strain used for vaccine development

auscultating—listening to sounds within the body

autonomic nervous system (ANS)—the branch of the peripheral nervous system that controls functions essential for survival

B

bacterial resistance—ability of bacteria to produce substances that inactivate or destroy impact of a drug

bactericidal—an agent or drug that destroys bacteria

bacteriostatic—drugs that slow or retard the multiplication of bacteria

bile acid sequestrants—these drugs bind to bile acids to form an insoluble substance that cannot be absorbed by the intestine, so it is excreted in the feces

biological standard unit—a specific amount of biologically active substance that is used pharmacologically or therapeutically

biotransformation—chemical alteration of a substance in the body occurring at some point between absorption into the general circulation and renal elimination

bipolar disorder—a psychiatric disorder characterized by severe mood swings from extreme hyperactivity to depression (manic–depressive disease)

blockade effect—the action of antiarrhythmic drugs blocking stimulation of beta receptors of the heart by adrenergic neurohormones

blood pressure—the force of the blood against the walls of the arteries

blood–brain barrier—a meshwork of tightly packed cells in the walls of the brain's capillaries that screen out certain substances

bone marrow suppression—a potentially dangerous adverse reaction to antineoplastic drugs, resulting in decreased production of blood cells

booster—the administration of an additional dose of the vaccine to "boost" the production of antibodies to a level that will maintain the desired immunity

bowel prep—the use of drugs preoperatively to reduce the number of bacteria normally present in the intestine

brachial plexus block—type of regional anesthesia produced by injection of a local anesthetic into the brachial plexus

bronchodilator—a drug used to relieve bronchospasm associated with respiratory disorders

buccal—within the cheek, between the cheek and gum

C

cardiac arrhythmia—irregular heartbeat

cardiac output—the amount of blood leaving the left ventricle with each contraction

catalyst—a substance that accelerates a chemical reaction without itself undergoing a change

cell-mediated immunity—the process of T lymphocytes and macrophages (large cells that surround, engulf, and digest microorganisms and cellular debris) working together to destroy an antigen

central nervous system (CNS)—consists of the brain and the spinal cord

chemoreceptor trigger zone (CTZ)—a group of nerve fibers in the brain that when stimulated by chemicals, such as drugs or toxic substances, sends impulses to the vomiting center of the brain

chemotherapy—drug therapy with antineoplastic drugs

cholesterol—one of the lipids in the blood

cholinergic blocking drugs—drugs that impede certain parasympathetic nervous system functions

cholinergic crisis—cholinergic drug toxicity

cholinergic drugs—drugs that mimic the activity of the parasympathetic nervous system

choreiform movements—the involuntary twitching of the limbs or facial muscles

chronic pain—pain that lasts longer than 6 months and ranges in intensity from mild to severe

chrysiasis—grey to blue pigmentation of the skin that may occur from gold deposits in tissues

cinchonism—a term for quinidine toxicity characterized by ringing in the ears (tinnitus), hearing loss, headache, nausea, dizziness, vertigo, and light-headedness

clearance—a measure of the body's ability to eliminate a substance or drug

colic—spasmodic pains in the abdomen; in infants, this often presents with crying and irritability due to a variety of causes, such as swallowing of air, emotional upset, or overfeeding

common (proper) fraction—a fraction with the numerator smaller than the denominator

complementary and alternative medicine (CAM)—a group of nontraditional therapies

complementary therapies—therapies such as relaxation techniques, massage, dietary supplements, healing touch, and herbal therapy used together or to "complement" traditional health care

conduction block—type of regional anesthesia produced by injection of a local anesthetic into or near a nerve trunk

constipation—a condition where bowel movements are infrequent or incomplete

controlled substances—drugs with a high potential for abuse and dependence that are regulated by the Drug Enforcement Agency (DEA)

convulsion—another term for seizure

corticosteroids—hormones secreted from the adrenal cortex that contain potent anti-inflammatory action; the collective name for the glucocorticoids and mineralocorticoids, hormones secreted by the adrenal cortex and essential to life

coughing—the forceful expulsion of air from the lungs

Crohn disease—chronic enteritis in the terminal ileum; symptoms include fever, diarrhea, cramping, abdominal pain, and weight loss

cross-allergenicity—allergy to drugs in the same or related group

cross-sensitivity—synonymous with cross-allergenicity

cryptorchism—failure of the testes to descend into the scrotum

culture and sensitivity tests—culturing performed to grow bacteria along with tests of their sensitivity to specific drugs

cumulative drug effect—a drug effect that occurs when the body has not fully metabolized a dose of a drug before the next dose is given

Cushing syndrome—a disease caused by the overproduction of endogenous glucocorticoids

cycloplegia—paralysis of the ciliary muscle, resulting in an inability to focus the eye

D

decongestant—a drug that reduces the swelling of nasal passages and relieves congestion

dehydration—loss of too much water from the body

dementia—decrease in cognitive functioning (memory, decision making, speech, etc.)

denominator—the divisor of a fraction written in the bottom half of a common fraction

depolarization—the movement of a stimulus passing along the nerve; the positive ions move from outside the cell into the cell, and the negative ions move from inside the cell to outside the cell

depression—a common psychiatric disorder characterized by feelings of intense sadness, helplessness, and worthlessness and by impaired functioning

dermis—the layer of skin below the epidermis that contains small capillaries, which supply nourishment to the dermis and epidermis

diabetes insipidus—a disease resulting from the failure of the posterior pituitary to secrete vasopressin or from surgical removal of the pituitary

diabetes mellitus—a chronic disorder characterized either by insufficient insulin production in the beta cells of the pancreas or by cellular resistance to insulin

diabetic ketoacidosis—a potentially life-threatening deficiency of insulin (hypoinsulinism), resulting in severe hyperglycemia and requiring prompt diagnosis and treatment

diarrhea—abnormally frequent discharge of semisolid or fluid stools from the bowel

dietary supplement—substances such as herbs, vitamins, minerals, amino acids, and other natural substances; also referred to as nutritional supplements

digitalization—a series of digitalis doses given until the drug begins to exert a full therapeutic effect

diuretic—a drug that increases the secretion of urine (water, electrolytes, and waste products) by the kidneys

dosage—the amount of a medication to be taken at a specific time

drug error—any incident in which a patient receives the wrong dose, the wrong drug, a drug by the wrong route, or a drug given at the incorrect time

drug idiosyncrasy—any unusual or abnormal reaction to a drug

drug tolerance—a decreased response to a drug, requiring an increase in dosage to achieve the desired effect

dyscrasia—a morbid general state, resulting from the presence of abnormal material in the blood

dysphoric—extreme or exaggerated sadness, anxiety, or unhappiness

dyspnea—shortness of breath

dystonia—facial grimacing and twisting of the neck into unnatural positions

dystonic movements—muscular spasms most often affecting the tongue, jaw, eyes, and neck

dysuria—burning and pain upon urination

E

edema—retention of excess fluid

efficacy—effectiveness

ejection fraction—the amount of blood that the ventricle ejects per beat in relationship to the amount of blood available to eject

electrolyte—an electrically charged particle (ion) that is essential for normal cell function and is involved in various metabolic activities

emesis—the expelled gastric contents; vomitus

emetic—a drug that induces vomiting

endogenous—made within the body; substances normally manufactured by the body

epidermis—the outermost layer of the skin

epidural block—type of regional anesthesia produced by injection of a local anesthetic into the space surrounding the dura of the spinal cord

epidural—drug administration is performed when a catheter is placed into the epidural space outside of the dura matter of the brain and spinal cord

epigastric distress—discomfort in the abdomen

epilepsy—a permanent, recurrent seizure disorder

epilepticus—an emergency situation characterized by continual seizure activity with no interruptions

ergotism—an overdose of ergonovine; characterized by necrosis of the extremities due to contraction of the peripheral vascular bed

essential hypertension—hypertension without a known cause

estradiol—the most potent of the three endogenous estrogens

estriol—one of three endogenous estrogens

estrogens—female hormones influenced by the anterior pituitary gland

estrone—one of three endogenous estrogens

euthyroid—a normal thyroid

expectorant—a drug that aids in raising thick, tenacious mucus from the respiratory passages

expectoration—the elimination of thick, tenacious mucus from the respiratory tract by spitting it up

extrapyramidal effects—a group of adverse reactions occurring in the extrapyramidal portion of the nervous system, causing abnormal muscle movements

extravasation—escape of fluid from a blood vessel into surrounding tissues

F

factors—any numbers multiplied together to form a product

fat-soluble vitamins—vitamins that are generally metabolized slowly and are stored in the liver

fibrinolytic drugs—another name for thrombolytic drugs

filtrate—fluid removed from the blood through kidney function

first-dose effect—an unusually strong therapeutic effect experienced by some patients with the first doses of a medication

first-pass effect—a process that may limit a drug's bioavailability whereby the drug is absorbed intact and transported to the liver via the portal circulation where it undergoes extensive metabolism

fluid overload—a condition when the body's fluid requirements are met and the administration of fluid occurs at a rate that is greater than the rate at which the body can use or eliminate the fluid

folinic acid or leucovorin rescue—the technique of administering leucovorin after a large dose of methotrexate to rescue normal cells and allow them to survive

fraction—a part of a whole containing a numerator and denominator

fungicidal—able to destroy fungi

fungistatic—able to slow or retard the multiplication of fungi

fungus—a colorless plant that lacks chlorophyll

G

gallstone-solubilizing—gallstone-dissolving

gastric stasis—failure to move food normally out of the stomach, also called gastroparesis

gastroesophageal reflux disease—a reflux or backup of gastric contents into the esophagus

general anesthesia—provision of a pain-free state for the entire body

germicide—a drug that kills bacteria

gingival hyperplasia—overgrowth of gum tissue

glaucoma—an eye condition in which a blockage of drainage channels within the eye results in increased intraocular pressure that may lead to blindness

globulin—proteins present in blood serum or plasma that contain antibodies

glucagon—a hormone produced by the alpha cells of the pancreas that increases blood sugar by stimulating the conversion of glycogen to glucose in the liver

glucocorticoids—a hormone essential to life produced by the adrenal cortex

glucometer—a device used to monitor blood glucose levels

goiter—enlargement of the thyroid gland

gonadotropins—hormones that promote growth and function of the gonads

gout—a form of arthritis in which uric acid accumulates in increased amounts in the blood and often is deposited in the joints

H

half-normal saline—solution containing 0.45% NaCl

heart failure—denoted by the area of the initial ventricle dysfunction: left-side (left-ventricular) dysfunction and right-side (right ventricular) dysfunction; because both sides work together, both sides are affected in heart failure

Helicobacter pylori—bacteria that causes a type of chronic gastritis and peptic and duodenal ulcers

helminthiasis—invasion of the body by helminths (worms)

helminths—worms

hemostasis—a process that stops bleeding in a blood vessel

hepatotoxic—capable of producing liver damage

herbal remedies—plants or herbs used to treat various disorders

herbal therapy—a type of complementary or alternative therapy that uses plants or herbs to treat various disorders; also called botanical medicine

herb—plant used in medicine or as seasoning

high-density lipoproteins (HDL)—carry cholesterol from peripheral cells to the liver, where it is metabolized and excreted

histamine—a substance in various body tissues, such as the heart, lungs, gastric mucosa, and skin, that is produced in response to injury

HMG-CoA reductase inhibitor—an enzyme that is a catalyst in the manufacture of cholesterol

human immunodeficiency virus (HIV)—a cytopathic retrovirus; human T-cell lymphotropic virus type III

humoral immunity—based on the antigen–antibody response, special lymphocytes (white blood cells) produce circulating antibodies to act against a foreign substance

hydrochloric acid—a substance the stomach secretes that aids in the digestive process

hyperglycemia—elevated blood glucose level

hyperkalemia—high blood level of potassium

hyperlipidemia—an increase (hyper) in lipids (lipid), which are fats or fat-like substances, in the blood (-emia)

hypersecretory—excessive gastric secretion of hydrochloric acid

hypersensitivity—allergic; being allergic to a drug

hyperstimulation syndrome—sudden ovarian enlargement with accumulation of serous fluid in the peritoneal cavity

hypertension—usually defined as a systolic pressure more than 140 mm Hg or a diastolic pressure more than 90 mm Hg

hyperthyroidism—an increase in the amount of thyroid hormones secreted

hypnotic—a drug that induces sleep

hypocalcemia—low blood calcium

hypoglycemia—low blood glucose level

hypokalemia—low blood level of potassium

hyponatremia—low blood sodium

hypothyroidism—a decrease in the amount of thyroid hormones secreted

I

immune globulin—solutions obtained from human blood containing antibodies that have been formed by the body to specific antigens

immunity—the ability of the body to identify and resist microorganisms that are potentially harmful

immunization—a form of artificial active immunity and an important method of controlling some infectious diseases that can cause serious and sometimes fatal consequences

immunocompromised—patients with an immune system not fully capable of fighting infection

improper fraction—fractions with the numerator larger than the denominator

induction drug—drug given at the beginning of an anesthesia process that results in a general anesthesia state

infiltration—the collection of fluid in a tissue

inhalation—route of administration in which drug droplets, vapor, or gas is inhaled and absorbed through the mucous membranes of the respiratory tract

insulin—a hormone produced by the pancreas that helps maintain blood glucose levels within normal limits

intermittent claudication—a group of symptoms characterized by pain in the calf muscle of one or both legs, caused by walking and relieved by rest

intradermal—route of administration in which the drug is injected into skin tissue

intramuscular—route of administration in which the drug is injected into muscle tissue

intraocular pressure—the pressure within the eye

intravenous—route of administration in which the drug is injected into a vein

intrinsic factor—a substance produced by cells in the stomach that is necessary for the absorption of vitamin B_{12} in the intestine

iodism—excessive amounts of iodine in the body

iron deficiency anemia—condition that results when the body does not have enough iron to supply the body's needs

ischemic—marked by reduced blood flow caused by arterial narrowing or blockage or other causes

isolated systolic hypertension—a condition of only an elevated systolic pressure

J

Jacksonian seizure—a focal seizure that begins with an uncontrolled stiffening or jerking of the body such as the finger, mouth, hand, or foot that may progress to a generalized seizure

K

keratolytic—a drug that removes excess growth of the epidermis (top layer of skin) in disorders such as warts

L

left ventricular dysfunction—also called left ventricular systolic dysfunction, the most common form of heart failure

leprosy—a chronic, communicable disease spread by prolonged intimate contact with an infected person

leukopenia—a decrease in the white blood cells or leukocytes; a symptom of bone marrow suppression

leukotrienes—substances that are released by the body during the inflammatory process and constrict the bronchia

lipids—fats or fat-like substances in the blood

lipodystrophy—atrophy of subcutaneous fat

lipoprotein—a lipid-containing protein

local anesthesia—provision of a pain-free state in a specific area

local infiltration anesthesia—anesthesia produced by injecting a local anesthetic drug into tissues

low-density lipoproteins (LDL)—transport cholesterol to peripheral cells

lumen—the inside diameter of a vessel such as an artery

M

malignant hypertension—hypertension in which the diastolic pressure usually exceeds 130 mm Hg

megaloblastic anemia—a type of anemia that results from a deficiency of folic acid and certain other causes

mineralocorticoids—a hormone essential to life produced by the adrenal cortex

minerals—in terms of nutrition, are inorganic nutrients necessary to maintain health in the human body

miosis—the contraction of the pupil of the eye; pinpoint pupils

miotics—drugs used to help contract the pupil of the eye

mixed number—fractions preceded by a whole number

mucolytic—a drug that loosens respiratory secretions

musculoskeletal—the bone and muscular structure of the body

myasthenia gravis—a disease that causes fatigue of skeletal muscles because of the lack of acetylcholine released at the nerve endings of parasympathetic nerve fibers

Mycobacterium leprae—the bacteria that cause leprosy

Mycobacterium tuberculosis—the bacteria that cause tuberculosis

mycotic infection—a superficial or deep infection caused by a fungal disease in humans that may be yeast-like or mold-like

mydriasis—dilation of the pupil

mydriatics—drugs that dilate the pupil, constrict superficial blood vessels of the sclera, and decrease the formation of aqueous humor

myoclonic seizures—sudden, forceful contractions involving the musculature of the trunk, neck, and extremities

myxedema—a severe hypothyroidism manifested by a variety of symptoms

N

narcolepsy—disorder causing an uncontrollable desire to sleep during normal waking hours

nausea—an unpleasant gastric sensation usually preceding vomiting

nebulization—the dispersing of liquid medication in a mist of extremely fine particles to be inhaled into the deeper parts of the respiratory tract

necrotic—dead, as in dead tissue

nephron—long tubular structure that is the functional part of the kidney

neurogenic bladder—altered bladder function caused by a nervous system abnormality

neuroleptanalgesia—a state of general quietness achieved through a combination of analgesic and neuroleptic drugs

neuroleptic drugs—another term for antipsychotic drugs

neuroleptic malignant syndrome—a rare reaction to antipsychotic drugs characterized by a combination of extrapyramidal effects, hyperthermia, and autonomic disturbance

neurotransmitter—a chemical substance, also called a neurohormone, released at nerve endings to help transmit nerve impulses

nomogram—a chart that is made up of several lines marked off to scale and arranged so that by using a straightedge to connect known values on two lines an unknown value can be read at the point of intersection with another line; used to calculate body surface area using a patient's height and weight

nonpathogenic—not disease causing

nonprescription drugs—drugs designated by the Food and Drug Administration (FDA) to be obtained without a prescription

nonproductive cough—a dry, hacking cough that produces no secretions

normal flora—nonpathogenic microorganisms within or on the body

normal saline—solution containing 0.9% NaCl

nosocomial pneumonia—hospital-acquired pneumonia

numerator—the top portion of a fraction

nutritional supplements—substances such as herbs, vitamins, minerals, amino acids, and other natural substances; also referred to as dietary supplements

nystagmus—constant, involuntary movement of the eyeball

O

on–off phenomenon—associated with long-term levodopa treatment, a patient may alternate suddenly between improved clinical status and loss of therapeutic effect

onychomycosis—nail fungus condition

ophthalmic—eye

opioids—narcotic analgesics obtained from the opium plant

oral mucositis—inflammation of the oral mucous membranes

orthostatic hypotension—a feeling of light-headedness and dizziness after suddenly changing position, caused by a decrease in blood pressure when a person sits or stands; also referred to as postural hypotension

osteoarthritis—a noninflammatory joint disease resulting in degeneration of the articular cartilage and changes in the synovial membrane

otic—ear

oxytocic drugs—used before birth to induce uterine contractions similar to those of normal labor

oxytocin—an endogenous hormone produced by the posterior pituitary gland

P

pain—an unpleasant sensory and emotional experience associated with actual or potential tissue damage

pancytopenia—a decrease in all of the cellular components of the blood

paralytic ileus—lack of peristalsis or movement of the intestines

parasite—an organism that lives in or on another organism (the host) without contributing to the survival or well-being of the host

parasympathetic nervous system—a branch of the autonomic nervous system partly responsible for activities such as slowing the heart rate, digesting food, and eliminating body wastes

parenteral—a general term for drug administration in which the drug is injected inside the body

Parkinson disease—a degenerative disorder of the central nervous system; also known as paralysis agitans

Parkinsonism—refers to the symptoms of Parkinson disease, as well as Parkinson-like symptoms that may be seen with the use of certain drugs, head injuries, and encephalitis

partial agonist—a category of narcotic analgesic that binds to a receptor, but the response is limited (i.e., is not as great as with the agonist)

passive immunity—a type of immunity occurring from the administration of ready-made antibodies from another individual or animal

patency—being open or exposed

pathogen—any virus, microorganism, or other substance that causes disease

patient-controlled analgesia—a method of pain relief that allows patients to administer their own analgesic by means of an intravenous pump system

penicillinase—an enzyme that inactivates penicillin

percent—a portion of a whole divided into 100 parts, means "per 100"

peripheral nervous system—all nerves outside of the brain and spinal cord, connecting all parts of the body with the central nervous system

pernicious anemia—a type of megaloblastic anemia that results from a deficiency of intrinsic factor

pharmaceutic phase—the dissolution of the drug

pharmacodynamics—a drug's actions and effects within the body

pharmacogenetic disorder—a genetically determined abnormal response to normal doses of a drug

pharmacokinetics—activities occurring within the body after a drug is administered, including absorption, distribution, metabolism, and excretion; the body's effect on the drug

pharmacology—the study of drugs and their action on living organisms

photophobia—an intolerance to light

photosensitivity—exaggerated or abnormally heightened response to brief exposure to the sun, resulting in moderate to severe sunburn

physical dependence—a compulsive need to use a substance repeatedly to avoid mild to severe withdrawal symptoms

polarization—the point at which positive ions on the outside and negative ions on the inside of the cell membrane are in equilibrium

polydipsia—increased thirst

polyphagia—increased appetite

polypharmacy—the taking of numerous drugs that can potentially react with one another

polyuria—increased urination

positive inotropic action—the increased force of the contraction of the muscle (myocardium) of the heart through the use of cardiotonic drugs

postural hypotension—a feeling of light-headedness and dizziness after suddenly changing position, caused by a decrease in blood pressure when a person sits or stands; also referred to as orthostatic hypotension

preanesthetic drug—a drug given before the administration of anesthesia

prescription drugs—drugs the FDA has designated as potentially harmful unless supervised by a licensed health care provider

priapism—prolonged erection accompanied by pain and tenderness

proarrhythmic effect—the development of a new arrhythmia or the worsening of an existing arrhythmia caused by an antiarrhythmic drug produce a therapeutic response

productive cough—a cough that expels secretions from the lower respiratory tract

progesterone—female hormones influenced by the anterior pituitary gland

progestins—natural or synthetic substances that cause changes similar to those of progesterone

prophylaxis—prevention; a drug or treatment designed for prevention of a condition or symptom

proportion—two ratios that are equal to each other

protein substrates—amino acid preparations that act to promote the production of proteins and are essential to life

proteolysis—the process of hastening the reduction of proteins into simpler substances

prothrombin—a substance that is essential for the clotting of blood

proton pump inhibitors—drugs with antisecretory properties

pseudomembranous colitis—a common bacterial superinfection

psychological dependence—a compulsion to use a substance to obtain a pleasurable experience

psychomotor seizures—most often occur in children younger than 3 years of age through adolescence; may involve an aura with perceptual alterations, such as hallucinations or a strong sense of fear

psychotherapeutic drug—used to treat disorders of the mind

psychotic disorder—a disorder, such as schizophrenia, characterized by extreme personality disorganization and a loss of contact with reality

psychotropic drug—another term for psychotherapeutic drugs

purulent exudates—pus-containing fluid

R

ratio—a comparison of two amounts which represents a constant relationship between two values, may be written with a color or as a fraction

rebound—causing the opposite of the desired effect

receptor sites—specific protein-like macromolecules required for a drug's action at the cellular level

receptor—a specialized macromolecule that binds to the drug molecule, altering the function of the cell and producing the therapeutic response

reciprocal—the inverse of a fraction

refractory period—the period between transmissions of nerve impulses along a nerve fiber

regional anesthesia—anesthesia produced by injecting a local anesthetic around nerves to limit the pain signals sent to the brain

repolarization—the movement back to the original state of positive and negative ions after a stimulus passes along the nerve fiber; the positive ions are on the outside and the negative ions on the inside of the nerve cell

Reye syndrome—a rare, life-threatening condition that occurs in children and is characterized by vomiting and lethargy, progressing to coma

rhabdomyolysis—a rare condition in which muscle damage results in the release of muscle cell contents into the bloodstream

rheumatoid arthritis—a chronic disease characterized by inflammatory changes within the body's connective tissue

rhinitis—nasal congestion, often referred to as a stuffy nose

rhinitis medicamentosa—rebound nasal congestion caused by extended use of topical nasal decongestants

S

salicylates—drugs that have analgesic, antipyretic, and anti-inflammatory effects

salicylism—a condition produced by salicylate toxicity

secondary failure—a gradual increase in blood sugar levels that can be caused by an increase in the severity of diabetes or a decreased response to a drug

secondary hypertension—hypertension in which a direct cause can be identified

sedative—a drug that produces a relaxing, calming effect

seizure—a periodic attack of disturbed cerebral function

shock—a life-threatening condition occurring when the supply of arterial blood flow and oxygen to the cells and tissues is inadequate

somatic nervous system—branch of the peripheral nervous system that controls sensation and voluntary movement

somatotropic hormone—a growth hormone secreted by the anterior pituitary

spinal anesthesia—a type of regional anesthesia produced by injecting a local anesthetic drug into the subarachnoid space of the spinal cord

standard (universal) precautions—a set of actions, such as wearing gloves or using other protective gear, recommended by CDC for preventing contact with potentially infectious blood or body fluids

status epilepticus—an emergency situation characterized by continual seizure activity with no interruptions

Stevens–Johnson syndrome—serious allergic reaction to a drug, which initially exhibits reactions easily confused with less severe disorders

stomatitis—inflammation of the mouth

subcutaneous—route of administration in which the drug is injected just below the layer of skin

sublingual—route of administration in which the drug is placed under the tongue for absorption

substrate—a substance that is the basic component of an organism

superinfection—an overgrowth of bacterial or fungal microorganisms not affected by the antibiotic being used for treatment

sympathetic nervous system—branch of the autonomic nervous system that regulates the expenditure of energy and has key effects in stressful situations

sympathomimetics—drugs that mimic the activities or actions of the sympathetic nervous system

synergism—a drug interaction that occurs when drugs produce an effect that is greater than the sum of their separate actions

T

tardive dyskinesia—a syndrome consisting of potentially irreversible, involuntary dyskinetic movements

teratogen—any substance that causes abnormal development of the fetus

testosterone—the most potent naturally occurring androgen

theophyllinization—process of giving the patient a higher initial dose, called a loading dose, of a prescription drug to bring blood levels of theophylline to a therapeutic range more quickly

therapeutic response—the intended (beneficial) effect of a drug

thrombocytopenia—a decrease in the thrombocytes; a symptom of bone marrow suppression

thrombolytic drugs—drugs designed to dissolve blood clots that have already formed within a blood vessel

thrombosis—the formation of a clot

thrombus—blood clot

thyroid storm—a severe form of hyperthyroidism also known as thyrotoxicosis

thyrotoxicosis—a severe form of hyperthyroidism, also known as thyroid storm

thyroxine—a hormone manufactured and secreted by the thyroid gland

tinea corporis—ringworm

tinea cruris—jock itch

tinea pedis—athlete's foot

tinnitus—ringing sound in the ear

tolerance—patient condition in which increasingly larger dosages are required to obtain the desired effect

tonic–clonic seizure—an alternate contraction (tonic phase) and relaxation (clonic phase) of muscles, a loss of consciousness, and abnormal behavior

toxic—harmful drug effect

toxin—a poisonous substance produced by some bacteria

toxoid—a toxin that is weakened but still capable of stimulating the formation of antitoxins

transdermal system—a convenient form of drug administration in which the drug is impregnated in a pad and absorbed through the skin

transdermal—route of administration in which the drug is absorbed through the skin from a patch

transsacral block—type of regional anesthesia produced by injection of a local anesthetic into the epidural space at the level of the sacrococcygeal notch

trichomonas—a parasitic protozoan

triglycerides—a type of lipids in the blood

triiodothyronine—a hormone manufactured and secreted by the thyroid gland

tuberculosis—a disease caused by *Mycobacterium tuberculosis*

U

ulcerative colitis—chronic disease characterized by ulceration of the colon and rectum; symptoms include rectal bleeding, abdominal pain, and diarrhea

unit dose—a single dose of a drug packaged ready for patient use

urge incontinence—accidental loss of urine caused by a sudden and unstoppable need to urinate

urinary frequency—frequent urination day and night

urinary tract infection—an infection caused by pathogenic microorganisms of one or more structures of the urinary tract; commonly abbreviated as UTI

urinary urgency—sudden strong need to urinate

uterine atony—marked relaxation of the uterine muscle

V

vaccine—artificial active immunity created with killed or weakened antigens for the purpose of creating resistance to disease

vasoconstriction—a narrowing of the blood vessel

vasodilation—an increase in the size of blood vessels, primarily small arteries and arterioles

vasopressor—a drug that raises the blood pressure because it constricts blood vessels

vertigo—an abnormal feeling of spinning or rotation-type motion that may occur with motion sickness and other disorders

vesicant—an adverse drug reaction resulting in tissue necrosis, which is caused by the infiltration or extravasation of the drug out of a blood vessel and into soft tissue

vestibular neuritis—inflammation of the vestibular nerve to the inner ear

viral load—the blood level of HIV viral RNA; used for monitoring the course of AIDS

virilization—acquisition of male sexual characteristics by a woman

virus—infectious agent that lacks independent metabolism and cannot grow or reproduce without a living cell

vitamin—organic substance needed by the body in small amounts for normal growth and nutrition

volatile liquid—a liquid that evaporates on exposure to the air

vomiting—forceful expulsion of gastric contents through the mouth

W

water-soluble vitamins—vitamins that are rapidly metabolized and are readily excreted in the urine

withdrawal—a syndrome of physical and psychological symptoms caused by abruptly stopping use of a drug in a dependent patient

word factors—the units used in a mathematical term

X

xanthine derivatives—drugs that stimulate the central nervous system and result in bronchodilation

Z

Z-track—a technique of intramuscular injection used with drugs that are irritating to subcutaneous tissues

B

Answers to Fact Check Questions

CHAPTER 4: Central Nervous System Stimulants

4-1 The actions of caffeine on the CNS include the following: respiratory stimulation, cardiac stimulation, dilation of coronary and peripheral blood vessels, constriction of cerebral blood vessels, skeletal muscle stimulation, and mild diuresis.

4-2 Central nervous system stimulants are used to treat respiratory depression, narcolepsy, obesity, and attention deficit hyperactivity disorder.

4-3 Common adverse reactions of CNS stimulants include headache, dizziness, apprehension, disorientation, nervousness, excitement, hyperactivity, nausea, vomiting, urinary retention, palpitations, tachycardia, anorexia, loss of appetite, and weight loss.

4-4 Central nervous system stimulants are used with caution or not used at all in patients with a known hypersensitivity, severe hypertension, epilepsy or convulsive states, pneumothorax, acute bronchial asthma, head injury, stroke, hyperthyroidism, glaucoma, or cardiovascular disease. These drugs also are used with caution or not at all in newborns, early in pregnancy, or in patients taking a monoamine oxidase inhibitor, a tricyclic antidepressant, and guanethidine.

4-5 Because CNS stimulants cause insomnia, they should be taken early in the day so that the effects are gone by the time the patient is ready for bedtime.

CHAPTER 5: Anticonvulsants and Antiparkinsonism Drugs

5-1 Anticonvulsants work by reducing the excitability of the neurons in the brain.

5-2 When anticonvulsant therapy is initiated, the starting drug and dosage will not be the same for all patients with a particular type of seizure. Some patients respond well to one drug, while others do not. Some patients require a combination of anticonvulsants. Dosage increases and decreases are often necessary in the beginning and during times of stress, severe illness, and when the patient is taking other drugs.

5-3 The most common adverse reaction of anticonvulsants is sedation, which can range from drowsiness to somnolence.

5-4 The most common adverse reactions of phenytoin are nystagmus, ataxia, slurred speech, and mental changes.

5-5 Because many of the anticonvulsants cause drowsiness or sedation, they should be used with caution when combined with central nervous system (CNS) depressants. Examples of CNS depressants are narcotic analgesics, antidepressants, and alcohol.

5-6 Anticonvulsants and CNS depressants should be used with caution when combined because when two drugs that cause sedation or drowsiness are combined, the result is increased sedation, drowsiness, and CNS depression, which could lead to death.

5-7 Examples of activities that might need to be restricted when seizure therapy is being initiated and adjusted include the following: A mother with a newborn infant will need help when caring for the child; a carpenter should not climb ladders or use power tools; all patients should avoid driving or operating heavy machinery.

5-8 The classic symptoms that characterize Parkinson disease are fine tremors and rigidity of some muscle groups and weakness of others.

5-9 None of the current therapies on the market cure Parkinson disease; they only treat the signs and symptoms of the disease.

5-10 The gold standard drug therapy for Parkinson disease is levodopa.

5-11 Levodopa's most common adverse effects are choreiform movements and dystonic movements.

5-12 The "on–off phenomenon" is a condition in which a patient may suddenly alternate between improved clinical status and loss of therapeutic effect of levodopa.

5-13 The anticholinergics are used in patients with Parkinson disease to help control the drug-induced extrapyramidal symptoms.

5-14 Anticholinergics should be used with caution in the elderly because they have an increased sensitivity to anticholinergics and their adverse effects.

5-15 The COMT inhibitors work with levodopa to prolong levodopa's effect by increasing the plasma concentration and duration of action of levodopa.

5-16 Hepatic (liver) damage and possibly failure is the adverse reaction that is a concern for patients taking tolcapone.

5-17 The exact mechanism of action of dopamine receptor agonists is unknown, but these drugs are thought to mimic the effects of dopamine in the brain.

5-18 If a family member informs you that the patient is experiencing dry mouth, you could recommend sucking on hard candy, preferably sugar-free, and frequent sips of water.

5-19 If a family member notices that the patient seems to be having difficulty walking, you could recommend using assistive devices such as a cane or walker, wearing rubber sole shoes, getting rid of rugs and other obstacles that could cause the patient to stumble, or installing hand rails in the bathroom.

CHAPTER 6: Cholinesterase Inhibitors

6-1 Cholinesterase inhibitors are the class of drugs used to treat Alzheimer disease.

6-2 Acetylcholine is the natural chemical in the brain that is lower in patients with Alzheimer disease.

6-3 The effectiveness of cholinesterase inhibitors varies from individual to individual.

6-4 Donepezil is the cholinesterase inhibitor that is considered the drug of first choice because it has fewer and milder side effects.

6-5 The common adverse reactions of cholinesterase inhibitors are anorexia, nausea, vomiting, diarrhea, weight loss, abdominal pain, dizziness, and headache.

6-6 Tacrine is a cholinesterase inhibitor that may cause liver damage.

6-7 For a patient with Alzheimer disease, the following items will be assessed after diagnosis and during treatment: cognitive ability and functional ability, confusion, agitation, impulsive behavior, speech, ability to perform the activities of daily living, and self-care abilities.

6-8 Drug therapy for Alzheimer disease is considered successful if the progression of symptoms is slowed.

CHAPTER 7: Psychiatric Drugs

7-1 The difference between a sedative and a hypnotic is that a sedative produces a relaxing, calming effect and a hypnotic induces sleep.

7-2 The barbiturates are divided into the following groups: ultrashort-acting, which have a duration of 20 minutes or less; short-acting, which have a duration of 3 to 4 hours; intermediate-acting, which have a duration of 6 to 8 hours; and long-acting, which have a duration of 10 to 16 hours.

7-3 The barbiturates produce central nervous system (CNS) depression and mood alteration, ranging from mild excitation to mild sedation, hypnosis (sleep), or deep coma.

7-4 The patient can take zaleplon later in the night if at least 4 hours remain before the patient will become active again.

7-5 Older adults are at greater risk for oversedation, dizziness, confusion, or ataxia (unsteady gait) when taking a sedative or hypnotic.

7-6 A patient taking a sedative or hypnotic should be warned to not combine it with alcohol, antidepressants, narcotic analgesics, antihistamines, and phenothiazines.

7-7 A barbiturate or miscellaneous sedative and hypnotic should not be given approximately 2 hours before or after administration of a narcotic analgesic or other CNS depressant.

7-8 Melatonin is a hormone produced by the pineal gland in the brain, and it is used mainly for the short-term treatment of insomnia in low doses.

7-9 Long-term use of benzodiazepines is not recommended because prolonged therapy can result in drug dependence and serious withdrawal symptoms.

7-10 Some of these drugs have additional uses as sedatives, muscle relaxants, or anticonvulsants and in the treatment of alcohol withdrawal.

7-11 Buspirone (Buspar) is the least addictive antianxiety drug.

7-12 Buspirone, unlike most of the benzodiazepines, must be taken regularly and is not effective on an as-needed basis. It also seems to have less abuse potential and less effect on motor ability and cognition than other antianxiety drugs.

7-13 Depression is characterized by feelings of intense sadness, helplessness, worthlessness, and impaired functioning.

7-14 The four types of antidepressants are tricyclics, monoamine oxidase inhibitors, selective serotonin reuptake inhibitors, and miscellaneous.

7-15 The antidepressants are used to manage major depression, depression accompanied by anxiety, and obsessive–compulsive disorder.

7-16 Older men with prostatic enlargement are at increased risk for urinary retention when taking a tricyclic antidepressant.

7-17 Tricyclic antidepressants may be administered in a single daily dose at night because the sedative effects promote sleep and adverse reactions are less troublesome.

7-18 Monoamine oxidase inhibitors are not widely used because of their potential for serious adverse reactions.

7-19 St. John's wort is a natural remedy for depression.

7-20 A psychotic disorder is characterized by extreme personality disorganization and the loss of contact with reality. The patient usually has hallucinations (a false perception having no basis in reality) or delusions (false beliefs that cannot be changed with reason).

7-21 Lithium is used to treat the manic phase of bipolar disorder.

7-22 Before antipsychotic therapy is started, patients and family members should be informed about extrapyramidal effects, tardive dyskinesia, and neuroleptic malignant syndrome.

CHAPTER 8: Analgesics and Antagonists

8-1 Three types of pain are acute pain, chronic pain associated with malignant disease, and chronic pain not associated with malignant disease. Acute pain is of short duration and lasts less than 3 to 6 months. Chronic pain lasts longer than 6 months and ranges in intensity from mild to severe. Chronic pain associated with a malignancy includes the pain of cancer, acquired immunodeficiency syndrome (AIDS), multiple sclerosis, sickle cell disease, and end-stage organ system failure. A patient's exact cause of chronic pain of a nonmalignant nature may or may not be known.

8-2 Drugs used in the management of pain include nonnarcotic analgesics and narcotic analgesics. The nonnarcotic analgesics include salicylates, nonsalicylates, and the nonsteroidal anti-inflammatory drugs (NSAIDs).

8-3 The salicylates have analgesic, antipyretic, and anti-inflammatory effects.

8-4 Aspirin has greater anti-inflammatory effects than other salicylates. It also has a greater effect of inhibiting platelet aggregation

8-5 Salicylate nonnarcotic analgesics are used to relieve mild to moderate pain, reduce elevated body temperature, treat inflammatory conditions, reduce the risk of myocardial infarction (MI) in those with unstable angina or previous MI, and reduce the risk of transient ischemic attacks or strokes in men who have had transient ischemia of the brain caused by fibrin platelet emboli.

8-6 Salicylates should be taken with food to prevent GI upset.

8-7 Salicylates are not recommended for children with chickenpox or influenza due to the risk of Reye syndrome.

8-8 No, patients should not take salicylates for at least 1 week before any type of major surgery. They should not use salicylates after surgery until complete healing has occurred.

8-9 Acetaminophen is used to treat pain and fever. It is the drug of choice for treating fever and flu-like symptoms.

8-10 The daily dose of acetaminophen should not exceed 4 g.

8-11 The signs of acute acetaminophen toxicity are nausea, vomiting, confusion, liver tenderness, hypotension, arrhythmias, jaundice, and acute hepatic and renal failure.

8-12 Patients who are malnourished or abuse alcohol are at risk for hepatotoxicity with the use of acetaminophen.

8-13 Nonsteroidal anti-inflammatory drugs are used to treat signs and symptoms of OA, RA, and other musculoskeletal disorders; mild to moderate pain; primary dysmenorrhea; and pain.

8-14 Celecoxib has less potential for adverse gastrointestinal reactions because it is considered a COX-2 inhibitor and the others inhibit both COX-1 and COX-2.

8-15 Before taking an over-the-counter NSAID, a patient should be educated about the drug's indication (what the drug is used for), dosage information, possible interactions, possible adverse effects, and the need to read the label before taking.

8-16 Nonsteroidal anti-inflammatory drugs may be taken with food or milk to prevent GI upset.

8-17 Narcotic analgesics are used to treat moderate to severe pain.

8-18 Other uses of narcotic analgesics include the following: lessen anxiety and sedate a patient before surgery, anesthesia, obstetrical analgesia, lessen anxiety in patients with dyspnea, detoxification, sedation, diarrhea, and cough.

8-19 Methadone is an opioid that is used in the treatment and management of opiate dependence.

8-20 One of the major hazards of narcotic administration is respiratory depression.

8-21 Older adults are especially prone to adverse reactions of narcotic analgesics, particularly respiratory depression, somnolence (sedation), and confusion.

8-22 Patient-controlled analgesia allows patients to administer their own analgesic by means of an intravenous pump system. The dose and the time interval permitted between doses are programmed into the device to prevent accidental overdosage.

8-23 Naltrexone is used to treat opioid dependence.

8-24 Naloxone is used to reverse the effects of narcotic depression or diagnose a suspected acute opioid overdose.

CHAPTER 9: Anesthetic Drugs

9-1   Three uses of local anesthetics include topical, local infiltration, and regional applications.

9-2   Benzocaine is a topical local anesthetic that may cause a hypersensitivity reaction.

9-3   A patient would need a preanesthetic drug to decrease anxiety and apprehension and to decrease secretions of the upper respiratory tract.

9-4   There is concern about the use of preanesthetic drugs in the elderly because many of the medical disorders for which these drugs are contraindicated occur in the elderly. Also, the adverse reactions from preanesthetic drugs may be more pronounced in the elderly.

9-5   General anesthesia is a condition of a pain-free state for the entire body where the patient loses consciousness.

9-6   General anesthesia is usually administered by intravenous injection or inhalation.

CHAPTER 10: Antiemetic and Antivertigo Drugs

10-1   Antiemetics are used to treat nausea and vomiting.

10-2   Antivertigo drugs are used to treat vertigo which may occur with motion sickness, Ménière disease of the ear, middle or inner ear surgery, and other disorders.

10-3   Antiemetics and antivertigo drugs act in the chemoreceptor trigger zone or by depressing the sensitivity of the vestibular apparatus of the inner ear.

10-4   Drowsiness is the most common adverse reaction of the antiemetic and antivertigo drugs.

10-5   A patient who is taking an antiemetic or antivertigo drug that causes drowsiness should avoid any central nervous system depressant (such as sedatives, hypnotics, antianxiety drugs, opiates, and antidepressants) and alcohol.

10-6   Dehydration is a concern for patients experiencing prolonged vomiting, especially among the elderly and chronically ill, infants, and children.

CHAPTER 11: Adrenergic Drugs

11-1   The autonomic nervous system is divided into the sympathetic and parasympathetic nervous systems.

11-2   The neurotransmitters of the sympathetic nervous system are epinephrine and norepinephrine.

11-3   The clinical manifestations of shock include the following:

- Pallor, cyanosis, cold and clammy skin, sweating
- Agitation, confusion, disorientation, coma
- Hypotension, tachycardia, arrhythmias, wide pulse pressure, gallop rhythm
- Tachypnea, pulmonary edema
- Urinary output less than 20 mL per hour</bl>
- Acidosis

11-4   An adrenergic drug improves a patient's hemodynamic status because it improves myocardial contractility and increases heart rate, which increase cardiac output. Peripheral resistance is increased by vasoconstriction, making more blood available for vital organs.

11-5   The more common adverse reactions associated with adrenergic drugs are cardiac arrhythmia, headache, insomnia, nervousness, anorexia, and increased blood pressure.

11-6   An adrenergic drug helps with the management of shock because it causes vasoconstriction, which increases blood pressure.

CHAPTER 12: Adrenergic Blocking Drugs

12-1   Vasodilation is the effect of blocking an α-adrenergic receptor.

12-2   The common adverse reactions of α-adrenergic blockers are weakness, orthostatic hypotension, cardiac arrhythmias, hypotension, and tachycardia.

12-3   The effect of β-adrenergic blocking drugs is a decrease in heart rate and vasodilation.

12-4   Beta-adrenergic blocking drugs are used to treat hypertension, cardiac arrhythmias, migraines, and angina and for heart attack prevention.

12-5   The two types of antiadrenergic drugs are peripherally acting and centrally acting.

12-6   Antiadrenergic drugs are used to treat cardiac arrhythmias and hypertension.

12-7   The two α-/β-adrenergic blocking drugs are carvedilol and labetalol.

12-8   The two α-/β-adrenergic blocking drugs, carvedilol and labetalol, are used to treat hypertension; carvedilol is also used to reduce progression to congestive heart failure.

12-9   The first-dose effect is when the patient experiences marked hypotension and syncope with the first few doses of the drug. To decrease the effect, decrease the initial dose and give it at bedtime.

12-10   Patients who need to monitor their blood pressure must know the following to ensure that they are taking it properly: Use the same arm and body position each time; know that blood pressure can vary slightly with emotion, time and day, and position of the body; and be aware that slight changes in readings are normal.

CHAPTER 13: Cholinergic Drugs

13-1   Cholinergic drugs act like the neurohormone acetylcholine.

13-2   The major uses of cholinergic drugs are to treat glaucoma, myasthenia gravis, and urinary retention.

13-3   Myopia (near-sightedness) may be caused cholinergic eyedrops cause.

13-4   The symptoms of a cholinergic crisis are severe abdominal cramping, diarrhea, excessive salivation, muscle weakness, rigidity and spasm, and clenching of the jaw.

CHAPTER 14: Cholinergic Blocking Drugs (Anticholinergics)

14-1   Cholinergic blocking drugs inhibit the action of acetylcholine in parasympathetic nerve fibers.

14-2 Cholinergic blocking drugs have a variety of uses because they have widespread effects on many organs and structures.

14-3 The most common adverse reactions of cholinergic blocking drugs are dry mouth with difficulty in swallowing, blurred vision, photophobia, constipation, and drowsiness.

14-4 Recommendations for a patient who is experiencing dry mouth include good dental hygiene, frequent water, ice chips or frozen ices, and chewing gum.

CHAPTER 15: Bronchodilators and Antiasthma Drugs

15-1 Theophyllinization is the process of giving the patient a higher initial dose, called a loading dose, of a prescription drug to bring blood levels of theophylline to a therapeutic range more quickly.

15-2 Common adverse reactions of xanthine derivatives include nausea, vomiting, restlessness, nervousness, tachycardia, tremors, headache, palpitations, increased respirations, fever, hyperglycemia, and electrocardiographic changes.

15-3 Corticosteroids work to treat asthma by decreasing the inflammatory process in the airways, which keeps the airways open and allows the patient to breathe more easily.

15-4 A patient who is using both a bronchodilator and a corticosteroid inhaler should use the bronchodilator first to open the airways and allow the corticosteroid to work more effectively.

15-5 The leukotriene receptor antagonists inhibit the leukotriene receptor sites in the respiratory tract, preventing airway edema and facilitating bronchodilation. The leukotriene formation inhibitor decreases the formation of leukotrienes.

15-6 It may take from 2 to 4 weeks for a patient to experience a therapeutic response to cromolyn.

CHAPTER 16: Antihistamines and Decongestants

16-1 An antihistamine competes with histamine at the receptor site, preventing histamine from entering the receptor site and producing its effect on body tissues.

16-2 The first-generation antihistamines readily cross the blood–brain barrier and have more adverse reactions than the second-generation antihistamines.

16-3 The most common adverse reactions for first-generation antihistamines are drowsiness and sedation.

16-4 First-generation antihistamines should be used with caution in the elderly because these patients are more likely to experience the adverse reactions (anticholinergic effects, dizziness, sedation, hypotension, confusion).

16-5 A decongestant relieves the nasal symptoms of rhinitis or congestion.

16-6 A decongestant is administered for nasal decongestion either topically in the form of a spray or drop or orally.

16-7 If a patient overuses a topical nasal decongestant, rebound congestion occurs, which means the congestion gets worse instead of better.

16-8 The most common adverse reactions of oral decongestants are tachycardia and other cardiac arrhythmias, nervousness, restlessness, insomnia, blurred vision, nausea, and vomiting.

CHAPTER 17: Antitussives, Mucolytics, and Expectorants

17-1 An antitussive is appropriate for a nonproductive cough.

17-2 Three types of antitussives and examples of each are centrally acting (codeine, dextromethorphan), peripherally acting (benzonatate), and antihistamine (diphenhydramine).

17-3 When a patient is suffering from a productive cough, the following needs to be noted about the cough and the patient's condition: lung sound, amount of dyspnea (if any), and consistency and description of sputum.

17-4 The most commonly used expectorant is guaifenesin.

CHAPTER 18: Cardiotonics and Miscellaneous Inotropic Drugs

18-1 Left ventricular dysfunction leads to pulmonary symptoms such as dyspnea and moist cough. Right ventricular dysfunction leads to neck vein distention, peripheral edema, weight gain, and hepatic engorgement.

18-2 Left ventricular dysfunction is the most common form of heart failure.

18-3 Digoxin is the most commonly used cardiotonic drug.

18-4 Cardiotonic drugs act in the following two ways: (1) increase cardiac output through positive inotropic activity and (2) decrease the conduction velocity through the atrioventricular (AV) and sinoatrial (SA) nodes in the heart

18-5 Cardiac output is the amount of blood that leaves the left ventricle with each contraction

18-6 Signs of digitalis toxicity:

   i. Gastrointestinal: anorexia (usually the first sign), nausea, vomiting, diarrhea
   ii. Muscular: weakness
   iii. Central nervous system: headache, apathy, drowsiness, visual disturbances, mental depression, confusion, disorientation, delirium
   iv. Cardiac: changes in pulse rate or rhythm, electrocardiographic changes, other arrhythmias (abnormal heart rhythms).

18-7 Cardiotonics are contraindicated in patients with known hypersensitivity, ventricular failure, ventricular tachycardia, or AV block and in the presence of digitalis toxicity.

18-8 The main use of inamrinone is short-term management of HF in patients with no response to digitalis, diuretics, or vasodilators.

18-9 Patients taking digoxin need to have their renal function checked because decreased renal function can affect the dosage of digoxin.

18-10 Digitalization involves a series of doses of digoxin given until the drug begins to exert a full therapeutic effect.

18-11 Digoxin injections are usually used for rapid digitalization; digoxin tablets or capsules are used for maintenance therapy.

CHAPTER 19: Antiarrhythmic Drugs

19-1 Cardiac arrhythmia is a disturbance or irregularity in the heart rate or rhythm, or both.

19-2 The most common types of arrhythmias are atrial flutter, atrial fibrillation, premature ventricular contractions (PVCs), ventricular tachycardia (VT), and ventricular fibrillation.

19-3 Ventricular fibrillation will result in death if not treated immediately because the heart is unable to pump any blood to the body.

19-4 The classes and subclasses of antiarrhythmic drugs are Class I, II, III, and IV and Class I-A, I-B, and I-C.

19-5 Calcium channel blockers produce antiarrhythmic actions by inhibiting the movement of calcium through channels across the myocardial cell membranes and vascular smooth muscle.

19-6 Antiarrhythmic drugs are generally used to prevent and treat PVCs, VT, premature atrial contractions, paroxysmal atrial tachycardia, atrial fibrillation, and atrial flutter.

19-7 The proarrhythmic effect is the development of a new arrhythmia or the worsening of an existing arrhythmia caused by an antiarrhythmic drug.

19-8 Renal or hepatic dysfunction may warrant a dosage reduction of an antiarrhythmic drug.

19-9 Hypokalemia, hyperkalemia, or hypomagnesemia are electrolyte disturbances that may alter the effects of antiarrhythmic drugs.

19-10 The following changes in a patient's condition should be reported to the health care provider: change in blood pressure, pulse, or rhythm; respiratory difficulty; change in respiratory rate or rhythm; and alteration in the patient's general condition.

CHAPTER 20: Antianginal and Peripheral Vasodilating Drugs

20-1 Antianginal drugs relieve chest pain by dilating the coronary arteries and increasing blood supply to the myocardium.

20-2 Antianginal drugs include nitrates and calcium channel blockers.

20-3 Nitrates are used to treat angina pectoris, as prophylaxis and long-term treatment of angina, and to relieve the pain of acute angina attacks.

20-4 Common adverse reactions of nitrates are headache, hypotension, dizziness, vertigo, weakness, and flushing.

20-5 Increased hypotensive effects may occur when nitrates are administered with antihypertensives, alcohol, calcium channel blockers, and phenothiazines.

20-6 It is important for the person applying nitroglycerin ointment to avoid contact with the fingers or hands because the drug will be absorbed through his or her skin.

20-7 Calcium channel blockers inhibit the movement of calcium ions across cell membranes.

20-8 The primary use of calcium channel blockers is to prevent angina pain associated with certain forms of angina, such as vasospastic angina and chronic stable angina.

20-9 Peripheral vasodilating drugs act on the smooth muscle layers of peripheral blood vessels, primarily by blocking α-adrenergic nerves and stimulating β-adrenergic nerves.

20-10 The chief use of peripheral vasodilating drugs is treatment of arteriosclerosis obliterans, Raynaud phenomenon, and spastic peripheral vascular disorders.

CHAPTER 21: Antihypertensive Drugs

21-1 Normal blood pressure for adults is <120 mm Hg systolic and <80 mm Hg diastolic.

21-2 The different levels of hypertension are as follows:
   a. Prehypertension: 120 to 139 mm Hg systolic or 80 to 89 mm Hg diastolic
   b. Stage 1 hypertension: 140 to 159 mm Hg systolic or 90 to 99 mm Hg diastolic
   c. Stage 2 hypertension: ≥160 mm Hg systolic or ≥100 mm Hg diastolic

21-3 Essential hypertension is hypertension that has no known cause. Secondary hypertension is hypertension in which a direct cause can be identified.

21-4 Antihypertensive drugs that have vasodilating activity are adrenergic blocking drugs, antiadrenergic blocking drugs, calcium channel blocking drugs, and vasodilating drugs.

21-5 Postural or orthostatic hypotension is a common adverse reaction of antihypertensive drugs.

21-6 Rebound hypertension (rapid rise in BP) may occur if an antihypertensive drug is withdrawn abruptly.

21-7 Hyponatremia and hypokalemia are two electrolyte imbalances that may commonly occur during diuretic therapy.

21-8 When antihypertensive drugs are given with diuretics or other antihypertensives, the hypotensive effects are increased.

CHAPTER 22: Antihyperlipidemic Drugs

22-1 Atherosclerosis is a disorder in which lipid deposits accumulate on the lining of blood vessels, eventually producing degenerative changes and obstructing blood flow.

22-2 Desirable total cholesterol is <200 mg/dL; optimal LDL cholesterol is <100 mg/dL.

22-3 Bile sequestrants bind to bile acids to form an insoluble substance that cannot be absorbed by the intestine, so it is excreted in the feces.

22-4 HMG-CoA reductase inhibitors appear to inhibit the manufacture of cholesterol or promote the breakdown of it.

22-5 The fibric acid derivative drugs clofibrate, fenofibrate, and gemfibrozil may increase cholesterol excretion into the bile.

22-6 The combination of ezetimibe with an HMG-CoA reductase inhibitor is contraindicated in patients with active liver disease or unexplained persistent elevations in serum transaminases.

22-7 Niacin is used as adjunctive therapy for treatment of very-high-serum triglyceride levels in patients who have a risk of pancreatitis and who do not adequately respond to dietary control.

22-8 Following recommended dietary guidelines is essential because drug therapy alone cannot significantly lower cholesterol and triglyceride levels.

CHAPTER 23: Anticoagulant and Thrombolytic Drugs

23-1 A thrombosis is the formation of a blood clot.

23-2 Anticoagulants are used to prevent the formation and extension of a blood clot, while thrombolytics are used to dissolve blood clots that have already formed within a blood vessel.

23-3 Because warfarin can be administered orally, it is the drug of choice for long-term therapy.

23-4 Oral contraceptives, ascorbic acid, barbiturates, diuretics, and vitamin K decrease the effects of warfarin.

23-5 Symptoms of warfarin overdosage include melena, petechiae, oozing from superficial injuries, and excessive menstrual bleeding.

23-6 Heparin inhibits the formation of fibrin clots and the conversion of fibrinogen to fibrin. It also inactivates several factors necessary for blood clotting.

23-7 Adverse reactions of heparin administration include hemorrhage (chief complication), thrombocytopenia, local irritation when the drug is given by subcutaneous injection, and hypersensitivity reactions.

23-8 Low-molecular-weight heparins are contraindicated in patients with a hypersensitivity to the drug, to heparin, or to pork products, and in hospitalized patients with active bleeding or thrombocytopenia.

23-9 Thrombolytic drugs are used to treat acute MI by lysing (dissolving) a blood clot in a coronary artery.

23-10 Bleeding is the most common adverse reaction of thrombolytic drugs.

CHAPTER 24: Antianemia Drugs

24-1 Iron deficiency anemia is characterized by insufficient iron in the body to produce hemoglobin.

24-2 Iron preparations given orally may cause constipation, while IV administration of iron salts may result in phlebitis at the injection site and IM injections may result in brown discoloration of the skin.

24-3 Epoetin alfa and darbepoetin alfa are produced using recombinant DNA technology and are used to treat anemia associated with chronic renal failure.

24-4 Megaloblastic anemia is characterized by the presence of large, abnormal, immature RBCs circulating in the blood.

24-5 Folic acid and leucovorin are contraindicated for treatment of pernicious anemia or other anemias in which vitamin B_{12} is deficient.

24-6 Recommended nutritional advice for a patient with pernicious anemia: Eat a balanced diet that includes seafood, eggs, meats, and dairy products.

CHAPTER 25: Diuretics

25-1 Edema is retention of excess fluid that can be caused by heart failure, endocrine disorders, and kidney and liver diseases.

25-2 Diuretic drugs reduce edema by increasing urine secretion by the kidneys.

25-3 Carbonic anhydrase inhibitors are used to treat glaucoma as well as edema due to CHF, drug-induced edema, and centrencephalic epilepsy.

25-4 Loop diuretics increase sodium and chloride excretion by inhibiting reabsorption of these ions in the distal and proximal tubules and in the loop of Henle.

25-5 Intravenous administration of osmotic diuretics may result in rapid fluid and electrolyte imbalance, especially when these drugs are given before surgery to a patient in a fasting state.

25-6 Triamterene and amiloride depress sodium reabsorption in the tubules, increasing sodium and water excretion. Spironolactone blocks the action of aldosterone, causing sodium and water to be excreted.

25-7 Patients taking potassium-sparing diuretics are at risk for hyperkalemia. Symptoms include paresthesia, muscle weakness, fatigue, flaccid paralysis of the extremities, bradycardia, shock, and electrocardiographic abnormalities.

25-8 Thiazides and related diuretics are used in the treatment of hypertension, edema caused by chronic heart failure, hepatitis cirrhosis, corticosteroid and estrogen therapy, and renal dysfunction.

CHAPTER 26: Urinary Anti-Infectives

26-1 Symptoms of urinary tract infection of the bladder include urinary urgency, urinary frequency, dysuria, a feeling of incomplete voiding after urination, and pain caused by spasm in the region of the bladder and lower abdominal area.

26-2 A bacteriostatic drug slows or retards bacteria, while a bactericidal drug kills bacteria. Nitrofurantoin may be bacteriostatic or bactericidal, depending on the concentration of the drug in the urine.

26-3 Signs and symptoms of chronic pulmonary reactions that may occur with prolonged use of nitrofurantoin are dyspnea, nonproductive cough, and malaise.

26-4 Advise a patient taking urinary anti-infectives to drink extra fluids and to continue increased fluid intake even after symptoms subside. Extra fluid intake helps in the physical removal of bacteria from the urinary tract.

26-5 Cranberries inhibit bacteria from attaching to the walls of the urinary tract.

CHAPTER 27: Miscellaneous Urinary Drugs

27-1 Anticholinergics counteract smooth muscle spasm of the urinary tract by relaxing the bladder muscle through action at the parasympathetic receptors.

27-2 The most common adverse effects associated with anticholinergics are dry mouth and constipation

27-3 Phenazopyridine exerts a topical analgesic effect on the urinary tract lining.

27-4 Patients taking Ditropan XL should know that the outer coating of the tablet does not disintegrate and may be seen in the stool. This is normal and is not a cause for concern.

27-5 Phenazopyridine may mask the symptoms of a more serious disorder if taken for more than 2 days.

CHAPTER 28: Drugs That Affect the Stomach and Pancreas

28-1 Antacids neutralize or reduce the acidity of stomach and duodenal contents by combining with hydrochloric acid and producing salt and water.

28-2 Because antacids may interfere with the activity of other oral drugs, they should not be given within 2 hours before or after administration of other oral drugs.

28-3 Antiflatulents are used to relieve painful symptoms of excess gas in the digestive tract.

28-4 Cimetidine, famotidine, nizatidine, and ranitidine are histamine H_2 antagonists.

28-5 Cimetidine has more drug interactions than the other H_2 antagonists.

28-6 Proton pump inhibitors are especially used in the treatment of *Helicobacter pylori* in patients with active duodenal ulcers.

28-7 Anticholinergics reduce gastric motility and decrease the amount of acid secreted by the stomach.

28-8 Gastrointestinal stimulants are used to treat gastroesophageal reflux disease and gastric stasis, to prevent nausea and vomiting associated with cancer chemotherapy and postoperatively, and to reduce the risk of paralytic ileus after major abdominal surgery.

28-9 High or prolonged doses of metoclopramide may cause extrapyramidal reactions or tardive dyskinesia.

28-10 Pancrelipase is an enzyme that breaks down and helps digest fats, starches, and proteins in food.

28-11 Ipecac causes vomiting because of its irritating effect on the stomach and its stimulation of the medulla's vomiting center.

28-12 Misoprostol is contraindicated in patients who are allergic to prostaglandins and during pregnancy and lactation.

CHAPTER 29: Drugs That Affect the Gallbladder and Intestines

29-1 Diarrhea, cramps, nausea, and vomiting are the most common adverse drug reactions of gallstone-solubilizing drugs.

29-2 Hepatotoxicity may result with prolonged use of gallstone-solubilizing drugs.

29-3 Antidiarrheal drugs decrease intestinal peristalsis, which is usually increased in a patient with diarrhea.

29-4 Antidiarrheal drugs are contraindicated in patients whose diarrhea is associated with organisms that can harm the intestinal mucosa (*Escherichia coli, Salmonella, Shigella*) and in patients with pseudomembranous colitis, abdominal pain of unknown origin, or obstructive jaundice. They are also contraindicated in children younger than 2 years.

29-5 The various types of laxatives include bulk-producing laxatives, emollient laxatives, fecal softeners, hyperosmolar drugs, irritant or stimulant laxatives, and saline laxatives.

29-6 Laxatives may reduce the absorption of other drugs present in the gastrointestinal tract by combining with them chemically or hastening their passage through the intestinal tract.

29-7 Bowel evacuants are used to treat constipation and to cleanse the bowel prior to a GI exam.

29-8 Drugs used to treat ulcerative colitis are olsalazine, sulfasalazine, balsalazide, and infliximab.

29-9 Mesalamine is used in the treatment of chronic inflammatory bowel disease.

29-10 Orlistat prevents the absorption of fat-soluble vitamins A, D, E, and K.

CHAPTER 30: Antidiabetic Drugs

30-1 Diabetes mellitus is a chronic disorder characterized by either insufficient insulin production by the pancreas or by cellular resistance to insulin.

30-2 Insulin helps the body to properly use glucose.

30-3 Insulin preparations are classified as rapid-acting, short-acting, intermediate-acting, or long-acting.

30-4 Hypoglycemia (low blood glucose) and hyperglycemia (elevated blue glucose) are the major adverse reactions of insulin administration.

30-5 A patient experiencing a hypoglycemic reaction could take one or more of the following actions: Drink orange juice or other fruit juice, suck on hard candy, eat honey, take a commercial glucose product, or use a glucagon product. Glucagon and glucose can also be given intravenously by a trained health care professional.

30-6 Diabetic ketoacidosis is a potentially life-threatening deficiency of insulin.

30-7 Site rotation is necessary to prevent injury to the skin and fatty tissue.

30-8 Types of antidiabetic drugs are sulfonylureas, biguanides, α-glucosidase inhibitors, meglitinides, thiazolidinediones, amylin analogs, dipeptidyl peptidase-4 inhibitors, and glucagon-like peptide 1 receptor agonists.

30-9 Sulfonylureas and meglitinides lower blood glucose by stimulating the pancreas to release insulin.

30-10 Dipeptidyl peptidase-4 inhibitors prevent the breakdown of incretin. Glucagon-like peptide 1 receptor agonists act on the same receptor as natural incretin.

30-11 Lactic acidosis, a buildup of lactic acid in the blood, can occur with metformin use.

30-12 The most common adverse reactions associated with the alpha-glucosidase inhibitors are bloating and flatulence.

30-13 Secondary failure is a gradual increase in blood glucose levels that can be caused by an increase in the severity of diabetes or a decreased response to the drug.

30-14 The glucagon-like peptide 1 receptor agonists are administered subcutaneously.

CHAPTER 31: Pituitary and Adrenocortical Hormones

31-1 Follicle-stimulating hormone, luteinizing hormone, growth hormone, adrenocorticotropic hormone, thyroid-stimulating hormone, and prolactin are secreted by the anterior pituitary gland.

31-2 Follicle-stimulating hormone and luteinizing hormone are called gonadotropins.

31-3 Follicle-stimulating hormone and luteinizing hormone influence the gonads or the reproductive organs.

31-4 Growth hormone therapy in children must occur before closure of the bone epiphyses. Once bone epiphyses close, growth in height can no longer occur.

31-5 Corticotropin (ACTH) has adverse effects similar to glucocorticoids because it stimulates the adrenal cortex to secrete glucocorticoids.

31-6 Vasopressin is produced in the posterior pituitary gland.

31-7 Vasopressin regulates the reabsorption of water by the kidneys.

31-8 Symptoms of water intoxication are drowsiness, listlessness, confusion, and headache.

31-9 The adrenal cortex lies on the superior surface of each kidney.

31-10 Glucocorticoids and mineralocorticoids are produced by the adrenal cortex.

31-11 Adrenal insufficiency is a critical lack of glucocorticoids and mineralocorticoids that requires immediate treatment.

31-12 Glucocorticoids are contraindicated in patients with infections such as tuberculosis and fungal and antibiotic-resistant infections.

31-13 Signs and symptoms of a cushingoid state include "buffalo" hump, moon face, oily skin and acne, osteoporosis, purple striae of the abdomen and hips, skin pigmentation, and weight gain.

31-14 Mineralocorticoid deficiency results in loss of sodium and water and retention of potassium.

CHAPTER 32: Thyroid and Antithyroid Drugs

32-1 The thyroid gland secretes thyroxine and triiodothyronine.

32-2 Hypothyroidism and hyperthyroidism are the two most common thyroid disorders.

32-3 Levothyroxine is the drug of choice for hypothyroidism.

32-4 Antithyroid drugs and iodine products are used to treat hyperthyroidism.

32-5 Agranulocytosis, a decrease in the number of WBCs, is a serious adverse reaction to methimazole.

32-6 Strong iodide is measured in drops, which are added to water or fruit juice. This drug has a strong, salty taste. The patient is allowed to experiment with various types of fruit juices to determine which one best disguises the taste of the drug. Iodine solutions should be drunk through a straw because they may cause tooth discoloration.

CHAPTER 33: Male and Female Hormones and Drugs for Erectile Dysfunction

33-1 Male hormones are androgens, anabolic steroids, and androgen hormone inhibitors.

33-2 In males, androgen therapy is used for testosterone deficiency. In postmenopausal women, it is used for inoperable metastatic breast carcinoma; in premenopausal women, for hormone-dependent breast carcinoma.

33-3 Adverse reactions of anabolic steroids include virilization (in women), acne, nausea, vomiting, diarrhea, fluid and electrolyte imbalances, testicular atrophy, jaundice, anorexia, and muscle cramps.

33-4 Androgens and anabolic steroids are contraindicated in patients with a known hypersensitivity, liver disorders, or serious cardiac disease and in men with prostate gland disorders.

33-5 The PDE5 inhibitors cause smooth muscle relaxation in the penis which allows for increased blood flow to the area resulting in an erection.

33-6 It is administered by either injection or urogenital insertion.

33-7 Estrogens and progesterone are the endogenous female hormones.

33-8 Estrogens are most commonly used as contraceptives (in combination with progestins) and as hormone replacement therapy in postmenopausal women. Progestins are used to treat amenorrhea, endometriosis, and uterine bleeding; they are also used alone or combined with an estrogen as oral contraceptives.

33-9 A history of thrombophlebitis or other vascular disorders, smoking history, and a history of liver diseases must be included for patients prescribed an estrogen.

33-10 Levonorgestrel is available as two 0.75 mg tablets under the trade names Next Choice and Plan B. These products are taken one tablet within 72 hours of unprotected intercourse, with the second tablet 12 hours after the first tablet. Levonorgestrel is also available as a single 0.15 mg tablet under the trade name Plan B One Step. It is to be taken one dose within 72 hours of unprotected intercourse.

CHAPTER 34: Uterine Drugs

34-1 Oxytocin is used to start or improve uterine contractions, manage incomplete abortion, control postpartum bleeding and hemorrhage, and stimulate milk letdown reflex.

34-2 Ergonovine and methylergonovine are used to prevent hemorrhage caused by uterine atony.

34-3 Carboprost, dinoprostone, and mifepristone are all used to terminate a pregnancy.

34-4 Water intoxication may occur with IV oxytocin administration because of the drug's antidiuretic effect.

34-5 Ergotism is an overdose of ergonovine. It is manifested by chest pain, muscle cramps or pain, weakness, numbness or tingling of the extremities, and an increased blood pressure.

34-6 Heavy and prolonged bleeding after use of mifepristone does not signify that an abortion has occurred.

34-7 In the event of a treatment failure with mifepristone, fetal malformation may result, and a surgical termination of pregnancy may be necessary.

CHAPTER 35: Antibacterial Drugs

35-1 Sulfonamides that are found in combination products are used to treat otitis media.

35-2 Mafenide and silver sulfadiazine are sulfonamides that are used to treat partial thickness and full thickness burns.

35-3 The following hematologic changes may occur during sulfonamide therapy: agranulocytosis, thrombocytopenia, aplastic anemia, and leukopenia.

35-4 Stevens–Johnson syndrome is manifested by fever, cough, muscular aches and pains, and headache. The appearance of lesions on the skin, mucous membranes, eyes, and other organs are diagnostically significant and may be the first conclusive signs of this syndrome.

35-5 Crystalluria is crystals in the urine. It can be prevented by drinking a lot of water, approximately 2,000 mL per day, during sulfonamide therapy.

35-6 Sulfonamides are usually taken on an empty stomach, 1 hour before or 2 hours after meals.

35-7 Examples of bacteria that may respond to penicillin therapy include gonococci, staphylococci, streptococci, and pneumococci.

35-8 Penicillins are used to treat infectious disease and as prophylaxis against potential secondary bacterial infections in patients with viral infections.

35-9 Pseudomembranous colitis and candidiasis are two common superinfections.

35-10 Signs and symptoms of *Clostridium difficile* include severe diarrhea with visible blood and mucus, fever, and abdominal cramps.

35-11 Penicillins may also be contraindicated in patients who are allergic to cephalosporins.

35-12 A woman taking an oral contraceptive containing estrogen should be told prior to starting penicillin therapy that the medication may interfere with the birth control pill making it less effective. An alternate form of birth control should be used while on the penicillin and until a new pack is started.

35-13 Progression from the first-generation cephalosporins to the second-generation and then to the third-generation drugs shows an increase in the sensitivity of gram-negative microorganisms and a decrease in the sensitivity of gram-positive microorganisms.

35-14 Cephalosporins make the bacteria cell wall defective and unstable.

35-15 Serious hypersensitivity reactions to cephalosporins include Stevens–Johnson syndrome, liver or kidney dysfunction, aplastic anemia, and epidermal necrolysis.

35-16 Cephalosporins and other anti-infectives are taken around the clock to provide adequate blood levels.

35-17 Tetracyclines inhibit bacterial protein synthesis, which ultimately either destroys the bacteria or slows their multiplication rate.

35-18 Lincosamides usually are used only for the treatment of serious infections in which penicillin or erythromycin (a macrolide) is not effective because of their high potential for toxicity.

35-19 Tetracyclines are not given to children under age 9 unless their use is absolutely necessary because these drugs may cause permanent yellow–gray–brown discoloration of the teeth.

35-20 The most frequent adverse reactions of macrolides are GI symptoms, including nausea, vomiting, diarrhea, and abdominal pain.

35-21 Fluoroquinolones interfere with an enzyme that is needed by bacteria for DNA synthesis.

35-22 Three serious adverse reactions of aminoglycosides are nephrotoxicity, ototoxicity, and neurotoxicity.

CHAPTER 36: Antimycobacterial Drugs

36-1 Antitubercular drugs are used to treat active tuberculosis and as prophylaxis against the disease.

36-2 Isoniazid is the only antitubercular drug to be prescribed alone.

36-3 Optic neuritis is a possible adverse reaction in patients receiving ethambutol.

36-4 Older adults are particularly susceptible to a potentially fatal hepatitis when taking isoniazid, especially if they consume alcohol on a regular basis. Two other antitubercular drugs, rifampin and pyrazinamide, can cause liver dysfunction in older adults.

36-5 For patients taking antitubercular drugs, directly observed therapy requires the patient to visit the health care provider's office and to be observed swallowing each medication dose by a health care worker.

36-6 Rifampin is an antitubercular agent that may cause a red–brown or red–orange discoloration of tears, sputum, urine, or sweat.

36-7 Dapsone is currently the only drug available to treat leprosy.

36-8 Substantial amounts of dapsone are excreted in breast milk and can cause hemolytic reactions in neonates, so it is contraindicated during lactation.

CHAPTER 37: Antiviral, Antiretroviral, and Antifungal Drugs

37-1 The herpes viruses that are treated with antivirals include herpes simplex (types 1 and 2), herpes zoster, and herpes varicella.

37-2 Most antiviral drugs act by inhibiting viral DNA or RNA replication in the virus, causing viral death.

37-3 Antiviral drugs used systemically may be administered orally or intravenously.

37-4 Crystalluria may occur with rapid IV administration of antiviral drugs.

37-5 All antiviral drugs are contraindicated in patients with previous hypersensitivity as well as in patients with congestive heart failure, seizures, or renal disease and during lactation.

37-6 When an antiviral drug is applied topically, gloves are used to avoid spreading the infection.

37-7 The antiretrovirals fall into one of six categories: cellular chemokine receptor antagonists, fusion inhibitors, integrase inhibitors, nonnucleoside reverse transcriptase inhibitors, nucleoside/nucleotide analog reverse transcriptase inhibitors, and protease inhibitors.

37-8 The goal of antiretroviral therapy is to decrease morbidity and mortality associated with HIV by preventing viral replication.

37-9 Fungicidal drugs can destroy fungi, and fungistatic drugs slow or retard the multiplication of fungi.

37-10 Amphotericin B is the most effective drug available for treating most systemic fungal infections. Kidney damage is its most serious adverse reaction.

37-11 Warfarin's anticoagulant effects may be decreased when given with griseofulvin. Warfarin's anticoagulant effects are increased when given with either itraconazole or ketoconazole.

37-12 The patient and family should be helped to understand that therapy must be continued until the infection is under control, which may take weeks or months.

CHAPTER 38: Antiparasitic Drugs

38-1 A parasite is an organism that lives in or on another organism (the host) without contributing to the survival or well-being of the host.

38-2 Roundworms, pinworms, whipworms, hookworms, and tapeworms are examples of helminths.

38-3 Albendazole and mebendazole have caused embryotoxic and teratogenic effects in animals.

38-4 Antimalarial drugs interfere with the lifecycle of the plasmodium, primarily when it is present in red blood cells.

38-5 Suppression prevents malaria from occurring, while treatment is the management of the malarial attack after infection has occurred.

38-6 Quinine use may result in cinchonism, hematologic changes, vertigo, and skin rash.

38-7 Iodoquinol, metronidazole, and paromomycin are used to treat intestinal amebiasis.

38-8 Chloroquine is used to treat extraintestinal amebiasis.

CHAPTER 39: Miscellaneous Anti-Infectives

39-1 Linezolid is used to treat nosocomial and community-acquired pneumonia.

39-2 Vancomycin acts against gram-positive bacteria by inhibiting bacterial cell wall synthesis and increasing cell wall permeability.

39-3 Blood dyscrasias are the chief adverse reaction that may occur with chloramphenicol use.

39-4 Meropenem can cause an abscess or phlebitis at the injection site.

39-5 Metronidazole should not be combined with alcohol because a disulfiram-like reaction may occur.

39-6 Patients receiving metronidazole for gynecologic infections should be told that sexual contact with infected partners may lead to reinfection, so sexual partners must also receive treatment.

CHAPTER 40: Immunologic Agents

40-1 The antigen–antibody response is a reaction that occurs when specific antibodies are formed in response to specific antigens.

40-2 An attenuated antigen is one that is weakened, not killed, for use in a vaccine.

40-3 Some antibodies have a short life, so booster injections may be needed to maintain sufficient immunity.

40-4 A toxin is a poisonous substance that is produced by some bacteria. Antitoxins are produced by the body in response to exposure to toxins and act similarly to antibodies.

40-5 Globulins are proteins that are found in blood serum or plasma that contain antibodies.

40-6 Because of the potential for hypersensitivity reactions, patients receiving immunologic agents may be observed for 30 minutes after administration of an immunologic agent.

CHAPTER 41: Antineoplastic Drugs

41-1 Antineoplastic drugs generally affect cells that divide and reproduce rapidly, which include cancer cells and some types of normal cells.

41-2 Types of antineoplastic drugs are alkylating drugs, antibiotics, antimetabolites, hormones, and mitotic inhibitors.

41-3 Common adverse reactions to antineoplastic drugs include bone marrow suppression, nausea, vomiting, stomatitis, diarrhea, and hair loss.

41-4 Antineoplastic drugs are used cautiously in patients with renal or hepatic impairment, active infection, or other debilitating illnesses or in those who have recently completed treatment with other antineoplastic drugs or radiation therapy.

41-5 A patient would likely have a complete blood count and liver function tests to determine if the drug is suppressing the bone marrow and to detect liver toxicity, both of which are common adverse reactions.

CHAPTER 42: Musculoskeletal System Drugs

42-1 Bisphosphonates act primarily on the bone by inhibiting normal and abnormal bone resorption, thus increasing bone mineral density and reversing the progression of osteoporosis.

42-2 Skeletal muscle relaxants are used with caution in patients with a history of cerebrovascular accident, cerebral palsy, Parkinsonism, or seizure disorders and during pregnancy and lactation.

42-3 Corticosteroids may be used to treat rheumatic disorders such as ankylosing spondylitis, rheumatoid arthritis, gout, bursitis, and osteoarthritis.

42-4 Allopurinol reduces uric acid production, colchicine reduces inflammation associated with the urate crystal deposits in the joints, and probenecid increases the excretion of uric acid by the kidneys.

42-5 Gold compounds are used to treat active juvenile and adult rheumatoid arthritis that are not controlled by other anti-inflammatory drugs.

42-6 Methotrexate is a pregnancy category X drug and may cause birth defects in a developing fetus. It is contraindicated during pregnancy.

CHAPTER 43: Integumentary System Topical Drugs

43-1 Topical anti-infectives include antibiotic, antifungal, and antiviral drugs.

43-2 Povidone–iodine is used instead of iodine solution or tincture because it is less irritating to the skin and areas treated with this drug may be bandaged or taped.

43-3 Topical corticosteroids are used to treat psoriasis, dermatitis, rashes, eczema, insect bite reactions, and burns.

43-4 Antipsoriatics may cause burning, itching, and skin irritation

43-5 Topical enzymes speed up proteolysis, which is the process by which proteins are reduced into simpler substances.

43-6 Keratolytics remove excess growth of the epidermis.

43-7 Topical anesthetics are used cautiously in patients receiving class I antiarrhythmic drugs.

CHAPTER 44: Otic and Ophthalmic Preparations

44-1 The three categories of drugs used to treat otic disorders are antibiotics, antibiotic and steroid combinations, and miscellaneous preparations.

44-2 Otic preparations are used to relieve pain, treat infection and inflammation, and to help remove earwax and water.

44-3 Intraocular pressure is the pressure within the eye. Glaucoma increases IOP and requires medication to lower it.

44-4 After instilling brimonidine, patients should wait at least 15 minutes before inserting soft contact lenses because the lenses may absorb the preservative in the drug.

44-5 Sympathomimetics lower IOP by increasing the outflow of aqueous humor in the eye.

44-6 Beta-adrenergic blocking drugs lower IOP by decreasing the rate of production of aqueous humor.

44-7 Common adverse reactions of direct acting miotics include stinging on instillation, burning, tearing, headache, brow ache, and decreased night vision.

44-8 Cholinesterase inhibitor miotics are used to treat open-angle glaucoma.

44-9 Carbonic anhydrase inhibitors block the enzyme carbonic anhydrase in the eye, which decreases aqueous humor secretion and thus decreases IOP.

44-10 Cycloplegia is paralysis of the ciliary muscle of the eye.

44-11 Antihistamines and mast cell stabilizers are used to treat the signs and symptoms of allergic conjunctivitis (excessive watering or tearing and itching) as well as ocular pruritus.

44-12 Antibiotics are used to treat eye infections.

44-13 Elevated IOP and optic nerve damage may occur with prolonged use of ophthalmic corticosteroids.

44-14 Diclofenac is used for inflammation after cataract surgery.

CHAPTER 45: Fluids, Electrolytes, and Total Parenteral Nutrition

45-1 Blood plasma is the liquid part of blood.

45-2 Plasma protein fractions are used to treat hypovolemic shock and hypoproteinemia.

45-3 Amino acids help with protein production, tissue repair, and wound healing and reduce the rate of protein breakdown.

45-4 Dextrose solutions and fat emulsion are energy substrates.

45-5 Hetastarch, low-molecular-weight dextran, and high-molecular-weight dextran are plasma expanders.

45-6 Sodium bicarbonate is given IV to treat metabolic acidosis.

45-7 Low blood calcium is called hypocalcemia.

45-8 Magnesium helps with nerve impulse transmission and with enzyme activity.

45-9 Hypokalemia is low blood potassium.

45-10 Normal saline solution contains 0.9% sodium chloride, while half-normal saline solution contains 0.45% sodium chloride.

45-11 Total parenteral nutrition may be administered through a peripheral vein or through a central venous catheter

CHAPTER 46: Complementary and Alternative Medicine

46-1 The Federal Food, Drug, and Cosmetic Act defines the following terms: cosmetics, devices, dietary supplements, drugs, foods, and food additives. CAM products that fall into these categories may be regulated under this act.

46-2 Biological products can include botanicals, animal-derived extracts, vitamins, minerals, fatty acids, amino acids, proteins, prebiotics and probiotics, whole diets, and functional foods.

46-3 The Food and Drug Administration is responsible for monitoring the safety of dietary supplements after they are marketed to the public.

46-4 The fat-soluble vitamins include vitamin A, D, E, and K.

46-5 Fat-soluble vitamins are generally metabolized slowly and are stored in the liver.

46-6 Water-soluble vitamins include all of the B vitamins and vitamin C.

46-7 Water-soluble vitamins are rapidly metabolized and are readily excreted in the urine.

46-8 Niacin (B_3) has been shown to lower LDL cholesterol.

46-9 Potassium is important for the heart to function properly. Too much potassium will cause the heart to stop.

46-10 Iron is essential for making hemoglobin and myoglobin

46-11 *Ginkgo biloba* is used to improve symptoms associated with reduced blood flow to the brain, including short-term memory loss and dizziness. It is also a frequent treatment for ringing in ears, headache, depression, erectile dysfunction, and anxiety. The potential adverse effects of regular use of ginkgo include mild gastrointestinal upset, headache, rash, muscle spasms, cramps, and bleeding. Large doses reportedly cause diarrhea, nausea, vomiting, and restlessness.

46-12 Ginseng is used for improving energy and mental performance. Ginseng is contraindicated in individuals with high blood pressure and during pregnancy.

C

Vaccine Adverse Event Reporting System Form

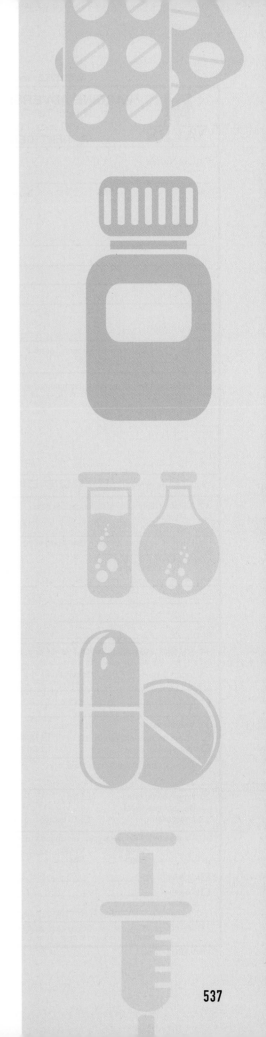

WEBSITE: www.vaers.hhs.gov   E-MAIL: info@vaers.org   FAX: 1-877-721-0366

VACCINE ADVERSE EVENT REPORTING SYSTEM
24 Hour Toll-Free Information 1-800-822-7967
P.O. Box 1100, Rockville, MD 20849-1100
PATIENT IDENTITY KEPT CONFIDENTIAL

VAERS

For CDC/FDA Use Only

VAERS Number _____

Date Received _____

Patient Name:	Vaccine administered by (Name):	Form completed by (Name):
Last First M.I.	Responsible Physician _____ Facility Name/Address	Relation ☐ Vaccine Provider ☐ Patient/Parent to Patient ☐ Manufacturer ☐ Other
Address		Address *(if different from patient or provider)*
City State Zip	City State Zip	City State Zip
Telephone no. (___) _____	Telephone no. (___) _____	Telephone no. (___) _____

1. State	2. County where administered	3. Date of birth ___/___/___ mm dd yy	4. Patient age	5. Sex ☐ M ☐ F	6. Date form completed ___/___/___ mm dd yy

7. Describe adverse events(s) (symptoms, signs, time course) and treatment, if any	8. Check all appropriate:
	☐ Patient died (date ___/___/___ mm dd yy) ☐ Life threatening illness ☐ Required emergency room/doctor visit ☐ Required hospitalization (_____ days) ☐ Resulted in prolongation of hospitalization ☐ Resulted in permanent disability ☐ None of the above

9. Patient recovered ☐ YES ☐ NO ☐ UNKNOWN	10. Date of vaccination ___/___/___ mm dd yy AM Time _____ PM	11. Adverse event onset ___/___/___ mm dd yy AM Time _____ PM
12. Relevant diagnostic tests/laboratory data		

13. Enter all vaccines given on date listed in no. 10

	Vaccine (type)	Manufacturer	Lot number	Route/Site	No. Previous Doses
a.					
b.					
c.					
d.					

14. Any other vaccinations within 4 weeks prior to the date listed in no. 10

	Vaccine (type)	Manufacturer	Lot number	Route/Site	No. Previous doses	Date given
a.						
b.						

15. Vaccinated at: ☐ Private doctor's office/hospital ☐ Military clinic/hospital ☐ Public health clinic/hospital ☐ Other/unknown	16. Vaccine purchased with: ☐ Private funds ☐ Military funds ☐ Public funds ☐ Other/unknown	17. Other medications

18. Illness at time of vaccination (specify)	19. Pre-existing physician-diagnosed allergies, birth defects, medical conditions (specify)

20. Have you reported this adverse event previously?	☐ No ☐ To health department ☐ To doctor ☐ To manufacturer	*Only for children 5 and under*
		22. Birth weight _____ lb. _____ oz.	23. No. of brothers and sisters

21. Adverse event following prior vaccination (check all applicable, specify)

	Adverse Event	Onset Age	Type Vaccine	Dose no. in series	*Only for reports submitted by manufacturer/immunization project*
☐ In patient					24. Mfr./imm. proj. report no. 25. Date received by mfr./imm.proj.
☐ In brother or sister					26. 15 day report? ☐ Yes ☐ No 27. Report type ☐ Initial ☐ Follow-Up

Health care providers and manufacturers are required by law (42 USC 300aa-25) to report reactions to vaccines listed in the Table of Reportable Events Following Immunization. Reports for reactions to other vaccines are voluntary except when required as a condition of immunization grant awards.

Form VAERS-1 (FDA)

"Fold in thirds, tape & mail — DO NOT STAPLE FORM"

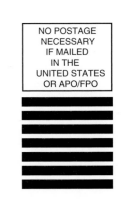

BUSINESS REPLY MAIL
FIRST-CLASS MAIL   PERMIT NO. 1895   ROCKVILLE, MD

POSTAGE WILL BE PAID BY ADDRESSEE

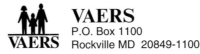 **VAERS**
P.O. Box 1100
Rockville MD 20849-1100

DIRECTIONS FOR COMPLETING FORM
(Additional pages may be attached if more space is needed.)

GENERAL

- Use a separate form for each patient. Complete the form to the best of your abilities. Items 3, 4, 7, 8, 10, 11, and 13 are considered essential and should be completed whenever possible. Parents/Guardians may need to consult the facility where the vaccine was administered for some of the information (such as manufacturer, lot number or laboratory data.)
- Refer to the Reportable Events Table (RET) for events mandated for reporting by law. Reporting for other serious events felt to be related but not on the RET is encouraged.
- Health care providers other than the vaccine administrator (VA) treating a patient for a suspected adverse event should notify the VA and provide the information about the adverse event to allow the VA to complete the form to meet the VA's legal responsibility.
- These data will be used to increase understanding of adverse events following vaccination and will become part of CDC Privacy Act System 09-20-0136, "Epidemiologic Studies and Surveillance of Disease Problems". Information identifying the person who received the vaccine or that person's legal representative will not be made available to the public, but may be available to the vaccinee or legal representative.
- Postage will be paid by addressee. Forms may be photocopied (must be front & back on same sheet).

SPECIFIC INSTRUCTIONS

Form Completed By: To be used by parents/guardians, vaccine manufacturers/distributors, vaccine administrators, and/or the person completing the form on behalf of the patient or the health professional who administered the vaccine.

Item 7:   Describe the suspected adverse event. Such things as temperature, local and general signs and symptoms, time course, duration of symptoms, diagnosis, treatment and recovery should be noted.

Item 9:   Check "YES" if the patient's health condition is the same as it was prior to the vaccine, "NO" if the patient has not returned to the pre-vaccination state of health, or "UNKNOWN" if the patient's condition is not known.

Item 10:   Give dates and times as specifically as you can remember. If you do not know the exact time, please
and 11:   indicate "AM" or "PM" when possible if this information is known. If more than one adverse event, give the onset date and time for the most serious event.

Item 12:   Include "negative" or "normal" results of any relevant tests performed as well as abnormal findings.

Item 13:   List ONLY those vaccines given on the day listed in Item 10.

Item 14:   List any other vaccines that the patient received within 4 weeks prior to the date listed in Item 10.

Item 16:   This section refers to how the person who gave the vaccine purchased it, not to the patient's insurance.

Item 17:   List any prescription or non-prescription medications the patient was taking when the vaccine(s) was given.

Item 18:   List any short term illnesses the patient had on the date the vaccine(s) was given (i.e., cold, flu, ear infection).

Item 19:   List any pre-existing physician-diagnosed allergies, birth defects, medical conditions (including developmental and/or neurologic disorders) for the patient.

Item 21:   List any suspected adverse events the patient, or the patient's brothers or sisters, may have had to previous vaccinations. If more than one brother or sister, or if the patient has reacted to more than one prior vaccine, use additional pages to explain completely. For the onset age of a patient, provide the age in months if less than two years old.

Item 26:   This space is for manufacturers' use only.

D

MedWatch Form

Next Page   Reset Form   Delete Page   Delete Multiple Pages

U.S. Department of Health and Human Services

MedWatch
The FDA Safety Information and Adverse Event Reporting Program   General Instructions

For VOLUNTARY reporting of adverse events, product problems and product use errors

Page 1 of____

Form Approved: OMB No. 0910-0291, Expires: 12/31/2011
See OMB statement on reverse.

FDA USE ONLY
Triage unit sequence #

PLEASE TYPE OR USE BLACK INK

A. PATIENT INFORMATION   Section A - Help

1. Patient Identifier	2. Age at Time of Event or Date of Birth:	3. Sex	4. Weight
In confidence		☐ Female ☐ Male	____ lb or ____ kg

B. ADVERSE EVENT, PRODUCT PROBLEM OR ERROR

Check all that apply: Section B - Help

1. ☐ **Adverse Event**   ☐ **Product Problem** (e.g., defects/malfunctions)
   ☐ **Product Use Error**   ☐ **Problem with Different Manufacturer of Same Medicine**

2. **Outcomes Attributed to Adverse Event**
   (Check all that apply)
   ☐ Death: _____ (mm/dd/yyyy)
   ☐ Life-threatening
   ☐ Hospitalization - initial or prolonged
   ☐ Required Intervention to Prevent Permanent Impairment/Damage (Devices)
   ☐ Disability or Permanent Damage
   ☐ Congenital Anomaly/Birth Defect
   ☐ Other Serious (Important Medical Events)

3. **Date of Event** (mm/dd/yyyy)   4. **Date of this Report** (mm/dd/yyyy)

5. **Describe Event, Problem or Product Use Error**

(Continue on page 3)

6. **Relevant Tests/Laboratory Data, Including Dates**

(Continue on page 3)

7. **Other Relevant History, Including Preexisting Medical Conditions** (e.g., allergies, race, pregnancy, smoking and alcohol use, liver/kidney problems, etc.)

(Continue on page 3)

C. PRODUCT AVAILABILITY   Section C - Help

Product Available for Evaluation? (Do not send product to FDA)

☐ Yes   ☐ No   ☐ Returned to Manufacturer on: _____
                                                    (mm/dd/yyyy)

D. SUSPECT PRODUCT(S)   Section D - Help

1. **Name, Strength, Manufacturer** (from product label)
#1 Name:
   Strength:
   Manufacturer:
#2 Name:
   Strength:
   Manufacturer:

2.	Dose or Amount	Frequency	Route
#1			
#2			

3. **Dates of Use** (If unknown, give duration) from/to (or best estimate)
#1
#2

4. **Diagnosis or Reason for Use** (Indication)
#1
#2

6. **Lot #**	7. **Expiration Date**
#1	#1
#2	#2

5. **Event Abated After Use Stopped or Dose Reduced?**
#1 ☐ Yes ☐ No ☐ Doesn't Apply
#2 ☐ Yes ☐ No ☐ Doesn't Apply

8. **Event Reappeared After Reintroduction?**
#1 ☐ Yes ☐ No ☐ Doesn't Apply
#2 ☐ Yes ☐ No ☐ Doesn't Apply

9. **NDC # or Unique ID**

E. SUSPECT MEDICAL DEVICE   Section E - Help

1. **Brand Name**

2. **Common Device Name**

3. **Manufacturer Name, City and State**

4. **Model #**	**Lot #**	5. **Operator of Device**
		☐ Health Professional
Catalog #	**Expiration Date** (mm/dd/yyyy)	☐ Lay User/Patient
		☐ Other:
Serial #	**Other #**	

6. **If Implanted, Give Date** (mm/dd/yyyy)	7. **If Explanted, Give Date** (mm/dd/yyyy)

8. **Is this a Single-use Device that was Reprocessed and Reused on a Patient?**
☐ Yes ☐ No

9. **If Yes to Item No. 8, Enter Name and Address of Reprocessor**

F. OTHER (CONCOMITANT) MEDICAL PRODUCTS

Product names and therapy dates (exclude treatment of event)   Section F - Help

(Continue on page 3)

G. REPORTER (See confidentiality section on back)

1. **Name and Address**   Section G - Help
   Name:
   Address:

   City: State: ZIP:

   Phone #   E-mail

2. **Health Professional?** 3. **Occupation**
   ☐ Yes ☐ No

4. **Also Reported to:**
   ☐ Manufacturer
   ☐ User Facility
   ☐ Distributor/Importer

5. **If you do NOT want your identity disclosed to the manufacturer, place an "X" in this box:** ☐

FORM FDA 3500 (1/09)   Submission of a report does not constitute an admission that medical personnel or the product caused or contributed to the event.

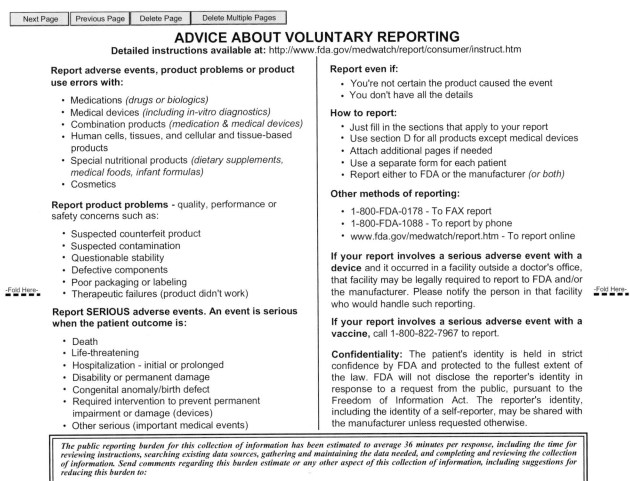

| Next Page | Previous Page | Delete Page | Delete Multiple Pages |

ADVICE ABOUT VOLUNTARY REPORTING

Detailed instructions available at: http://www.fda.gov/medwatch/report/consumer/instruct.htm

Report adverse events, product problems or product use errors with:

- Medications *(drugs or biologics)*
- Medical devices *(including in-vitro diagnostics)*
- Combination products *(medication & medical devices)*
- Human cells, tissues, and cellular and tissue-based products
- Special nutritional products *(dietary supplements, medical foods, infant formulas)*
- Cosmetics

Report product problems - quality, performance or safety concerns such as:

- Suspected counterfeit product
- Suspected contamination
- Questionable stability
- Defective components
- Poor packaging or labeling
- Therapeutic failures (product didn't work)

Report SERIOUS adverse events. An event is serious when the patient outcome is:

- Death
- Life-threatening
- Hospitalization - initial or prolonged
- Disability or permanent damage
- Congenital anomaly/birth defect
- Required intervention to prevent permanent impairment or damage (devices)
- Other serious (important medical events)

Report even if:

- You're not certain the product caused the event
- You don't have all the details

How to report:

- Just fill in the sections that apply to your report
- Use section D for all products except medical devices
- Attach additional pages if needed
- Use a separate form for each patient
- Report either to FDA or the manufacturer *(or both)*

Other methods of reporting:

- 1-800-FDA-0178 - To FAX report
- 1-800-FDA-1088 - To report by phone
- www.fda.gov/medwatch/report.htm - To report online

If your report involves a serious adverse event with a device and it occurred in a facility outside a doctor's office, that facility may be legally required to report to FDA and/or the manufacturer. Please notify the person in that facility who would handle such reporting.

If your report involves a serious adverse event with a vaccine, call 1-800-822-7967 to report.

Confidentiality: The patient's identity is held in strict confidence by FDA and protected to the fullest extent of the law. FDA will not disclose the reporter's identity in response to a request from the public, pursuant to the Freedom of Information Act. The reporter's identity, including the identity of a self-reporter, may be shared with the manufacturer unless requested otherwise.

-Fold Here-

-Fold Here-

The public reporting burden for this collection of information has been estimated to average 36 minutes per response, including the time for reviewing instructions, searching existing data sources, gathering and maintaining the data needed, and completing and reviewing the collection of information. Send comments regarding this burden estimate or any other aspect of this collection of information, including suggestions for reducing this burden to:

Department of Health and Human Services
Food and Drug Administration
Office of Chief Information Officer
1350 Piccard Drive, Room 400
Rockville, MD 20850

Please DO NOT
RETURN this form
to this address.

OMB statement:
"An agency may not conduct or sponsor, and a person is not required to respond to, a collection of information unless it displays a currently valid OMB control number."

U.S. DEPARTMENT OF HEALTH AND HUMAN SERVICES
Food and Drug Administration

FORM FDA 3500 (1/09) (Back)   Please Use Address Provided Below -- Fold in Thirds, Tape and Mail

DEPARTMENT OF
HEALTH & HUMAN SERVICES

Public Health Service
Food and Drug Administration
Rockville, MD 20857

Official Business
Penalty for Private Use $300

NO POSTAGE
NECESSARY
IF MAILED
IN THE
UNITED STATES
OR APO/FPO

BUSINESS REPLY MAIL

FIRST CLASS MAIL PERMIT NO. 946 ROCKVILLE MD

POSTAGE WILL BE PAID BY FOOD AND DRUG ADMINISTRATION

MEDWATCH
The FDA Safety Information and Adverse Event Reporting Program
Food and Drug Administration
5600 Fishers Lane
Rockville, MD 20852-9787

| Next Page | Previous Page | Reset Form | Delete Page | Delete Multiple Pages |

U.S. Department of Health and Human Services

MEDWATCH
**The FDA Safety Information and
Adverse Event Reporting Program**

(CONTINUATION PAGE)
**For VOLUNTARY reporting of
adverse events and product problems**

Page 3 of____

B.5. Describe Event or Problem *(continued)*

Back to Form

B.6. Relevant Tests/Laboratory Data, Including Dates *(continued)*

Back to Form

B.7. Other Relevant History, Including Preexisting Medical Conditions *(e.g., allergies, race, pregnancy, smoking and alcohol use, hepatic/renal dysfunction, etc.) (continued)*

Back to Form

F. Concomitant Medical Products and Therapy Dates *(Exclude treatment of event) (continued)*

Back to Form

| Next Page | Previous Page | Delete Page | Delete Multiple Pages |

General Instructions for Completing the MedWatch Form FDA 3500

For use by health professionals and consumers for **VOLUNTARY** reporting of adverse events, product use errors and product quality problems with:

- Drugs

- Biologics (including blood components, blood derivatives, allergenics, human cells, tissues, and cellular and tissue-based products (HCT/Ps)

- Medical devices (including *in-vitro* diagnostics)

- Combination products (e.g. drug-device, biologic-device)

- Special nutritional products (dietary supplements, infant formulas, medical foods)

- Cosmetics

Adverse events involving **vaccines** should be reported to the Vaccine Adverse Event Reporting System (VAERS), http://vaers.hhs.gov/pdf/vaers_form.pdf Adverse events involving **investigational (study) drugs, such as those relating to Investigational New Drug (IND) applications**, should be reported as required in the study protocol and sent to the address and contact person listed in the study protocol. They should generally not be submitted to FDA MedWatch as voluntary reports.

Note for consumers: If possible, please take the 3500 form to your health professional (e.g., doctor or pharmacist) so that information based on your medical record that can help in the evaluation of your report will be provided. If, for whatever reason, you do not wish to have your health professional fill out the form, you are welcome to do so yourself.

GENERAL INSTRUCTIONS

- Please make sure that all entries are either typed, printed in a font no smaller than 8 point, or written using black ink.

- Please complete all sections that apply to your report.

- Dates should be entered as mm/dd/yyyy (e.g., June 3, 2005 = 06/03/2005). If exact dates are unknown, please provide the best estimate (see block **B3**).

- For narrative entries, if the fields do not provide adequate space, attach additional pages as needed.

- If attaching additional pages, please do the following:

  - Identify all attached pages as Page __ of __

  - Indicate the appropriate section and block number next to the narrative continuation.

- Include the phrase continued at the end of each field that has additional information continued on to another page.

- **Section D,** Suspect product(s), should be used to report on special nutritional products and cosmetics as well as drugs or biologics, including human cells, tissues, and cellular and tissue-based products (HCT/Ps).

- If your report involves a serious adverse event with a device and it occurred in a facility other than a doctor's office, that facility may be legally required to report to FDA and/or the manufacturer. Please notify the person in that facility who would handle such reporting.

| Next Page | Previous Page | Delete Page | Delete Multiple Pages |

SECTION A: PATIENT INFORMATION

Complete a separate form for each patient, unless the report involves a medical device where multiple patients were adversely affected through the use of the same device. In that case, please indicate the number of patients in block **B5** (Describe event or problem) and complete Section A and blocks **B2**, **B5**, **B6**, **B7**, and **F** for each patient. Enter the corresponding patient identifier in block **A1** for each patient involved in the event.

Parent-child/fetus report(s) are those cases in which either a fetus/breast-feeding infant or the mother, or both have an adverse event that is possibly associated with a product administered to the mother during pregnancy. Several general principles are used for filing these reports:

- If there has been no event affecting the child/fetus, report only on the parent.
- For those cases describing fetal death, miscarriage or abortion, report the parent as the patient in the report.
- When only the child/fetus has an adverse reaction/event (other than fetal death, miscarriage or abortion), the information provided in **Section A** applies to the child/fetus. However, the information in **Section D** would apply to the parent who was the source of exposure to the product.
- When a newborn baby is found to have a birth defect/congenital anomaly that the initial reporter considers possibly associated with a product administered to the mother during pregnancy, the patient is the newborn baby.
- If both the parent and the child/fetus have adverse events, separate reports should be submitted for each patient.

A1:   Patient Identifier

Please provide the patient's initials or some other type of identifier that will allow you, the reporter, to readily locate the case if you are contacted for more information. Do not use the patient's name or social security number.

The patient's identity is held in strict confidence by FDA and protected to the fullest extent of the law. FDA will not disclose the reporter's identity in response to a request from the public, pursuant to the Freedom of Information Act.

If no patient was involved (such as may be the case with a product problem), enter none.

A2:   Age at Time of Event or Date of Birth

Provide the most precise information available. Enter the patient's birth date, if known, or the patient's age at the time of event onset. For age, indicate time units used (e.g., years, months, days):

- If the patient is 3 years or older, use years (e.g., 4 years).
- If the patient is less than 3 years old, use month (e.g., 24 months).
- If the patient is less than 1 month old, use days (e.g., 5 days).
- Provide the best estimate if exact age is unknown.

A3:   Sex

Enter the patient's gender. If the adverse event is a congenital anomaly/birth defect, report the sex of the child.

A4:   Weight

Indicate whether the weight is in pounds (lb) or kilograms (kg). Make a best estimate if exact weight is unknown.

Next Page | Previous Page | Delete Page | Delete Multiple Pages

SECTION B: ADVERSE EVENT, PRODUCT PROBLEM, PRODUCT USE ERROR

B1: Adverse Event, Product Problem, Product Use Error, or Problem with Different Manufacturer of Same Medicine.

Choose the appropriate box(es). If a product problem may have caused or contributed to the adverse event, check both boxes.

Adverse event: Any incident where the use of a medication (drug or biologic, including HCT/P), at any dose, a medical device (including *in-vitro* diagnostics) or a special nutritional product (e.g., dietary supplement, infant formula or medical food) is suspected to have resulted in an adverse outcome in a patient.

To report, it is not necessary to be certain of a cause/effect relationship between the adverse event and the use of the medical product(s) in question. Suspicion of an association is sufficient reason to report. Submission of a report does not constitute an admission that medical personnel or the product caused or contributed to the event.

Please limit your submissions to those events that are serious. An event is classified as serious when the patient outcome is:

- Death
- Life-threatening
- Hospitalization (initial or prolonged)
- Disability or Permanent Damage
- Congenital Anomaly/Birth Defect
- Required Medical or Surgical Intervention to Prevent Permanent Impairment or Damage (Devices)
- Other Serious (Important Medical Events)

Please see instructions for block **B2** for further information on each of these criteria.

Product problem (e.g., defects/malfunctions): Any report regarding the quality, performance, or safety of any medication, medical device or special nutritional product. In addition, please select this category when reporting device malfunctions that could lead to a death or serious injury if the malfunction were to recur. Product problems include, but are not limited to, such concerns as:

- Suspected counterfeit product
- Suspected contamination
- Questionable stability
- Defective components
- Therapeutic failures (product didn't work)
- Product confusion (caused by name, labeling, design or packaging)
- Suspected superpotent or subpotent medication
- Labeling problems caused by printing errors/omissions

Product Use Error:

Medication Use Error: Any report of a medication error regardless of patient involvement or outcome. Also report circumstances or events that have the capacity to cause error (e.g., similar product appearance, similar packaging and labeling, sound-alike/look-alike names, etc.).

Medication errors can and do originate in all stages of the medication use system, which includes selecting and procuring drugs, prescribing, preparing and dispensing, administering and monitoring. A medication error is defined as "any preventable event that may cause or lead to inappropriate medication use or patient harm while the medication is in the control of the health care professional, patient, or consumer. Such events may be related to professional practice, health care products, procedures, and systems, including prescribing, order communication, product labeling, packaging, nomenclature, compounding, dispensing, distribution, administration, education, monitoring and use."

Medical Device Use Error: Health care professionals, patients, and consumers can unintentionally cause harm to patients or to themselves when using medical devices. These problems can often arise due to problems with the design of the medical device or the manner in which the device is used. Often, use errors are caught and prevented before they can do harm (close call). Report use errors regardless of patient involvement or outcome. Also report circumstances or events that could cause use errors. Medical device use errors usually occur for one or more of the following reasons:

- Users expect devices to operate differently than they do.
- Product use is inconsistent with use's expectations or intuition.
- Product use requires physical, perceptual, or cognitive abilities that exceed those of the user.
- Devices are used in ways not anticipated by the manufacturer.
- Product labeling or packaging is confusing or inadequate.
- The environment adversely affects or influences device use.

Problem with Different Manufacturer of Same Medicine: Any incident, to include, but not be limited to, differences in noted therapeutic response, suspected to have resulted from a switch, or change, from one manufacturer to another manufacturer of the **same** medicine or drug product. This could be changes from a brand name drug product to a generic manufacturer's same product, or from a generic manufacturer's product to the same

(continued on next page)

Next Page | Previous Page | Delete Page | Delete Multiple Pages

SECTION B: ADVERSE EVENT, PRODUCT PROBLEM, PRODUCT USE ERROR *(continued)*

product as supplied by a different generic manufacturer, or from a generic manufacturer's product to a brand name manufacturer of the same product. In order to fully evaluate the incident, please include in **Section B5**, if available, specific information relative to the switch between different manufacturers of the same medicine, to include, but not be limited to, the names of the manufacturers, length of treatment on each manufacturer's product, product strength, and any relevant clinical data.

B2: Outcomes Attributed to Adverse Event: Indicate all that apply to the reported event:

Death: Check ony if you suspect that the death was an outcome of the adverse event, and include the date if known.

Do not check if:

- The patient died while using a medical product, but there was no suspected association between the death and the use of the product
- A fetus is aborted because of a congenital anomaly (birth defect), or is miscarried

Life-threatening: Check if suspected that:

- The patient was at substantial risk of dying at the time of the adverse event, or
- Use or continued use of the device or other medical product might have resulted in the death of the patient

Hospitalization (initial or prolonged): Check if admission to the hospital or prolongation of hospitalization was a result of the adverse event.

Do not check if:

- A patient in the hospital received a medical product and subsequently developed an otherwise nonserious adverse event, unless the adverse event prolonged the hospital stay

Do check if:

- A patient is admitted to the hospital for one or more days, even if released on the same day
- An emergency room visit results in admission to the hospital. Emergency room visits that do not result in admission to the hospital should be evaluated for one of the other serious outcomes (e.g., life-threatening; required intervention to prevent permanent impairment or damage; other serious (medically important event)

Disability or Permanent Damage: Check if the adverse event resulted in a substantial disruption of a person's ability to conduct normal life functions. Such would be the case if the adverse event resulted in a significant, persistent or permanent change, impairment, damage or disruption in the patient's body function/structure, physical activities and/or quality of life.

Congenital Anomaly/Birth Defect: Check if you suspect that exposure to a medical product prior to conception or during pregnancy may have resulted in an adverse outcome in the child.

Required Intervention to Prevent Permanent Impairment or Damage (Devices): Check if you believe that medical or surgical intervention was necessary to preclude permanent impairment of a body function, or prevent permanent damage to a body structure, either situation suspected to be due to the use of a medical product.

Other Serious (Important Medical Events): Check when the event does not fit the other outcomes, but the event may jeopardize the patient and may require medical or surgical intervention (treatment) to prevent one of the other outcomes. Examples include allergic brochospasm (a serious problem with breathing) requiring treatment in an emergency room, serious blood dyscrasias (blood disorders) or seizures/convulsions that do not result in hospitalization. The development of drug dependence or drug abuse would also be examples of important medical events.

B3: Date of Event

Provide the actual or best estimate of the date of first onset of the adverse event. If day is unknown, month and year are acceptable. If day and month are unknown, year is acceptable.

- When a newborn baby is found to have a congenital anomaly, the event onset date is the date of birth of the child.
- When a fetus is aborted because of a congenital anomaly, or is miscarried, the event onset date is the date pregnancy is terminated.
- If information is available as to time during pregnancy when exposure occurred, indicate that information in narrative block **B5**.

B4: Date of this Report

The date the report is filled out.

B5: Describe Event, Problem or Product Use Error

For an **adverse event:**

Describe the event in detail, including a description of what happened and a summary of all relevant clinical information (medical status prior to the event; signs and/or symptoms; differential diagnosis for the event in question; clinical course; treatment; outcome, etc.). If available and if relevant, include synopses of any office visit notes or the hospital discharge summary. To save time and space (and if permitted by your institution), please attach copies of these records with any confidential information deleted. **Do not identify any patient, physician, or institution by name. The reporter's identity should be provided in full in Section G.**

(continued on next page)

| Next Page | Previous Page | Delete Page | Delete Multiple Pages |

SECTION B: ADVERSE EVENT, PRODUCT PROBLEM, PRODUCT USE ERROR *(continued)*

Information as to any environmental conditions that may have influenced the event should be included, particularly when (but not exclusive to) reporting about a device.

- Results of relevant tests and laboratory data should be entered in block **B6**. (See instructions for **B6**.)
- Preexisting medical conditions and other relevant history belong in block **B7**. Be as complete as possible, including time courses for preexisting diagnoses (see instructions for **B7**).

If it is determined that reuse of a medical device labeled for single use may have caused or contributed to an adverse patient outcome, please report in block **B5** the facts of the incident and the perceived contribution of reuse to the occurrence.

For a product problem: Describe the problem (quality, performance, or safety concern) in sufficient detail so that the circumstances surrounding the defect or malfunction of the medical product can be understood.

- If available, the results of any evaluation of a malfunctioning device and, if known, any relevant maintenance/service information should be included in this section.
- For a medication or special nutritional product problem, please indicate if you have retained a sample that would be available to FDA.

For a product use error: Describe the sequence of events leading up to the error in sufficient detail so that the circumstances surrounding the error can be understood.

- **For Medication Use Errors:** Include a description of the error, type of staff involved, work environment in which the error occurred, indicate causes or contributing factors to the error, location of the error, names of the products involved (including the trade (proprietary) and established (proper) name), manufacturer, dosage form, strength, concentration, and type and size of container.

- **For Medical Device Use Errors:** Report circumstances or events that could cause use errors. Medical device use errors usually occur for one or more of the following reasons:

  - Users expect devices to operate differently than they do.
  - Product use is inconsistent with user's expectations or intuition.
  - Product use requires physical, perceptual, or cognitive abilities that exceed those of the user.
  - Devices are used in ways not anticipated by the manufacturer.
  - Product labeling or packaging is confusing or inadequate.
  - The environment adversely affects or influences device use.

For a problem with a different manufacturer of the same medicine:

Please include specific information relative to the switch between different manufacturers of the same medicine, to include, but not be limited to, the names of the manufacturers, length of treatment on each manufacturer's product, product strength, and any relevant clinical data.

B6: Relevant Tests/Laboratory Data, Including Dates

Please provide all appropriate information, including relevant negative test and laboratory findings, in order to most completely convey how the medical work-up/assessment led to strong consideration of medical product-induced disease as etiology for clinical status, as other differential diagnostic considerations were being eliminated.

Please include:

- Any relevant baseline laboratory data prior to the administration or use of the medical product
- All laboratory data used in diagnosing the event
- Any available laboratory data/engineering analyses (for devices) that provide further information on the course of the event

If available, please include:

- Any pre- and post-event medication levels and dates (if applicable)
- Synopses of any relevant autopsy, pathology, engineering, or lab reports

If preferred, copies of any reports may be submitted as attachments, with all confidential information deleted. **Do not identify any patient, physician or institution by name.** The initial reporter's identity should be provided in full in **Section G.**

B7: Other Relevant History, Including Preexisting Medical Conditions

Knowledge of other risk factors can help in the evaluation of a reported adverse event. If available, provide information on:

- **Other known conditions in the patient, e.g.,**
  - Hypertension (high blood pressure)
  - Diabetes mellitus
  - Liver or kidney problems

- **Significant history**
  - Race
  - Allergies
  - Pregnancy history
  - Smoking and alcohol use, drug abuse
  - Setting

| Next Page | Previous Page | Delete Page | Delete Multiple Pages |

SECTION C: PRODUCT AVAILABILITY

Product available for evaluation? (Do not send the product to FDA.)
To evaluate a reported problem with a medical product, it is often critical to be able to examine the product. Please indicate whether the product is available for evaluation. Also indicate if the product was returned to the manufacturer and, if so, the date of the return.

SECTION D: SUSPECT PRODUCT(S)

For adverse event reporting:

A suspect product is one that you suspect is associated with the adverse event. In **Section F** enter other concomitant medical products (drugs, biologics including human cells, tissues, and cellular and tissue-based products (HCT/Ps), medical devices, etc.) that the patient was using at the time of the event but which you do not think were involved in the event.

Up to two (2) suspect products may be reported on one form (#1=first suspect product, #2=second suspect product). Attach an additional form if there were more than two suspect products associated with the reported adverse event.

For product quality problem reporting:

A suspect product is the product that is the subject of the report. A separate form should be submitted for each individual product problem report.

Identification of the labeler/distributor and pharmaceutical manufacturer and labeled strength of the product is important for prescription or non-prescription products.

This section may also be used to report on special nutritional products (e.g., dietary supplements, infant formula or medical foods), cosmetics, human cells, tissues, or cellular and tissue-based products (HCT/Ps) or other products regulated by FDA.

If reporting on a special nutritional or drug product quality problem, please attach labeling/packaging if available.

If reporting on a special nutritional product only, please provide directions for use as listed on the product labeling.

D1:   Name, Strength, Manufacturer

Use the trade/brand name. If the trade/brand name is not known or if there is no trade/brand name, use the generic product name and the name of the manufacturer or labeler. These names are usually found on the product packaging or labeling. Strength is the amount in each tablet or capsule, the concentration of an injectable, etc. (such as "10mg", "100 units/cc", etc.).

For human cells, tissues, and cellular and tissue-based products (HCT/Ps), please provide the common name of the HCT/P. You can also indicate if the HCT/P has a proprietary or trade name. Examples: Achilles tendon, Iliac crest bone or Islet cells.

D2:   Dose or Amount, Frequency, Route

Describe how the product was used by the patient (e.g., 500 mg QID orally or 10 mg every other day IV). For reports involving overdoses, the amount of product used in the overdose should be listed, not the prescribed amount. (See **APPENDIX** for list of **Routes of Administration** on the next page.)

D3:   Dates of Use

Provide the date administration was started (or best estimate) and the date stopped (or best estimate). If no dates are known, an estimated duration is acceptable (e.g., 2 years) or if therapy was less than one day, then duration is appropriate (e.g., 1 dose or 1 hour for an IV).

For human cells, tissues, and cellular and tissue-based products, provide the date of transplant and if applicable, the date of explanation.

D4:   Diagnosis or Reason for Use (Indication)

Provide the reason or indication for which the product was prescribed or used in this particular patient.

D5:   Event Abated After Use Stopped or Dose Reduced

If available, this information is particularly useful in the evaluation of a suspected adverse event. In addition to checking the appropriate box, please provide supporting lab tests and dates, if available, in block **B6**.

D6:   Lot #

If known, include the lot number(s) with all product quality problem reports, or any adverse event report with a biologic, or medication.

D7:   Expiration Date

Please include if available.

(continued on next page)

| Next Page | Previous Page | Delete Page | Delete Multiple Pages |

SECTION D: SUSPECT PRODUCT(S) *(continued)*

D8: Event Reappeared After Reintroduction

This information is particularly useful in the evaluation of a suspected adverse event. In addition to checking the appropriate box, please provide a description of what happened when the drug was stopped and then restarted in block **B5**, and any supporting lab tests and dates in block **B6**.

D9: NDC # or Unique ID

The national drug code (NDC #) is requested only when reporting a drug product problem. Zeros and dashes should be included as they appear on the label. NDC # can be found on the original product label and/or packaging, but is usually not found on dispensed pharmacy prescriptions.

If the product has a unique or distinct identification code, please provide this here. This is applicable to human cells, tissues, and cellular and tissue-based products (HCT/Ps).

Appendix - Routes of Administration

Auricular (otic) 001	Intracerebral 018	Intrasynovial 035	Perineural 052
Buccal 002	Intracervical 019	Intratumor 036	Rectal 053
Cutaneous 003	Intracisternal 020	Intrathecal 037	Respiratory (inhalation) 054
Dental 004	Intracorneal 021	Intrathoracic 038	Retrobulbar 055
Endocervical 005	Intracoronary 022	Intratracheal 039	Subconjunctival 056
Endosinusial 006	Intradermal 023	Intravenous bolus 040	Subcutaneous 057
Endotracheal 007	Intradiscal (intraspinal) 024	Intravenous drip 041	Subdermal 058
Epidural 008	Intrahepatic 025	Intravenous (not otherwise specified) 042	Sublingual 059
Extra-amniotic 009	Intralesional 026	Intravesical 043	Topical 060
Hemodialysis 010	Intralymphatic 027	Iontophoresis 044	Transdermal 061
Intra corpus cavernosum 011	Intramedullar (bone marrow) 028	Occlusive dressing technique 045	Transmammary 062
Intra-amniotic 012	Intrameningeal 029	Ophthalmic 046	Transplacental 063
Intra-arterial 013	Intramuscular 030	Oral 047	Unknown 064
Intra-articular 014	Intraocular 031	Oropharyngeal 048	Urethral 065
Intra-uterine 015	Intrapericardial 032	Other 049	Vaginal 066
Intracardiac 016	Intraperitoneal 033	Parenteral 050	
Intracavernous 017	Intrapleural 034	Periarticular 051	

| Next Page | Previous Page | Delete Page | Delete Multiple Pages |

SECTION E: SUSPECT MEDICAL DEVICE

The suspect medical device is 1) the device that may have caused or contributed to the adverse event or 2) the device that malfunctioned.

In **Section F**, report other concomitant medical products (drugs, biologics including HCT/Ps, medical devices, etc.) that the patient was using at the time of the event but which you do not think were involved in the event.

If more than one suspect medical device was involved in the event, complete all of **Section E** for the first device and attach a separate completed **Section E** for each additional device.

If the suspect medical device is a single-use device that has been reprocessed, then the reprocessor is now the device manufacturer.

E1: Brand Name

The trade or proprietary name of the suspect medical device as used in product labeling or in the catalog (e.g., Flo-Easy Catheter, Reliable Heart Pacemaker, etc.). This information may 1) be on a label attached to a durable device, 2) be on a package of a disposable device, or 3) appear in labeling materials of an implantable device. Reprocessed single-use devices may bear the Original Equipment Manufacturer (OEM) brand name. If the suspect device is a reprocessed single-use device, enter "NA".

E2: Common Device Name

The generic or common name of the suspect medical device or a generally descriptive name (e.g., urological catheter, heart pacemaker, patient restraint, etc.). Please do not use broad generic terms such as "catheter", "valve", "screw", etc.

E3: Manufacturer Name, City and State

If available, list the full name, city and state of the manufacturer of the suspected medical device. If the answer of block **E8** is "yes", then enter the name, city and state of the reprocessor.

E4: Model #, Catalog #, Serial #, Lot #, Expiration Date, Other

If available, provide any or all identification numbers associated with the suspect medical device exactly as they appear on the device or device labeling. This includes spaces, hyphens, etc.

Model #:

The exact model number found on the device label or accompanying packaging.

Catalog #:

The exact number as it appears in the manufacturer's catalog, device labeling, or accompanying packaging.

Serial #:

This number can be found on the device label or accompanying packaging; it is assigned by the manufacturer, and should be specific to each device.

Lot #:

This number can be found on the label or packaging material.

Expiration Date (mm/dd/yyyy):

If available, this date can often be found on the device itself or printed on the accompanying packaging.

Other #:

Any other applicable identification number (e.g., component number, product number, part bar-coded product ID, etc.)

E5: Operator of Device

Indicate the type (not the name) of person operating or using the suspect medical device on the patient at the time of the event as follows:

- Health professional = physician, nurse, respiratory therapist, etc.
- Lay user/patient = person being treated, parent/spouse/friend of the patient
- Other = nurses aide, orderly, etc.

E6: If Implanted, Give Gate (mm/dd/yyyy)

For medical devices that are implanted in the patient, provide the implant date or your best estimate. If day is unknown, month and year are acceptable. If month and day are unknown, year is acceptable.

E7: If Explanted, Give Date (mm/dd/yyyy)

If an implanted device was removed from the patient, provide the explantation date or your best estimate. If day is unknown, month and year are acceptable. If month and day are unknown, year is acceptable.

E8: Is this a Single-use Device that was returned before Reprocessed and Reused on a Patient?

Indicate "Yes" or "No".

E9: If Yes to Item No. 8, Enter Name and Address of Reprocessor

Enter the name and address of the reprocessor of the single-use device. Anyone who reprocesses single-use devices for reuse in humans is the manufacturer of the reprocessed device.

Previous Page | Delete Page | Delete Multiple Pages

SECTION F: OTHER (CONCOMITANT) MEDICAL PRODUCTS

Product names and therapy dates (exclude treatment of event)

Information on the use of concomitant medical products can frequently provide insight into previously unknown interactions between products, or provide an alternative explanation for the observed adverse event. Please list and provide product names and therapy dates for any other medical products (drugs, biologics including HCT/Ps, medical devices, etc.) that the patient was using at the time of the event. Do not include products used to treat the event.

SECTION G: REPORTER

FDA recognizes that confidentiality is an important concern in the context of adverse event reporting. The patient's identity is held in strict confidence by FDA and protected to the fullest extent of the law. However, to allow for timely follow-up in serious cases, the reporter's identity may be shared with the manufacturer unless specifically requested otherwise in block G5. FDA will not disclose the reporter's identity in response to a request from the public, pursuant to the Freedom of Information Act.

G1:   Name, Address, Phone #, E-mail

Please provide the name, mailing address, phone number and E-mail address of the person who can be contacted to provide information on the event if follow-up is necessary. While optional, providing the fax number would be most helpful, if available. This person will also receive an acknowledgment letter from FDA on receipt of the report.

G2:   Health Professional?

Please indicate whether you are a health professional (e.g., physician, pharmacist, nurse, etc.) or not.

G3:   Occupation:

Please indicate your occupation (particularly type of health professional), and include specialty, if appropriate.

G4:   Also Reported to:

Please indicate whether you have also notified or submitted a copy of this report to the manufacturer and/or distributor of the product, or, in the case of medical device reports only, to the user facility (institution) in which the event occurred. This information helps to track duplicate reports in the FDA database.

G5:   Release of reporter's Identity to the manufacturer

In the case of a serious adverse event, FDA may provide name, address and phone number of the reporter denoted in block **G1** to the manufacturer of the suspect product. If you do not want your identity released to the manufacturer, please put an X in this box.

E

Drugs and Health Care Information Sources on the World Wide Web

AIDS.gov	http://www.aids.gov
Agency for Healthcare Research and Quality	http://www.ahrq.gov
Alzheimer's Association	http://www.alz.org
Alzheimer's Disease Education & Referral Center	http://www.nia.nih.gov/alzheimers
American Academy of Allergy, Asthma and Immunology	http://www.aaaai.org
American Academy of Pediatric Dentistry Web site	http://www.aapd.org
American Association of Poison Control Centers	www.aapcc.org
American Congress of Obstetricians and Gynecologists	www.acog.org
American Diabetes Association	http://www.diabetes.org
American Heart Association (AHA)	http://www. heart.org
American Optometric Association	http://www.aoa.org
American Society for Parenteral and Enteral Nutrition	http://www.nutritioncare.org
Centers for Disease Control and Prevention	http://www.cdc.gov
Centers for Disease Control Travel's Health	http://www.cdc.gov/travel
Clinical Trials	http://ClinicalTrials.gov
Cystic Fibrosis Foundation	http://www.cff.org
Epilepsy Foundation of America	http://www.efa.org
Hospice	http://www.hospicenet.org
Institute of Medicine	http://www.iom.edu
Institute for Safe Medication Practices	http://www.ismp.org
Kids Health	http://www.kidshealth.org
Mayo Clinic's public health information	http://www.mayoclinic.com
Medline Plus (NIH)	http://medlineplus.gov
MedWatch	http://www.fda.gov/Safety/MedWatch/default.htm
Merck Manuals	http://www.merckmanuals.com/
National Cancer Institute	http://www.cancer.gov

National Center for Complementary and Alternative Medicine	http://nccam.nih.gov
National Center for Health Statistics	http://www.cdc.gov/nchs/fastats
National Comprehensive Cancer Network	http://www.nccn.org
National Digestive Diseases Information Clearinghouse	http://www.digestive.niddk.nih.gov
National Guideline Clearinghouse	http://www.guideline.gov
National Heart Lung and Blood Institute	http://www.nhlbi.nih.gov
National High Blood Pressure Education Program (NHBPEP)	http://www.nhlbi.nih.gov/about/nhbpep/index.htm
National Institute of Diabetes and Digestive and . Kidney Diseases (NIDDK)	http://www2.niddk.nih.gov/
National Institute on Drug Abuse	http://www.steroidabuse.org
National Institutes of Health	http://www.health.nih.gov
National Institute of Mental Health	http://www.nimh.nih.gov
National Institute of Neurological Disorders and Stroke	http://www.ninds.nih.gov/
National Kidney and Urologic Disease Information Clearinghouse	http://www.kidney.niddk.nih.gov
National Library of Medicine	http://www.nlm.nih.gov
NIH SeniorHealth	http://nihseniorhealth.gov/
National Parkinson Foundation	http://www.parkinson.org
National Psoriasis Foundation	http://www.psoriasis.org
National Sleep Foundation	http://www.sleepfoundation.org
Office of Dietary Supplements	http://ods.od.nih.gov
Spina Bifida Association	http://www.spinabifidaassociation.org
U.S. Department of Health and Human Services, Health Information Privacy	http://www.hhs.gov/ocr/privacy/
U.S. Department of Labor Occupational Safety & Health Administration (OSHA)	http://www.osha.gov
U.S. Food and Drug Administration	http://www.fda.gov
Vaccine Adverse Event Reporting System	http://vaers.hhs.gov

Drug Indications for Nursing Mothers

Drugs and Lactation Database (LactMed)	http://Toxnet.nlm.nih.gov/cgi-bin/sis/htmlgen?LACT
American Academy of Pediatrics	http://aap.org/healthtopics/breastfeeding.cfm

F

Abbreviations

A

aa	of each
abd	abdomen, abdominal
ABG	arterial blood gas
ac	before meals
ADH	antidiuretic hormone
ADL	activities of daily living
ad lib	as much as desired
ADT	alternate-day therapy
AIDS	acquired immunodeficiency syndrome
ALT	alanine aminotransferase
AMA	against medical advice
AMI	acute myocardial infarction
AODM	adult-onset diabetes mellitus
ARC	AIDS-related complex
ASAP	as soon as possible
ASHD	arteriosclerotic heart disease
AST	aspartate aminotransferase

B

BE	barium enema; base excess
bid	twice a day
bili	bilirubin
BM	bowel movement
BMR	basal metabolic rate
B&O	belladonna and opium
BP	blood pressure
BPH	benign prostatic hypertrophy
BRP	bathroom privileges
BUN	blood urea nitrogen

C

c̄	with
Ca	cancer; calcium
C&A	Clinitest and Acetest

CAD	coronary artery disease	
caps	capsules	
CBC	complete blood count	
CC	chief complaint	
CCU	Coronary Care Unit	
CHF	congestive heart failure	
CHO	carbohydrate	
chol	cholesterol	
CLL	chronic lymphocytic leukemia	
CNS	central nervous system	
C/O	complains of	
COPD	chronic obstructive pulmonary disease	
CPK	creatine phosphokinase	
CRF	chronic renal failure	
C&S	culture and sensitivity	
CTZ	chemoreceptor trigger zone	
CVA	cerebrovascular accident	
CVP	central venous pressure	
CXR	chest x-ray	

D

/d	per day
d	daily
DC (D/C)	discontinue
Diff	differential blood count
DJD	degenerative joint disease
DM	diabetes mellitus
DOE	dyspnea on exertion
DT	delirium tremens
Dx	diagnosis

E

ECG	electrocardiogram
ECT	electroconvulsive therapy
EENT	eyes, ears, nose, and throat
EKG	electrocardiogram
ENT	eyes, nose, and throat
ER	emergency room
ESR	erythrocyte sedimentation rate (sed rate)
et	and

F

F	Fahrenheit
FBS	fasting blood sugar
fl	fluid
fx	fracture; fraction

G

g	gram
GB	gallbladder
GERD	gastroesophageal reflux disease
GFR	glomerular filtration rate
GI	gastrointestinal
gtt	drop
GU	genitourinary

H

h	hour
HA	headache
Hct	hematocrit
Hgb	hemoglobin
hs	hour of sleep

HTN	hypertension
Hx	history

I

ICU	intensive care unit
IM	intramuscular
I&O	intake and output
IOP	intraocular pressure
IPPB	intermittent positive pressure breathing
IU	international units
IV	intravenous
IVP	intravenous pyelogram
IVPB	intravenous piggyback

J

JRA	juvenile rheumatoid arthritis

K

K	potassium
KUB	kidney, ureters, and bladder
KVO	keep vein open

L

L	liter
LDH	lactic dehydrogenase
LDL	low-density lipoproteins
LOC	level of consciousness
LP	lumbar puncture
lytes	electrolytes

M

mg	milligram
mcg	microgram
MI	myocardial infarction (heart attack)
mL	milliliter
MOM	milk of magnesia
MS	morphine sulfate; multiple sclerosis; mitral steno

N

N	normal
NG	nasogastric
NGT	nitroglycerin
NPO	nothing by mouth
NS	normal saline
NVD	nausea, vomiting, diarrhea; neck vein distension

O

O_2	oxygen
OD	right eye
OOB	out of bed
OR	operating room
OS	left eye
OTC	over the counter (nonprescription)
OU	both eyes

P

PAT	paroxysmal atrial tachycardia
PBI	protein-bound iodine
PC	after meals
PERRLA	pupils equal, round, react to light and accommodation
PERL	pupils equal and react to light
PID	pelvic inflammatory disease

PKU	phenylketonuria		SR	sedimentation rate (ESR)
PND	paroxysmal nocturnal dyspnea		STAT	as soon as possible
PO	by mouth			
postop	after surgery		**T**	
preop	before surgery		t	temperature
prn	as needed		T_3	triiodothyronine
PT	physical therapy; prothrombin time		T_4	thyroxine
PZI	protamine zinc insulin		T&A	tonsillectomy and adenoidectomy
			TB	tuberculosis
Q			TEDS	elastic stockings
qd	every day		TIA	transient ischemic attack
qh	every hour (q2h, q3h, etc.—every 2 hours, every 3 hours, etc.)		tid	three times per day
			TKO	to keep open
qid	four times per day		TLC	tender loving care
qod	every other day		TM	tympanic membrane
			TPN	total parenteral nutrition
R			TPR	temperature, pulse, and respiration
RA	rheumatoid arthritis; right atrium		TSH	thyroid-stimulating hormone
RBC	red blood cell			
REM	rapid eye movement		**U**	
RF	rheumatoid factor		UGI	upper gastrointestinal
RHD	rheumatic heart disease; renal hypertensive disease		ung	ointment
			URI	upper respiratory infection
ROM	range of motion		UTI	urinary tract infection
RR	recovery room			
			V	
S			VS	vital signs
s̄	without			
sed. rate	erythrocyte sedimentation rate (ESR)		**W**	
SGOT	serum glutamic oxaloacetic transaminase		WNL	within normal limits
SGPT	serum glutamic pyruvic transaminase		Wt	weight
SL	sublingual			
SOB	shortness of breath			

INDEX

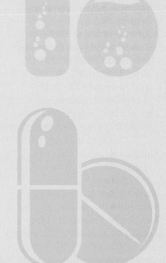

Page numbers followed by b indicate box; those followed by t indicate table; those in *italics* indicate figure.